www.harcourt-international.com

Bringing you products from all companies including Baillère T Mosby and W.B. Saunders

○ **Browse** for latest information on new books, journals and electronic products

○ **Search** for information on over 20 000 published titles with full product information including tables of contents and sample chapters

○ **Keep up to date** with our extensive publishing programme in your field by registering with eAlert or requesting postal updates

○ **Secure online ordering** with prompt delivery, as well as full contact details to order by phone, fax or post

○ **News** of special features and promotions

If you are based in the following countries, please visit the country-specific site to receive full details of product availability and local ordering information

USA: www.harcourthealth.com

Canada: www.harcourtcanada.com

Australia: www.harcourt.com.au

Baillière Tindall · CHURCHILL LIVINGSTONE · Mosby · W.B. SAUNDERS

Nursing Journals from Churchill Livingstone

Accident and Emergency Nursing
Editor: Bob Wright, Leeds, UK
ISSN 0965 2302 • 4 issues
www.harcourt-international.com/journals/aaen

Clinical Effectiveness in Nursing
Editor: Dr Rob Newell, Bradford, UK
ISSN 1361-9004 • 4 issues
www.harcourt-international.com/journals/cein

Complementary Therapies in Nursing & Midwifery
Editor: Denise Rankin-Box, Cheshire, UK
ISSN 1353 6117 • 4 issues
www.harcourt-international.com/journals/ctnm

European Journal of Oncology Nursing
The Official Journal of the EUROPEAN ONCOLO-GY NURSING SOCIETY

Editor: Professor Alison Richardson, London, UK
ISSN 1462-3889 • 4 issues
www.harcourt-international.com/journals/ejon

Intensive and Critical Care Nursing
Editor-in-Chief: Dr Carol Ball, London, UK
ISSN 0964-3397 • 6 issues
www.harcourt-international.com/journals/iccn

Journal of Orthopaedic Nursing
Official journal of the Canadian Orthopaedic Nurses Association
Editor-in-Chief: Peter Davis, Nottingham, UK
ISSN 1361-3111 • 4 issues
www.harcourt-international.com/journals/joon

Midwifery
Editor-in-Chief:
Professor Ann M. Thomson, Manchester, UK
ISSN 0266-6138 • 4 issues
www.harcourt-international.com/journals/midw

Nurse Education Today
Editor-in-Chief:
Professor Peter Birchenall, York, UK
ISSN 0260 6917 • 8 issues
www.harcourt-international.com/journals/nedt

Nurse Education in Practice
Editor: Karen Holland, Salford, UK
ISSN 1471-5953 • 4 issues
www.harcourt-international.com/journals/nepr

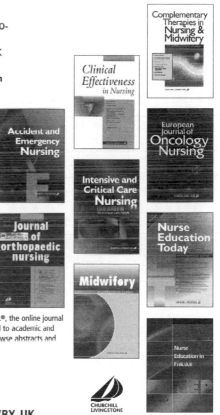

IDEAL®   IDEAL'Alert

All of the above titles are available electronically on IDEAL®, the online journal library. IDEAL® features over 200 full text journals licensed to academic and industrial library consortia worldwide. Guest users may browse abstracts and tables of contents at www.idealibrary.com
IDEAL® is a registered trademark of Harcourt Inc.

**Journals Marketing Department,
Harcourt Publishers Ltd,
32 Jamestown Road, London NW1 7BY, UK
tel: +44 (0)20 8308 5700   fax: +44 (0)20 7424 4433
e-mail: journals@harcourt.com • www.harcourt-international.com**

CHURCHILL
LIVINGSTONE

PERSONAL INFORMATION

Name

Address

Job/Course Title

Work/University/College Address

National Insurance No.

RCN Membership No.

NMC/UKCC PIN No.

Date of Registration

Date for Reregistration

Churchill Livingstone's

Dictionary
of Nursing

For Churchill Livingstone:

Senior Commissioning Editor: Jacqueline Curthoys
Project Manager: Gail Murray
Designer: George Ajayi
Illustrators: Robert Britton and Paul Richardson

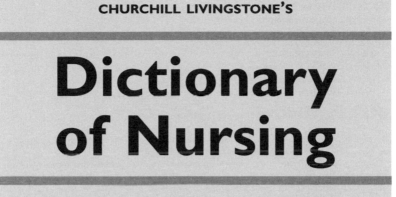

CHURCHILL LIVINGSTONE'S

Dictionary of Nursing

EIGHTEENTH EDITION

Edited by
Chris Brooker BSc RGN MSc CM RNT
Author and Lecturer, Norfolk, UK

Foreword by
Sarah Mullally
Chief Nursing Officer, Department of Health, London, UK

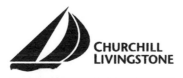

CHURCHILL
LIVINGSTONE

EDINBURGH LONDON NEW YORK PHILADELPHIA ST LOUIS SYDNEY TORONTO 2002

CHURCHILL LIVINGSTONE
An imprint of Harcourt Publishers Limited

© E. & S. Livingstone Ltd 1961, 1966, 1969
© Longman Group Limited 1973, 1978
© Longman Group UK Limited 1989
© Pearson Professional Limited 1996
© Harcourt Publishers Limited 2002

First edition 1932
Second edition 1933
Third edition 1934
Fourth edition 1936
Fifth edition 1938
Sixth edition 1940
Seventh edition 1941
Eighth edition 1943
Ninth edition 1946

Tenth edition 1949
Eleventh edition 1961
Twelfth edition 1966
Thirteenth edition 1969
Fourteenth edition 1973
Fifteenth edition 1978
Sixteenth edition 1989
Seventeenth edition 1996
Eighteenth edition published 2002

ISBN 0 443 06483 0

British Library Cataloguing in Publication Data
A catalogue record for this book is available from the British Library

Library of Congress Cataloging in Publication Data
A catalog record for this book is available from the Library of Congress

Note
Medical knowledge is constantly changing. As new information becomes available, changes in treatment, procedures, equipment and the use of drugs become necessary. The editor, advisers and the publishers have taken care to ensure that the information given in this text is accurate and up to date. However, readers are strongly advised to confirm that the information, especially with regard to drug usage, complies with the latest legislation and standards of practice.

The
publisher's
policy is to use
**paper manufactured
from sustainable forests**

Printed in China by RDC Group Limited

CONTENTS

FOREWORD

Communication is vital to good nursing care. Much communication is non-verbal – the smile, the comforting touch, a procedure handled speedily and competently, a gesture of support or sympathy. Whilst non-verbal skills are important, an essential part of a nurse's communication skills are verbal – in both speech and writing. A dictionary is therefore an essential tool for any nurse, midwife or health visitor. It helps the nurse to learn and understand clinical conditions, pharmacology, anatomy and physiology. It provides a useful reference guide to the growing technical terminology of medicine, and the growing language of nursing interventions, with which as a profession we must all become familiar.

Nurses must be able to adapt their language to their circumstances. Patients often turn to the nurse to help them understand their condition, to explain complex procedures and treatments in plain and simple language. Just as importantly, the nurse is now expected to hold her own in multidisciplinary discussion where technical and professional jargon are the order of the day. This ability to 'translate' language and adapt to different audiences is a critically important skill that nurses themselves sometimes overlook and undervalue.

Increasingly the nurse, midwife or health visitor also needs to gain an insight into emerging health policy. It is part of a professional approach to the practice of health care to understand the context in which you work, and the impact of health systems and organizations on patient care. The new edition of the dictionary offers a comprehensive overview of the new language of policy – from clinical governance to NICE, from nurse consultants to Primary Care Trusts. This is knowledge to underpin the practice of every health professional.

The importance of practice is matched by the importance of continuous professional development. Appendices in this dictionary that guide the development of effective curriculum vitae, personal development plans, mentorship and professional networking provide tools that both support the individual and enhance professional practice. Every nurse, midwife and health visitor should value their own development and recognize the contribution it makes to better patient care.

Nursing is a rooted profession: rooted in the development of understanding about health, about illness, about treatments and about the relief of suffering. Only with strong and secure roots in that knowledge can the practice of nursing flourish. This new edition of *Churchill Livingstone's Dictionary of Nursing* will provide an essential reference for trained staff and new students alike. I commend it to you.

Sarah Mullally

PREFACE

Nursing practice continues to change at a rapid pace and nurses need easy access to information from many areas of nursing and other healthcare disciplines. This well-established dictionary was due for a major revision and the opportunity has been taken to increase its size in terms of both breadth and depth of information. A team of advisers from academic institutions and many areas of clinical practice have revised existing entries, removed those no longer relevant, added new entries and written expanded entries.

The many new subject areas include: ethics, research, management, quality issues, information technology and health promotion. The number of longer, in-depth entries has been increased to over one hundred, covering a variety of topics from many disciplines. These are displayed in boxes so that they can be found easily. Another improvement is an increase in the number of clear and informative illustrations to seventy-five. The appendices have been completely revised and new topics relevant to students and registered nurses have been added in the areas of career and professional development and research. These topics include enhancing and developing your career via your CV, personal development planning and networking (all covered in Appendix 8); and research, evidence-based practice, libraries, literature searching, reference and citation systems, and referencing and web sources (all covered in Appendix 9).

The advisers and I hope that the dictionary will continue to be a valuable resource for students, registered nurses and others with an interest in health and health care, and that it will help nurses to fulfil their professional development responsibilities.

Norfolk 2002   *Chris Brooker*

ACKNOWLEDGEMENTS

The editor would like to thank the advisers as well as Christine Barnes, Maggie Nicol, David Llewellyn, Jacqueline Curthoys and Gail Murray.

The following figures have been reproduced with permission from these publications: Bale S, Jones V 1997 Wound Care Nursing. A patient-centred approach. London, Baillière Tindall, Figure 68; Brooker C (ed.) 1996 Nurse's Pocket Dictionary, 31st edn. London, Mosby, Figures 1, 4, 7, 9, 11, 17, 19, 23, 24, 29, 33, 34, 35, 39, 41, 51, 53, 54, 62 and 69; Brooker C 1998 Human Structure and Function. Nursing Applications in Clinical Practice, 2nd edn. London, Mosby, Figures 3, 5, 6, 13, 14, 21, 22, 27, 30, 31, 36, 37, 38, 42, 48, 49, 50 and 61; Bruce L, Finlay T M D (eds) 1997 Nursing in Gastroenterology. Edinburgh, Churchill Livingstone, Figures 57 and 67; Heath H B M (ed) 1995 Potter and Perry's Foundations in Nursing Theory and Practice. London, Mosby, Figure 58; Hinchliff S, Montague S, Watson R 1996 Physiology for Nursing Practice, 2nd edn. London, Baillière Tindall, Figure 15; Macleod J, Edwards C, Bouchier I (eds) 1987 Davidson's Principles and Practice of Medicine. Edinburgh, Churchill Livingstone, Figure 56; Nicol M, Bavin C, Bedford-Turner S, Cronin P, Rawlings-Anderson K 2000 Essential Nursing Skills. Edinburgh, Mosby, Figures 2, 20, 25, 28, 46, 47, 52, 59, 60, 63, 64 and 66; Westwood O M R 1999 The Scientific Basis for Health Care. Edinburgh, Mosby, Figures 12B, 26 and 32; Wilson J 1995 Infection Control in Clinical Practice. Edinburgh, Baillière Tindall, Figure 8.

PANEL OF ADVISERS

Denis Anthony BA(Hons) MSc PhD RMN RGN RN (Canada)
Professor of Nursing Informatics, Mary Seacole Research Centre, School of Nursing and Midwifery, De Montfort University, Leicester, UK

Helen Barker BSc SRD MPH
Senior Lecturer in Dietetics, School of Health and Social Sciences, Coventry University, Coventry, UK

Gaëtan Béphage BA(Hons) RGN RMN DipN(Lond) FETC CertEd Cert Social Studies RNT
Lecturer, School of Nursing, Hull University, Hull, UK

Tanya Campbell BSc(Hons) PGDip (Post Compulsory Education RGN)
Lecturer in Oncology Care Nursing, Institute of Health and Community Studies, Bournemouth University, Bournemouth, UK

Bridgit Dimond MA LLB DSA AHSM Barrister-at-Law
Emeritus Professor, University of Glamorgan, Pontypridd, UK

Anne Eaton BSc RN RM RCNT RNT CertEd
Education/Vocational Qualifications Adviser, Royal College of Nursing, London, UK

Catherine Gamble BA(Hons) RMN RGN RNT
Senior Lecturer in Mental Health, RCN Development Centre, South Bank University, London, UK

Rosemary Hagedorn DipCOT DipTCDHEd MSc(AOT) FCOT
Retired Occupational Therapist; Freelance Author and Lecturer, Arundel, UK

Julie Hyde BA(Hons) RGN RCNT RNT CertEd(FE) CertHSM FRSH MIHM MIMgt ILTM
Education, Policy and Management Consultant, Leeds, UK

Jennifer Kelly BA(Hons) MSc RGN DipN DipNEd
Senior Lecturer, Homerton School of Health Studies, Cambridge, UK

David C M Llewellyn
Computer Consultant, Norfolk, UK

Catherine Meredith BA MPH DCR(t)
Senior Lecturer, Department of Physiotherapy, Podiatry and Radiography, Glasgow Caledonian University, Glasgow, UK

Anne Parry PhD MCSP DipTP
Professor of Physiotherapy and Senior Research Fellow, Professions Allied to Medicine, School of Health and Social Care, Sheffield Hallam University, Sheffield, UK

Joan Ramsay MSc RGN RSCN RNT DN(Lond)
Lead Paediatric Nurse, Taunton and Somerset NHS Trust, Taunton, UK

HOW TO USE THIS DICTIONARY

Main entries
These are listed in alphabetical order and appear in bold type. Derivative forms of the main entry also appear in bold type and along with their parts of speech are to be found at the end of the definition.

Separate meanings of main entry
Different meanings of the same word are separated by means of a bold Arabic numeral before each meaning. For example:

acme *n* **1.** highest point. **2.** crisis or critical state of a disease.

Subentries
Subentries relating to the defined headword are listed in alphabetical order and appear in italic type following the main definition. For example:

intelligence *n* inborn mental ability. *intelligence quotient (IQ)* the ratio of mental age to chronological (actual) age. *intelligence tests* designed to determine the level of intelligence.

Parts of speech
The part of speech follows many of the single word main entries and derivative forms of the main entry and appears in italic type. The parts of speech used in the dictionary are:

abbr	abbreviation
acr	acronym
adj	adjective
adv	adverb
ant	antonym
n	noun
npl	plural noun
pl	plural
sing	singular
syn	synonym
v	verb
vi	intransitive verb
vt	transitive verb

Cross-references

Cross-references alert the reader to related words and additional information elsewhere in the dictionary. A single symbol has been used for this purpose: an arrow =>. Either within or at the end of a definition, the arrow indicates the word(s) you can then look up for related subject matter.

For example:

hyperparathyroidism *n* excessive secretion of the parathyroid glands due to adenoma or hyperplasia. The resultant increase in serum calcium levels may result in osteitis fibrosa cystica with decalcification, leading to backache, joint and bone pain and possible spontaneous fracture of bones. The increase in urinary excretion of calcium leads to renal damage. => hypercalcaemia. => hypercalciuria. => von Recklinghausen's disease.

Technical words within a definition are explained, or have a main entry or subentry elsewhere in the text.

For example:

In the definition for **hyperparathyroidism** the technical words adenoma, decalcification, hyperplasia, osteitis fibrosa cystica, parathyroid glands, renal and urinary are all defined in the dictionary.

Expanded entries (boxes)

These are longer entries covering a variety of topics relevant to nurses. They are displayed in separate boxes so that they can be found easily. All are cross-referenced in the main entries and many of the boxed entries provide useful references and suggestions for further reading. For example:

Ageism

A discriminatory attitude which disadvantages older adults on the basis of chronological age. Ageism is also interpreted to be stigmatizing and to demarcate the older person from others who are younger. Further, ageism can affect people of any age. The practice of ageist behaviours is often demonstrated in the choice of words used. For example, 'senile' and 'geriatric' are terms which have become derogatory (Behrens 1998). In addition the media often reinforce this negative stereotyping. Ageist attitude could have developed from the process of socialization: parental behaviours; peer influences; teachers' attitude.

A balanced approach to healthy ageing is adopted by professionals to promote antiageist behaviours across boundaries. The co-ordination between care services to promote a positive image of older people is perceived to be the way forward in the 21st century (Pulford 2000). It is recommended that in developing an assessment of needs tool a positive attitude toward ageing is essential (Vernon et al 2000). Healthcare professionals can reduce the impact of ageism by exercising sensitivity in daily interactions with clients and promoting a positive image of ageing.

References
Behrens H 1998 Ageism real or imagined? Elderly Care. 10(2):10–13
Pulford E 2000 A balanced approach to healthy ageing in the 21st century. Geriatric Medicine. 30(1):9
Veron S, Ross F, Gould M A 2000 Assessment of older people: politics and practice in primary care. Journal of Advanced Nursing. 31(2):282–287

PREFIXES

Prefixes which can be used as combining forms in compounded words

Prefix	Meaning
a-	without, not
ab-	away from
abdo-/abdomino-	abdominal
acro-	extremity
ad-	towards
adeno-	glandular
adip-	fat
aer-	air
amb-/ambi-	both, on both sides
amido-	NH$_2$ group united to an acid radical
amino-	NH$_2$ united to a radical other than an acid radical
amphi-	on both sides, around
amyl-	starch
an-	not, without
ana-	up
andro-	male
angi-	vessel (blood)
aniso-	unequal
ant-/anti-	against, counteracting
ante-/antero-	before
antro-	antrum
aorto-	aorta
app-	away, from
arachn-	spider
arthro-	joint
auto-	self
bi-	twice, two
bili-	bile
bio-	life
blenno-	mucus
bleph-	eyelid
brachio-	arm
brachy-	short
brady-	slow
broncho-	bronchi

Prefix	Meaning
bucc-	cheek
calc-	chalk
carcin-	cancer
cardio-	heart
cárpo-	wrist
cata-	down
cav-	hollow
centi-	a hundredth
cephal-	head
cerebro-	brain
cervic-	neck
cheil-	lip
cheir-	hand
chemo-	chemical
chlor-	green
chol-	bile
cholecysto-	gall bladder
choledocho-	bile duct
chondro-	cartilage
chrom-	colour
cine-	film, motion
circum-	around
co-/col-/com-/con-	together
coli-	bowel
colpo-	vagina
contra-	against
costo-	rib
cox-	hip
crani-/cranio-	skull
cryo-	cold
crypt-	hidden, concealed
cyan-	blue
cysto-	bladder
cyto-	cell
dacryo-	tear
dactyl-	finger
de-	away, from, reversing
deca-	ten

Prefix	Meaning	Prefix	Meaning
deci-	tenth	hexa-	six
demi-	half	histo-	tissue
dent-	tooth	homeo-	like
derma-/dermat-	skin	homo-	same
dextro	to the right	hydro-	water
di-/dip-	twos, double	hygro-	moisture
dia-	through	hyper-	above
dis-	separation, against	hypno-	sleep
dors-	the back	hypo-	below
dys-	difficult, painful, abnormal	hystero-	uterus
		iatro-	physician
ec-	out from	idio-	peculiar to the individual
ecto-	outside, without, external	ileo-	ileum
electro-	electricity	ilio-	ilium
em-	in	immuno-	immunity
en-/end-/endo-	in, into, within	in-	not, in, into, within
ent-	within	infra-	below
entero-	intestine	inter-	between
epi-	on, above, upon	intra	within
erythr-	red	intro-	inward
eu	well, normal	ischio-	ischium
ex-/exo-	away from, out, out of	iso-	equal, same
extra-	outside	karyo-	nucleus
		kerato-	horn, skin, cornea
faci-	face	kin-	movement, motion
ferri-/ferro-	iron	kypho-	rounded, humped
feto-	fetus		
fibro-	fibre, fibrous tissue	lacri-	tears
flav-	yellow	lact-	milk
fore-	before, in front of	laparo	abdomen, flank
		laryngo-	larynx
gala-	milk	later-	side
gastr-/gastro-	stomach	lepto-	thin, soft
genito-	genitals, reproductive	leuco-/leuko-	white
		lip-/lipo-	fat
ger-	old age	litho-	stones
gloss-/glosso-	tongue	lympho-	lymphatic
glyco-	sugar		
gnatho-	jaw	macro-	large
gynae-	female	macul-	spot
		mal-	abnormal, poor
haema-/haemo-	blood	mamm-/mast-	breast
hemi-	half	medi-	middle
hepa-/hepatico-/ hepato-	liver	mega-	large
		melano-	black, dark
hetero-	unlikeness, dissimilarity	meso-	middle
		meta-	after, between

SUFFIXES

Suffixes which can be used as combining forms in compounded words

Suffix	Meaning	Suffix	Meaning
-able	able to, capable of	-gogue	increasing flow
-aemia	blood	-gram	a tracing
-aesthesia	sensibility, sense-perception	-graph	instrument for writing or recording
-agra	attack, severe pain		
-al	characterized by, pertaining to	-ia/-iasis	condition of, state
-algia	pain	-iatric	practice of healing
-an	belonging to, pertaining to	-ism	condition, state
		-itis	inflammation of
-ase	catalyst, enzyme		
-asis	state of	-kinesis/-kinetic	motion
-blast	cell	-lith	calculus, stone
		-lithiasis	presence of stones
-caval	pertaining to venae cavae	-logy	science of, study of
		-lysis/-lytic	breaking down, disintegration
-cele	tumour, swelling		
-centesis	to puncture		
-cide	destructive, killing	-malacia	softening
-cle/-cule	small	-megaly	enlargement
-clysis	infusion, injection	-meter	measure
-coccus	spherical cell	-morph	shape, form
-cyte	cell		
		-odynia	pain
-derm	skin	-ogen	precursor
-desis	to bind or fix together	-oid	likeness, resemblance
-dynia	pain	-ol	alcohol
		-ology	the study of
-ectasis	dilation, extension	-oma	tumour
-ectomy	removal of	-opia	eye
-emesis	vomiting	-opsy	looking
		-ose	sugar
-facient	making	-osis	condition, disease, excess
-ferent	carry		
-form	having the form of	-ostomy	to form an opening or outlet
-fuge	expelling		
		-otomy	incision of
-genesis/-genetic	formation, origin	-ous	like, having the nature of
-genic	capable of causing		

Suffix	Meaning	Suffix	Meaning
-pathy	disease	-scopy	to examine visually
-penia	lack of	-soma/-somatic	body
-pexy	fixation	-somy	pertaining to
-phage	ingesting		chromosomes
-phagia	swallowing	-sonic	sound
-phasia	speech	-stasis	stagnation,
-phil/-philia	affinity for, loving		cessation of
-phobia	fear		movement
-phylaxis	protection	-sthenia	strength
-plasty	reconstruct	-stomy	to form an opening
-plegia	paralysis		or outlet
-pnoea	breathing		
-poiesis	making	-taxia/-taxis/-taxy	arrangement,
-ptosis	falling		coordination,
			order
-rhythmia	rhythm	-tome	cutting
-rrhage/-rrhagia	to burst forth,		instrument
	pour, excessive	-tomy	incision of
-rrhaphy	repair	-trophy	growth,
-rrhoea	flow, discharge		nourishment
		-tropic	turning, influencing
-saccharide	carbohydrate		
-scope	instrument for	-uria	urine
	visual examination		

A

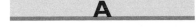

AA *abbr* Alcoholics Anonymous.

abdomen *n* the largest body cavity, immediately below the thorax, from which it is separated by the diaphragm. It is enclosed largely by muscle and fascia, and is therefore capable of change in size and shape. Contains many important organs, including the liver, spleen, pancreas, lower oesophagus, stomach and intestines. It is lined with a serous membrane, the peritoneum, which is reflected as a covering over most of the organs. *acute abdomen* pathological condition within the abdomen requiring immediate surgical intervention. *pendulous abdomen* a relaxed condition of the anterior wall, allowing it to hang down over the pubis.

abdominal *adj* pertaining to the abdomen. *abdominal aortic aneurysm (AAA)* a dilatation in the abdominal part of the aorta. → aneurysm. *abdominal breathing* more than usual use of the diaphragm and abdominal muscles to increase the input of air to and output from the lungs. It can be done voluntarily in the form of exercises. When it occurs in disease it is a compensatory mechanism for inadequate oxygenation. *abdominal excision of the rectum*, normally for a tumour the rectum is mobilized through an abdominal incision. The bowel is divided well proximal to the tumour. The proximal end is brought out as a permanent colostomy. Excision of the distal bowel containing the tumour, together with the anal canal, is completed through a perineal incision. *abdominal pregnancy* condition where the embryo/fetus develops in the abdominal cavity, the placenta adhering to the gut, peritoneum and other organs. Rare, occasionally results in the operative birth of a live baby but normally the fetus will die. ⇒ lithopaedion. *abdominal reflex* a superficial reflex where the abdominal muscles contract when the skin is stroked. *abdominal regions* where the surface anatomy is divided into nine regions used to describe the location of organs or symptoms, such as pain (see Figure 1). *abdominal thrust* ⇒ Heimlich manoeuvre.

abdominocentesis *n* aspiration of the peritoneal cavity. ⇒ amniocentesis. ⇒ colpocentesis. ⇒ thoracentesis.

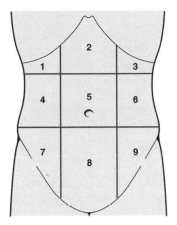

Figure 1 Abdominal regions.
1. Right hypochondrium. 2. Epigastrium. 3. Left hypochondrium. 4. Right lumbar. 5. Umbilical. 6. Left lumbar. 7. Right iliac. 8. Hypogastrium. 9. Left iliac. (Reproduced from Brooker 1996 with permission.)

abdominopelvic *adj* pertaining to the abdomen and pelvis or pelvic cavity.

abdominoperineal *adj* pertaining to the abdomen and perineum.

abduct *vt* to draw away from the midline of the body. ⇒ adduct *ant*.

abduction *n* the act of abducting away from the midline. → adduction *ant*.

abductor *n* a muscle, e.g. the deltoid, which contracts to move a part away from the midline of the body. ⇒ adductor *ant*.

aberrant *adj* abnormal; usually applied to a blood vessel or nerve which does not follow the normal course.

aberration *n* a deviation from normal. *chromosomal aberration* loss, gain or exchange of genetic material in the chromosomes of a cell, resulting in deletion, duplication, inversion or translocation of genes. *mental aberration* ⇒ mental. *optical aberration* imperfect focus of light rays by a lens — **aberrant** *adj*.

ability *n* the physical and mental capacity to perform skills, such as the functional ability required for the activities of daily living.

ablation *n* removal. In surgery, the word means excision, amputation or destruction, such as in endometrial ablation with laser therapy. *transvenous catheter radiofrequency ablation* a technique used to destroy the abnormal atrial tissue that forms a bypass tract responsible for Wolff-Parkinson-White syndrome — **ablative** *adj*.

ABO groups *n* ⇒ blood groups.

abort *vt, vi* to terminate before full development, especially applied to pregnancy.

abortifacient *adj* causing abortion. A drug or agent that induces abortion, e.g. mifepristone.

abortion *n* 1. abrupt termination of a process. 2. expulsion from a uterus of the products of conception before the fetus is viable, i.e. developed sufficiently to be capable of a separate existence. In English law, a fetus is viable at 24 weeks gestation, but some infants born before this survive because of advances in neonatal intensive care. Abortion may be spontaneous, when it is generally termed miscarriage, or therapeutic, where the pregnancy is intentionally terminated. ⇒ abortus. *complete abortion* the entire contents of the uterus are expelled. *criminal abortion* intentional evacuation of uterus by other than trained, licensed medical personnel, and/or when abortion is prohibited by law. *habitual abortion* (preferable *syn*) *recurrent abortion* term used when abortion recurs in successive pregnancies. *incomplete abortion* part of the products of conception; fetus or placenta are retained within the uterus. *induced abortion* (also called 'artificial') intentional evacuation of uterus. *inevitable abortion* one which has advanced to a stage where spontaneous loss is imminent and cannot be prevented. *missed abortion* early signs and symptoms of pregnancy disappear and the fetus dies, but is not expelled for some time. ⇒ carneous mole. *septic abortion* one associated with uterine infection, rise in body temperature and possible overwhelming infection and shock. *spontaneous abortion* a miscarriage. One which occurs naturally without intervention. *therapeutic abortion* intentional termination of a pregnancy. ⇒ termination of pregnancy. *threatened abortion* slight vaginal bleeding whilst the cervix remains closed. May be accompanied by abdominal pain. *tubal abortion* an ectopic pregnancy where the embryo is expelled from the fimbriated end of the uterine tube into the peritoneal cavity — **abortive** *adj*.

abortus *n* an aborted fetus weighing less than 500 g. It is either dead or incapable of surviving.

abortus fever *n* ⇒ brucellosis.

ABPI *abbr* ankle brachial pressure index.

abrasion *n* 1. superficial injury to skin or mucous membrane from scraping or rubbing; excoriation. 2. can be used therapeutically for removal of scar tissue (dermabrasion).

abreaction *n* an emotional reaction resulting from recall of past painful experiences, relived in speech and action during psychoanalysis, or under the influence of light anaesthesia or drugs. ⇒ catharsis. ⇒ narcoanalysis.

abscess *n* localized collection of pus produced by pyogenic organisms. May be acute or chronic. Surgical incision and drainage may be required before healing can occur. *alveolar abscess* at the root of a tooth. *cold abscess* one occurring with few signs of inflammation and may be due to *Mycobacterium tuberculosis*. ⇒ psoas abscess.

absolute threshold the smallest stimulus that can be detected.

absorption *n* 1. movement of substances across membranes or surfaces into body fluids or cells, e.g. water and nutrients into cells. 2. the take-up of a substance by another, such as gas absorption by a liquid. 3. transfer of energy to the tissues during exposure to ionizing radiation.

absorption rate constant *n* the amount of drug absorbed in a unit of time.

absorptive state *n* the fed state. Metabolic state that exists immediately following a meal and lasting for around four hours. The nutrients absorbed are used for instant energy or in anabolic processes such as lipogenesis and glycogenesis. ⇒ postabsorptive state.

abuse *n* 1. deliberate injury to another person – either physical, sexual, psychological or through neglect, such as failure to feed or clothe. The term can apply to any group of people, especially the most vulnerable in society, such as children, people with learning disabilities, women and older people. *child abuse* physical, sexual or emotional abuse or neglect of children by relatives or health and social care staff. ⇒ neglect. ⇒ nonaccidental injuries. *elder* *abuse* physical, sexual, psychological or financial abuse of older people. May be carried out by those relatives and friends responsible for their care or by health and social care staff. 2. misuse of equipment, drugs and other substances, authority, power and position.

acalculia *n* inability to do simple arithmetic.

acanthosis *n* thickening of the prickle-cell layer of the skin, such as in psoriasis and eczema. *acanthosis nigricans* thickened, pigmented skin seen in the groin, axillae and perianal areas.

acatalasaemia *n* rare genetic disorder transmitted as an autosomal recessive. Results in a deficiency of the enzyme catalase in red blood cells and tissues and is characterized by ulcerating oral lesions.

access to obtain sight of, used in connection with health records, or to a child, such as after a divorce.

Access to Health Records Act (1990) *n* allows access to both paper and computerized health records made after 1991, with certain exceptions, e.g. where they may cause serious mental or physical harm to a person.

accident form also called untoward incident form. A form designed by a Health Authority or NHS Trust to be used as soon as possible after an accident to any person on its premises. The signed forms (data) are collected centrally and analysed to provide information such as the most common type of accident, to whom it occurred, where and when and so on. Such factual information is essential to the trade union Health and Safety Representatives as well as to managers. There is a legal requirement to report serious accidents to the Health and Safety executive. ⇒ accidents – prevention of.

accidents, prevention of part of the nursing role. Nurses must ensure that their fear of accidents does not prevent patients, especially those who are older, from taking reasonable risk, thereby lowering their level of independence. ⇒ accident form. ⇒ manual handling. ⇒ risk assessment. ⇒ risk management.

accommodation *n* 1. adjustment, e.g. the power of the eye to alter the convexity of the lens, so that distinct images are achieved of objects at different distances.

2. process by which individuals and groups adapt or modify activity to meet social requirements. It does not always resolve basic conflicts between different groups — **accommodative** *adj*.

accountability *n* a nurse has a duty to care according to law. In some countries the statutory body, and/or the professional organisation, elaborate a code of conduct via which each qualified nurse can accept responsibility and accountability for the nursing service delivered to each patient/client. ⇒ duty of care. ⇒ malpractice. ⇒ negligence. ⇒ NMC. ⇒ UKCC.

Accreditation (Assessment) of Prior Experiential Learning (APEL) see Box – APEL, APL and CATS.

Accreditation (Assessment) of Prior Learning (APL) see Box – APEL, APL and CATS.

accretion *n* an increase of substance or deposit round a central object; in dentistry, an accumulation of tartar or calculus around the teeth — **accretive** *adj*.

ACE *abbr* angiotensin-converting enzyme.

acetabuloplasty *n* an operation to improve the depth and shape of the hip socket (acetabulum); necessary in such conditions as developmental dysplasia of the hip (congenital dislocation of the hip) and osteoarthritis of the hip.

acetabulum *n* a cup-like socket on the innominate bone or hip into which the head of the femur fits to form the hip joint — **acetabula** *pl*.

acetate *n* a salt of acetic acid.

acetic acid *n* an organic acid. Found in vinegar.

acetic acids *npl* a group of nonsteroidal anti-inflammatory drugs, e.g. indometacin (indomethacin).

acetoacetate *n* an acidic ketone formed during an intermediate stage in the oxidation of fats in the human body. It can be used as a fuel molecule by some tissues, such as the kidney. Where carbohydrates are not available for metabolism, such as in starvation and diabetes mellitus, there is an excess which leads to high levels in the blood and ketoacidosis with severe disturbances of pH, fluid and electrolyte imbalance and altered consciousness.

acetonaemia *n* ⇒ acidosis. ⇒ ketoacidosis. ⇒ ketonaemia — **acetonaemic** *adj*.

acetone *n* inflammable liquid with characteristic 'pear drops' odour; valuable as a solvent. *ketone bodies* ⇒ ketones.

acetonuria *n* ⇒ ketonuria — **acetonuric** *adj*.

acetylcholine (ACh) *n* a chemical neurotransmitter that facilitates the passage of a nerve impulse across synapses in parasympathetic nerves and at the neuromuscular junction in skeletal muscles. The nerve fibres releasing this chemical are termed 'cholinergic'. Hydrolysed into choline and acetate by the enzyme acetylcholinesterase. ⇒ anticholinergic. ⇒ myasthenia gravis.

acetylcholinesterase *n* the enzyme that inactivates acetylcholine after the nerve impulse has passed across the synapse. Its presence in the synaptic gap/cleft ensures that only one action potential crosses the synapse and prevents continuous muscle contraction.

acetylcoenzyme A *n* also known as acetyl Co A. An important metabolic molecule involved in many cellular processes, e.g. Krebs' citric acid cycle, glycolysis.

achalasia *n* failure of a muscle sphincter to relax. Applied particularly to the cardiac (gastro-oesophageal) sphincter. ⇒ cardia. ⇒ cardiomyotomy. ⇒ Heller's operation.

Achilles tendon *n* tendon of the calf muscles (gastrocnemius and soleus) situated at the back of the ankle and attached to the calcaneus bone of the heel. Named after the figure in Greek mythology who could only be wounded in the heel.

achlorhydria *n* the absence of free hydrochloric acid in the gastric juice. May occur in pernicious anaemia and gastric cancer. ⇒ anaemia — **achlorhydric** *adj*.

acholia *n* the absence of bile — **acholic** *adj*.

acholuria *n* the absence of bile pigment from the urine. ⇒ jaundice — **acholuric** *adj*.

achondroplasia *n* a genetically inherited disorder characterized by arrested growth of the long bones due to premature ossification of the episphyseal plates. It results in short stature of varying degrees because the long bones are abnormally 'short', but the trunk and most of the skull develop normally. Inheritance is dominant — **achondroplastic** *adj*.

achromatopsia *n* colour blindness.

achylia *n* absence of chyle — **achylic** *adj*.

acid *n* substances having an excess of hydrogen ions over hydroxyl ions, e.g. hydrochloric acid. They release hydrogen ions on dissociation in solution. Acids are hydrogen ion (proton) donators. Acids have a pH below 7, turn blue litmus paper red and are neutralized by alkalis. Acids combine with alkalis to form salts and water. *acid phosphatase* an enzyme requiring an acid medium that acts in several metabolic reactions involving phosphates. Found in the prostate gland, semen, kidney and serum. Levels in serum rise in prostatic cancers with bone spread. *acid rebound* hypersecretion of gastric acid after the buffering effects of an antacid have disappeared.

acid-alcohol fast *adj* in microbiology, describes an organism which, when stained, is resistant to decolourization by alcohol as well as acid, e.g. *Mycobacterium tuberculosis*. ⇒ Ziehl-Neelsen technique.

acid-base balance equilibrium between the acid and base elements of the blood and body fluids which determine the pH of body fluids. Normal pH range for blood is 7.35–7.45. ⇒ acidosis. ⇒ alkalosis.

acid-fast *adj* in microbiology, describes an organism which, when stained, is able to retain dyes despite washing with acid. *acid-fast bacilli (AFB)* bacteria that can be identified in the laboratory by use of acid-fast staining techniques.

acidity *n* the state of being acid or sour. The degree of acidity can be determined and interpreted on the pH scale where a pH below 7 is acid.

acidosis *n* depletion of the body's alkali reserve, with resulting disturbance of the acid-base balance. The hydrogen ion concentration in the blood increases and the blood pH falls. *metabolic acidosis* caused by diabetic ketoacidosis, increased lactic acid production in muscles and loss of alkali, such as in severe diarrhoea. ⇒ ketosis. *respiratory acidosis* may result from hypoventilation, e.g. respiratory failure — **acidotic** *adj*.

Acinetobacter *n* a genus of Gram-negative aerobic bacteria of the family Neisseriaceae. It causes a range of infections, e.g. pneumonia, wound infection and meningitis. It has developed drug resistance and is a particular hazard to very ill patients in intensive care or high dependency settings.

acini *npl* minute saccules or alveoli, lined or filled with secreting cells, as in the breast. Several acini combine to form a lobule — **acinous, acinar** *adj*.

acme *n* 1. highest point. 2. crisis or critical state of a disease.

acne, acne vulgaris *n* inflammation and overstimulation of the pilosebaceous glands associated with high levels of androgen hormones. Occurs during adolescence and is usually worse in males, but later onset does occur. It is characterized by comedones, papules, pustules, pitting and scars, especially on the face and back. Excessive sebum is trapped by a plug of keratin, one of the protein constituents of human hair. Skin bacteria then colonize the glands and convert the trapped sebum into irritant fatty acids responsible for the swelling and inflammation (pustules) which follow.

acneiform *adj* resembling acne.

acoustic neuroma benign tumour of the auditory nerve.

acquired immune deficiency syndrome (AIDS) a complex syndrome caused by Human Immunodeficiency Virus (HIV), which belongs to the retrovirus group. The virus damages the immune system, especially the CD4 (T-helper) lymphocytes which are concerned with cell mediated immunity. The virus is spread by contact with infected blood and other body fluids. This may occur through sexual contact, drug misusers sharing equipment such as syringes, vertical transmission from mother to fetus (via the placenta, at delivery or via breast milk), transmission to health workers, such as through 'needlestick' injuries or by the transfusion of infected blood/blood products. Management involves the use of antiviral drugs, usually in combination to prevent resistance, and antimicrobial drugs to reduce the risk of opportunistic infection. Prophylactic drug therapy is offered after occupational exposure. Drug therapy can be offered to women found to be HIV positive during pregnancy to reduce the risk of vertical transmission to the fetus. HIV disease can be classified into three groups: (a) acute HIV infection which has a latent period followed by seroconversion (antibody production) during which some people experiece a mild illness with fever, rash, joint pain and headache. An asymptomatic phase following seroconversion that may last several years, or accompanied by persistent generalized lymphadenopathy (PGL); (b) an early symptomatic stage, also known as AIDS-related complex (ARC), when patients have symptoms, such as weight loss, fever, diarrhoea, fatigue and infections, e.g. herpes zoster, but without any AIDS defining conditions; (c) fully developed AIDS with weight loss etc as for ARC and a range of AIDS defining opportunistic infections, such as *Pneumocystis carinii* pneumonia (PCP), oesophageal candidiasis and chronic cryptosporidiosis. Some individuals will develop secondary neoplasms, e.g. Kaposi's sarcoma and nonHodgkin's lymphoma.

acrocyanosis *n* coldness and blueness of the extremities due to circulatory disorder — **acrocyanotic** *adj*.

acrodynia *n* painful reddening of the extremities

acromegaly *n* condition caused by oversecretion of growth hormone by the pituitary gland after fusion of the epiphyses. It causes enlargement of the bones of the hands, face and feet and also the heart and liver. ⇒ gigantism. ⇒ growth hormone test — **acromegalic** *adj*.

acromicria *n* smallness of the hands, feet and facial features.

acromioclavicular *adj* pertaining to the acromion process (of scapula) and the clavicle. *acromioclavicular joint* the synovial joint between the acromion and the clavicle.

acromion *n* the point or summit of the shoulder; the triangular process at the extreme outer end of the spine of the scapula — **acromial** *adj*.

acroparaesthesia *n* tingling and numbness of the hands.

acrophobia *n* irrational fear of being at a height.

acrosome *n* the structure situated on the head of the spermatozoon. It contains lytic enzymes required for spermatozoa to penetrate the cervical mucus and the oocyte.

Act of Parliament statute, legislation.

ACTH *abbr* adrenocorticotrophic hormone. ⇒ corticotrophin.

ACTH stimulation test measurement of cortisol level in the blood after the administration of tetracosactide (tetracosactrin), the active part of ACTH. Normally this produces pituitary stimulation for increased secretion of corticosteroid hormones by the adrenal cortex. Lack of response denotes inactivity of adrenal cortex as in Addison's disease and other forms of adrenal insufficiency.

actin *n* a contractile protein, one of the component filaments of a muscle myofibril. It reacts with myosin to cause contraction.

acting out *n* reduction of emotional distress by the release of disturbed or violent behaviour, which is unconsciously determined and reflects previous unresolved conflicts and attitudes.

actinic dermatoses skin conditions in which the integument is abnormally sensitive to ultraviolet light.

Actinomyces *n* a genus of branching micro-organisms. *Actinomyces israeli* is the cause of actinomycosis in humans.

actinomycosis *n* a disease caused by the micro-organism *Actinomyces israeli*. It commonly affects the face and neck, lungs or abdomen with the formation of pus containing yellowish 'sulphur' granules, abscesses, sinuses and necrosis. Sites most affected being the lung, jaw and intestine — **actinomycotic** *adj*.

action *n* process of activity or functioning. *action potential* the change in electrical potential and charge that occurs across cell membranes when muscles contract or nerve impulses are conducted. *antagonistic action* performed by those muscles which limit the movement of an opposing group. ⇒ antagonist. *compulsive action* an overwhelming need to perform an act which is not necessarily rational. *impulsive action* resulting from a sudden urge rather than the will. *reflex action* ⇒ reflex. *synergistic action* ⇒ synergy — **active** *adj active immunity* ⇒ immunity. *active movements* where the individual performs movements unaided, as in physiotherapy. ⇒ passive *ant*. *active transport* is the use of metabolic energy to move substances across cell membranes. ⇒ adenosine triphosphate.

active *adj* energetic. ⇒ passive *ant*. *active hyperaemia* ⇒ hyperaemia. *active immunity* ⇒ immunity. *active movements* those produced by the patient using his neuromuscular mechanism. *active principle* an ingredient which gives a complex drug its chief therapeutic value, e.g. atropine is the active principle in belladonna.

Activities of Daily Living (ADLs) most nurses include the usual hygiene activities associated with washing and dressing, and maintenance activities such as eating and drinking. Occupational therapists recognize the activities and tasks that are essential for self-care or home management. They include Personal Activities of Daily Living (PADL): washing, dressing, personal hygiene and eating; Domestic Activities of Daily Living (DADL): cooking, laundry and cleaning; and Instrumental Activities of Daily Living (IADL), sometimes used synonomously with DADL, but including a wider range of activities, such as using means of communication, shopping, using transport, maintaining home and garden. Competence and independence in ADLs is essential for personal survival, health and well-being. Persons who are unable to cope with the necessary range of activities are likely to be at risk and require care services of various kinds. *ADL assessment and training* an occupational therapy technique where a period of objective appraisal of a person's ability to perform ADLs is followed by a training programme to improve function.

Activities of Living (ALs) on the grounds that not all activities are carried out daily, some nurses prefer the term 'activities of living' to that of 'activities of daily living'. Roper, Logan and Tierney selected 12 ALs as the focus for their model for nursing based on a model of living; they are: maintaining a safe environment, communicating, breathing, eating and drinking, eliminating, personal cleansing and dressing, controlling body temperature, mobilising, working and playing, expressing sexuality, sleeping and dying.

activity a specific action or function. *activity analysis* breaking down an activity into its component parts (tasks) so as to identify the skills needed by an individual to perform the activity. *activity programme* in occupational therapy, a programme designed to encourage groups or individuals to maintain or improve skills, interactions and roles. *activity synthesis* bringing together and adapting the components of an activity with those of the environment to assess existing performance and improve skills.

activity theory *n* a psychosocial theory of ageing. It describes the view that those individuals who remain socially active into old age and develop new roles, derive benefit and satisfaction. ⇒ disengagement theory.

activity tolerance the amount of physical activity tolerated by a patient. It may be assessed in patients with angina or following myocardial infarction. Graded exercise, including walking, cycling and going up stairs, may be used to rebuild confidence during the convalescent phase after any serious illness or injury – an important aspect of any rehabilitation programme.

actomyosin *n* protein complex formed by the contractile proteins actin and myosin during muscle fibre contraction.

acuity *n* sharpness, clearness, keenness, distinctness. *auditory acuity* ability to hear clearly and distinctly. Tests include the use of tuning fork, whispered voice and audiometry. Neonatal hearing screening can be performed by otoacoustic emission testing (OAE). ⇒ neonatal hearing screening. *visual acuity* the extent of visual perception is dependent on the clarity of retinal focus, integrity of nervous elements and cerebral interpretation of the stimulus. Usually tested by Snellen's test types at 6 metres.

acupuncture *n* an ancient system of healthcare practice which aims to treat illness and maintain health by stimulating the body's self-healing powers. Can

---

Acupuncture

Acupuncture forms part of Chinese medical care, which may also include diet, nutrition, herbal medicine and environmental issues. Whilst it has been used in China for over 3000 years acupuncture has become increasingly used as a discrete medical technique in the West (Downey 1995).

The word acupuncture is derived from the Latin acus (needle) and punctura (puncture). The technique is rooted in a rich and complex theoretical system derived from Confucian and Taoist philosophy. Although acupuncture has gained prominence in the West as a method of pain relief, its efficacy also extends to disorders of the nervous, digestive and respiratory systems as well as emotional and psychological problems (Downey 1995).

Acupuncture is based upon a set of principles which see the body as inseparable from the environment, universe and permeated with the same energy. In the human body this energy is referred to as *Qi* which flows through twelve main channels (meridians) and two further channels, the *conception* and *governing* channels. The dynamic balance of energy seen as central to acupuncture is expressed by the concepts Yin and Yang. These are relative rather than absolute terms. Yang is characterized by heat, activity and movement; Yin refers to cold, sluggishness and inactivity. There should be an equal balance of Yin and Yang energy for health. Yin and Yang are further refined into five elements or phases that link organs to meridians, emotions, seasons and to

the elements of fire, earth, metal, water and wood, creating a dynamic interactive cycle.

Illness is said to occur when there is excess, deficiency or obstruction of the energy within the organs or meridian pathways (Downey 1995). Acupuncture treatment involves the insertion of fine needles into specific parts of the body. In some instances the herb moxa is also used to warm and stimulate certain points. This is known as moxibustion. There are approximately 365 points along meridians at which needles can be inserted into the body to stimulate or suppress the flow of energy (Woodham & Peters 1997).

Whilst there is an increasing body of evidence to support the use of acupuncture to treat a number of conditions, it is argued that accurate diagnosis focuses upon a recognition of the uniqueness of each individual's condition. Thus two people presenting with the diagnostic label of arthritis may experience differing types of symptoms requiring treatment of disparate acupuncture points.

By restoring the flow of Qi in the channels, the vital energy (⇒ Complementary Medicine) is restored.

References

Downey S 1995 Acupuncture. In: Rankin-Box D (ed) The Nurses' Handbook of Complementary Therapies. Churchill Livingstone, Edinburgh

Woodham A, Peters D (eds) 1997 Encyclopedia of Complementary medicine. Dorling Kindersley, London also be used for the relief of pain or production of anaesthesia. See Box – Acupuncture.

acute *adj* short and severe; not long, drawn out or chronic. *acute abdomen* ⇒ abdomen. *acute confusional state* ⇒ confusion. *acute defibrination syndrome (ADS)* ⇒ afibriongenaemia. ⇒ disseminated intravascular coagulation. *acute dilatation of the stomach* sudden enlargement of this organ due to paralysis of the muscular wall. ⇒ ileus. ⇒ paralytic ileus. *acute haemorrhagic fevers* also called viral haemorrhagic fevers. ⇒ Ebola. ⇒ Lassa fever. ⇒ Marburg disease. *acute heart failure* ⇒ cardiac failure. *acute lymphoblastic leukaemia (ALL)* ⇒ leukaemia. *acute myeloblastic leukaemia* ⇒ leukaemia. *acute rheumatism* ⇒ rheumatic fever. *acute yellow atrophy* massive necrosis of liver associated with severe infection, pregnancy or ingested poisons.

acute respiratory distress syndrome (ARDS) *n* acute respiratory failure associated with multiple organ dysfunction syndrome. It is characterized by tachypnoea, dyspnoea and tachycardia, and analysis of arterial blood gases shows a reduced PaO_2 and eventually an increase in $PaCO_2$ with a fall in pH. Patients are treated with increased oxygen and respiratory support. ⇒ mechanical ventilation. ⇒ neonatal respiratory distress syndrome.

acute wounds *npl* those associated with trauma and or surgery. They usually heal quickly. ⇒ chronic wounds. ⇒ wound healing.

acyanosis *n* without cyanosis — **acyanotic** *adj* used to differentiate congenital cardiovascular defects.

acyesis *n* absence of pregnancy — **acyetic** *adj*.

acystia *n* congenital absence of the bladder — **acystic** *adj*.

Adam's apple *n* the laryngeal prominence in front of the neck, especially in the adult male, formed by the junction of the two wings of the thyroid cartilage.

adaptability *n* the capacity to adjust mentally and physically to circumstances in a flexible way.

adaptation *n* **1.** the ability to cope with new challenges in the environment. *home adaptations* the design and physical alterations to a person's home to enhance independent living. **2.** changes made by an occupational therapist to specific objects or the environment to provide therapy or to enhance the client's functional ability. *environmental adaptation* changes made to the social or physical environment in order to improve performance, increase or decrease a behaviour or for therapy.

adaptive behaviour beneficial or appropriate behaviour in response to a change.

addiction *n* craving for chemical substances, such as drugs, alcohol and tobacco, which the addicted person finds difficult to control. ⇒ dependence. ⇒ drug dependence.

Addison's disease a condition caused by a failure of adrenocortical hormone secretion due to disease affecting the adrenal glands, e.g. autoimmune failure, tuberculosis. The deficiency of glucocorticoids (cortisol) and mineralocorticoids (aldosterone) results in a serious condition characterized by wasting, weight loss, muscle weakness, hypoglycaemia, bronze skin pigmentation, gastrointestinal disturbances, fluid and electrolyte imbalance and hypotension. Lack of adrenal androgens causes a decrease in body hair. Management involves replacement of deficient hormones, correction of fluid and electrolyte imbalances and, where possible, treatment of the cause.

additive *n* any substance added to another in order to perform a specific quality, e.g. food additives that enhance flavour, texture or appearance, and those that act to stop food spoiling, e.g. preservatives or antioxidants. ⇒ E-number.

adduct *vt* to draw towards the midline of the body. ⇒ abduct *ant.*

adduction *n* the act of adducting, drawing towards the midline. ⇒ abduction *ant.*

adductor *n* any muscle which moves a part toward the midline of the body, e.g. the adductor muscles of the thigh. ⇒ abductor *ant.*

adenectomy *n* surgical removal of a gland.

adenine *n* nitrogenous base derived from purine. A component of nucleic acids (DNA, RNA).

adenitis *n* inflammation of a gland or lymph node.

adenocarcinoma *n* a malignant growth of glandular epithelium — **adenocarcinomatous** *adj*.

adenohypophysis ⇒ pituitary gland.

adenoid *adj* resembling a gland. ⇒ adenoids.

adenoidectomy *n* surgical removal of enlarged pharyngeal tonsil (adenoid tissue) from nasopharynx.

adenoids *npl* enlarged pharyngeal tonsils. The mass of lymphoid tissue in the nasopharynx can obstruct breathing and interfere with hearing.

adenoma *n* a benign tumour of glandular epithelium — **adenomatous** *adj*.

adenomyoma *n* a benign tumour composed of muscle and glandular epithelium, usually applied to benign growths of the uterus — **adenomyomatous** *adj*.

adenopathy *n* any disease or enlargement of a gland — **adenopathic** *adj*.

adenosine *n* a nucleoside formed from ribose (a pentose sugar) and adenine; with the addition of one, two or three phosphate groups it forms the nucleotides adenosine monophosphate, adenosine diphosphate and adenosine triphosphate. These molecules are vital in cellular energetic processes.

adenosine diphosphate (ADP) *n* an important cellular metabolite involved in energy exchange within the cell. Chemical energy is conserved in the cell, by the oxidative phosphorylation of ADP to ATP primarily in the mitochondrion, as a high energy phosphate bond.

adenosine monophosphate (AMP) *n* an important cellular metabolite involved in the release of energy for cell use. *cyclic adenosine monophosphate (cAMP)* an important metabolic molecule that functions as a 'second messenger' for many hormones, e.g. glucagon, and in biochemical process where many reactions are catalysed simultaneously (enzyme cascade).

adenosine triphosphate (ATP) *n* a high energy compound which, on hydrolysis to ADP, releases chemically useful energy. ATP is generated during the catabolism of organic fuel molecules, such as glucose. ATP molecules are generated during glycolysis, in the reactions of Krebs' citric acid cycle, but most are produced during oxidative phosphorylation of ADP in the electron transfer chain (during a series of oxidation-reduction reactions), situated in the inner mitochondrial membrane. The energy from ATP is used to drive metabolic processes, such as active transport of substances across cell membranes, synthesis of molecules and muscle fibre contraction.

adenotonsillectomy *n* surgical removal of the adenoids and palatine tonsils.

adenovirus *n* a group of DNA viruses of the Adenoviridae family. They cause conjunctivitis, respiratory and gastrointestinal infections.

adenylate cyclase *n* enzyme that catalyses the conversion of adenosine triphosphate (ATP) to cyclic adenosine monophosphate (cAMP).

ADH *abbr* antidiuretic hormone. ⇒ vasopressin.

ADHD *abbr* attention deficit hyperactivity disorder.

adhesion *n* abnormal union of two parts, occurring after inflammation; a band of fibrous tissue which joins such parts. In the abdomen, such a band may cause intestinal obstruction; in joints, it restricts movement; between two surfaces of pleura, it prevents complete pneumothorax — **adhere** *vi*.

adipocyte *n* a fat cell.

adipose *n, adj* fat; of a fatty nature. *adipose tissue* connective tissue containing fat cells in a matrix. The cells constituting adipose tissue contain either white or brown fat. → adipocyte.

adiposity *n* excessive accumulation of fat in the body.

aditus an opening; especially that between the mastoid antrum and the middle ear.

adjustment *n* stability within an individual and a satisfactory relationship between the individual and his environment.

adjuvant *n* a substance included in a prescription to aid the action of other drugs. *adjuvant therapy* a treatment (usually refers to a cancer treatment) given in conjunction with another, usually after any obvious tumour has been removed, either by surgery or radiotherapy. The aim is to improve cure rate and prevent recurrence. ⇒ neo-adjuvant therapy.

Adler, Alfred Austrian psychiatrist (1870–1937). ⇒ Adler's theory.

Adler's theory the theory that people develop neuroses to compensate for feelings of inferiority.

ADLs *abbr* Activities of Daily Living.

admissions *npl* the word is usually reserved for admission to a hospital. The admission may be planned, from a waiting list, or as an emergency, e.g. from an outpatient clinic or via the Accident and Emergency Department.

adolescence *n* the period between the onset of puberty and full maturity; youth. The special needs of this age group as patients are being increasingly recognized, with the provision, in some hospitals, of special facilities and/or separate units — **adolescent** *adj, n.*

adoption *n* the acquisition of legal responsibility for a child who is not a natural offspring of the adopter.

ADP *abbr* adenosine diphosphate.

adrenal *adj* near the kidney, by custom referring to the adrenal glands, one lying above each kidney (suprarenal). Each gland has a cortex and medulla. The cortex secretes glucocorticoids, mineralocorticoids and sex hormones which control metabolism, chemical constitution of body fluids, sustained stress responses and secondary sexual characteristics. Secretion is controlled by the pituitary hormone corticotrophin which is also known as adrenocorticotrophic hormone (ACTH), and changes in body chemistry in conjunction with other hormones. The adrenal medulla secretes the catecholamines adrenaline (epinephrine) and noradrenaline (norepinephrine). These hormones are involved in the initial response to stress.

adrenal function tests abnormal adrenocortical function can be detected by measuring plasma cortisol and ACTH levels at 08.00 hours. If undersecretion (hypoadrenalism) is suspected, the measurement is repeated following the administration of tetracosactide (tetracosactrin). ⇒ ACTH stimulation test. Urinary cortisol levels can be measured where oversecretion, such as in Cushing's syndrome, is suspected. A suppression test can be used to detect Cushing's syndrome; cortisol levels are not suppressed by a small dose of dexamethasone, a synthetic corticosteroid. Increased adrenal medullary secretion

may be detected by measuring the urinary excretion of vanyl mandelic acid (VMA), free catecholamines and other metabolites. ⇒ phaeochromocytoma.

adrenalectomy *n* removal of an adrenal gland, usually due to a tumour. If both adrenal glands are removed, replacement administration of cortical hormones is required.

adrenaline (epinephrine) *n* a catecholamine hormone, produced by the adrenal medulla from the amino acid tyrosine. It augments the effects of the sympathetic nervous system during times of physiological stress by preparing the body for 'fight or flight' responses. These include bronchodilation and increased respiratory rate, increased heart rate and glucose release. Adrenaline (epinephrine) is used therapeutically as a sympathomimetic in situations that include: acute allergic reactions, cardiac arrest, as eye drops to reduce the production of aqueous humor and in local anaesthetic to prolong the anaesthetic effects. ⇒ alpha (α)-adrenoceptor agonist. ⇒ alpha (α)-adrenoceptor antagonist. ⇒ beta (β)-adrenoceptor agonist. ⇒ beta (β)-adrenoceptor antagonist. ⇒ monoamine. ⇒ noradrenaline (norepinephrine).

adrenergic *adj* describes the sympathetic nerves that use noradrenaline (norepinephrine) as their neurotransmitter. *adrenergic receptor (adrenoceptor)* receptor sites on the effector structures innervated by sympathetic nerves. These receptors are of two main types: alpha (α) and beta (β). Both receptor types, which respond differently to neurotransmitters, are further subdivided into: α_1, α_2, α_3, β_1 and β_2. ⇒ cholinergic *ant.* ⇒ muscarinic. ⇒ nicotinic.

adrenocorticotrophic hormone (ACTH) hormone produced by the anterior pituitary. It stimulates the release of glucocorticoid hormones, such as cortisol, by the adrenal cortex. Also known as corticotrophin.

adrenogenital syndrome also called adrenal virilism. In female infants there is pseudohermaphrodism present at birth, and male children exhibit precocious penile development with small testes. In both male and female there is rapid growth, muscularity and advanced bone age. Adult females become masculinized and males show feminization. These effects are due to overproduction of androgenic hormones caused by hyperplasia or adenoma of the adrenal cortex. ⇒ pseudohermaphrodite.

adrenoleucodystrophy (ALD) rare hereditary disease transmitted as a recessive sex-linked condition affecting male children. It is characterized by demyelination in the brain, leading to spasticity, optic neuritis and blindness, adrenal insufficiency and mental deterioration.

ADRs *abbr* adverse drug reactions.

adsorbents *npl* solids which bind gases or dissolved substances on their surfaces. Charcoal adsorbs gases and acts as a deodorant. Kaolin adsorbs bacterial and other toxins, hence used in cases of food poisoning.

adsorption *n* the property of a substance to attract and to hold to its surface a gas, liquid or solid in solution or suspension — **adsorb** *vt*.

advance directive a written declaration made by a mentally competent person, which sets out their wishes with regard to life-prolonging medical interventions if they are incapacitated by an irreversible disease or are terminally ill, which prevents them making their wishes known to health professionals at the time. It is legally binding if it is in the form of an advanced refusal and the maker is competent at the time. Also called a living will.

advanced life support (ALS) resuscitation techniques used during a cardiac arrest that follow on from basic life support. They include defibrillation and the administration of drugs appropriate to the type of cardiac arrest, e.g. adrenaline (epinephrine), atropine etc. *paediatric advanced life support (PALS)* involves the use of techniques, equipment and drug doses appropriate for each child according to body weight and surface area. ⇒ Broselow paediatric resuscitation system.

adventitia *n* the external coat, especially of an artery or vein — **adventitious** *adj*.

adverse drug reactions (ADRs) *npl* any unwanted effect from a drug. ⇒ side-effect. ⇒ yellow card reporting. See Box – Adverse drug reactions.

advocacy *n* process by which a person supports or argues for the needs of another. Nurses may act as advocate for their patients or clients. There are variations, such as individuals are helped to develop the skills of self-advocacy. See Box – Advocacy.

Aedes *n* a genus of mosquito which includes *Aedes aegypti*, the principal vector of yellow fever and dengue.

aerobe *n* a micro-organism that will grow in the presence of oxygen. *strict or obligate aerobe* a micro-organism that must have oxygen to grow and survive — **aerobic** *adj*.

aerobic *adj* needing free oxygen or air to support life. *aerobic exercise* physical activity which causes the lungs and heart

---

Adverse drug reactions

Adverse drug reactions (ADRs) are any unwanted drug effects. They range from minor side-effects through to harmful or seriously unpleasant effects and can be classified into five groups.

Classification of ADRs

- Type A or augmented effects are adverse effects that occur as a result of the drug's pharmacology. They are also referred to as side-effects, for example the constipation caused by morphine;
- Type B or bizarre effects are unpredictable adverse effects that are not dose-related, for example hypersensitivity reactions to penicillin. They are relatively uncommon, but they have a high morbidity and mortality rate;

- Type C or chronic effects occur after prolonged drug usage, for example parkinsonism, that occurs with phenothiazines used to treat psychoses;
- Type D or delayed effects occur years after the original drug therapy, for example cancers caused by the use of cytotoxic drugs in leukaemia treatment. In some cases, the adverse effect may affect the next generation, as in the case of vaginal cancer occurring in the daughters of women who took diethylstilbestrol (a sex hormone) during pregnancy;
- Type E or ending-of use effects are adverse effects that occur when the drug is stopped suddenly, i.e. withdrawal effects, illustrated by delirium tremors which occurs when a person stops misusing alcohol.

Advocacy

Advocacy means speaking up for people who have difficulty doing this for themselves. However, an important variant in health and social care is self-advocacy which involves teaching and supporting disadvantaged individuals in putting forward their own case. In contrast, the terms *citizen advocacy* or *independent advocacy* are often used when someone outside the main support agency speaks up on behalf of a client. Formal advocacy services tend to be funded most frequently in support of those with learning disabilities or mental illnesses. A further variant is *class advocacy* or *collective advocacy*, where a group of people try to win rights or change attitudes on behalf of a cause rather than specific individual clients. The work of Help the Aged, Mencap and other campaigning charities tends to fall into this category. Many healthcare professionals also regard themselves as advocates for their patients or clients, although external advocacy services are frequently critical of the ability of paid staff to be sufficiently independent of the employing organization to act as true advocates.

to work harder in order to obtain and circulate the extra oxygen needed for contracting skeletal muscles.

aerogenous *adj* gas producing.

aerophagia, aerophagy *n* excessive air swallowing.

aerosol *n* finely atomized droplets or small solid particles finely dispersed in a gas phase. Commercial aerosol sprays may be used: (a) as inhalation drug therapy (b) to sterilize the air (c) in insect control (d) for skin application. Some aerosol sources (e.g. sneezing) are responsible for the spread of infection.

aetiology *n* (etiology) a science dealing with the causation of disease — **aetiologically** *adv*.

AFB *n* acid-fast bacillus.

afebrile *adj* without fever.

affect *n* emotion or mood.

affection *n* the feeling or emotional aspect of mind; one of the three aspects. ⇒ cognition. ⇒ conation.

affective *adj* pertaining to emotions or moods. *affective psychosis* major mental illness in which there is grave disturbance of the emotions or mood, with psychotic features such as hallucinations or delusions. ⇒ psychosis.

afferent *adj* conducting inward to a part or organ; used to describe nerves, blood and lymphatic vessels. ⇒ efferent *ant. afferent degeneration* that which spreads up sensory nerves.

affiliation *n* settling of the paternity of an illegitimate child on the putative father.

affinity *n* attraction. In chemistry, a chemical attraction between two substances, e.g. oxygen and haemoglobin.

afibrinogenaemia *n* a relative lack or complete deficiency of fibrinogen in the blood, leading to serious impairment of normal blood coagulation. It may be primary, as in a rare genetic disorder in which fibrinogen is not produced, or secondary to conditions such as severe trauma, sepsis and amniotic fluid embolus, that cause disseminated intravascular coagulation (DIC). ⇒ multiple organ dysfunction syndrome — **afibrinogenaemic** *adj*.

aflatoxin *n* carcinogenic metabolites of certain strains of *Aspergillus flavus* which can infect peanuts and carbohydrate foods stored in warm humid climates. Four major aflatoxins: B_1, B_2, G_1 and G_2. Human liver cells contain the enzymes necessary to produce the metabolites of aflatoxins which predispose to liver cancer.

AFP *abbr* alpha-fetoprotein.

afterbirth *n* the placenta, cord and membranes (amnion and chorion) which are expelled from the uterus during the third stage of labour.

aftereffect *n* a response which occurs after the initial effect of a stimulus.

afterimage *n* a visual impression of an object which persists after the object has been removed. This is called 'positive' when the image is seen in its natural bright colours; 'negative' when the bright parts become dark, while the dark parts become light.

afterload the backpressure of blood in the aorta and pulmonary artery that creates the resistance that ventricular contraction must overcome to pump blood into the circulation. A high afterload, such as that caused by hypertension, increases the work required by the heart muscle. ⇒ preload. ⇒ stroke volume.

afterpains *npl* the pains felt after childbirth, due to contraction and retraction of the uterine muscle fibres. Also associated with breast feeding, caused by the release of the hormone oxytocin.

agammaglobulinaemia *n* absence of gammaglobulin in the plasma proteins of the blood, with consequent inability to produce immunity to infection. ⇒ dysgammaglobulinaemia. ⇒ globulins — **agammaglobulinaemic** *adj*.

aganglionosis *n* absence of ganglia, as those of the bowel. ⇒ Hirschsprung's disease. ⇒ megacolon.

agar *n* a polysaccharide obtained from certain seaweeds. It is used as a bulk-increasing laxative and as a solidifying agent in bacterial culture media.

age *n* ⇒ mental age.

age associated memory impairment *n* short-term memory declines with age, but usually older people learn to compensate for these changes. However, for some older people age associated memory impairment causes great inconvenience, problems and distress. Memory loss is a cardinal characteristic of dementia. → Alzheimer's disease.

ageism *n* stereotyping people according to chronological age; overemphasizing negative aspects to the detriment of positive aspects. See Box — Ageism.

agenesis *n* incomplete and imperfect development — **agenetic** *adj*.

agglutination *n* the clumping of bacteria, red blood cells or antigen-coated particles by antibodies called 'agglutinins', developed in the blood serum of a previously infected or sensitized person or animal. Agglutination forms the basis of many laboratory tests — **agglutinate** *vt, vi*.

agglutinins *npl* antibodies which agglutinate or clump organisms or particles on contact with an antigen.

agglutinogen *n* antigenic substance which stimulates production of antibodies (agglutinins) that cause agglutination. Used in the production of immunity, e.g. dead bacteria as in vaccine, particulate protein as in toxoid.

aggregate *v* to group together; unite.

aggression *n* a feeling of anger or hostility — **aggressive** *adj*.

agitated depression persistent restlessness, with deep depression and apprehension. Occurs in affective psychoses.

aglossia *n* absence of the tongue — **aglossic** *adj*.

aglutition *n* dysphagia.

agnosia *n* inability to organise sensory information so as to recognise objects (visual agnosia) or parts of the body (somatoagnosia) — **agnosic** *adj*.

agonist *n* 1. a muscle which contracts and shortens to perform a movement. It is opposed by the action of another muscle

---

Ageism

A discriminatory attitude which disadvantages older adults on the basis of chronological age. Ageism is also interpreted to be stigmatizing and to demarcate the older person from others who are younger. Further, ageism can affect people of any age. The practice of ageist behaviours is often demonstrated in the choice of words used. For example, 'senile' and 'geriatric' are terms which have become derogatory (Behrens 1998). In addition the media often reinforce this negative stereotyping. Ageist attitude could have developed from the process of socialization: parental behaviours; peer influences; teachers' attitude.

A balanced approach to healthy ageing is adopted by professionals to promote antiageist behaviours across boundaries. The co-ordination between care services to promote a positive image of older people is perceived to be the way forward in the 21st century (Pulford 2000). It is recommended that in developing an assessment of needs tool a positive attitude toward ageing is essential (Vernon et al 2000). Healthcare professionals can reduce the impact of ageism by exercising sensitivity in daily interactions with clients and promoting a positive image of ageing.

References
Behrens H 1998 Ageism real or imagined? Elderly Care. 10(2):10–13
Pulford E 2000 A balanced approach to healthy ageing in the 21st century. Geriatric Medicine. 30(1):9
Veron S, Ross F, Gould M A 2000 Assessment of older people: politics and practice in primary care. Journal of Advanced Nursing. 31(2):282–287

2. a drug or other substance that imitates the response of the natural chemical at a receptor site. ⇒ antagonist *ant.*

agoraphobia *n* irrational fear of being alone in large open places or in places from which escape might be difficult or embarrassing, e.g. on public transport or in a supermarket queue — **agoraphobic** *adj.*

agranulocyte *n* a nongranular leucocyte (white blood cell), e.g. lymphocyte.

agranulocytosis *n* marked reduction in or complete absence of granulocytes. Usually results from bone marrow depression caused by (a) hypersensitivity to drugs; (b) cytotoxic drugs or (c) irradiation. It is characterized by fever, ulceration of the mouth and throat and may be fatal — **agranulocytic** *adj.*

agraphia *n* loss of language facility. *motor agraphia* inability to express thoughts in writing, usually due to left precentral cerebral lesions. *sensory agraphia* inability to interpret the written word, due to lesions in the posterior part of the left parieto-occipital region of the brain — **agraphic** *adj.*

ague *n* ⇒ malaria.

AHF *abbr* antihaemophilic factor.

AID *abbr* artificial insemination of a female with donor semen. More often now known as donor insemination (DI).

AIDS *acr* acquired immune deficiency syndrome.

AIDS-related complex (ARC) also known as early symptomatic disease. Individuals display symptoms, but without any of the AIDS-defining conditions. ⇒ acquired immune deficiency syndrome.

aids to independence any articles which enable a person to retain or regain independence. They include those used for preparation, cooking, serving and eating food, as well as swallowing liquids; those used for personal hygiene, dressing and undressing; those used to accomplish walking, ascending stairs and so on; and those used for transit. Their use is explicit in the concept 'aided independence'. ⇒walking aids.

AIH *abbr* artificial insemination of a female with her husband's (or partner's) semen.

air *n* ⇒ atmosphere. *air-bed* a mattress inflated with air. *air embolism* caused by an air bubble entering the circulation. *air hunger* a type of respiratory distress characterized by deep indrawing of breath and gasping. It is caused by a lack of available oxygen, such as in severe uncontrolled haemorrhage. *air swallowing* swallowing of excessive air particularly when eating; it may result in belching or expulsion of gas via the anus. ⇒ aerophagia. *tidal air* ⇒ tidal volume.

airway *n* a word used to describe the entry to the larynx from the pharynx. *Brook airway* an oropharyngeal airway used in expired air resuscitation. It has a one-way protective valve. *Dual Aid airway* designed for both nasal and oral application in expired air resuscitation. It, too, has a one-way protective valve; it has a longer mouthpiece than the Brook airway, allowing good support for the tongue when used orally. It is unique in that a self-inflating bag such as an Ambubag can be attached to it for inflation of the lungs. *ororpharyngeal airway* a flexible oval tube, (e.g. Guedel airway),which can be placed along the upper surface of the tongue; it is held in position by a metal ending which rests between the front teeth and the lips. It prevents a flaccid tongue from resting against the posterior pharyngeal wall, thereby obstructing the airway, and is commonly used during general anaesthesia. Also used during cardiopulmonary resuscitation. (See Figure 2).

akathisia *n* a state of persistent motor restlessness; it can occur as a side-effect of neuroleptic drugs.

akinetic *adj* literally 'without movement'. A word applied to states or conditions where there is lack of movement — **akinesia** *n.*

Albers-Schönberg disease ⇒ osteopetrosis.

albinism *n* congenital absence, either partial or complete, of normal pigmentation, so that the skin is fair, the hair white and the eyes pink: due to a defect in melanin synthesis.

albino *n* a person affected with albinism — **albinotic** *adj.*

albumin *n* a variety of protein found in animal and vegetable matter. It is soluble in water and coagulates on heating. *serum albumin* the chief protein of blood plasma and other serous fluids. It is produced by the liver. ⇒ lactalbumin — **albuminous, albuminoid** *adj.*

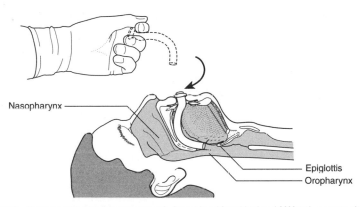

Nasopharynx

Epiglottis
Oropharynx

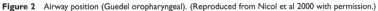

Figure 2 Airway position (Guedel oropharyngeal). (Reproduced from Nicol et al 2000 with permission.)

albuminuria *n* the presence of the albumin (protein) in the urine. Also known as proteinuria. The condition is frequently benign and temporary, as in many febrile states, but it may be an indication of renal disease. *chronic albuminuria* prolonged loss of protein, such as occurs in the nephrotic syndrome, may lead to hypoproteinaemia. ⇒ orthostatic albuminuria — **albuminuric** *adj.*

albumose *n* an early product of proteolysis. It resembles albumin, but is not coagulated by heat.

albumosuria *n* the presence of albumose in the urine — **albumosuric** *adj.*

alcohol *n* a group of organic compounds containing hydroxyl groups (OH). Ethyl alcohol (*syn* ethanol) is the intoxicating constituent of alcoholic drinks: beer, wines and spirits. It potentiates the action of many drugs including hypnotics and tranquillizers. *alcohol misuse* ⇒ alcoholism. *alcohol psychosis* ⇒ Korsakoff's psychosis, syndrome.

alcohol-fast *adj* in microbiology, describes an organism which, when stained, is resistant to decolourization by alcohol.

Alcoholics Anonymous (AA) a voluntary, locally based organization which helps people with alcohol dependency deal with their urge to drink, particularly through a system of mutual support.

alcoholism *n* a morbid state of dependence upon an excessive intake of alcohol. Poisoning resulting from alcoholic addiction may be acute or chronic. In its chronic form it causes severe damage to most body systems, e.g. the liver, digestive organs with malnutrition, the heart and nervous system. Longterm alcohol misuse is associated with: hepatitis, cirrhosis, portal hypertension, varices and gastrointestinal haemorrhage, gastritis, iron overload, primary liver cancer, other cancers, e.g. head and neck, pancreatitis, arterial hypertension, ischaemic heart disease and neurological problems caused by alcohol toxicity or B vitamin deficiency. ⇒ fetal alcohol syndrome. ⇒ hypertension. ⇒ Korsakoff's psychosis, syndrome. ⇒ Wernicke's encephalopathy. In addition there are social, emotional and psychological problems, such as relationship difficulties, financial problems and unemployment.

alcoholuria *n* alcohol in the urine.

ALD *abbr* adrenoleucodystrophy.

aldehyde *n* a group of organic compounds containing a carbonyl group (-CHO). They are formed by the oxidation of an alcohol. For example, acetaldehyde is formed from ethyl alcohol.

aldolase *n* an enzyme found in muscle, it is involved in glycolysis. Increased levels of aldolase and other enzymes in the blood are indicative of certain diseases affecting muscle, such as severe muscular dystrophy.

aldosterone *n* a mineralocorticoid hormone produced by the adrenal cortex. It enhances the reabsorption of sodium accompanied by water and the excretion of potassium by the renal tubules. Secretion is regulated by the action of renin and angiotensin.

aldosteronism *n* ⇒ hyperaldosteronism.

Aleppo boil ⇒ leishmaniasis.

Alexander technique a series of techniques with the aim of improving the functioning of a person's mind and body in movement known as 'psychophysical' re-education. It is based on the theory that poor body posture can contribute towards ill health, injury and chronic pain. The technique aims to promote postural improvement through self-awareness.

algesia *n* excessive sensitivity to pain; hyperaesthesia. ⇒ analgesia *ant* — **algesic** *adj*.

alginates *npl* seaweed derivatives used in some wound dressings. Their properties include: high absorbency, haemostatic, and removal without tissue damage. They can be used on wounds with moderate to heavy exudate, infected wounds and for wet wound debridement.

alienation *n* in psychology and sociology, estrangement from self or other people. People feel powerless and isolated. It may be a feature of mental illness such as schizophrenia.

alimentary *adj* pertaining to food. *alimentary canal/tract* the whole digestive tract from mouth to anus. It comprises the mouth, oesophagus, stomach, small and large intestine.

alimentation *n* the act of nourishing with food; feeding. ⇒ enteral. ⇒ parenteral.

alkali *n* also known as bases. Substances having an excess of hydroxyl ions over hydrogen ions, e.g. sodium bicarbonate (hydrogen carbonate). Alkalis are hydrogen ion (proton) acceptors. Alkalis have a pH greater than 7, turn red litmus blue and are neutralized by acids. They combine with acids to form salts and water, and combine with fats to form soaps. *alkaline reserve* a biochemical term denoting the amount of alkali, normally bicarbonate (hydrogen carbonate), available in the blood for buffering acids (normally dissolved CO_2) and preventing pH changes in the blood. The amount is regulated by the kidney. ⇒ buffer.

alkaline *adj* 1. possessing the properties of or pertaining to an alkali. 2. containing an alkali, having a pH greater than 7. *alkaline phosphatase* an enzyme produced by several tissues including liver, kidney and bone. An increase in the enzyme alkaline phosphatase in the blood is indicative of such conditions as obstructive jaundice and is also indicative of osteoblastic activity.

alkalinuria *n* alkalinity of urine — **alkalinuric** *adj*.

alkaloid *n* resembling an alkali. A name often applied to a large group of organic bases found in plants and which possess important physiological actions. Morphine, quinine, caffeine, atropine and strychnine are well-known examples of alkaloids. ⇒ vinca alkaloids — **alkaloidal** *adj*.

alkalosis *n* excess of alkali or reductions of acid in the body, with resulting disturbance of acid-base balance. The alkali reserve in the blood increases or the hydrogen ion concentration in the blood falls and the pH rises. *metabolic alkalosis* caused by overdosage with alkali, such as indigestion mixtures or acid loss with excessive vomiting. *respiratory alkalosis* caused by hyperventilation.

alkaptonuria *n* the presence of alkaptone (homogentisic acid) in the urine due to a rare inherited disorder of amino acid metabolism, where the absence of an enzyme results in the partial oxidation of phenylalanine and tyrosine. It is characterized by darkly stained urine which is usually noticed in the nappies, or when urine is left to stand. Apart from this, and a tendency to arthritis in later life, there are no ill-effects from alkaptonuria.

alkylating agents organic compounds containing alkyl groups. They disrupt the process of cell division by binding to DNA in the nucleus and preventing replication. Some are useful in the treatment of cancer, e.g. chlorambucil, cyclophosphamide and busulfan (busulphan). ⇒ chemotherapy. ⇒ cytotoxic.

ALL *acr* acute lymphoblastic leukaemia.

all-or-none phenomenon *n* relates to the conduction of an action potential in excitable tissue, e.g. nerve or muscle fibres. The action potential in a particular neuron is always of the same size and duration regardless of the intensity of the stimulus. There are only two possible responses to a stimulus: either a full response or no response. There is no partial response to reduced stimuli.

allantois *n* a ventral outgrowth of the hindgut of the early embryo which becomes a small vestigial structure in the developing fetus. Stretching from the urachus at the apex of the bladder to the umbilicus, its blood vessels develop into those of the umbilical cord and, later, the placenta — **allantoic, allantoid** *adj*.

alleles *npl* originally used to denote inherited characteristics that are alternative and contrasting, such as normal colour vision contrasting with colour blindness, or the ability to taste or not to taste certain substances, or different blood groups. The basis of Mendelian inheritance of dominants and recessives. In modern usage allelomorph(s) is equivalent to allele(s), namely alternative forms of a gene at the same chromosomal location (locus). ⇒ Mendel's law.

allelomorph ⇒ allele.

allergen *n* an antigen capable of producing an allergic reaction (type I hypersensitivity reaction). The substance, e.g. proteins found in pollen, foods, drugs, house dust and animal hair/fur, is said to be allergenic. ⇒ hypersensitivity — **allergenicity** *n*.

allergic rhinitis inflammation of the nasal mucosa caused by an allergy, e.g. to pollen (hay fever), house dust or animal dander. Affected individuals often have associated conjunctivitis with sore and watery eyes.

allergy *n* an altered or exaggerated susceptibility to various foreign substances or physical agents. Colloquially, implies that an individual has become over-reactive to an allergen (antigen) which would not normally produce an adverse response. Sometimes caused by the interaction of an allergen (antigen) with IgE antibody (immunoglobulin) on the surface of mast cells. Scientifically, describes disorders due to an altered immune response, a state of altered reactivity. Some food and drug reactions, hay fever, insect bite reactions, urticarial reactions and allergic asthma are classed as allergic diseases. ⇒ anaphylactic. ⇒ sensitization — **allergic** *adj* pertaining to allergy. *allergic reaction* the reaction caused by hypersentivity to an allergen. It is caused by the release of various chemical mediators, e.g. histamine, inflammation and an anaphylactic reaction. The effects may be local, such as rhinitis, skin rashes or bronchospasm, or more unusually

there are systemic effects that result in anaphylaxis (anaphylactic shock).

Allitt Inquiry (Clothier Report 1994) the report of an independent inquiry team into the events surrounding deaths and injuries to children in the care of one particular nurse in an English hospital. It includes recommendations designed to strengthen procedures that safeguard children in hospital and prevent any repetition.

alloantibody *n* ⇒ isoantibody.

allocation *n* 1. the allocation of patients who are assigned to one nurse or a nursing team for a spell of duty or as part of a caseload. The nurse is able to address the total care needs of each patient. 2. task allocation is the term used when one nurse is allocated to carry out one nursing activity for all patients. This method of organizing care is no longer considered to be in the patient's best interests and individualized nursing is preferred. 3. ward allocation. ⇒ placement.

allograft *n* tissue or organ which is transplanted from a donor of dissimilar geno type, but of the same species. Also known as homograft.

allopathy *n* conventional medical health care. ⇒ homeopathy — **allopathic** *adj*.

alogia poverty of thought. A negative symptom associated with mental illness such as schizophrenia. It is characterized by: little or no spontaneous speech; little said during interactions; speech conveys little actual information; stopping in middle of conversation and forgetting what was said.

alopecia *n* baldness, which can be congenital, premature or age related. *alopecia areata* a patchy baldness, usually of a temporary nature. Cause unknown, probably autoimmune, but shock and anxiety are common precipitating factors. Exclamation mark hairs are diagnostic. *cicatrical alopecia* progressive alopecia of the scalp in which tufts of normal hair occur between many bald patches. Folliculitis decalvans is an alopecia of the scalp characterized by pustulation and scars.

alpha (α) first letter of the Greek alphabet. *alpha antitrypsin* a protein, made in the liver, that normally opposes trypsin; low blood levels are associated with a genetic predisposition to emphysema and liver disease. *alpha cells* ⇒ islets of Langerhans. *alpha rays* a type of ionizing radiation emitted as a radioactive isotope disintegrates. It has very limited penetrating ability and is rarely used for therapeutic purposes. *alpha receptor* ⇒ adrenergic receptor (adrenoceptor). *alpha redistribution phase* the point following an intravenous injection when blood concentrations of the drug will start to fall below the peak levels achieved. *alpha state* relaxed wakefulness without stimulation or concentration. *alpha wave (rhythm)* a brain wave pattern recorded during the alpha state. They are slow, synchronous waves which typically have a frequency between 8–13 Hz.

alpha (α)-adrenoceptor agonists *npl* also known as α stimulants. A group of drugs that stimulate α-adrenoceptors, e.g. adrenaline (epinephrine), which produces vasoconstriction and a rise in blood pressure, is used in anaphylactic shock and cardiac arrest (NB adrenaline (epinephrine) is also a beta (β)-adrenoceptor agonist), and methoxamine, used to treat hypotension and as a nasal decongestant.

alpha (α)-adrenoceptor antagonists *npl* also known as α blockers. A group of drugs which prevent stimulation of the α-adrenoceptors, e.g. doxazosin, prazosin. They are vasodilators and are used as long-acting antihypertensive drugs and may be useful in reducing urinary obstruction in benign prostatic hyperplasia.

alpha-fetoprotein *n* present in maternal serum and amniotic fluid in some types of fetal abnormality. Also a tumour marker for hepatocellular cancer and testicular cancer.

ALS *abbr* advanced life support.

ALs *abbr* Activities of Living.

ALT *abbr* alanine aminotransferase. ⇒ aminotransferases.

altered consciousness the level of consciousness is normally changed during sleep; it can also be altered by some drugs, alcohol, general anaesthesia, head injuries, strokes and other neurological diseases. ⇒ coma. ⇒ Glasgow coma scale. ⇒ stupor.

altruism unselfish behaviour aimed at helping others.

alveolar *adj* pertaining to alveoli. *alveolar ventilation rate* the volume of inspired air reaching the alveoli in one minute available for gaseous exchange.

alveolar abscess ⇒ abscess.

alveolitis *n* inflammation of alveoli, by custom usually referring to those in the lung; when caused by inhalation of an organic dust, such as from mouldy hay or bird excreta, it is termed *extrinsic allergic alveolitis.*

alveolus *n* 1. an air sac in the lung. 2. bone of the tooth socket, providing support for the tooth, partially absorbed when the teeth are lost. 3. a gland follicle or acinus. ⇒ acini — **alveoli** *pl.*

Alzheimer's disease *n* a degenerative neurological disorder affecting the brain. It is the most common cause of presenile dementia (occurring before 65 years of age) and is possibly associated with the inheritance of a gene that codes for apolipoprotein E (a transport protein). There are specific brain abnormalities including: loss of neurons, brain shrinkage and the presence of neurofibrillary tangles. The onset is insidious and is characterized by progressive memory loss (particularly short term or recent), failing intellectual ability, confusion, restlessness, speech problems, motor retardation, depression and personality changes. Eventually the person becomes bed-bound and totally dependent upon others for every need. It may start in late middle age but is primarily a problem associated with older people.

amalgam *n* a mixture or combination. *dental amalgam* an alloy of mercury and another metal or metals, used for filling cavities in teeth.

amastia *n* congenital absence of the breasts.

amaurosis *n* blindness caused by an extraocular cause, such as optic nerve damage, brain lesions, diabetes or renal disease.

ambidextrous *adj* able to perform skilled movements, such as writing, with either hand, equally well — **ambidexterity** *n.*

ambiopia *n* ⇒ diplopia.

ambisexual *adj* denoting sexual characteristics common to both sexes before sexual differentiation occurs at about 7 weeks after fertilization in male embryos and week 8 in females.

ambivalence *n* coexistence of opposite feelings at the same time in one person, e.g. love and hate — **ambivalent** *adj.*

amblyopia *n* defective vision in a structurally normal eye. *toxic amblyopia* caused by toxins, such as nicotine, quinine and lead, that cause neuritis — **amblyopic** *adj.*

ambulant *adj* able to walk. ⇒ ambulation.

ambulation a term which was introduced in the 1950s and 60s after identification of complications associated with bedrest. Patients are encouraged to mobilize soon after surgery to prevent complications such as deep vein thrombosis (DVT). Where patients are required to stay in bed or are unable to mobilize, the nurse, in conjunction with the physiotherapist, plans and encourages a set of exercises that can be undertaken.

ambulatory *adj* mobile, walking about. *ambulatory ECG* ➡ electrocardiogram. *ambulatory surgery (day case surgery)* patients have minor surgery on the day of admission and, where no problems exist, they are discharged home on the same day. *ambulatory treatment* interventions, such as cancer chemotherapy, provided for patients on a day care basis. ⇒ continuous ambulatory peritoneal dialysis.

amelia *n* congenital absence of a limb or limbs. *complete amelia* absence of both arms and legs. ⇒ phocomelia.

amelioration *n* reduction of the severity of symptoms.

amenorrhoea *n* absence of the menses. There is amenorrhoea during pregnancy, but it may occur in a variety of disorders that include anorexia nervosa and endocrine disorders. *primary amenorrhoea* menstruation has not been established at the time when it should have been. *secondary amenorrhoea* absence of the menstruation after it had once commenced — **amenorrhoeal** *adj.*

amentia *n* old term. Learning disability from birth; to be distinguished from dementia, which is acquired mental impairment.

ametria *n* congenital absence of the uterus.

ametropia *n* defective sight due to imperfect refractive power of the eye — **ametrope** *n.*

amfetamine (amphetamine) *n* a sympathomimetic agent which is a potent CNS stimulant. The stimulant action of amfetamine (amphetamine) has led to considerable misuse and dependence. It has very limited use in clincal situations.

amines *npl* a group of organic compounds containing amine (NH_2) groups. They include several important biochemical molecules, e.g. dopamine and histamine.

amino acids *npl* nitrogenous organic acids from which all proteins are formed. They contain an amine (NH_2) group and a carboxyl (COOH) group. There are twenty common amino acids, of which eight are considered essential or indispensable in adults as they are not synthesized by the body in sufficient quantities: isoleucine, leucine, lysine, methionine, phenylalanine, threonine, tryptophan and valine; during childhood, histidine is essential and arginine is also considered to be essential because it is only synthesized in small amounts. They must be obtained from the dietary intake of high quality protein. The remaining ten can be synthesized by the body from essential amino acids: alanine, asparagine, aspartate, cysteine, glutamate, glutamine, glycine, proline, serine and tyrosine. (See Figure 3).

aminoaciduria *n* the abnormal presence of amino acids in the urine; it usually indicates an inborn error of metabolism as in cystinosis and Fanconi syndrome — **aminoaciduric** *adj.*

aminoglycosides *npl* bactericidal antibiotics that act against a wide range of Gram-negative bacteria and some Gram-positive bacteria, e.g. gentamicin, streptomycin etc. This group of drugs have toxic side-effects on kidney function and hearing.

aminopeptidases *npl* intestinal enzymes that act upon the amine end of the peptide chain during protein digestion.

aminotransferases *npl* transaminases. A group of enzymes that facilitate the transfer of amine (NH_2) groups between amino acids. *alanine aminotransferase (ALT)* formerly called glutamic pyruvic transaminase (SGPT). *aspartate aminotransferase (AST)* formerly called serum glutamic oxalacetic transaminase (SGOT).The enzymes are released by certain damaged cells and when blood levels are measured may be useful in the

Indispensable/essential (must be taken in the diet)	Dispensable/non-essential (can be synthesized in the body)
Isoleucine	Alanine
Leucine	Arginine (semi-essential)
Lysine	Asparagine
Methionine	Aspartate (aspartic acid)
Phenylalanine	Cysteine
Threonine	Glutamate (glutamic acid)
Tryptophan	Glutamine
Valine	Glycine
	Proline
Note: during childhood, histidine is indispensable	Serine
	Tyrosine

Figure 3   Amino acids. (Reproduced from Brooker 1998 with permission.)

diagnosis of liver disease (ALT) and heart disease (AST). Liver disease is also characterized by increased activity of both ALT and AST.

ammonia *n* a naturally occurring compound of nitrogen and hydrogen. In the human, several inborn errors of ammonia metabolism can cause learning disability, neurological signs and seizures. *ammonia solution* (liq. ammon) colourless liquid with a characteristic pungent odour — **ammoniated, ammoniacal** *adj.*

amnesia *n* complete loss of memory; can occur after concussion, in dementia, hysterical neurosis and following electroconvulsive therapy (ECT). The term *anterograde amnesia* is used when there is impairment of memory for recent events, after an accident etc, and *retrograde amnesia* when the impairment is for past events — **amnesic** *adj.*

amniocentesis *n* aspiration of amniotic fluid from the uterus for the prenatal diagnosis of fetal abnormalities and haemolytic disease. Many single gene and chromosome abnormalities can be diagnosed from testing amniotic fluid and fetal cells shed into the amniotic fluid surrounding the fetus. The sample is obtained using a wide-bore needle which is passed into the amniotic sac via the abdominal wall (suitably anaesthetized). Fetal cells obtained from the fluid are grown and examined for chromosomal abnormalities such as Down's syndrome. The amniotic fluid may contain chemical markers for a particular abnormality, e.g. presence of alpha-fetoproteins may indicate neural tube defects. Amniocentesis is usually performed at 16–18 weeks gestation after which a further wait for the chromosome tests is required. It is not without risk and may cause miscarriage. Earlier amniocentesis at 10–14 weeks may be developed as an alternative to CVS.

amniochorial *adj* pertaining to the amnion and chorion.

amniogenesis *n* development of the amnion.

amniography *n* radiographic examination of the amniotic sac after injection of opaque medium — **amniographically** *adv.*

amnion *n* the inner fetal membrane enclosing the developing fetus and containing the amniotic fluid. It ensheaths the umbilical cord and is connected with the fetus at the umbilicus — **amnionic, amniotic** *adj.*

amnion nodosum a nodular condition of the fetal surface of the amnion, observed in oligohydramnios, which may be associated with the absence of kidneys in the fetus.

amnionitis *n* inflammation of the amnion.

amniorrhoea *n* escape of amniotic fluid.

amniorrhoexia *n* rupture of the amnion.

amnioscopy *n* amnioscope (endoscope) passed through the abdominal wall enables viewing of the fetus and amniotic fluid. Clear, colourless fluid is normal; yellow or green staining is due to meconium and occurs in cases of fetal hypoxia. *cervical amnioscopy* can be performed late in pregnancy. A different instrument is inserted via the vagina and cervix for the same reasons — **amnioscopically** *adv.*

amniotic cavity the fluid-filled cavity between the embryo/fetus and the amnion.

amniotic fluid a fluid produced by the amnion (inner fetal membrane) and the fetus which surrounds the fetus throughout pregnancy. It protects the fetus from physical trauma and variations in temperature and allows movement. It is secreted and reabsorbed by cells lining the amniotic cavity and is swallowed and excreted as fetal urine. ⇒ amniocentesis. ⇒ amnioscopy. *amniotic fluid embolism* the formation of an embolus caused by amniotic fluid entering the maternal circulation. A rare, but extremely serious, complication of pregnancy with a high mortality. ⇒ disseminated intravascular coagulation.

amniotome *n* an instrument for rupturing the fetal membranes.

amniotomy *n* artificial rupture of the fetal membranes to induce or expedite labour.

amoeba *n* a unicellular protozoon. Some strains are human parasites, e.g. *Entamoeba histolytica*, which produces amoebic dysentery (intestinal amoebiasis). ⇒ protozoa — **amoebic** *adj*.

amoebiasis *n* disease caused by parasitic amoeba, such as *Entamoeba histolytica*, which infects the intestine by cysts spread via uncooked food, such as salads or water contaminated with human faeces. It causes ulceration of the large intestine mucosa. This results in pain, diarrhoea alternating with constipation and the passage per rectum of mucus and blood, hence the term 'amoebic dysentery'. If the amoebae enter the hepatic portal circulation they may cause a liver abscess. Diagnosis is by isolating the amoebae in the stools and the detection of antibodies by immunofluorescence techniques. Cutaneous amoebiasis, causing genital or perianal ulceration, may occur in homosexual men. Treatment is with amoebicidal drugs that include: metronidazole and diloxanide furoate to deal with the cysts.

amoebicide *n* an agent which kills amoebae, e.g. metronidazole — **amoebicidal** *adj*.

amoeboid *adj* resembling an amoeba in shape or in mode of movement, e.g. white blood cells.

amoeboma *n* a localized granuloma in the rectum caused by *Entamoeba hystolytica*. Fibrosis may occur and obstruct the bowel.

amorph *n* an inactive gene. One that does not express a trait.

amorphous *adj* having no regular shape.

AMP *abbr* adenosine monophosphate.

ampere (A) *n* a measurement of electric current. One of the seven base units of the International System of Units (SI).

amphiarthrosis a cartilaginous, slightly movable joint. ⇒ joint.

amphipathic a molecule that has parts with very different properties, such as having a polar (hydrophilic) end and a non-polar (hydrophobic) end.

ampoule *n* a sealed glass or plastic phial containing a single sterile dose of a drug.

ampulla *n* any flask-like dilatation. *ampulla of Vater* the enlargement formed by the union of the common bile duct with the pancreatic duct where they enter the duodenum. Now known as the hepatopancreatic ampulla — **ampullar, ampullary, ampullate** *adj*.

amputation *n* removal of an appending part, e.g. breast, limb.

amputee *n* a person who has undergone amputation.

amylase *n* any enzyme which converts starches into sugars. Present in saliva and pancreatic juice; it converts starchy foods to maltose. *serum amylase* the amount of amylase in the blood. The level is elevated in pancreatic disorders, such as pancreatitis.

amylin a peptide secreted by the beta cells of the pancreas that inhibits the secretion of insulin and opposes its effects (it is unclear whether amylin is of physiological significance).

amyloid *n* a glycoprotein. ⇒ amyloidosis.

amyloid disease *n* ⇒ amyloidosis.

amyloidosis *n* amyloid disease. Formation and deposit of amyloid (a glycoprotein) in any organ, notably the liver, heart and kidney, where it disrupts normal function. It may be: *primary amyloidosis* with no apparent cause, or *secondary amyloidosis* which is associated with malignancy and any chronic inflammatory or infectious disease, such as rheumatoid arthritis, Crohn's disease, tuberculosis and leprosy.

amylolysis *n* the digestion of starch — **amylolytic** *adj*.

anabolic steroids *npl* a group of androgens that have marked anabolic effects, e.g. nandralone, stanozolol etc. They increase protein synthesis and increase weight and muscle mass. They are used clinically in the treatment of some breast cancers, and sometimes to increase appetite and a feeling of well-being in patients with terminal cancer. They are subject to considerable misuse by athletes and body builders, who may take many times the therapeutic dose.

anabolism *n* the series of chemical reactions in the living body requiring energy to build up or synthesize other molecules. ⇒ adenosine diphosphate. ⇒ adenosine triphosphate. ⇒ catabolism. ⇒ metabolism — **anabolic** *adj* pertaining to anabolism. A feature of the absorptive state (or fed state) where absorbed nutrients are used for instant energy or used in anabolic processes.

anacidity *n* lack of normal acidity, especially in the gastric juice. ⇒ achlorhydria.

anacrotism *n* an oscillation in the ascending curve of a sphygmographic pulse tracing, occurring in aortic stenosis — **anacrotic** *adj.*

anaemia *n* diminished oxygen-carrying capacity of the blood, due to a reduction in the number of red blood cells or the amount of haemoglobin, or both. May produce clinical manifestations arising from hypoxaemia, such as lassitude and breathlessness on exertion. The cause may be due to: (a) blood loss; (b) deficiency of substances required for the production of red blood cells and haemoglobin, e.g. iron, vitamin B_{12} and folic acid; (c) failure of the bone marrow; (d) excessive breakdown of red blood cells (haemolysis); (e) abnormalities of erythropoiesis and the metabolism of iron. Treatment is according to the cause and severity and includes oral iron and blood transfusion. The specific anaemias include: *aplastic anaemia* the result of complete bone marrow failure that may be primary or result from cancer chemotherapy, some antibiotics, antirheumatic drugs, toxic chemicals, viral hepatitis and radiotherapy. *anaemia of chronic disease (ACD)* associated with cancer and chronic inflammation or infection. *haemolytic anaemia* results from premature destruction of red blood cells, as in some inherited red cell disorders and haemoglobinopathies, the presence of abnormal antibodies, e.g.

autoimmune antibodies, as a response to drugs or toxic agents, infection or mechanical trauma, such as artificial heart valves. *iron deficiency anaemia* the commonest form of anaemia; due to lack of absorbable iron in the diet, poor absorption of dietary iron or chronic bleeding. Oral iron-containing medications usually correct the condition. *megaloblastic anaemia* a form of anaemia caused by a deficiency of vitamin B_{12} or folic acid. It is characterized by the presence of large red blood cells known as megaloblasts. *microcytic anaemia* characterized by small red blood cells commonly associated with iron deficiency. *pernicious anaemia* the megaloblastic anaemia that results from a deficiency of the intrinsic factor (secreted by gastric oxyntic cells), which is necessary for the absorption of dietary vitamin B_{12} in the ileum. It is an autoimmune disorder. *sickle-cell anaemia* ⇒ sickle cell disease. ⇒ blood count. ⇒ haemoglobinopathies. ⇒ haemolytic disease of the newborn. ⇒ thalassaemia — **anaemic** *adj.*

anaerobe *n* a micro-organism that is able to grow in the absence of oxygen. Strict or *obligate anaerobes* cannot grow in the presence of oxygen. The majority of pathogens are indifferent to atmospheric conditions and will grow in the presence or absence of oxygen and are therefore termed *facultative anaerobes* — **anaerobic** *adj anaerobic infection* infection with anaerobes, such as *Clostridium perfringens*, that causes gas gangrene in wounds contaminated with soil or faeces.

anaerobic *adj* pertaining to the absence of oxygen. Also used to describe the ability to survive without air or oxygen, such as certain micro-organisms. ⇒ anareobe. ⇒ anaerobic infection. *anaerobic exercise* vigorous physical exercise where oxygen supplies to contracting skeletal muscle is inadequate. Metabolic fuel molecules are broken down anaerobically with the formation of lactic acid.

anaesthesia *n* loss of sensation. *epidural anaesthesia* achieving lower body anaesthesia with drugs injected into the epidural space. *general anaesthesia* loss of sensation with loss of consciousness. In *local anaesthesia* the nerve conduction is blocked directly and painful impulses fail to reach the brain. *spinal anaesthesia* may be caused by (a) injection of a local anaesthetic into the spinal subarachnoid space (b) a lesion of the spinal cord. ⇒ epidural.

anaesthesiology *n* the science dealing with anaesthetics, their administration and effect.

anaesthetic *n* insensible to stimuli. *general anaesthetic* a drug which produces general anaesthesia by inhalation or injection. ⇒ inhalation anaesthetic. ⇒ intravenous anaesthetic. *local anaesthetic* a drug which injected into the tissues or applied topically causes local insensibility to pain. *rectal anaesthetic* rectal administration of anaesthetic drugs. *spinal anaesthetic* local anaesthetic solution injected into the subarachnoid space to produce insensitivity in the area supplied by the selected spinal nerves. ⇒ spinal— **anaesthetize** *vt*.

anaesthetist *n* a person who is medically qualified to administer anaesthetics.

anakastic personality disorder tends to be characterized by perfectionism and a person who is extremely conscientious in the work situation. They may find it hard to relax, and personal relationships can suffer. The person may be obstinate and cautious with inflexible thinking.

anal *adj* pertaining to the anus. *anal canal* 3.8 cm long, forming the terminal part of the gastrointestinal tract. The internal anal sphincter muscle is covered by mucous membrane and controlled by the autonomic nervous system. The external anal sphincter muscle is covered by skin and is under voluntary nerve control. The tissues are puckered so that they can distend for the passing of faeces. ⇒ haemorrhoids. An electronic probe can be placed in the anal canal to measure the body's core temperature, by custom inaccurately called rectal temperature. *anal eroticism* sexual pleasure derived from stimulation and possible penetration of the anus. *anal fissure* → fissure. *anal fistula* ⇒ fistula.

anal stage the second stage of psychosexual development, characterized by a child's sensual interest in the anal area and passing or retaining faeces.

analeptic *adj, n* restorative. Drugs that stimulate the central nervous system, e.g. caffeine, amfetamines (amphetamines), cocaine etc.

analgesia *n* loss of painful impressions without loss of tactile sense. *patient controlled analgesia* patients use a push button system to self-administer a preset dose of pain-relieving drug. Safety precautions prevent overdose. ⇒ algesia *ant* — **analgesic** *adj*.

analgesic *n* a drug which relieves pain. Can be administered locally, topically or systemically, e.g. aspirin, paracetamol, morphine.

analogous *adj* similar in function but not in origin — **analogue** *n*.

analysis *n* a term used in chemistry to denote the determination of the composition of a compound substance — **analytically** *adv*.

analysis of variance (ANOVA) a statistical method of comparing sample means. It can be used to compare more than two means.

anaphase the third stage of mitosis and meiosis.

anaphylactic *adj* pertaining to anaphylaxis. *anaphylactic shock* ⇒ anaphylaxis.

anaphylactoid *adj* pertaining to or resembling anaphylaxis.

anaphylaxis *n* a life-threatening condition resulting from an extreme systemic hypersensitivity reaction to a previously encountered allergen, e.g. foreign protein in penicillin, bee stings etc. It is characterized by laryngeal oedema, bronchospasm, extreme dyspnoea and vasodilation leading to hypovolaemia and shock. Life-saving interventions include: administration of adrenaline (epinephrine), provision of an airway, e.g. by tracheostomy, and antihistamines, such as chlorphenamine (chlorpheniramine).

anaplasia *n* reversal of the distinctive characteristics of a special tissue or cells to a less differentiated type. A feature of malignancy — **anaplastic** *adj*.

anarthria *n* a severe form of dysarthria. Loss of ability to produce the motor movements for speech. Muscle weakness involves the respiratory, phonatory, articulatory and resonatory systems of speech.

anasarca *n* massive generalized oedema, often associated with renal disease — **anasarcous** *adj*.

anastomosis *n* 1. the intercommunication of the branches of two or more arteries or veins. 2. in surgery, the establishment of an intercommunication between two hollow organs, vessels or nerves — **anastomose** *vt*.

anatomy *n* the science which deals with the structure of the body — **anatomical** *adj* pertaining to anatomy. *anatomical dead space* the conducting part of the respiratory tract containing air (around 150 mL) that is not involved in gaseous exchange. Generally *anatomical position* for the purpose of accurate description the anterior view is of the upright body facing forward, hands by the sides with palms facing forwards. The posterior view is of the back of the upright body in that position.

Ancylostoma *n* (*syn* hookworm) a genus of nematode worm. *Ancylostoma duodenale* is parasitic in the human duodenum and jejunum. It is predominantly found in southern Europe and the Middle and Far East and Africa. *Necator americanus* is found in the Central and South America, the Far East and tropical Africa. Mixed infections are not uncommon. Only clinically significant when infestation is moderate or heavy. Worms inhabit the duodenum and upper jejunum, eggs are passed in stools, hatch in moist soil and produce larvae which can penetrate bare feet and reinfect people. Prevention is by wearing shoes and using latrines. ⇒ ancylostomiasis.

ancylostomiasis *n* (*syn* hookworm disease) infestation of the human intestine with Ancylostoma, giving rise to malnutrition and severe anaemia. Treatment is with anthelmintic drugs, e.g. mebendazole, pyrantel, and appropriate measures for the degree of anaemia.

androblastoma *n* (*syn* arrhenoblastoma) a tumour of the ovary that produces androgens (male hormones). The abnormal hormone production causes defeminization followed by virilization (masculinization).

androgens *npl* a group of steroid hormones, e.g. testosterone, derived from cholesterol. They are secreted by the testes and the adrenal cortex in both sexes. They produce the male secondary sexual characteristics, e.g. male distribution of hair and deepening of voice, influence spermatogenesis and exert widespread anabolic effects — **androgenic, androgenous** *adj*.

anencephaly *n* absence of the brain. Cerebral hemispheres completely or partially missing. The condition is incompatible with life — **anencephalous, anencephalic** *adj*.

aneuploidy an abnormal chromosome number that is not a multiple of the normal haploid number (23). Examples include; monosomy where there are 45 chromosomes, e.g. Turner's syndrome and trisomy, such as Down's syndrome, where there are 47 chromosomes. ⇒ polyploidy.

aneurysm *n* a permanent, abnormal dilatation of an artery, that may be congenital or more usually due to degenerative arterial disease. It may be fusiform, sacculated or dissecting through the layers of the arterial wall. (See Figure 4). *aortic aneurysm* one affecting the aorta. ⇒ abdominal aortic aneurysm. *arteriovenous aneurysm* a communication between an artery and a vein, usually the result of injury. *berry aneurysm* congenital condition of the cerebral blood vessels; may rupture, causing subarachnoid haemorrhage.

angiectasis *n* abnormal dilatation of blood vessels. ⇒ telangiectasis — **angiectatic** *adj*.

angiitis *n* inflammation of a blood or lymph vessel. ⇒ vasculitis — **angiitic** *adj*.

angina *n* sense of suffocation or constriction. *angina pectoris* severe but transient attack of chest pain which may radiate to the arms (especially the left), abdomen, jaw, neck and throat. Results from myocardial ischaemia, mainly caused by narrowing of the coronary arteries by atheroma but there are other causes, such

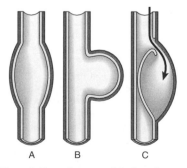

Figure 4 Types of aneurysm. A Fusiform. B Sacculated. C Dissecting. (Reproduced from Brooker 1996 with permission.)

as coronary artery spasm. ⇒ myocardial infarction. Often the pain is induced by exertion, cold weather and wind, emotional stress and sometimes following a large meal. The pain is promptly relieved by rest. Management involves: (a) lifestyle changes, such as smoking cessation; (b) low dose aspirin daily; (c) nitrates, such as glyceryl trinitrate (GTN) given transdermally or sublingually; (d) beta (β)-adrenoceptor antagonists, e.g. atenolol; (e) calcium antagonists, such as nifedipine and verapamil and (f) surgical treatment. → angioplasty. ⇒ coronary — **anginal** *adj.*

angioblast *n* the earliest formative tissue from which blood vessels develop.

angiocardiography *n* demonstration of the chambers of the heart and great vessels after injection of a contrast medium — **angiocardiographically** *adv.*

angiofibroma *n* benign tumour arising from nasopharynx, most commonly seen in young males.

angiogenesis *n* vascularization (formation of new blood vessels, such as, during wound healing). Also seen in oncology when new blood vessels may develop to supply a tumour.

angiography *n* demonstration of vessels (arteries, veins) after injection of a contrast medium. *digital subtraction angiography (DSA)* an image subtraction technique which produces clean, clear views of flowing blood, or its blockage by narrowed vessels, and demonstrates stenosed or occluded vessels — **angiographically** *adv*

angiology *n* the science dealing with blood and lymphatic vessels — **angiologically** *adv.*

angioma *n* a tumour of blood vessels → naevus.

angioneurotic oedema → angio-oedema.

angio-oedema *n* (*syn* angioneurotic oedema) a severe form of urticaria which may involve the skin of the face, hands or genitals and the mucous membrane of the mouth and throat; oedema of the glottis may be fatal. Immediately there is an abrupt local increase in vascular permeability, as a result of which fluid escapes from blood vessels into surrounding tissues. Swelling may be due to an allergic

hypersensitivity reaction to drugs, pollens or other known allergens, but in many cases no cause can be found.

angioplasty *n* surgical reconstruction of blood vessels. *balloon angioplasty* a catheter with an inflatable balloon is passed into a stenosed blood vessel, e.g. coronary, femoral, iliac or renal arteries. The balloon is inflated to dilate the stenosis. When the technique is used on the coronary arteries it is termed percutaneous transluminal coronary angioplasty (PTCA) **angioplastic** *adj.*

angiosarcoma *n* a malignant tumour arising from blood vessels — **angiosarcomatous** *adj.*

angiospasm *n* constricting spasm of blood vessels — **angiospastic** *adj.*

angiotensin a polypeptide formed by the action of renin on a precursor protein in the blood plasma. *angiotensin-aldosterone response* in the lungs, angiotensin I is converted into angiotensin II, a highly active substance which constricts blood vessels and causes release of aldosterone from the adrenal cortex.

angiotensin-converting enzyme (ACE) inhibitors *npl* drugs, such as captopril and enalapril maleate, that block the angiotensin aldosterone response. They are used in the treatment of hypertension and heart failure.

Angleman syndrome an inherited condition that arises from mutations in the maternal chromosome 15 during gametogenesis. It is characterized by severe learning disability, poor muscle tone and ataxia. ⇒ genetic imprinting. ⇒ Prader-Willi syndrome.

angular stomatitis ⇒ stomatitis.

anhendonia diminished capacity to experience pleasure. A negative symptom associated with mental illness. It is characterized by: lack of enjoyment from recreational activities; inability to feel close to others, such as family and friends; and difficulty experiencing pleasure from anything.

anhidrosis *n* deficient sweat secretion — **anhidrotic** *adj.*

anhidrotics *n* any agent which reduces perspiration.

anhydrous *adj* entirely without water, dry.

anion *n* an ion with a negative charge, such as chloride (Cl⁻). Anions are attracted to the positive electrode (anode) during electrolysis. *anion gap* the difference between the anions and cations in the blood. ⇒ cation. ⇒ ion.

aniridia *n* lack or defect of the iris; usually congenital.

anisocoria *n* inequality in diameter of the pupils.

anisocytosis *n* variation in size of red blood cells. Often seen on blood film in cases of anaemia.

anisomelia *n* unequal length of limbs — **anisomelous** *adj*.

anisometropia *n* a difference in the refraction of the two eyes — **anisometropic** *adj*.

ankle brachial pressure index (ABPI) an investigation used as part of leg ulcer assessment to confirm the diagnosis and inform decisions regarding the use of compression therapy. The systolic blood pressure at the ankle is divided by the brachial systolic blood pressure to give the ankle brachial pressure index.

ankylosing spondylitis ⇒ spondylitis.

ankylosis *n* 1. stiffness or fixation and immobility of a joint as a result of disease. ⇒ spondylitis. 2. surgical fixation of a joint. ⇒ arthrodesis — **ankylose** *vt, vi*.

annual budget the amount of money allocated to a department at the start of the financial year. ⇒ budget holder. ⇒ cost centre.

annular *adj* ring-shaped. *annular ligaments* hold two long bones in proximity, as in the wrist and ankle joints.

anogenital *adj* pertaining to the anus and the genital region.

anomaly *n* that which is unusual or differs from the normal — **anomalous** *adj*.

anomia *n* a difficulty in word finding occurring in many aphasic patients. Most often demonstrated in naming tasks but also evident by the use of circumlocutions in spontaneous speech samples.

anomie *n* sociological term applied to a situation where the norms guiding behaviour are not present. The situation of 'normlessness' caused by weak social controls and moral obligations leads to a disturbance in social behaviour. ⇒ social norms.

anonychia *n* absence of nails.

anoperineal *adj* pertaining to the anus and perineum.

Anopheles *n* a genus of mosquito. The females of some species are the host of the malarial parasite, and their bite is the means of transmitting malaria to humans.

anophthalmos *n* congenital absence of a true eyeball.

anoplasty *n* plastic reconstructive surgery of the anus — **anoplastic** *adj*.

anorchism *n* congenital absence of one or both testes — **anorchic** *adj*.

anorectal *adj* pertaining to the anus and rectum, e.g. a fissure.

anorexia *n* loss of or impaired appetite for food. *anorexia nervosa* a serious psychological illness with a complex aetiology that may include an association with poor self esteem, distorted body image, fear of obesity and an obsession with thinness. Most common in female adolescents but affects males and adults. It is characterized by a refusal to eat, self-induced vomiting, misuse of laxatives and excessive exercise. Can progress to severe emaciation and life threatening metabolic consequences. ⇒ bulimia nervosa. ⇒ eating disorders — **anorexic** *adj*.

anosmia *n* absence of sense of smell — **anosmic** *adj*.

ANOVA *abbr* analysis of variance.

anovular *n* absence of ovulation, especially a menstrual cycle where ovulation does not occur, such as with some types of oral contraceptives. *anovular cycle* shows no progestational changes.

anoxia *n* literally, no oxygen in the tissues. Usually used to signify hypoxia — **anoxic** *adj*.

ANP *abbr* atrial natriuretic peptide.

antacid *n* a substance which neutralizes or counteracts acidity. Commonly used in alkaline indigestion remedies, e.g. aluminium hydroxide and magnesium trisilicate. They are available as tablets, powders and mixtures.

antagonist *n* 1. a muscle that reverses or opposes the action of an agonist muscle. 2. a drug or substance that opposes or blocks the action of another substance; e.g. naloxone is a narcotic antagonist and reverses the action of opioid drugs. ⇒ agonist *ant*. ⇒ opioid.

anteflexion *n* the bending forward of an organ, commonly applied to the position of the uterus. ⇒ retroflexion *ant*.

antemortem *adj* before death. ⇒ postmortem *ant*.

antenatal *adj* prenatal. Before birth; the time from conception to birth. *antenatal care* regular care and monitoring of the woman and fetus. ⇒ postnatal *ant* — **antenatally** *adj*.

antepartum *adj* before birth. More generally confined to the 3 months preceding full-term delivery, i.e. the 6th to 9th month. ⇒ postpartum *ant*. *antepartum haemorrhage* bleeding from the genital tract (for any reason) occurring after 24 weeks of pregnancy and before labour. May be due to placenta praevia, placental abruption or other causes.

anterior *adj* in front of; the front surface of; ventral. ⇒ posterior *ant*. *anterior chamber of the eye* the space between the posterior surface of the cornea and the anterior surface of the iris. ⇒ aqueous. *anterior fontanelle* ⇒ fontanelle. *anterior tibial syndrome* severe pain and inflammation over anterior tibial muscle group, with inability to dorsiflex the foot — **anteriorly** *adv*.

anterograde *adj* proceeding forward. *anterograde amnesia* ⇒ amnesia. *anterograde urography/pyelography* ⇒ urography. ⇒ retrograde *ant*.

anterolateral in front and to the side.

anteversion *n* the normal forward tilting, or displacement forward, of an organ or part, such as the uterus → retroversion *ant* — **antevert** *vt*.

anthelmintic *adj* (describes) any remedy for the destruction or elimination of parasitic worms, e.g. mebendazole.

anthracosis *n* lung disease of coal-workers. An accumulation of carbon in the lungs due to inhalation of coal dust may cause fibrotic reaction. A form of pneumoconiosis — **anthracotic** *adj*.

anthrax *n* a contagious disease of domestic animals, e.g. cattle and sheep, which may be transmitted to humans by inoculation, inhalation and ingestion, causing malignant pustule (skin lesion) with toxaemia and septicaemia, woolsorter's disease (haemorrhagic bronchopneumonia), severe gastroenteritis and meningitis. Causative organism is *Bacillus anthracis*.

Preventive measures include strict import controls on potentially infected animals or material, destruction and proper disposal of infected animals, prophylactic immunization of cattle and humans. Certain occupations are at high risk: livestock farmers, butchers, veterinary surgeons and those working with wool and hides.

anthropoid *adj* resembling man. Used to describe a pelvis that is narrow from side to side. ⇒ cephalopelvic.

anthropology *n* the science and study of mankind. Subdivided into several specialities. ⇒ ethnology.

anthropometry *n* comparative measurement of the human body and its parts, such as weight, height, skin fold thickness etc — **anthropometric** *adj*.

antiadrenergic *adj* neutralizing or lessening the effects of impulses produced by adrenergic postganglionic fibres of the sympathetic nervous system,

antiallergic *adj* preventing or lessening allergy.

antiarrhythmic *adj* describes drugs and treatments used in a variety of cardiac rhythm disorders. ⇒ arrhythmia. Antiarrhythmic drugs are divided into four classes: (a) class I drugs act by reducing excitability in the heart muscle and slow conduction, e.g. quinidine, disopyramide, lidocaine (lignocaine), flecainide; (b) class II drugs are the beta (β)-adrenoreceptor antagonists, e.g. atenolol; (c) class III drugs act by prolonging the action potential, e.g. amiodarone; (d) class IV drugs act by blocking calcium channels (calcium antagonists) in the muscle and preventing abnormal conduction, e.g. verapamil. ⇒ cardioversion. ⇒ glycosides.

antibacterial *adj* describes any agent which destroys bacteria or inhibits their growth. ⇒ antibiotic. ⇒ antiseptics. ⇒ bactericide. → bacteriostasis. → disinfectants.

antibilharzial *adj* against Bilharzia. ⇒ *Schistosoma*.

antibiosis *n* an association between organisms which is harmful to one of them. ⇒ symbiosis *ant* — **antibiotic** *adj*.

antibiotics *npl* strictly speaking, they are antibacterial substances derived from fungi and bacteria, exemplified by the penicillins.

The term is generally used to describe all antibacterial drugs. There are many groups of drugs that act against bacteria; some have a narrow spectrum of activity, whereas others are wide (broad) spectrum drugs that can be used to treat a wide range of infections. ⇒ aminoglycosides. ⇒ antituberculosis drugs. ⇒ β-lactam antibiotics. ⇒ cephalosporins. ⇒ macrolides. ⇒ penicillins. ⇒ fluoroquinolones. ⇒ sulphonamides. ⇒ tetracyclines.

antibodies *npl* ⇒ immunoglobulins.

anticholinergic *adj* term applied to agents that inhibit cholinergic nerve impulse transmission by their action on the functioning of the neurotransmitter acetylcholine. ⇒ muscarinic antagonists (antimuscarinic drugs).

anticholinesterase *n* enzyme that destroys/neutralizes cholinesterase enabling acetylcholine to accumulate at nerve endings, thus permitting resumption of normal muscle contraction.

anticoagulant *n* an agent which prevents or delays the clotting of blood. Uses: (a) to obtain specimens suitable for pathological investigation and chemical analyses where whole blood or plasma is required instead of serum; the anticoagulant is usually oxalate; (b) to obtain blood suitable for transfusion, the anticoagulant usually being sodium citrate; (c) as a therapeutic agent in the prophylaxis and treatment of thromboembolic conditions, e.g. heparin, warfarin.

anticodon *n* in genetics, the triplet of bases in tRNA (transfer ribonucleic acis) involved in the translation stage of protein synthesis. ⇒ codon.

anticonvulsives ⇒ antiepileptic drugs.

anti-D *n* antibody formed when rhesus negative individuals are exposed to rhesus positive blood. ⇒ blood groups. *anti-D (Rh₀) immunoglobulin* sterile solution of globulins derived from human plasma containing antibody to the erythrocyte factor Rh(D); used to prevent the formation of the anti-D antibody by rhesus negative women during pregnancy, after delivery or following a spontaneous miscarriage or termination of pregnancy. ⇒ haemolytic disease of the newborn.

antidepressants *npl* drugs which relieve depression. There are three main types: ⇒ monoamine oxidase inhibitors (MAOIs). ⇒ selective serotonin re-uptake inhibitors (SSRIs). ⇒ tricyclic antidepressants (TCAs).

antidiabetic *adj* literally 'against diabetes'. Describes the therapeutic measures used in diabetes mellitus to lower and control blood glucose. ⇒ hypoglycaemic drugs. ⇒ insulin.

antidiarrhoeals *npl* agents that relieve diarrhoea, e.g. codeine phosphate, loperamide etc.

antidiphtheritic *adj* against diphtheria. Describes preventive measures such as immunization with diphtheria toxoid to produce active immunity; therapeutic measures, e.g. diphtheria antitoxin, used to provide passive immunity.

antidiuretic *adj* reducing the volume of urine. *antidiuretic hormone (ADH)* vasopressin.

antidiuretic hormone *n* ⇒ vasopressin.

antidote *n* a drug or agent that opposes the action of a poison, e.g. naloxone is the antidote for opioid (opiate) drugs.

antiembolic *adj* against embolism. *antiembolic hose* stockings worn to decrease the risk of deep vein thrombosis, especially after surgery. Also known as thromboembolic deterrents (TEDs).

antiemetic *adj* against emesis. Any agent which prevents nausea and vomiting. *antiemetic drugs* several groups of drugs that act in a variety of ways to prevent nausea and vomiting caused by different conditions, such as motion sickness. ⇒ cannabinoids. ⇒ D_2-receptor antagonists. ⇒ H_1-receptor antagonists. ⇒ $5\text{-}HT_3$-receptor antagonists. ⇒ muscarinic antagonists.

antienzyme *n* a substance which exerts a specific inhibiting action on an enzyme. Found in the digestive tract to prevent digestion of its lining, and in blood where they act as immunoglobulins.

antiepileptic drugs *npl* also known as anticonvulsives. They are used to prevent seizures (convulsions), e.g. phenytoin, carbamazepine, valporate, ethosuximide and vigabatrin. The drugs used to control a seizure include: a benzodiazepine, such as diazepam, or phenytoin. ⇒ status epilepticus.

antifibrinolytic *adj* describes any agent which prevents fibrinolysis, e.g. tranexamic acid.

antifungal *adj* describes any agent which destroys fungi, e.g. nystatin, griseofulvin etc.

antigen *n* any substance, usually a protein, which is capable, under appropriate conditions, of inducing a specific immune response and of reacting with the products of that response: that is with specific antibody or specifically sensitized T-lymphocytes, or both. ⇒ hapten. — **antigenic** *adj*.

antigen presenting cell (APC) *n* immune cells of the mononuclear phagocytic system, such as macrophages, that are able to alert other immune cells to the presence of a foreign antigen. ⇒ antigen. ⇒ macrophage.

antigenic determinant *n* the area on an antigen where the specific antibody or T-lymphocyte binds and interacts. Also known as an epitope.

antigenic drift *n* the mutations occuring in micro-organisms over time that change their antigenic properties, such as those occurring in the influenza virus. This property complicates the production of effective vaccines and antimicrobial drugs.

antigenicity the ability or power of micro-organisms and their products to stimulate antibody production, as in a vaccine.

anti-HBc *abbr* antibody against the hepatitis B core antigen (HBcAg).

anti-HBe *abbr* antibody against the e antigen (HBeAg) associated with the core of the hepatitis B virus.

anti-HBs *abbr* antibody against the hepatitis B surface antigen (HBsAg).

antihaemophilic factor (AHF) factor VIII involved in blood clotting, deficiency of which produces haemophilia (classical or Type A).

antihaemophilic factor B ⇒ Christmas factor.

antihaemorrhagic *adj* describes any agent which prevents haemorrhage; used to describe vitamin K.

antihistamines *npl* histamine antagonists. Drugs which suppress some of the effects of released histamine, e.g. chlorphenamine (chlorpheniramine). They are widely used in the palliative treatment of hay fever, urticaria, angio-oedema (angioneurotic oedema) and some forms of pruritus. They also have antiemetic properties, and are effective in motion and radiation sickness. Side-effects include drowsiness, tinnitus and dizziness.

antihypertensive *adj* describes any agent which reduces high blood pressure, e.g. propranolol. ⇒ beta (β)-adrenoceptor antagonists. ⇒ angiotensin-converting enzyme (ACE) inhibitors. ⇒ calcium antagonists (channel blockers). ⇒ diuretics.

anti-inflammatory *adj* tending to reduce or prevent inflammation. ⇒ nonsteroidal anti-inflammatory drugs.

antilymphocyte immunoglobulin immunoglobulin containing antibodies that inhibit lymphocyte function. It is occasionally used as an immunosuppressive agent to prevent rejection of transplanted organs. Also known as antilymphocyte serum.

antimalarial *adj* against malaria. Drugs used for prophylaxis and for treatment of an attack include: chloroquine, proguanil etc.

antimetabolites *npl* chemicals which prevent cell division. They are similar to essential metabolites and are able to interfere with the metabolic pathways needed for their use by cells. Examples are methotrexate, a folic acid antagonist, mercaptopurine, which is analogous with purines, and 5-fluorouracil, which is analogous with pyrimidines. Antimetabolites are used in the treatment of cancer.

antimicrobial *adj* against microbes. ⇒ antibiotics. ⇒ antiseptics. ⇒ disinfectants.

antimitotic *adj* preventing cell replication by mitosis. Describes many of the drugs used to treat cancer.

antimutagen *n* a substance which nullifies the action of a mutagen — **antimutagenic** *adj*.

antimycotic *adj* ⇒ antifungal.

antineoplastic *adj* describes any substance or procedure that kills or slows the growth of cancer cells (neoplasms), such as chemotherapy with cytotoxic drugs and radiotherapy, which act directly to kill cancer cells, and therapies that work indirectly: biological response modifier therapy and hormonal therapy.

antineuritic *adj* describes any agent which prevents neuritis. Specially applied to vitamin B complex.

antinuclear antibodies *npl* autoantibodies detected in conditions such as rheumatoid arthritis and systemic lupus erythematosus. They specifically attack the cell nucleus.

antioestrogens *npl* oestrogen antagonist drugs that block oestrogen receptors, thereby preventing the binding of oestrogen to the receptors. Some, such as clomifene (clomiphene), are used in certain types of infertility, whereas others, e.g. tamoxifen, are used in the management of breast cancer and prevention of breast cancer in high risk women. ⇒ selective (o)estrogen receptor modulators (SERMS).

antioxidants *npl* describes any substances which delay the process of oxidation. Certain vitamins, such as vitamins A, C and E, as part of a balanced healthy diet, act as antioxidants and help to prevent free radical oxidative damage to cells. Some minerals, such as copper, zinc and selenium, also act as antioxidants.

antiparasitic *adj* describes any agent which prevents or destroys parasites.

antiparkinson(ism) drugs *npl* drugs used in the treatment of parkinsonism include: (a) muscarinic antagonists, e.g. benzatropine (benztropine) to reduce tremor and rigidity (b) dopaminergic drugs that enhance endogenous dopamine, e.g. amantidine that reduces hypokinesis, and those that replace dopamine production, e.g. L-dopa (combined with an enzyme inhibitor, such as carbidopa, to prevent L-dopa being broken down before it reaches the brain), and drugs such as bromocriptine that mimic dopamine.

antiperistalsis *n* reversal of the normal peristaltic action — **antiperistaltic** *adj*.

antiprostaglandins *npl* group of drugs that inhibit the formation of prostaglandins. They include most of the NSAIDs.

antiprothrombin *n* arrests blood clotting by preventing conversion of prothrombin into thrombin. Anticoagulant.

antipruritic *adj* describes any agent which relieves or prevents itching.

antipsychotic *adj* literally, against psychosis. ⇒ neuroleptics.

antipyretic *adj* describes any agent which allays or reduces fever, e.g. paracetamol.

antirabic *adj* describes any agent which prevents or cures rabies.

antireflux *adj* against backward flow. Usually refers to reimplantation of ureters into bladder in cases of chronic pyelonephritis associated with vesicoureteric reflux.

antischistosomal *adj* describes any agent which works against *Schistosoma*, e.g. praziquantel.

antisepsis *n* prevention of infection of tissues or body surfaces by the application of nonantibiotic chemicals (antiseptics). Introduced into surgery in 1880 by Lord Lister, who used carbolic acid — **antiseptic** *adj*.

antiseptics *npl* substances which destroy or inhibit the growth of micro-organisms. They can be applied to living tissues and are used in hand decontamination and for preparing the skin prior to invasive procedures and surgery, e.g. 4% chlorhexidine.

antiserum *n* a substance prepared from the blood of an animal which has been immunized by the requisite antigen; it contains a high concentration of antibodies (immunoglobulins). Previously used to provide passive immunity, but now replaced by the administration of human immunoglobulins.

antisocial *adj* against society. A term used to denote a psychopathic state in which the individual cannot accept the obligations and restraints imposed on a community by its members. *antisocial personality disorder* ⇒ psychopathic personality — **antisocialism** *n*.

antispasmodic *adj* (*syn* spasmolytic). Describes any measure used to relieve spasm in muscle, such as diazepam and baclofen used to reduce muscle spasticity, and drugs that reduce intestinal spasm, e.g. mebeverine hydrochloride etc.

antistatic *adj* preventing the accumulation of static electricity.

antistreptolysin *adj* against streptolysins. A raised antistreptolysin titre in the blood is indicative of recent streptococcal infection.

antisyphilitic *adj* describes any measures taken to combat syphilis.

antitetanus toxoid *n* ⇒ ATT.

antithrombin III *n* a protease inhibitor of coagulation, synthesized in the liver. Normally present in the blood where it limits coagulation to areas where it is needed. It reacts with several clotting factors and is the cofactor for heparin. ⇒ thrombin.

antithrombotic *adj* describes any measures that prevent or cure thrombosis. ⇒ anticoagulant. ⇒ antiembolism hose.

antithymocyte globulin (ATG) an immunoglobulin which binds to antigens on thymic lymphocytes (T-lymphocytes) and inhibits lymphocyte-dependent immune responses.

antithyroid *n* any agent used to decrease the activity of the thyroid gland and production of thyroid hormones, e.g. carbimazole. ⇒ iodine.

antitoxin *n* a specific antibody which neutralizes a given toxin. Made in response to the invasion by toxin-producing bacteria, or the injection of toxoids — **antitoxic** *adj*.

antitreponemal *adj* describes any measures used against infections caused by *Treponema*.

antituberculosis drugs *npl* drugs that are effective against tuberculosis, e.g. rifampicin, ethambutal, isoniazid, pyrazinamide etc.

antitumour antibiotics *npl* cytotoxic antibiotics disrupt DNA and the cell membrane, e.g. doxorubicin, bleomycin etc. Used in the treatment of solid cancers, leukaemia and lymphoma.

antitussive *adj* describes any measures which suppress cough, e.g. codeine phosphate, morphine in terminal illness.

antiviral *adj* acting against viruses. Antiviral drugs include: aciclovir, idoxuridine, ganciclovir, zidovudine, ritonavir etc.

antrectomy *n* excision of an antrum, e.g. maxillary antrum or pyloric antrum of stomach.

antrochoanal polyp nasal polyp arising from the maxillary antrum (sinus), presenting in the nasopharynx.

antro-oral *adj* pertaining to the maxillary antrum and the mouth. *antro-oral fistula* can occur after extraction of an upper molar tooth, the root of which has protruded into the floor of the antrum.

antrostomy *n* operation to enlarge the natural ostium or to create an artificial opening from nasal cavity to maxillary antrum

(sinus) for the purpose of drainage. ⇒ sinusitis.

antrum *n* a cavity, especially in bone. *antrum of Highmore* ⇒ maxillary antrum — **antral** *adj*.

anuria *n* cessation of urine secretion by the kidneys. Also called suppression. ⇒ oliguria — **anuric** *adj*.

anus *n* the end of the canal/tract, at the extreme termination of the rectum. It is formed of a sphincter muscle which relaxes to allow the passage of faeces. *artificial anus* → colostomy. *imperforate anus* → imperforate — **anal** *adj*.

anxiety *n* a normal reaction to stress or threat. 'Clinical' anxiety is said to be present if the threat is minimal or nonexistent. Anxiety may occur in discrete attacks ('panic' attacks) or as a persistent state (anxiety state). *free-floating anxiety* psychological and physical symptoms occur, unrelated to any event or circumstance; generalized and pervasive feelings of fear may be present for most of the time ⇒ Beck Anxiety Inventory. ⇒ Fear Questionnaire. → panic attacks.

anxiolytics *npl* agents which reduce anxiety, such as the benzodiazepines, e.g. diazepam. ⇒ hypnotics. ⇒ sedatives. ⇒ tranquillizers.

aorta *n* the main artery arising out of the left ventricle of the heart. It supplies oxygenated blood to all parts of the body.

aortic *adj* pertaining to the aorta. *aortic murmur* abnormal heart sound heard over aortic area. *aortic regurgitation* blood from the aorta flows back into the left ventricle. Usually caused by bicuspid valve, rheumatic heart disease, endocarditis and aortic dilatation. *aortic stenosis* narrowing of aortic valve. This is usually due to rheumatic heart disease, congenital valve disorders, calcification or age-related valvular degeneration. *aortic valve* the three cusp semilunar valve between the left ventricle and the aorta.

aortitis *n* inflammation of the aorta.

aortography *n* demonstration of the aorta after introduction of a contrast medium, either via a catheter passed along the femoral or brachial artery or by direct translumbar injection.

apathy *n* 1. abnormal listlessness and lack of activity. 2. attitude of indifference — **apathetic** *adj*.

APEL *abbr* Accreditation (Assessment) of Prior Experiential Learning. See Box – APEL, APL and CATS.

aperients *npl* ⇒ laxatives.

aperistalsis *n* absence of peristaltic movement in the bowel. Characterizes the condition of paralytic ileus — **aperistaltic** *adj*.

apex *n* the narrowest part of anything which is cone-shaped, e.g. the heart or lung. *apex beat* left ventricular contraction felt, seen or heard against the chest. Usually situated at the level of the fifth intercostal space in the mid-clavicular line — **apical** *adj*.

Apgar score a measure used to evaluate the general condition of a newborn baby, developed by an American anaesthetist, Dr Virginia Apgar. A score of 0, 1, or 2 is given to each of the criteria – heart rate, respiratory effort, skin colour, muscle tone and reflex response to a nasal catheter. A score of between 8 and 10 would indicate a baby in excellent condition, whereas a score of below 7 would cause concern. (See Figure 5).

aphagia *n* inability to swallow — **aphagic** *adj*.

aphakia *n* absence of the crystalline lens. Describes the eye after removal of a cataract — **aphakic** *adj*.

aphasia *n* a disorder of language following brain damage, due primarily to impairment to the linguistic system. The term does not include disorders in language comprehension or expression that are primarily due to mental disorders, including psychosis, dementia and confusion, or to hearing impairment or muscle weakness. There are several classification systems but the most commonly used terms are *expressive aphasia* and *receptive aphasia*, although patients may exhibit difficulties in both language comprehension and expression. ⇒ dysarthria. ⇒ expressive aphasia. ⇒ receptive aphasia — **aphasic** *adj*.

apheresis *n* the process whereby blood is drawn from a donor into a blood cell separator which collects the required components, plasma (plasmapheresis) or platelets (plateletpheresis), and returns the remainder to the donor. Plasmapheresis may be

---

APEL, APL, CATS

(otherwise known as Accreditation(Assessment) of Prior Experiential Learning, Accreditation (Assessment) of Prior Learning, and Credit Accumulation and Transfer System.)

It has long been suggested that employers and educational establishments should acknowledge and, where possible, credit learning that has already taken place and where evidence of that learning can be demonstrated, e.g. with a personal professional profile. This credit should not only apply to academic learning, with or without qualifications such as a diploma or degree, but also to the acquisition of experience and expertise through practice, often gained through normal working roles and individual personal development.

Universities, colleges and employers now recognize the need to give appropriate credit to individuals in certain circumstances, e.g. when applying to undertake a programme of learning and some of the content has already been accredited, or when applying for a post and prior experience can be acknowledged.

Within the further and higher education institutions a process of credit accumulation and transfer has been established and certain programmes attract 'points'. Those points are at distinct levels; level 1 denoting certificate level achievement, level 2 indicating diploma level work, and level 3 identifying achievement at first degree level. Masters level work is accredited at that level.

Unfortunately, different universities allot different credit ratings to potentially the same programmes, and within nursing, the English National Board programme – Teaching and assessing in practice (ENB 998) will be awarded different credit ratings by different universities. The ENB is not allowed to set the credit rating at a national level. This system means that the currency value of certain programmes is not standard and universities may not accept the credit rating given by a different establishment. Individuals looking to gain credit therefore may need to submit their claim to a university to allot their own rating.

Accreditation of practice needs to be done on a much more individual approach, and the claimant will need to submit evidence, usually in the form of a profile or portfolio, for individual assessment to be made of the claim and credit awarded accordingly.

In other countries, for example the United States of America, credentialing is a similar process with similar outcomes.

Signs/Criteria	Score		
	0	1	2
Heart rate	Absent	Slow, below 100/min	Over 100/min
Respiratory effort	Absent	Slow, weak, irregular	Good chest movements or crying
Muscle tone	Limp	Poor tone, some movement	Active resistance, strong movement
Reflex irritability (response to stimulation such as sole flicks)	None	Slight withdrawal	Vigorous movement, cries
Colour (Note: designed for Caucasian newborns)	Pale or blue	Extremities blue	Completely normal colour

Figure 5 Apgar score. (Reproduced from Brooker 1998 with permission.)

used in the treatment of some diseases caused by antibodies or immune complexes circulating in the patient's plasma, e.g. myasthenia gravis.

aphonia *n* loss of voice due to organic, neurological, behavioural or psychogenic causes. ⇒ dysphonia — **aphonic** *adj*.

aphrodisiac *n* an agent which stimulates sexual excitement.

aphthae *npl* small ulcers of the oral mucosa surrounded by a ring of erythema — **aphthous** *sing*.

aphthous stomatitis ⇒ stomatitis.

apicectomy *n* excision of the apex of the root of a tooth.

APKD *abbr* adult polycystic kidney disease. ⇒ polycystic kidneys.

APL *abbr* Accreditation (assessment) of Prior Learning. See Box – APEL, APL and CATS.

aplasia *n* nondevelopment of an organ or tissue.

aplastic *adj* **1.** without structure or form. **2.** incapable of forming new tissue. *aplastic anaemia* ⇒ anaemia.

apneustic centre *n* a respiratory centre in the brain that ensures a smooth respiratory rhythm. → pneumotaxic centre.

apnoea *n* cessation of spontaneous breathing as seen, e.g. in Cheyne-Stokes respiration. *apnoea mattress* a mattress which gives an auditory alarm signal when a baby has not breathed for a preset time, usually 15 to 20 seconds. The baby can then be stimulated to breathe before he or she becomes hypoxic. ⇒ sudden infant death syndrome. *apnoea of the newborn*

⇒ periodic breathing. *apnoea of prematurity* commonly occurs in preterm babies of less than 34 weeks gestation: due to immaturity of both the respiratory centre and chemoreceptors. *sleep apnoea* breathing pauses (and near pauses as in hypopnoea) due to periodic upper airway closure during sleep. This results in a cycle of apnoea-awakenings-apnoea etc throughout the night, disturbing sleep, and also in daytime sleeping and risk of accidents. The sudden awakenings are associated with a sudden increase in blood pressure that may eventually lead to an increased risk of high blood pressure, strokes and ischaemic heart disease. The condition is more common in men and in people who are overweight. ⇒ continuous positive airway pressure. — **apnoeic** *adj*.

apocrine glands modified sweat glands, especially in axillae, genital and perineal regions. Responsible, after puberty, for body odour, hormone dependent. ⇒ eccrine.

apodia *n* congenital absence of the feet.

apolipoproteins *npl* special proteins that coat lipoproteins during transportation in the plasma. They act as recognition sites for the cell receptors and enzymes that deal with the lipoprotein.

aponeurosis *n* a broad glistening sheet of white fibrous tissue which serves to invest and attach muscles to each other, and also to the parts which they move. ⇒ tendon — **aponeurotic** *adj*.

aponeurositis *n* inflammation of an aponeurosis.

apophysis *n* a projection, protuberance or outgrowth. Usually used in connection with bone.

apoplexy *n* obsolete term for cerebrovascular accident or stroke — **apoplectic, apoplectiform** *adj*.

apoprotein *n* a protein prior to it binding with the prosthetic group needed for biological activity.

apoptosis *n* programmed cell death. For example, immune cells (many lymphocytes) that would react against body tissues are destroyed in the thymus gland during the maturation of immune cells.

appendicectomy *n* excision of the appendix vermiformis. *laparoscopic appendicectomy* excision of the appendix via a laparoscope, using a minimally invasive approach.

appendicitis *n* inflammation of the appendix vermiformis.

appendix *n* an appendage. *appendix vermiformis* a worm-like appendage of the caecum about the thickness of the little finger and usually measuring around 5 cm in length. Its position is variable and it contains considerable lymphoid tissue — **appendicular** *adj*.

apperception *n* clear perception of a sensory stimulus, in particular where there is identification or recognition — **apperceptive** *adj*.

appetite *n* pleasant anticipation of taking food and fluid; it can become fickle in illness; maintaining oral hygiene, hydration and offering small attractive portions will be helpful. *appetite suppressant* drugs sometimes used in the management of severe obesity, e.g. dexfenfluramine, diethylpropion. Dependence and misuse are particular problems. Appetite may also be suppressed with the use of bulk-forming drugs, such as methylcellulose.

application *n* in computing the programs that allow a PC to perform a specific function, such as word processing.

applicator *n* an instrument for local application of remedies.

apposition *n* the approximation or bringing together of two surfaces or edges.

appraisal *n* the process of making a valuation. *performance appraisal or performance review* a formal procedure where an appraiser (manager) systematically reviews the role performance of the appraisee and they jointly set goals for the future. There are many different systems of appraisal but common features include: separate preparation by appraiser and appraisee, the review meeting and some form of follow-up.

approved name the nonproprietary (generic) name for a drug, e.g. nifedipine. The approved name should be used in all prescribing except in cases where the bioavailability may vary between brands. ⇒ Recommended International Nonproprietary Name.

apraxia *n* a disorder, resulting from brain damage, in the ability to control motor movements. Involuntary movements may be relatively normal but more deliberate or voluntary movements are affected. *constructional apraxia* inability to arrange objects to a plan. ⇒ dyspraxia — **apraxic, apractic** *adj*.

aptitude *n* natural ability and facility in performing tasks, either mental or physical.

apyrexia *n* absence of fever — **apyrexial** *adj*.

aqueous *adj* watery. *aqueous humor* the fluid contained in the anterior and posterior chambers of the eye.

arachidonic acid a polyunsaturated fatty acid with four double bonds. Used in the body for the synthesis of important regulatory lipids that include: prostaglandins and thromboxanes. It can be synthesized from linoleic acid in the body, but may be considered to be an essential fatty acid (EFA) when linoleic acid is deficient in the diet.

arachnodactyly *n* congenital abnormality resulting in excessively long, thin fingers and toes ('spider fingers').

arachnoid *adj* resembling a spider's web. *arachnoid mater* a delicate membrane enveloping the brain and spinal cord, lying between the pia mater internally and the dura mater externally; the middle membrane of the meninges. ⇒ phobia — **arachnoidal** *adj*.

arborization *n* an arrangement resembling the branching of a tree. Characterizes both ends of a neuron, i.e. the dendrons and the axon.

arboviruses *abbr* abbreviation for ARthropod-BOrne viruses. Various RNA viruses are transmitted by arthropods: mosquitos, sandflies, ticks and biting midges. The diseases transmitted include: some haemorrhagic fevers, e.g. yellow fever, dengue, several types of encephalitis and sandfly fever.

ARC *acr* AIDS-related complex.

arcus a ring or arch. *arcus senilis* an opaque ring round the edge of the cornea, seen in older people.

ARDS *abbr* acute respiratory distress syndrome.

arenaviruses *npl* a family of RNA viruses that includes the Lassa fever virus.

areola *n* the pigmented area round the nipple of the breast. A *secondary areola* surrounds the primary areola in pregnancy — **areolar** *adj* areolar tissue a loose woven connective tissue with a matrix, fibres and cells.

ARF *abbr* 1. acute renal failure. ⇒ renal. 2. acute respiratory failure. ⇒ acute respiratory distress syndrome. → respiratory failure.

arginase *n* an enzyme found in the liver, kidney and spleen. It splits arginine into ornithine and urea during the reactions of the urea cycle.

arginine *n* an amino acid. Used in treatment of acute liver failure to tide patient over acute ammonia intoxication.

argininosuccinic acidaemia *n* an inherited disorder of amino acid metabolism. Deficiency of an enzyme leads to high levels of argininosuccinic acid in the blood. Affected individuals have learning disability and are prone to seizures.

argininosuccinuria *n* presence of argininosuccinic acid in the urine. ⇒ argininosuccinic acidaemia.

Argyll Robertson pupil one which reacts to accommodation, but not to light. Diagnostic sign in neurosyphilis, but other important causes include multiple sclerosis and diabetes mellitus. In the non-syphilitic group the pupil is not small, but often dilated and unequal and is called atypical.

ariboflavinosis *n* a deficiency state caused by lack of riboflavin and other members of the vitamin B complex. Characterized by cheilosis, seborrhoea, angular stomatitis, glossitis and photophobia.

Arnold Chiari malformation a group of disorders affecting the base of the brain. Commonly occurs in hydrocephalus associated with meningocele and meningomyelocele. There are degrees of severity but usually there is some 'kinking' or 'buckling' of the brainstem with cerebellar tissue herniating through the foramen magnum at the base of the skull.

aromatherapy *n* a therapy involving the therapeutic use of fragrances derived from essential oils. These may be combined with a base oil, inhaled or massaged into the skin.

arrectores pilorum *n* involuntary muscles attached to hair follicles, which, by contraction, erect the follicles, causing 'gooseflesh' — **arrector pili** *sing*.

arrhenoblastoma *n* ⇒ androblastoma.

arrhythmia *n* any deviation from the normal rhythm, usually referring to the heartbeat. (See Figure 6). ⇒ asystole. ⇒ atrial fibrillation. ⇒ atrial flutter. → bradycardia. ⇒ extrasystole (ectopics). ⇒ fibrillation. ⇒ heart block. ⇒ Stokes-Adams syndrome. ⇒ supraventricular tachycardia. ⇒ tachycardia. ⇒ ventricular fibrillation. ⇒ ventricular tachycardia. ⇒ Wolff-Parkinson-White syndrome.

arsenic (As) *n* a poisonous metallic element present in preparations which include: pesticides and herbicides. Small amounts may be present in fruit, vegetables and other foods. In some forms it is a potent toxin, causing malaise, anaemia, gastrointestinal symptoms, abnormal skin pigmentation and nervous symptoms.

art therapy the therapeutic use of painting, drawing, modelling or sculpture to express emotions and stimulate a mood. The use of certain colours is thought to promote particular emotions, affecting breathing and circulatory rhythms. Sculpture and modelling therapy may be used in certain psychiatric conditions involving loss of orientation in space, giddiness and lack of concentration.

artefact *n* any artificial product resulting from a physical or chemical agent; an unnatural change in a structure or tissue.

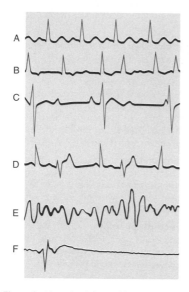

Figure 6 Normal and abnormal heart rhythms. A Sinus rhythm. B Atrial fibrillation: atrial rate is rapid and irregular, with no proper P wave. Ventricular rate is irregular and produces an irregular pulse. C Complete heart block (third-degree AV block): no impulses from the AV node reach the ventricles. Atrial contraction is regular but the slower ventricular contraction is initiated by fibres in the AV bundle or ventricle. D Ventricular ectopic beats: these are wide QRS complexes without a P wave. They can occur in healthy people, being associated with an excess of tea, coffee or alcohol. They may also be a feature of disease such as myocardial infarction. E Ventricular fibrillation: a completely disordered pattern of irregular QRS complexes which produce no cardiac output. This is the usual reason for cardiac arrest and is the commonest cause of sudden death. It requires the commencement of immediate resuscitation. F Asystole: in this case no QRS complexes are seen. Again, this is a cardiac arrest situation which requires immediate resuscitation. (Reproduced from Brooker 1998 with permission.)

arterial blood gases (ABGs) the measurement of arterial blood gases: PaO_2, $PaCO_2$ and pH. It provides information on arterial haemoglobin oxygen saturation and the acid-base status as affected by respiratory and metabolic function. Commonly performed in critical care situations, such as patients with severe asthma, shock and those requiring respiratory support. A sample of arterial blood is obtained from a suitable vessel, such as the radial or femoral artery. ⇒ oxygenation.

arterial cannula n a cannula inserted into an artery, used for continuous monitoring of blood pressure in shocked patients. It also enables repeated sampling of arterial blood for gas analysis. They are generally only used in specialist units (ITU, HDU) because of the potential risk of accidental removal or disconnection with severe blood loss. They should always be attached to a pressure transducer and monitor, and have an alarm that indicates any disconnection.

arterial ulcer n a leg ulcer with an arterial aetiology. They are usually on the foot, near the ankle or between the toes; the surrounding skin is discoloured (pale, dusky or purple), shiny and hairless; and the ulcer is small and deep with some exudate. Patients often have a history of cardiovascular disease or diabetes, and complain of leg pain on exertion and rest pain at night. ⇒ claudication.

arteriography n demonstration of the arterial system after injection of a contrast medium — **arteriographically** *adv*.

arteriole n a small artery, joining an artery to a capillary. ⇒ peripheral resistance.

arteriopathy n disease of any artery — **arteriopathic** *adj*.

arterioplasty n plastic surgery applied to an artery — **arterioplastic** *adj*.

arteriosclerosis n common degenerative disorder of arteries characterized by hardening of the walls with calcification, narrowing of the lumen and loss of elasticity, which results in decreased blood flow. Commonly affects the cerebral vessels and those of the lower extremities. It is associated with increasing age, hypertension and hyperlipidaemia. ⇒ atheroma. ⇒ atherosclerosis — **arteriosclerotic** *adj*.

arteriotomy n incision or needle puncture of an artery.

arteriovenous *adj* pertaining to an artery and a vein, e.g. an arteriovenous aneurysm, fistula, anastomosis, or shunt for haemodialysis. *arteriovenous filtration* haemofiltration.

arteritis n an inflammatory disease affecting the walls of the arteries. It may be caused by infection, radiation, chemicals and trauma, or as part of a systemic disease, such as autoimmune thyroiditis and systemic lupus erythematosus. *giant cell arteritis* occurs in older people and mainly affects the external carotid artery and its branches, such as the temporal arteries of the scalp. There is severe headache, scalp tenderness, pyrexia, anorexia and weight loss. Visual impairment can ensue if there is thrombosis of the ophthalmic artery. Treatment with corticosteroids is effective. ⇒ polymyalgia rheumatica — **arteritic** adj.

artery n a vessel carrying blood away from the heart. The internal endothelial lining provides a smooth surface to prevent clotting of blood. The middle layer of plain muscle and elastic fibres (in large arteries) allows for distension as blood is pumped from the heart. The outer, mainly connective tissue, layer prevents overdistension. artery forceps forceps used to secure haemostasis — **arterial** adj pertaining to arteries. arterial disease ⇒ atheroma. ⇒ arteriosclerosis. ⇒ peripheral.

arthralgia n (syn arthrodynia) pain in a joint, used especially when there is no inflammation — **arthralgic** adj.

arthrectomy n surgical excision of a joint.

arthritis n inflammation of one or more joints which swell, become warm to touch, are painful and are restricted in movement. There are many causes and the treatment varies according to the cause. ⇒ arthropathy. ⇒ gout. ⇒ juvenile chronic arthritis (JCA). ⇒ osteoarthritis. ⇒ rheumatoid arthritis. ⇒ septic arthritis. ⇒ Still's disease — **arthritic** adj.

arthrocentesis n aspiration of fluid from within a joint for diagnostic purposes.

arthroclasia n operation to break up an ankylosed joint to allow free movement.

arthrodesis n the fixation or stiffening of a joint by operative means.

arthrodynia n ⇒ arthralgia — **arthrodynic** adj.

arthrography n a radiographic examination to determine the internal structure of a joint, outlined by contrast media – either a gas or a liquid contrast medium or both — **arthrographically** adv.

arthrology n the science which studies the structure and function of joints, their diseases and treatment.

arthropathy n any joint disease.

arthroplasty n surgical remodelling or replacement of a joint. Commonly performed on the hip, knee and other joints, where plastic, carbon fibre, metal or biological materials are used to refashion or replace diseased or damaged structures. cup arthroplasty articular surface is reconstructed and covered with a cup. excision arthroplasty gap is filled with fibrous tissue as in Keller's operation. Girdlestone arthroplasty excision arthroplasty of the hip. replacement arthroplasty insertion of a prosthesis of similar shape. total replacement arthroplasty replacement of the head of femur and the acetabulum, both being cemented into the bone — **arthroplastic** adj.

arthroscope n an endoscope used for the visualization of the interior of a joint cavity. Used for diagnosis and operative procedures. ⇒ endoscope — **arthroscopic** adj.

arthroscopy n endoscopic examination of the interior of a joint cavity using an arthroscope — **arthroscopic** adj.

arthrosis n degeneration in a joint.

arthrotomy n incision into a joint.

Arthus reaction n localized hypersensitivity (type III) reaction involving immune complexes. It occurs at the site of antigen injection. ⇒ hypersensitivity.

articular adj pertaining to a joint or articulation. Applied to cartilage, surface, capsule, etc.

articulation 1. the junction of two or more bones; a joint. 2. enunciation of speech **articular** adj pertaining to a joint or joint structures. articular cartilage the hyaline cartilage covering the articular surfaces of a synovial joint.

artificial feeding ⇒ enteral. ⇒ nutritional support. ⇒ parenteral.

artificial insemination ⇒ insemination.

artificial limb ⇒ prosthesis.

artificial lung ⇒ respirator.

artificial pacemaker cardiac pacemaker. ⇒ cardiac.

artificial pneumothorax ⇒ pneumothorax.

artificial respiration any method used to support life when spontaneous breathing has ceased or is failing to maintain the blood gases within the normal range.

It includes emergency mouth-to-mouth respiration and various levels of support with ventilation equipment. ⇒ resuscitation. ⇒ ventilation.

artificial sweetener *n* food additives, such as saccharine, acesulfame K and aspartame, used to sweeten processed food or to reduce sugar intake.

arytenoid *n* two funnel-shaped cartilages of the larynx.

asbestos *n* a fibrous, mineral substance which does not conduct heat and is incombustible. There are several forms including white and blue asbestos. It has many uses, including brake linings, asbestos textiles and asbestos-cement sheeting. The use of asbestos has declined, and in many countries there is strict health and safety legislation controlling its use or removal. Contact with asbestos may cause asbestosis, bronchial cancer, laryngeal cancer and mesothelioma.

asbestosis *n* a pneumoconiosis. A chronic pulmonary and/or pleura fibrosis caused by the inhalation of asbestos dust and fibre. It may be seen in people who mine or process asbestos; those working in demolition and the manufacture of asbestos products; and in people living near factories dealing with asbestos. In the UK asbestosis is a prescribed industrial disease. ⇒ mesothelioma.

ascariasis *n* infestation by nematodes (roundworms) of the genus Ascaris, such as *Ascaris lumbricoides*. The ova are ingested. Hatching occurs in the duodenum and the larvae pass to the lungs, via the blood, from where they ascend to be swallowed and returned to the small bowel. The mature worms (20–35 cm in length) cause colicky abdominal pain and may be passed rectally or vomited. Occasionally they cause intestinal obstruction and can migrate to block the bile ducts. Treatment is with anthelmintic drugs, e.g. mebendazole, levamisole, piperazine.

ascaricide *n* a substance lethal to ascarides, e.g. levamisole — **ascaricidal** *adj.*

ascarides *n* nematode worms of the family Ascaridae, such as the large roundworm *Ascaris lumbricoides*. ⇒ ascariasis.

Aschoff's nodules the focal necrotic lesions found in the heart tissues in rheumatic fever.

ASCII *abbr* for American Standard Code for Information Interchange. In computing a coding system where each character is represented by a number between 0 and 256. ASCII files are often used to transfer data between different applications. Known colloquially as 'askey'.

ascites *n* (*syn* hydroperitoneum) free fluid in the peritoneal cavity producing abdominal distension. May have benign or malignant causes, including renal failure, cirrhosis of the liver and right-sided heart failure. Ascites is associated with cancers of the ovary, gastrointestinal tract and metastatic cancers of the breast and lung — **ascitic** *adj.*

ascorbic acid vitamin C. A water-soluble vitamin which is necessary for healthy connective tissue, particularly the collagen fibres and cell membranes. It is present in fresh fruits and vegetables, especially citrus fruit, blackcurrants and potatoes. It is destroyed by cooking in the presence of air and by plant enzymes released when cutting and grating food; it is also lost by storage. Deficiency causes scurvy.

ASD *abbr* atrial septal defect.

asepsis *n* the state of being free from living pathogenic micro-organisms — **aseptic** *adj.*

aseptic technique describes procedures which exclude pathogenic micro-organisms from an environment, such as non-touch technique and the use of sterilized equipment. Used where there is a possibility of introducing micro-organisms into the patient's body.

asparaginase *n* an enzyme, in the form of crisantaspase, used pharmacologically to treat cancers, e.g. acute lymphoblastic leukaemia.

aspartame *n* an artificial sweetener. It should be avoided by individuals with phenylketonuria as it is metabolized by the body to a form of phenylalanine.

Asperger's syndrome *n* a syndrome classified as part of the autistic disorders. Diagnosed during childhood, it is associated with various problems with communication, social interaction, expressing emotions and clumsiness. See Box – Asperger's syndrome.

aspergillosis *n* fungal infection, usually bronchopulmonary, caused by any species of the genus Aspergillus, such as *Aspergillus fumigatus*. ⇒ bronchomycosis.

Aspergillus *n* a genus of fungi; some species are pathogenic. The spores are present in air and are therefore continuously inhaled. They are found in soil, manure and on various grains.

aspermia *n* **1.** inability to produce or ejaculate semen. **2.** lack of spermatozoa in semen — **aspermic** *adj*.

asphyxia *n* suffocation; cessation of breathing. The O_2 content of the air in the lungs falls while the CO_2 rises and similar changes follow rapidly in the arterial blood. *blue asphyxia, asphyxia livida* deep blue appearance of a newborn baby which otherwise has good muscle tone and is responsive to stimuli. *white (pale) asphyxia, asphyxia pallida* more severe condition of newborn: pale, flaccid, unresponsive to stimuli. ⇒ acute respiratory distress syndrome. ⇒ Apgar. ⇒ neonatal respiratory distress syndrome.

aspiration *n* **1.** (*syn* paracentesis, tapping) the withdrawal of fluids from a body cavity by means of suction or siphonage apparatus. Examples include aspiration of a pleural effusion, gastric aspiration following surgery or the aspiration of mucus from a newborn's oropharynx. **2.** the entry of fluids or solids into the airway. *aspiration pneumonia* inflammation of lung from inhalation of foreign body, usually fluid or food particles. → Heimlich manoeuvre. ⇒ recovery position — **aspirate** *vt*.

aspirator *n* a negative pressure apparatus for withdrawing fluids from cavities.

aspirin *n* → nonsteroidal anti-inflammatory drugs.

assault a threat of unlawful contact. ⇒ trespass against the person.

assay *n* a quantitative test used to determine the amount of a substance present or its activity, such as drugs or hormones.

assertiveness training aims at developing self-confidence in personal relationships. It focuses on the honest expression of feelings, both negative and positive; the technique is learned by role playing in a therapeutic setting, followed by practice in actual situations.

assessment *n* **1.** the collection by the nurse of relevant data about a patient or client in order to enable individualized nursing. The most detailed information is usually ascertained at the initial interview. Assessment is an ongoing activity, however, and nursing interventions and the goals of patient care should constantly be re-evaluated in the light of this. ⇒ biographical and health data. ⇒ interviewing. **2.** the measurement of a candidate's level of competence in theoretical and practical nursing skills.

assimilation *n* the process whereby the already digested foodstuffs are absorbed and utilized by the tissues — **assimilate** *vt, vi*.

assisted fertility/conception *n* the techniques which aim to assist infertile couples achieve conception and a successful pregnancy, e.g. fertility drugs, in vitro fertilization.

association *n* a word used in psychology. *association of ideas* the principle by which ideas, emotions and movements are connected so that their succession in the mind occurs *controlled association* ideas called up in consciousness in response to words spoken by the examiner. *free association* ideas arising spontaneously when censorship is removed; an important feature of psychoanalysis.

Asperger's syndrome

Asperger's syndrome was first described in 1944 by Hans Asperger. It is characterized by six features:

- difficulties in interacting with other children;
- exclusive absorption in one topic or hobby;
- close adherence to routines in daily life;
- problems in understanding figurative language or jokes;
- clumsiness;
- inappropriate facial expressions or gestures.

The condition is now regarded as part of the autistic spectrum of disorders, with the problems in interacting with others frequently continuing into adult life. However, supportive teaching of language and communication skills, as well as behaviour therapy to deal with the obsessional behaviour that can develop in relation to daily routines, are seen as important in limiting the effects that persist into adulthood. Early recognition of the syndrome with information and support for parents is also very important.

AST *abbr* aspartate aminotransferase. ⇒ aminotransferases.

astereognosis *n* loss of ability to recognize the shape and consistency of objects.

asthenia *n* lack of strength; weakness, debility — **asthenic** *adj*.

asthenopia *n* weakness of vision.

asthma *n* bronchial asthma. Reversible air-flow obstruction precipitated by intake of allergens or drugs, infection, vigorous exercise, temperature/weather changes or emotional stress. It is generally classified as being either early onset (atopic) type, where there is a family history of asthma and other atopic conditions, e.g. eczema, or late onset (nonatopic) type. Asthma is characterized by paroxysmal dyspnoea, expiratory wheeze, cough and difficulty in expiration because of bronchospasm. Management involves: (a) avoidance of allergens (b) inhaled beta (β)$_2$-adrenoceptor agonist bronchodilator drugs, such as short-acting salbutamol or terbutaline or longer-acting salmeterol, other bronchodilators, such as theophylline, inhaled muscarinic-receptor antagonist bronchodilators, e.g. ipratropium bromide (c) inhaled or oral anti-inflammatory drugs that include corticosteroids, e.g. beclometasone (beclomethasone), and prophylactic drugs such as sodium cromoglicate (cromoglycate) that prevent mast cell breakdown and act to block allergic mechanisms. ⇒ severe acute asthma (*syn* status asthmaticus) — **asthmatic** *adj*.

astigmatism *n* defective vision caused by inequality of one or more refractive surfaces, usually the corneal, so that the light rays do not converge to a point on the retina. May be congenital or acquired. Individuals find it difficult to focus on horizontal and vertical lines at the same time without blurring. Corrected by the use of suitable spectacles or contact lenses — **astigmatic, astigmic** *adj*.

astringent *adj* describes an agent which contracts organic tissue and causes local vasoconstriction, thus lessening secretion. Used on heavily exudating wounds, e.g. potassium permanganate — **astringency, astringent** *n*.

astrocyte n a type of neuroglial cell (supporting cells) of the central nervous system. The star-shaped cells contribute to the blood-brain barrier. ⇒ neuroglia.

astrocytoma *n* a slowly growing tumour of the glial tissue of brain and spinal cord. A glioma.

asymmetry *n* lack of similarity of the organs or parts on each side.

asymptomatic *adj* symptomless.

asystole *n* one form of cardiac arrest where the heart ceases to contract. No PQRST complexes are seen on ECG. ⇒ cardiac arrest.

atavism *n* the reappearance of a hereditary trait which has skipped one or more generations — **atavic, atavistic** *adj*.

ataxia, ataxy *n* literally, a disorder. Applied to defective muscular control resulting in irregular and jerky movements; staggering. ⇒ Friedreich's ataxia. ⇒ locomotor ataxia — **ataxic** *adj* pertaining to ataxia. *ataxic gait* ⇒ gait.

ATD *abbr* Alzheimer's type dementia.

atelectasis *n* collapse of lung tissue with consequent reduction in gas exchange because a number of pulmonary alveoli do not contain air. This may be due to failure of expansion (congenital atelectasis) or resorption of air from the alveoli (collapse) — **atelectatic** *adj*.

atherogenic *adj* capable of producing atheroma — **atherogenesis** *n*.

atheroma *n* plaques of fatty (lipid) material deposited in the lining (tunica intima) of arteries. It commences with fatty streaks on the intima, low density lipoprotein is deposited and a plaque forms which eventually disrupts the middle layer (tunica media). The lumen of the vessel is eventually reduced which leads to ischaemia. A plaque may rupture with the formation of a thrombus which will further occlude the vessel. ⇒ atherosclerosis — **atheromatous** *adj*.

atherosclerosis *n* coexisting atheroma and arteriosclerosis, extremely common degenerative arterial disease. It is characterized by the deposition of atheromatous plaques with damage, calcification and hardening of the walls of large and medium sized arteries. These changes lead to narrowing of the vessel lumen and reduced blood flow. A major cause of coronary heart disease: angina pectoris and myocardial infarction — **atherosclerotic** *adj*.

athetosis *n* a condition marked by purposeless movements of the hands and feet and generally due to a brain lesion — **athetoid, athetotic** *adj.*

athlete's foot tinea pedis. ⇒ tinea.

atlas *n* the first cervical vertebra.

atmosphere *n* 1. the air surrounding the Earth; consists of nitrogen (78%), oxygen (20%), carbon dioxide (0.04%) and inert gases with variable amounts of water vapour. 2. a unit of gas pressure which is equal to average atmospheric pressure at sea level – 101.3 kPa (760 mm of mercury pressure). Atmospheric pressure decreases with altitude and increases with depth, e.g. deep mines or under the sea.

atom *n* the smallest particle of an element that exhibits the characteristics of that element and is capable of existing individually, or in combination with one or more atoms of the same or another element — **atomic** *adj* pertaining to atoms *atomic mass unit (amu)* or *Dalton* a relative weight used to measure atoms and subatomic particles. The weight of a neutron and proton have both been designated as being 1 amu. *atomic number* the number of protons in the nucleus or the number of electrons, e.g. hydrogen with one of each has an atomic number of 1. *atomic weight or mass* also known as *relative atomic mass* the relative average mass of an atom based on the mass of an atom of carbon-12.

atomizer *n* nebulizer.

atonic *adj* without tone; weak — **atonia, atony, atonicity** *n.*

atonic bladder urinary bladder with no tone – the detrusor has lost its contractility, resulting in incomplete voiding or inability to void at all. It may be a temporary or permanent condition. ⇒ incontinence.

atopic syndrome an inherited tendency to develop infantile eczema, asthma, hay fever or all three when there is a positive family history.

atopy the clinical presentation of allergic (type I hypersensitivity) reactions. It includes: eczema, allergic rhinitis (hay fever), allergic asthma and food allergies. ⇒ hypersensitivity.

ATP *abbr* adenosine triphosphate.

atresia *n* imperforation or closure of a normal body opening, duct or canal, such as of the oesphagus, anus or bile duct etc — **atresic, atretic** *adj.*

atrial fibrillation a cardiac arrhythmia caused by the independent contraction of the muscle bundles in the atrial walls. It is characterized by a chaotic irregularity of atrial rhythm without any semblance of order. The ventricular rhythm, depending on conduction through the atrioventricular node, is irregular. Commonly associated with mitral stenosis or hyperthyroidism.

atrial flutter a cardiac arrhythmia characterized by rapid, but regular, atrial contraction. It is caused by an irritable focus in the atrial muscle and is usually associated with organic heart disease. The atrial contraction rate may be between 260 and 340 per minute. The ventricles respond variably to every second, third or fourth beat.

atrial natriuretic peptides *npl* peptides produced by the cardiac atria. They help to control blood pressure by inhibiting the release of vasopressin (ADH) and aldosterone when the blood pressure rises. This increases sodium and water loss by the kidneys.

atrial septal defect (ASD) an abnormal communication between right and left atria, commonly due to nonclosure of foramen ovale at birth.

atrioventricular (A-V) *adj* pertaining to the atria and the ventricles of the heart. Applied to a node, bundle and valves. *atrioventricular (A-V) bundle* part of the conducting system of the heart. A mass of neuromuscular fibres in the ventricular septum which conduct impulses from the atrioventricular node to the ventricles. Branches into right and left bundle branches which carry the impulse to the apex of each ventricle to terminate in Purkinje's fibres. Also known as the bundle of His. *atrioventricular (A-V) node* specialized cells, located at the bottom of the right atrium, which carry impulses from the sinoatrial node to the A-V bundle. *atrioventricular valves* ⇒ bicuspid. ⇒ tricuspid.

atrium *n* cavity, entrance or passage. One of the two upper chambers of the heart — **atrial** *adj* pertaining to the atrium. *atrial arrhythmias (fibrillation, flutter)* ⇒ arrhythmia.

atrophic rhinitis a type of rhinitis characterized by atrophy (wasting) of the nasal tissues with the development of foul-smelling crusts in the nose. The nasal cavity is widened and there is atrophy of the inferior turbinate bone.

atrophy *n* wasting, emaciation, diminution in size and function. It may be a normal feature, as in normal age changes, or pathological, such as disuse atrophy associated with poor mobility — **atrophied, atrophic** *adj*.

atropine *n* principal alkaloid of belladonna. ⇒ muscarinic antagonists.

ATT *abbr* antitetanus toxoid. Contains inactivated but antigenically intact tetanus toxins. Produces active immunity. ⇒ DTPer.

attachment state of being joined. In psychology, the dependent relationship which one person forms with another, originating from the unique bonding between infant and parent figure.

attempted suicide ⇒ parasuicide.

attention ability to select some stimuli for closer inspection while discarding others deemed less important.

attention deficit hyperactivity disorder (ADHD) a behavioural disorder of children. It is characterized by poor attention/concentration, increased motor activity (hyperkinesia) and impulsive behaviour. It is more common in boys, and is managed by supporting and working with the family and teachers, behaviour therapy and medication with methylphenidate hydrochloride. Also known as attention deficit syndrome.

attenuation *n* the process by which pathogenic micro-organisms are induced to develop or show less virulent characteristics. Thus they retain antigenicity without pathogenicity. They can then be used in the preparation of vaccines — **attenuate** *vt, vi*.

attitudes personal evaluations of and reactions to people, situations and objects. They may be positive, e.g. like, or negative, e.g. dislike.

attribution in psychology, the theory that deals with the inferences that people make about the causes of their own and other peoples' behaviour.

attrition *n* wearing down by friction, such as the erosion of the occlusal surfaces of the teeth by use.

atypical *adj* not typical; unusual, irregular; not conforming to type, e.g. atypical pneumonia.

audiogram *n* a visual record of the acuity of hearing tested with an audiometer. ⇒ audiometry.

audiology *n* the scientific study of hearing — **audiologically** *adv*.

audiometry measurement of hearing acuity. Using an audiometer, the results are plotted on an audiogram to record how the ear responds to different sound frequencies tested at varying intensities measured in decibels (dB). ⇒ acuity.

audit investigative methods used to systematically measure outcomes and review performance. *medical audit* systematic and critical review of medical care, including diagnosis and treatment, outcomes and quality of life. *nursing audit* systematic investigation into outcomes and standards and quality of nursing care. It may be concurrent or retrospective. ⇒ audit trail. ⇒ clinical audit. ⇒ concurrent audit. ⇒ Monitor. ⇒ Qualpacs. ⇒ retrospective audit.

Audit Commission originally set up to appoint and regulate external auditors of local authorities in England and Wales. Since 1990 the responsibilities now include the NHS. The main role of the Audit Commission is to promote 'best practice' in terms of economy, effectiveness and efficiency.

audit trail a way of working and record keeping that allows the processes to be transparent and clear.

auditory *adj* pertaining to the sense of hearing. *auditory acuity* ⇒ acuity. *auditory area* that portion of the temporal lobe of the cerebral cortex which interprets sound. *auditory canal or meatus* the canal between the pinna and eardrum. Generally known as the external auditory canal. *auditory nerve* the vestibulocochlear nerve. The eighth cranial nerve. *auditory ossicles* the three small bones in the middle ear – malleus, incus and stapes.

aura *n* **1.** a premonition; a peculiar sensation or warning of an impending attack, such as occurs in migraine or epilepsy. It may be auditory, optic, olfactory or gustatory. 2. one of several terms used in complementary medicine to describe the individual's innate energy. ⇒ Qi energy.

aural *adj* pertaining to the ear.

aural toilet a procedure used to clean, dry and remove debris from the external auditory canal.

auricle *n* 1. the pinna of the outer (external) ear. 2. an appendage to the cardiac atrium. → atrium — **auricular** *adj.*

auriscope *n* ⇒ otoscope.

auscultation *n* a method of listening to the body sounds, particularly the heart, lungs and fetal circulation for diagnostic purposes. It may be: (a) immediate, by placing the ear directly against the body (b) mediate, by the use of a stethoscope — **auscult, auscultate** *v.*

Australia antigen term previously used to describe hepatitis B surface antigen (HBsAg).

autism *n* a condition usually first recognized in childhood. ⇒ Asperger's syndrome ⇒ autistic disorders — **autistic** *adj.*

autistic disorders *npl* a spectrum of disorders usually first recognized in children. Characterized by an inability to interact with poor social skills, communication difficulties, poor language development, fantasies, withdrawal, isolation and a preoccupation with routine and a specific activity, such as rocking. ⇒ Asperger's syndrome.

autoagglutination *n* the clumping together of the body's own red blood cells caused by autoantibodies; this occurs in acquired autoimmune haemolytic anaemia. ⇒ anaemia.

autoantibody *n* immunoglobulins which destroy part of the body to cause an autoimmune disease, e.g. red blood cells in autoimmune haemolytic anaemia.

autoantigen *n* antigens in normal tissues which can bind to autoantibodies.

autoclave 1. *n* an apparatus for high-pressure steam sterilization. 2. *vt* sterilize in an autoclave.

autodigestion *n* self-digestion of tissues within the living body. ⇒ autolysis.

autoeroticism *n* self-gratification of the sex instinct. ⇒ masturbation — **autoerotic** *adj.*

autogenic therapy a complementary therapy which combines relaxation and self-hypnosis. The client is 'trained' to enter a relaxed, receptive state to which certain conditions, such as indigestion or cardiac arrhythmias, may be susceptible. Autogenic modification amplifies the training and directs it to certain areas.

autograft *n* a graft using tissue transplanted from one site to another in the same person, such as a skin graft.

autoimmune the production of immunoglobulins (autoantibodies) or cell mediated immunity against some body component. *autoimmune diseases* diverse group of diseases where body cell antigens stimulate an immunological reaction within the body. They include: Hashimoto's disease/thyroiditis, rheumatoid arthritis, haemolytic anaemia, Addison's disease, gastritis and pernicious anaemia, and insulin-dependent diabetes mellitus.

autoimmunization *n* the process which leads to an autoimmune disease.

autoinfection *n* one caused by microorganisms already present on or in the body. ⇒ infection.

autointoxication *n* poisoning from faulty or excessive metabolic products elaborated within the body. Such products may be derived from infected or dead tissue.

autologous blood transfusion (ABT) a patient donates their own blood or blood products prior to elective surgery to be transfused postoperatively. Cross-matching and compatibility problems are avoided as is the risk of receiving infected blood or blood products.

autolysis *n* a process of tissue digestion by enzymes produced by the body. It occurs as a physiological process, e.g. of the uterus during the puerperium or pathologically if digestive enzymes escape into surrounding tissues — **autolytic** *adj.*

automatic *adj* performed without the influence of the will; spontaneous; nonvolitional acts; involuntary acts.

automatism *n* organized behaviour which occurs without subsequent awareness of it. ⇒ epilepsy. ⇒ somnambulism.

autonomic *adj* independent; self-governing. *autonomic nervous system (ANS)* is divided into parasympathetic and sympathetic portions. They are involuntary and are concerned with reflex control of bodily functions. ⇒ central nervous system.

autonomic dysreflexia syndrome occurring in people with spinal cord injuries (above the level of the 7th thoracic vertebra) as a result of a life-threatening sympathetic response to noxious stimuli. Includes headache, tachycardia, hypertension, sweating and flushing above the lesion, fits, exaggerated reflex and bladder or bowel distension.

autopeep otherwise known as air-trapping or intrinsic PEEP. Incomplete exhalation resulting in a pressure being maintained in the lungs at the end of each expiration. In some circumstances this can accumulate with deleterious effects.

autopsy *n* postmortem examination of a body (cadaver) for diagnostic purposes.

autoregulation the homeostatic mechanisms by which certain organs control their immediate environment, e.g. renal blood flow is regulated by mechanisms initiated by the kidney.

autorhythmic describes cells such as those in the sinoatrial node, capable of producing an action potential without innervation.

autosome *n* a chromosome other than a sex chromosome. One of 44 (22 pairs) of non-sex chromosomes. With the 2 sex chromosomes they make up the full chromosome complement of 46 (23 pairs) found in somatic cells — **autosomal** *adj* pertaining to autosomes. *autosomal inheritance* occurs through the expression or not of genes on the autosomes. Autosomal inheritance may be dominant or recessive.

autosuggestion *n* self-suggestion; uncritical acceptance of ideas arising in the individual's own mind. Occurs in hysterical neurosis.

autotransfusion *n* the infusion into a patient of the actual blood lost by haemorrhage, especially when haemorrhage occurs into a sterile site.

A-V *abbr* atrioventricular.

avascular *adj* bloodless; not vascular, i.e. without blood supply, such as the heart valves. *avascular necrosis* death of tissue, such as bone, when deprived of blood, as in the femoral head following some types of the femoral neck fracture — **avascularize** *vt, vi.*

aversion therapy a method of treatment by deconditioning. Effective in some forms of addiction and abnormal behaviour.

avian *adj* pertaining to birds. *avium tubercle* or *Mycobacterium avium intracellulare (MAI)* an atypical mycobacterium that causes infection in humans.

avidin *n* a high molecular weight protein with a high affinity for biotin, which can interfere with the absorption of biotin. Found in raw egg white.

avidity *n* an imprecise measure of the strength of antigen-antibody binding based on the rate at which the complex is formed.

Avogadro's number ⇒ mole.

avoidance the use of a defence mechanism to avoid feelings, thoughts or situations that the person finds difficult.

avoidant personality disorder tends to be characterized by feelings of anxiety created by fears of rejection and critical comments from others. They may feel inferior, unattractive and socially isolated, and find it difficult to engage with their peer group.

avolition loss of motivation and drive. A negative symptom associated with mental illness such as schizophrenia. It is characterized by: difficulty in following through on activities; lack of interest in doing things; sitting around doing little, or engaged in activities requiring little effort, such as watching television.

avulsion *n* a forcible wrenching away, as of a limb, nerve or polypus.

axilla *n* the armpit — **axillary** *adj* applied to nerves, blood and lymphatic vessels and nodes, of the axilla.

axis *n* 1. the second cervical vertebra. 2. an imaginary line passing through the centre (midline); the median line of the body — **axial** *adj.*

axon *n* that process of a nerve cell conveying impulses away from the cell; a direct prolongation of the nerve cell — **axonal** *adj* pertaining to an axon. *axonal transport* carries organelles, enzymes and other substances away from the nerve cell body, and organelles back to the nerve cell body for destruction. Harmful agents, such as viruses, may utilize axonal transport.

axon reflex *n* a reflex dilatation of the arterioles occurring when sensory nerves in the skin are stimulated by injury or massage manipulations. ⇒ inflammation.

axonotmesis *n* (*syn* neuronotmesis, neurotmesis) peripheral degeneration as a result of damage to the axons of a nerve. The internal architecture is preserved and recovery depends upon regeneration of the axons, and may take many months. Such a lesion may result from pinching, crushing or prolonged pressure.

azoospermia *n* absence of viable spermatozoa in the semen, causing male sterility.

azotaemia *n* excessive amounts of nitrogenous compounds, such as urea, in the blood.

azoturia *n* excretion of abnormal amounts of nitrogenous compounds, such as urea, in the urine — **azoturic** *adj.*

azygos *adj* occurring singly, not paired. *azygos veins* three unpaired veins of the abdomen and thorax which empty into the vena cava — **azygous** *adj.*

B

Babinski's reflex, or sign movement of the great toe upwards (dorsiflexion) instead of downwards (plantar flexion) on stroking the sole of the foot. It is indicative of disease or injury to upper motor neurons. Infants exhibit dorsiflexion, but after learning to walk they show the normal plantar flexion response.

Bacille-Calmette-Guérin *n* ⇒ BCG.

bacilluria *n* the presence of bacilli in the urine — **bacilluric** *adj.*

Bacillus *n* a genus of bacteria consisting of aerobic, Gram-positive, rod-shaped cells which produce endospores. The majority are motile by means of flagella. These organisms are saprophytes and their spores are common in soil, dust and water. Colloquially, the word is still used to describe any rod-shaped micro-organism. *Bacillus anthracis* causes anthrax in animals, such as cattle and sheep. It may also affect people who have contact with infected animals, animal products, e.g. hides, or contaminated soil, where the

spores remain viable for many years. *Bacillus cerus* produces exotoxins that give rise to food poisoning. It often occurs after eating foods, such as cooked rice which is stored overnight (when toxins are produced) and reheated.

back up *v* a computer term meaning to store data by copying from the hard disk to a removable disk or tape. Regular back ups should be made as routine, and stored safely in case the original data are lost.

backache *n* describes a chronic low grade sensation of pain, usually in the lower back. It is estimated that 1 in 20 adults visiting their general practitioner each year do so because of low back pain; the most common causes are degenerative disease of the spine, prolapsed intervertebral disc and nerve entrapment syndrome. Healthcare workers, including nurses and other carers, are at special risk and should follow local moving and handling policies. ⇒ manual handling. ⇒ prolapse. ⇒ sciatica.

bacteraemia *n* the presence of bacteria in the blood — **bacteraemic** *adj.*

bacteria *npl* microscopic unicellular organisms widely distributed in a variety of different environments. They may be free living, sacrophytic or parasitic. May be pathogenic (disease producing) in humans, other animals and plants, or nonpathogenic; some serve useful functions, e.g. production of an environment which is hostile to pathogens such as commensal lactobacilli in the adult vaginal flora. Some pathogens are particularly virulent and exposure will nearly always lead to infection, but others with a low pathogenicity, known as opportunists, usually only cause infection when the host defences are impaired, such as occurs in illness. Nonpathogens may become pathogenic if they move from their normal site, a common example being a urinary infection caused by organisms normally found in the gut flora. Bacteria generally multiply by simple binary fission when environmental conditions are suitable. Some types have developed various physical and biochemical adaptations which allow them to exploit environments and survive hostile conditions, e.g. flagella, pili, waxy outer capsules, spore formation and enzymes which destroy antibacterial drugs. Bacteria are classified and identified by criteria which include: shape and outer coat staining characteristics with Gram stain (positive or negative). The main forms are: (a) cocci, round in shape; some are paired – diplococci; some form chains – streptococci; and others bunches – staphylococci. Some important pathogenic cocci include: *Staphylococcus aureus, Streptococcus pyogenes* and *Neisseria meningitidis*; (b) bacilli, rod-shaped. Important pathogenic bacilli include: *Escherichia coli, Haemophilus influenzae, Clostridium tetani* and *Mycobacterium tuberculosis* (acid-fast bacilli); (c) spiral forms – curved vibrios, spirilla and spirochaetes, which are corkscrew-shaped. This group includes: *Vibrio cholerae, Treponema pallidum* and *Leptospira icterohaemorrhagiae*. (See Figure 7) — **bacterial** *adj*.

bactericide *n* any agent which destroys bacteria, such as some antibiotic drugs — **bactericidal** *adj*.

bactericidin *n* an antibody which kills bacteria.

bacteriologist *n* a person who is an expert in bacteriology.

bacteriology *n* the scientific study of bacteria — **bacteriologically** *adv*.

bacteriolysin *n* a specific antibody formed in the blood which causes dissolution (break-up) of bacteria.

bacteriolysis *n* the disintegration and dissolution of bacteria — **bacteriolytic** *adj*.

bacteriophage *n* a virus parasitic on bacteria. They are specific to a particular strain and may be used to identify certain bacteria, e.g. phage-typing staphylococci etc.

bacteriostasis *n* arrest or hindrance of bacterial growth — **bacteriostatic** *adj*.

bacteriuria *n* the presence of bacteria in the urine (100 000 or more pathogenic micro-organisms per mL). Acute urinary tract infection may be preceded by, and active pyelonephritis may be associated with, asymptomatic bacteriuria.

BAI *abbr* Beck Anxiety Inventory.

Bainbridge reflex *n* a cardiac mechanism. Stretch receptors in the right atrium can increase heart rate through sympathetic stimulation when venous return increases.

baker's itch 1. contact dermatitis resulting from flour or sugar. Also called grocer's itch. 2. itchy papules from the bite of the flour mite.

balance of probabilities the standard of proof required in civil proceedings.

balanced diet *n* a varied diet that provides the individual with sufficient energy, macronutrients and micronutrients. The balance depends on choosing food from five broad groups: (a) cereals, bread and potatoes; (b) fruit and vegetables; (c) meat, fish or protein alternatives, e.g. nuts; (d) milk and dairy products, such as cheese; (e) food containing fat and sugar.

balanitis *n* inflammation of the glans penis.

balanus *n* the glans of the penis or clitoris.

baldness *n* ⇒ alopecia.

Balkan beam/frame overhead beam attached to a hospital bed that may hold suspension and traction pulleys.

balloon angioplasty ⇒ angioplasty.

ballottement *n* testing for a floating object, especially used to diagnose pregnancy. A finger is inserted into the vagina and the uterus is pushed forward; if a fetus is present it will fall back again, bouncing in its bath of fluid. External ballottement may be used to determine per abdomen whether the fetal presenting part has entered the pelvis — **ballottable** *adj*.

bandage *n* a piece of material applied to a wound or used to bind an injured part of the body. Available in strips or circular form in a range of different materials and applying varying levels of pressure. Compression bandages are widely used in the management of venous leg ulceration.

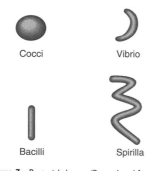

Cocci   Vibrio

Bacilli   Spirilla

Figure 7 Bacterial shapes. (Reproduced from Brooker 1996 with permission.)

Bankart's operation capsular repair in the glenoid cavity, for recurrent dislocation of shoulder joint.

Barbados leg (*syn* elephant leg) ⇒ elephantiasis.

barber's itch ⇒ sycosis barbae.

barbiturates *npl* a group of hypnotic/sedative drugs derived from barbituric acid; use is limited to general anaesthesia and epilepsy due to serious addiction problems.

barium enema *n* a radiographic examination of the large bowel using barium sulphate as the contrast medium. The barium sulphate suspension, plus a quantity of air, is introduced into the large bowel via a rectal catheter, during fluoroscopy. Used for diagnostic purposes in conjunction with endoscopy. The bowel is emptied prior to the examination, with laxatives such as sodium picosulfate (picosulphate). ⇒ barium sulphate. ⇒ colonoscopy. → laxatives.

barium meal, swallow a radiographic examination of the upper gastrointestinal tract (oesophagus and stomach) and the small intestine with follow-through X-rays, using barium sulphate as the contrast medium. The barium sulphate suspension (several flavours) is swallowed and X-rays are taken of successive parts of the gastrointestinal tract. Preparation is important and involves a period without food or drink, and stopping medicines that may interfere with the examination, such as some antacids. Patients may be required to continue nil orally until certain follow through X rays are taken and, because instructions may vary according to particular circumstances, the patient, nurses and other health professionals should ensure they are fully informed. ⇒ barium sulphate.

barium sulphate a barium salt that is insoluble in water and opaque to X-rays. It is used in an aqueous suspension, as a contrast medium for radiographic examination of the gastrointestinal tract. ⇒ barium enema. ⇒ barium meal, swallow.

Barlow's disease infantile scurvy.

Barlow's sign/test *n* a test performed, by an experienced clinician, soon after birth for the diagnosis of developmental dysplasia of the hip (congenital dislocation). Often used in conjunction with Ortolani's test.

baroreceptors *npl* sensory nerve endings which respond to changes in pressure; they are present in the cardiac atria, venae cavae, aortic arch, carotid sinus and the internal ear.

barotrauma *n* injury due to a change in atmospheric or water pressure, e.g. ruptured eardrum.

Barr body *n* ⇒ chromatin.

barrier nursing a method of preventing the spread of infection from an infectious patient to others. It is achieved by isolation techniques. → containment isolation. ⇒ isolation. ⇒ protective isolation. ⇒ source isolation.

Barthel index *n* a disability profile score developed in the 1960s. A person's ability to selfcare is assessed in ten areas including walking, feeding, bladder and bowel control, hygiene and dressing etc.

bartholinitis *n* inflammation of Bartholin's glands.

Bartholin's glands *npl* two small glands situated at each side of the external orifice of the vagina. Their ducts open into the vaginal orifice. They produce lubricating mucus, that increases during sexual stimulation to facilitate coitus. Also known as greater vestibular glands. ⇒ Skene's glands. → vestibule.

basal cell carcinoma *n* the most common skin cancer. Generally occurs in middle age and later life; it is due to the cumulative damage from sun exposure over many years. Found on the face or scalp which, although locally invasive, rarely gives rise to metastases. Also known as a rodent ulcer.

basal ganglia → basal nuclei.

basal metabolic rate (BMR) the energy consumed at complete rest for the essential physiological functions, e.g. respiration. It depends on age, size and gender. BMR is calculated indirectly by measuring the amount of oxygen used over a given time, and is expressed as kJ or kcal per square metre body surface area per hour (kJ or kcal/m^2/h). Adult males need about 40 kcal/m^2/h and females 37 kcal/m^2/h.

basal narcosis the preanaesthetic administration of narcotic drugs which reduce fear and anxiety, induce sleep and thereby minimize perioperative and postoperative complications. Used less frequently with the advent of day surgery. ⇒ premedication.

basal nuclei *npl* isolated grey cells deep within the cerebral hemispheres concerned with modifying and coordinating voluntary muscle movement. Their proper functioning requires the release of the neurotransmitter dopamine. Sometimes erroneously referred to as ganglia which more properly describes structures in the peripheral nervous system. Site of degeneration in Parkinson's disease. ⇒ dopamine.

base *n* the **1.** lowest part. **2.** the main part of a compound. **3.** an alkali. In chemistry, the substance which combines with an acid to form a salt — **basal, basic** *adj*.

base excess *n* the number of millimoles of acid needed to titrate 1 L of blood to pH 7.4 at 37°C at a PCO_2 of 5.3 kPa. A positive value suggests a relative deficit of blood acid (noncarbonic acid), whereas a negative value suggests a relative excess of acid (noncarbonic acid).

basement membrane *n* a two part membrane that separates epithelial tissue from underlying connective tissue.

BASIC *acr* for Beginner's All-purpose Symbolic Instruction Code. A computer language still sometimes used for writing programs although it has been largely superseded by a version known as Visual Basic.

basic life support (BLS) a term which describes maintenance of a clear airway and cardiopulmonary resuscitation.

basilar *adj* pertaining to the base. *basilar artery* formed by the two vertebral arteries. *basilar membrane* part of the cochlea.

basilar-vertebral insufficiency ⇒ vertebrobasilar insufficiency.

basilic *adj* prominent. *basilic vein* on the inner side of the arm. *median basilic* a vein at the bend of the elbow which is generally chosen for venepuncture.

basophil *n* **1.** a cell which has an affinity for basic dyes. **2.** a granulocytic polymorphonuclear leucocyte (white blood cell) which takes up a particular dye; its cytoplasm contains blue-staining granules, which contain the important chemical mediators (e.g. histamine) of acute inflammation. Basophils are concerned with the inflammatory response and anaphylaxis. Those that migrate into the tissues are known as mast cells. ⇒ eosinophil. ⇒ inflammatory. ⇒ neutrophil.

basophilia *n* **1.** ncrease of basophils in the blood. **2.** basophilic staining of red blood cells, occurring in conditions such as lead poisoning.

Batchelor plaster a type of double abduction plaster, with the legs encased from groins to ankles, in full abduction and medial rotation. The feet are then attached to a wooden pole or 'broomstick'. Alternative to frog plaster, but the hips are free.

battery an unlawful touching. ⇒ trespass against the person.

Bazin's disease (*syn* erythema induratum) a recurrent tuberculous infection, involving the skin of the legs of women. There are reddish or purple deep-seated nodules which later ulcerate.

BBA *abbr* born before arrival.

BBB *abbr* **1.** blood-brain barrier. **2.** bundle branch block.

BBVs *abbr* blood-borne viruses, such as hepatitis B, hepatitis C and HIV, that are transmitted in the blood and body fluids. ⇒ biohazard.

BCG *abbr* Bacille-Calmette-Guérin. Live attenuated strain of mycobacterium bovis that has lost its power to cause tuberculosis (pathogenicity), but retains its antigenic function; it is the base of a vaccine used for immunization against tuberculosis.

BDI *abbr* Beck Depression Inventory.

beacon sites *npl* NHS Trusts and general practices identified as examples of 'best practice'. They will receive funding to facilitate sharing of best practice initiatives. ⇒ benchmarking.

bearing-down *n* **1.** a popular term for the expulsive contractions in the second stage of labour. **2.** a feeling of weight and descent in the pelvis associated with uterine prolapse or pelvic tumours.

beat *n* pulsation of the blood in the heart and blood vessels brought about by cardiac contraction. *apex beat* ⇒ apex. *dropped beat* refers to the loss of an occasional ventricular beat as occurs in extrasystoles. *premature beat* an extrasystole.

Beck Anxiety Inventory (BAI) a questionnaire that measures the degree of anxiety felt by clients. It includes an evaluation of both cognitive and physical manifestations of anxiety.

Beck Depression Inventory (BDI) a self-administered inventory for measuring depression.

Beck Hopelessness Scale (BHS) an assessment instrument designed to identify suicidality/risk.

Beck Scale for Suicide Ideation (BSS) an assessment instrument designed to identify suicidality/risk.

becquerel (Bq) *n* the derived SI unit (International System of Units) for radioactivity. It equals the amount of a radioactive substance undergoing one nuclear disintegration per second. This unit has replaced the curie.

bed bath bathing a patient in bed. Includes mouth care, teeth/denture cleaning, making sure that spectacles are clean, care of nails, hair and shaving male patients as appropriate. It provides an opportunity to assess the condition of the patient's skin, especially the pressure areas, and other features such as breathlessness or mobility problems. Following the bed bath, the bed is remade with fresh linen as required and the patient is left comfortable in bed or a chair with call system, drink (if not contraindicated) and belongings within reach.

bedbug *n* a blood-sucking insect belonging to the genus Cimex. *Cimex lecturlarius* is the most common species in temperate and C. *hemipterus* in tropical zones. They live and lay eggs in bedding, cracks and crevices of furniture and walls. They are nocturnal in habit and their bites leave a route for secondary infection.

bedrest *n* confinement of a person to bed for most of each 24 hours with the prime objective of rest and minimal functioning of body systems. To avoid the complications of bedrest, it is only used when absolutely necessary. ⇒ boredom, prevention of. ⇒ bedrest, complications of. ⇒ constipation. ⇒ deep vein thrombosis. ⇒ pressure ulcers.

bedrest, complications of potential problems associated with confinement to bed. They include loss of interest, depression, anorexia and weight loss, chest infection due to stagnant secretions, kidney stones (renal calculi), cystitis from stagnation of urine in bladder, pressure ulcers (sores), muscle wastage, bone thinning (osteoporosis), foot drop, deep vein thrombosis, constipation and abdominal distension. ⇒ bedrest.

bedsore obsolete term. ⇒ pressure ulcer.

bedwetting *n* ⇒ enuresis.

behaviour the observable behavioural response of a person to an internal or external stimulus. *behaviour modification* in a general sense, an inevitable part of living, resulting from the consistent rewarding or punishing of response to a stimulus, whether that response is negative or positive. Some education systems deliberately employ a behaviour modification approach to maximize learning. *behaviour therapy* a kind of psychotherapy to modify observable, maladjusted patterns of behaviour by the substitution of a learned response or set of responses to a stimulus. The treatment is designed for a particular patient and not for the particular diagnostic label which has been attached to him. Such treatment includes assertiveness training, aversion therapy, conditioning and desensitization.

behaviour change health education approach that encourages individuals to make changes to their lifestyle such as dietary changes or smoking cessation through the provision of information, examination of existing health beliefs and values and building self confidence.

behaviourism *n* a word used in psychology to describe an approach which studies and interprets behaviour by objective observation of that behaviour, without reference to the underlying subjective mental phenomena such as ideas, emotions and will. Behaviour is seen as a series of conditioned responses.

Behçet syndrome an inflammatory disorder characterized by aphthous stomatitis, iritis, skin lesions and ulcers on the genitalia. There may also be arthritis of one or more of the large joints, gastrointestinal ulceration, thrombophlebitis, epididymitis and meningoencephalitis. The aetiology may be an abnormal response to an infection in genetically susceptible individuals. Management involves symptomatic treatment with NSAIDs and, in more severe cases, the administration of corticosteroids or immunosuppression.

bejel *n* nonvenereal syphilis found in the Middle East, Asia, sub-Saharan Africa and Australia. It is caused by *Treponema pallidum*, and the lesions affect the skin, mucosae and bones. ⇒ pinta. ⇒ yaws.

beliefs *npl* a set of ideas and thoughts which an individual uses to construct their views and behaviour. They are formed by culture, family, life experiences and many other factors.

belladonna *n* deadly nightshade. The alkaloid from belladonna is poisonous but from it atropine and hyoscine are extracted. ⇒ muscarinic antagonists.

'belle indifference' the incongruous lack of appropriate emotion in the presence of incapacitating symptoms commonly shown by patients with conversion hysteria. First noted by Janet in 1893. ⇒ conversion disorder.

Bell's palsy paralysis of the facial nerve (VIIth cranial). The cause is unknown, but may be due to: viral infection, trauma, exposure to cold or vascular disturbance. It is characterized by facial muscle weakness, failure of eye closure, the mouth drawn to the unaffected side with drooling of saliva. The management includes protecting the eye that does not close and possibly the corticosteroid dexamethasone.

Bence-Jones protein an abnormal protein produced by myeloma cells and excreted in the urine in some cases of malignant myeloma. ⇒ multiple myeloma.

benchmarking *n* a quality assurance process. It involves identifying examples of best practice from others engaged in similar practice. From this, best practice benchmark scores in agreed areas of care are identified, against which individual units can compare their own performance.

bends *npl* ⇒ caisson disease.

beneficence ethical principle of doing good. An ideal that also involves avoiding, removing and preventing harm and promoting good. Problems and dilemmas may arise when the common good conflicts with that for individuals. ⇒ nonmaleficence.

benign *adj* **1.** noninvasive, noncancerous (of a growth). **2.** describes a condition or illness which is not serious and does not usually have harmful consequences.

benign hypotonia term applied to infants who are initially floppy but otherwise healthy. Improvement occurs and the infant regains normal tone and motor development.

benign prostatic hyperplasia *n* ⇒ prostate.

Bennett's fracture fracture of proximal end of first metacarpal involving the articular surface.

benzamides a group of neuroleptic drugs, e.g. sulpiride.

benzene *n* a toxic hydrocarbon derived from coal tar. Extensively used as a solvent. Continued exposure to it results in aplastic anaemia and leukaemia.

benzodiazepines *npl* a large group of anxiolytic drugs widely used to reduce anxiety, e.g. diazepam, and as hypnotics, e.g. temazepam. They can be used with caution to reduce anxiety, relax muscles, sedate and help to alleviate short-term insomnia. They should not be described by the misleading term of 'minor tranquilizers'. Dependence and withdrawal symptoms may occur and they are subject to considerable misuse.

bereavement *n* a response to a life event involving loss. Includes that which happens to a person after the death of another person who has been important in his or her life. It also occurs in other situations of loss, such as redundancy, loss of home, divorce or loss of a body part, e.g. mastectomy, amputation etc. ⇒ grieving process. *bereavement counsellors* those who work in a professional capacity helping bereaved people to work through the emotions which they are experiencing during bereavement. Nurses need to be aware of the availability of skilled bereavement counsellors, yet, at the same time, they need to develop the necessary skills to help a person who is bereaved who may be encountered in both hospital and the community, as well as in school and at work. There are also various groups available to those whose loved one has died from a particular disease or in particular circumstances. Some are voluntary organizations; some are led by a professional person who enhances the skills of the volunteers.

beri-beri *n* a deficiency disease caused by lack of vitamin B_1 (thiamine). It occurs mainly in those countries where the staple diet is polished rice. It is characterized by polyneuropathy, muscular wasting, progressive oedema, dyspnoea and, finally, heart failure. ⇒ Korsakoff's psychosis, syndrome. ⇒ Wernicke's encephalopathy.

berylliosis *n* an industrial disease; there is impaired lung function because of interstitial fibrosis from inhalation of beryllium. It may affect workers in the atomic, aircraft and electronic industries.

beta (β) second letter of Greek alphabet. *beta cells* → islets of Langerhans. *beta oxidation* a process by which fatty acids are converted to acetyl CoA prior to the production of energy (ATP). *beta phase* the period which follows the alpha redistribution phase of drug administration; it is characterized by a slow decline in drug blood levels during its metabolism and excretion. *beta rays* a type of ionizing radiation emitted as a radioactive isotope disintegrates. They consist of electrons which penetrate tissue to a greater depth than alpha rays. *beta receptors* → adrenergic receptors (adrenoceptors) *beta state* alert wakefulness associated with thinking and concentration. *beta wave (rhythm)* brain wave pattern seen when the individual is in the beta state. The waves are more irregular than alpha waves and have a frequency between 14–25 Hz.

beta (β)-adrenoceptor agonists *npl* also known as β stimulants. A group of drugs that stimulate β-adrenoceptors (adrenergic receptors), e.g. dobutamine, which acts selectively on β_1-adrenoceptors and is used in acute reversible heart failure and cardiogenic shock, and terbutaline, which acts selectively on β_2-adrenoceptors to relieve brochospasm in asthma. Non-selective β adrenoceptor agonists, such as isoprenaline, are not used for treating asthma because they cause cardiac arrhythmias and other side effects.

beta (β)-adrenoceptor antagonists *npl* also known as β blockers. A group of drugs which prevent stimulation of the β-adrenoceptors (adrenergic receptors) in the myocardium and other sites, e.g. propranolol, atenolol etc. They reduce myocardial contractility and are described as being negative inotropes. As they reduce heart rate and blood pressure, they are used in the management of angina, post myocardial infarction and hypertension. Other uses include: controlling some arrhythmias, preoperatively in hyperthyroidism, anxiety, topically for glaucoma, e.g. timolol, and in the prophylaxis of migraine. They may cause bronchospasm and should not be taken by people with asthma or obstructive pulmonary disease, except where no other suitable drug is available. ⇒ inotropes.

beta (β)-lactam antibiotics *npl* the antibiotics that contain a β-lactam ring in their chemical structure. (See Figure 8). They include the penicillins, the cephalosporins and others used less commonly, such as the carbapenems, e.g. imipenem. Many bacteria produce beta (β)-lactamases, e.g staphylococcal strains, that destroy the β-lactam ring and stop the antibiotic working properly. Some of the antibiotics are combined with a beta (β)-lactamase inhibitor, e.g. clavulanic acid, to overcome this problem.

beta (β)-lactamases *npl* enzymes produced by many bacteria, notably over 90% of staphylococci, many *Escherichia coli* and some strains of *Neisseria gonorrhoeae*, which allow them to destroy antibiotics containing a β-lactam ring. Previously called penicillinases.

Betz cells pyramidal cells. Neurons in the motor cortex that control voluntary muscle contraction

BHS *abbr* Beck Hopelessness Scale.

bibliographical databases details of papers etc, but abstracts and full articles sometimes available electronically via CD-ROM or the internet, e.g. CINAHL, Medline.

bibliotherapy *n* literally 'book therapy'. Extracts from books are used to help patients gain insight into their problems and promote communication with therapist. In a group situation, making a positive contribution helps to maintain self-esteem. Also used for encouraging older people to talk about their lives.

bicarbonate (hydrogen carbonate) *n* a salt of carbonic acid. *serum bicarbonate* that in the blood indicating the alkali reserve. Also called 'plasma bicarbonate'.

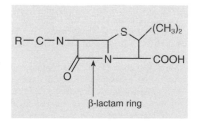

Figure 8 Structure of a beta lactam antibiotic. (Reproduced from Wilson 1995 with permission.)

biceps brachii *n* the two-headed muscle on the front of the upper arm. It flexes and supinates the forearm; flexes and abducts the arm.

biconcave *adj* concave or hollow on both surfaces, such as a red blood cell.

biconvex *adj* convex on both surfaces, such as a lens.

bicornuate *adj* having two horns, generally applied to a double uterus, or a single uterus possessing two horns.

bicuspid *adj* having two cusps or points. *bicuspid teeth* the premolars. *bicuspid valve* the mitral valve between the left atrium and ventricle of the heart. ⇒ atrioventricular.

BID *abbr* **1.** brought in (to hospital) dead. **2.** Latin abbreviation previously used in prescriptions. It means twice daily administration, as of medication. Also known as BD.

bifid *adj* divided into two parts. Cleft or forked.

bifocal *adj* having a double focus. *bifocal spectacles* can be used for near and distant vision.

bifurcation *n* division into two branches, such as the bifurcation of the trachea to form the two main bronchi — **bifurcate** *adj, vi, vt.*

biguanides *npl* ⇒ hypoglycaemic drugs.

bilateral *adj* pertaining to both sides — **bilaterally** *adv.*

bile *n* a green-yellow, alkaline, viscid fluid secreted by the liver and stored in the gallbladder. Between 500–1000 mL of bile is produced daily. It consists of water, mucin, lecithin, bile acids, bile salts, bile pigments, cholesterol, enzymes, electrolytes and molecules for excretion such as drug metabolites. Bile drains into the intestine where it helps to provide an alkaline environment, emulsifies fat globules prior to their digestion, facilitates the absorption of fat soluble vitamins, stimulates peristalsis and deodorizes faeces. *bile acids* organic acids, cholic and chenodeoxycholic, found in bile. *bile ducts* the hepatic, cystic and common bile ducts that convey bile from the liver, via the gallbladder, to the duodenum. *bile pigments* ⇒ bilirubin. ⇒ biliverdin. *bile salts* emulsifying agents, sodium glycocholate and taurocholate. Conjugated bile acids (joined with glycine and tau-

rine) form these sodium salts — **bilious, biliary** *adj.*

Bilharzia *n* ⇒ Schistosoma.

bilharziasis *n* ⇒ schistosomiasis.

biliary *adj* pertaining to bile. *biliary atresia* congenital narrowing or absence of a bile duct or other biliary structure. It causes jaundice and liver damage. Treatment is surgical and includes liver transplant. *biliary calculus* a stone formed in the gallbladder or biliary tract. ⇒ gallstones. *biliary colic* severe pain in the right upper quadrant of abdomen caused by the movement of a gallstone within the biliary tract. Vomiting may occur. *biliary fistula* an abnormal track conveying bile to the surface or to some other organ.

bilious *adj* **1.** a word usually used to signify vomit containing bile. **2.** a nonmedical term, usually meaning 'suffering from indigestion'.

bilirubin *n* a red bile pigment, largely derived from the haem molecule during red blood cell breakdown by macrophages. Unconjugated, fat-soluble bilirubin, which is toxic to cells, is transported in the blood bound to albumen which makes it less likely to enter and damage brain cells. Unconjugated bilirubin in the blood is potentially harmful to metabolically active tissues in the body, particularly the basal nuclei of the immature brain. ⇒ haemolytic disease of the newborn. ⇒ kernicterus. ⇒ jaundice. Once in the liver, it is conjugated with glucuronic acid in an enzyme catalysed reaction and the less toxic water-soluble bilirubin is excreted in bile.

bilirubinuria *n* the presence of bilirubin in the urine.

biliuria *n* (choluria) the presence of bile in the urine — **biliuric** *adj.*

biliverdin *n* the green bile pigment formed during red cell breakdown. ⇒ bilirubin.

Billroth's operation ⇒ gastrectomy.

bilobate *adj* having two lobes.

bilobular *adj* having two small lobes or lobules.

bimanual *adj* performed with both hands. A method of examination used in gynaecology, whereby the internal genital organs are examined between one hand on the abdomen and the other hand or finger within the vagina.

binary *adj* the base 2 system of numbers where digits are either 0 or 1. For example, decimal 1, 2, 3, 4, 5, 6, 7 become 1, 10, 11, 100, 101, 110, 111. Used in digital computer processes. *binary digit* ⇒ bit. ⇒ byte.

binary fission cell division that results in two equal 'daughter' cells.

binge-purge syndrome ⇒ bulimia nervosa.

binocular relating to both eyes. *binocular vision* the focusing of both eyes on one object at the same time, in such a way that only one image of the object is seen. ⇒ stereoscopic vision.

binovular *adj* derived from two separate ova. Binovular twins may be of different sexes. ⇒ uniovular *ant.*

bioassay *n* ⇒ assay.

bioavailability the proportion of a drug that enters the circulation in an active form. It can also be applied to a nutrient. See Box – Bioavailability.

biochemistry *n* the chemistry of living organisms and organic molecules — **biochemical** *adj.*

bioengineering *n* manipulating living cells so as to promote their growth in a desired way.

bioethics *n* the application of ethics to biological problems.

biofeedback *n* physiological activities, such as excessive muscle tension, raised blood pressure and heart rate, are measured graphically and presented to the patient. Either by trial and error or by operant conditioning, a person can learn to repeat behaviour which relaxes muscles or lowers blood pressure, etc.

biofilm the collection of micro-organisms and their protein products adhering to a surface, such as an indwelling urinary catheter.

bioflavenoid *n* general term for the coloured substances found in many fruits and vegetables, such as citrus fruits, rosehips, plums, grapes, cherries, blackcurrants, broccoli and tomatoes. They are also present in red wine and tea. Many have antibacterial properties and may be protective against cancer and heart disease.

biographical and health data a term usually applied to information collected at the initial assessment of a patient after admission to the healthcare service, whether in hospital or in the community. Most of the biographical data will not change but it will be helpful to all health professionals involved in care and treatment, enabling them to individualize conversation with the person. The health data, particularly those about dependence/independence for carrying out everyday living activities, may well change during the patient's contact with the healthcare service. All data will be useful when planning the person's discharge from the service.

biohazard *n* any hazard to health arising from inadvertent human biological processes. It includes accidental contact with body fluids, such as with cadaver bags, linen, needlestick injury and spills.

biological engineering provision of aids, electrical or electronic, to aid functioning of the body, e.g. hearing aids, pacemakers.

biological response modifier (BRM) *n* cancer therapies based on the manipulation of the person's immune system. Substances, such as interferons, interleukins and colony stimulating factors, are used to stimulate the person's immune cells to attack the cancer cells.

Bioavailability

Bioavailabilty is the amount of drug that reaches the systemic circulation. It is related to the route of administration, absorption, and any presystemic metabolism. Thus if a drug is given intravenously bioavailability will be 100%. However, drugs taken orally may be only partially absorbed from the gut into the blood due to interactions with food, e.g. tetracyclines are not effectively absorbed if taken with dairy products. Furthermore, drugs taken orally enter the hepatic portal circulation and are taken to the liver where they undergo first-pass metabolism, i.e. they are metabolized before entering the systemic circulation. The degree of metabolism is variable. For example, if glyceryl trinitrate is taken orally the hepatic enzymes metabolize it totally, so no active drug enters the systemic circulation and bioavailability is zero. For this reason glyceryl trinitrate is taken sublingually as the veins draining the mouth return the blood directly to the heart, without passing through the liver.

biology *n* the science of life, dealing with the structure, function and organization of all living things — **biologically** *adv*.

bionursing *n* direct application of knowledge from the life sciences to the theory and practice of nursing.

biopsy *n* **1.** excision of tissue from a living body for microscopic examination to establish diagnosis. Methods of obtaining tissue include: via a needle, aspiration and punch biopsy. **2.** the tissue excised for examination.

biopsychosocial pertaining to biological, psychological and social perspectives. A psychological approach that may be used to explain behaviour.

biorhythm *n* any of the cyclical patterns of biological functions unique to each individual, such as variations in body temperature, sleep-wake cycles and menstrual cycle — **biorhythmic** *adj*.

BIOS *acr* for Basic Input/Output System. BIOS describes computer programs which are permanently embedded in a chip (ROM). They are used by the computer operating system to perform fundamental input/output tasks. ⇒ chip. ⇒ ROM.

biosensors *npl* noninvasive instruments which measure the result of biological processes, e.g. local skin temperature and humidity; or biological response to, e.g. external pressure.

biotechnology *n* the use of biological knowledge in the scientific study of technology and vice versa — **biotechnically** *adv*.

biotin *n* a member of vitamin B complex; functions as a coenzyme. Synthesized by intestinal flora. Deficiency is rare, but it may cause dermatitis, anorexia, nausea, fatigue and muscular pains.

bipolar *adj* having two poles. *bipolar version* ⇒ version.

bipolar affective disorder an affective disorder characterized by both manic and depressive features. ⇒ depression. ⇒ manic depressive psychosis/manic depression.

bipolar depression ⇒ depression. ⇒ manic depressive psychosis/manic depression.

bird fancier's lung a form of extrinsic alveolitis due to allergy to avian proteins found in bird excreta, feathers and protein. Management includes: avoiding the allergen, corticosteroids and oxygen in patients with hypoxia. ⇒ extrinsic allergic alveolitis.

birth *n* the act of expelling the young from the mother's body; delivery; being born. *birth canal* the cavity or canal of the pelvis through which the baby passes during labour. *birth certificate* a legal document given on registration, within 42 days of a birth in the UK. *birth control* prevention or regulation of conception by any means; contraception. *birth injury* any injury occurring during parturition, e.g. fracture of a bone, subluxation of a joint, injury to peripheral nerve, intracranial haemorrhage. *birth mark* naevus. *birth rate* the number of births as a proportion of a population. Expressed as number of live births per 1000 population in one year. It can be applied to women aged 15–44 years to calculate a fertility rate. *premature birth* one occurring after the 24th week of pregnancy, but before term.

bisexual *adj* **1.** describes a person who is sexually attracted to both men and women. **2.** having some of the physical genital characteristics of both sexes; a hermaphrodite. When there is gonadal tissue of both sexes in the same person, that person is a true hermaphrodite.

bistoury *n* a long narrow knife, straight or curved, used for cutting from within outwards in the opening of a hernial sac, an abscess, sinus or fistula.

bit *acr* binary digit. In computing the smallest unit of data storage. A bit is represented by 1 or 0 and can be viewed as an electronic on/off switch. There are eight bits in a byte. ⇒ binary. ⇒ byte.

Bitôt's spots white plaques of dried epithelium present on the cornea. A manifestation of vitamin A deficiency. ⇒ xerophthalmia. ⇒ xerosis conjunctivae.

bivalent *n* **1.** formed by the pairing (or synapsis) of homologous chromosomes during meiosis. Also known as divalent. **2.** in chemistry, a substance with a valence of two.

bivalve *adj* having two valves or blades, such as in some types of vaginal speculum. The division of a plaster cast into two portions – an anterior and posterior half.

bivariate statistics descriptive statistics that compare the relationship between two variables. May be used to inform decisions regarding the need to use multivariate statistics.

blackhead *n* ⇒ comedone.

blackwater fever complication of the type of malaria caused by infection with *Plasmodium falciparum*. It is characterized by haemolysis of red blood cells. There is pyrexia, haemoglobinuria, which causes dark coloured urine, jaundice and renal failure.

bladder *n* a membranous sac containing fluid or gas. ⇒ atonic bladder. ⇒ bladder retraining. ⇒ gallbladder. ⇒ neurogenic bladder. ⇒ urinary bladder.

bladder retraining a nursing intervention to prevent episodes of urinary incontinence and to reduce symptoms of frequency and urgency by gradually increasing the time interval between voiding. Time intervals may be mandatory or self-scheduled. → incontinence. → habit retraining.

Blalock-Taussig procedure formation of a temporary shunt used to overcome congenital pulmonary stenosis and atrial septal defect in infants with Fallot's tetralogy. It involves an anastomosis between the pulmonary artery (distal to obstruction to the right ventricular outflow) and the subclavian artery. Surgical correction of the basic defects takes place during early childhood.

blanket bath obsolete term. ⇒ bed bath.

blast cell *n* immature cell.

blastocyst *n* early embryonic stage, it follows the morula. Consists of the trophoblast cells surrounding a fluid-filled cavity and inner cell mass. ⇒ gastrula.

blastoderm *n* layer of cells forming the blastocyst. It eventually gives rise to the primary germ layers, ectoderm, endoderm and mesoderm, from which the embryo will develop.

Blastomyces *n* a genus of pathogenic fungi. *Blastomyces dermatitidis* causes blastomycosis in humans — **blastomycetic** *adj*.

blastomycosis *n* granulomatous condition caused by *Blastomyces dermatitidis*. The systemic infection starts in the lungs and lymph nodes and has similarities with tuberculosis. It also affects the skin, viscera, bones and joints. Treatment is with the antifungal drug amphotericin — **blastomycotic** *adj*.

blastula *n* ⇒ blastocyst.

bleb *n* a large blister. ⇒ bulla. ⇒ vesicle.

blennorrhagia *n* **1.** a copious discharge of mucus, particularly from the vagina or male urethra. Also called blennorrhoea. **2.** obsolete term for gonorrhoea.

blennorrhoea *n* blennorrhagia.

blepharitis *n* inflammation of the eyelids, particularly the edges — **blepharitic** *adj*.

blepharon *n* the eyelid; palpebra — **blephara** *pl*.

blepharoplasty *n* (*syn* tarsoplasty) plastic surgery to the eyelid.

blepharospasm *n* spasm of the muscles in the eyelid, causing rapid involuntary blinking — **blepharospastic** *adj*.

blind loop syndrome associated with situations leading to intestinal stasis, such as surgical anastomosis, small bowel abnormalities and intestinal obstruction. Excessive bacterial growth occurs, causing diarrhoea, steatorrhoea and malabsorption of nutrients. Also called stagnant loop syndrome.

blind spot *n* the spot at which the optic nerve leaves the retina; without cones and rods it is insensitive to light.

blindness lack of sight or visual impairment. Causes worldwide include: macular degeneration, retinopathy, glaucoma, cataracts, infections such as trachoma, trauma, vitamin A deficiency and tumours. *cortical blindness* blindness due to a lesion of the visual centre in the cerebral cortex of the brain. *word blindness* inability to recognize familiar written words due to a brain lesion. → colour blindness. → night blindness.

blister *n* separation of the epidermis from the dermis by a collection of fluid, usually serum or blood.

blood *n* a fluid connective tissue, it consists of a pale yellow fluid, plasma, in which are suspended the red blood cells or erythrocytes, the white blood cells or leucocytes and the blood platelets or thrombocytes. The plasma contains many substances, including protein clotting factors, nutrients (amino acids, glucose, lipids, minerals and vitamins), enzymes, hormones, gases, drugs and metabolic waste. Blood volume is proportional to size and adults usually have 4–6 litres circulating. Cells form around 45% of blood volume with plasma forming the remaining 55%. In health the pH of blood remains within the range 7.35–7.45.

blood bank a special refrigerator in which blood is kept after withdrawal from donors until required for transfusion.

blood-brain barrier (BBB) the protective barrier between the circulating blood and the brain that assists the brain to maintain a stable environment. It consists of a special structural arrangement of capillary endothelial cells and astrocytes which makes the capillaries relatively impermeable. Nutrients pass through, but harmful substances are generally prevented from doing so. Certain drugs can pass from the blood through this barrier to the cerebrospinal fluid, e.g. some antibiotics which can be used to treat meningitis. Alcohol also passes through the barrier. The barrier is less effective in infants and children and allows the passage of harmful substances, such as bile pigments and lead. ⇒ astrocyte.

blood casts casts of red blood cells, formed in the renal tubules. They are found in the urine in some kidney diseases.

blood clotting ⇒ coagulation.

blood coagulation *n* ⇒ coagulation.

blood count examination of a sample of venous blood to determine the types, numbers and condition of red cells, white cells and platelets (thrombocytes) using an automated counter or haemocytometer. A typical count for a healthy adult would be: red cells 3.8–6.5 × 10^{12}/litre, white cells 4.0–11.0 × 10^9/litre and platelets 150–400 × 10^9/litre. *differential blood count* the estimation of the relative proportions of the different white blood cells in the blood. The normal differential count is: neutrophils 40–75%, lymphocytes 20–45%, monocytes 2–10%, eosinophils 1–6%, basophils 0–1%.

blood culture a venous blood sample is incubated in a suitable medium at an optimum temperature, so that any contained organisms can multiply and so be isolated and identified under the microscope. ⇒ septicaemia.

blood formation ⇒ haemopoiesis.

blood gases *n* ⇒ arterial blood gases.

blood glucose profiles used to make rational adjustments to treatment of individual diabetic patients. They can show the peaks and troughs and the duration of action of a given insulin preparation, which can vary from patient to patient. Blood samples are taken on fasting, 2 h after breakfast, before lunch, 2 h after lunch, before the evening meal, at bedtime and possibly during the night. Many patients are independent for collecting these profiles and do so at home.

blood groups the ABO blood groups are genetically determined by the presence or not of certain antigens (agglutinogens) on the surface of the red cells. In 1900 Landsteiner discovered that human blood can be classified into four groups: A, B, AB and O, according to the presence of A and B antigens. Group A has the A antigen, group B the B antigen, group AB has both antigens and group O has neither antigen. In the plasma there are antibodies (agglutinins) that are specific to the antigen not carried by the person's red cells; group A has anti-B, group B has anti-A, group AB has neither and group O has both anti-A and anti-B. It is these antibodies that cause agglutination (clumping) of donor red cells if incompatible blood is transfused. Blood grouping is determined by: (a) testing a suspension of red cells with anti-A and anti-B serum or (b) testing serum with known cells. Transfusion with an incompatible ABO group will cause agglutination and a severe haemolytic reaction and may lead to death. For most transfusion purposes, group A can receive groups A and O, group B can receive groups B and O, group AB can have blood of any group and group O can only have group O. (See Figure 9). The terms universal donor and

	Recipient			
Group	A	B	O	AB
A	+	–	–	+
B	–	+	–	+
AB	–	–	–	+
O	+	+	+	+

+ = compatible
– = non-compatible

Figure 9 Blood group compatibility. (Reproduced from Brooker 1996 with permission.)

recipient are outdated and confusing because many other blood groups exist, such as Rhesus and Kell factor. *Rhesus (Rh) blood group* a further three pairs of antigens coded for by genes designated the letters Cc, Dd and Ee were discovered by Landsteiner and Wiener in 1943. The letters denote allelomorphic genes which are present in all cells except the sex cells where a chromosome can carry C or c, but not both. In this way the Rhesus genes and blood groups are derived equally from each parent. When the cells contain only the cde groups, then the blood is said to be Rhesus negative (Rh-); when the cells contain C, D or E singly or in combination with cde, then the blood is Rhesus positive (Rh+). For general purposes only, the Dd antigens are of clinical significance. About 85% of the Caucasian population have the D antigen. In contrast to the ABO system, there are no preformed antibodies to the D antigen. They are produced by (a) transfusion of Rhesus positive blood to a Rhesus negative person; (b) immunization during pregnancy by Rhesus positive fetal red cells, with the D antigen, entering the maternal circulation where the women is Rhesus negative. This can cause haemolytic disease of the newborn (erythroblastosis fetalis). ⇒ anti-D. ⇒ haemolytic diease of the newborn. ⇒ Rhesus incompatibility.

blood-letting venesection.

blood plasma ⇒ plasma.

blood pressure the pressure exerted by the blood on the blood vessel walls. Usually refers to the pressure within the arteries as the left ventricle pumps blood into the aorta. The pressure is produced when flow meets resistance: blood pressure = peripheral resistance × cardiac output. Factors contributing to blood pressure include: peripheral resistance, cardiac output, blood volume, venous return, blood viscosity and the elasticity of arterial walls. The arterial blood pressure has two readings: the systolic, which represents the highest pressure in the left ventricle during systole when blood is ejected from the heart; and the diastolic, which is the lowest pressure as the ventricles fill during diastole when the aortic and pulmonary valves are closed. It is generally measured indirectly in the brachial artery using a stethoscope and sphygmomanometer and recorded in millimetres of mercury pressure (mm Hg). A typical blood pressure for a young adult would be 120/70 mm Hg. Usually values for both systolic and diastolic pressures are recorded (e.g. 138/88), and blood pressure may be measured with the person lying, sitting or standing. Arterial blood pressure may also be recorded directly by the use of an arterial pressure transducer. ⇒ hypertension. ⇒ hypotension. ⇒ Korotkoff sounds.

blood sedimentation rate (BSR) ⇒ erythrocyte sedimentation rate.

blood serum ⇒ serum.

blood sugar the amount of sugar (glucose) in the circulating blood; varies within a normal homeostatic range that is controlled by hormones that include: insulin, glucagon, catecholamines, thyroid hormones, cortisol and growth hormone. ⇒ hyperglycaemia. ⇒ hypoglycaemia.

blood transfusion ⇒ transfusion.

blood urea the amount of urea in the blood; varies within the normal range. This is virtually unaffected by the amount of protein in the diet when the kidneys, which are the main organs of urea excretion, are normal. When they are diseased the blood urea quickly rises. The blood urea may be abnormally low in serious liver disease. ⇒ uraemia.

BLS *abbr* basic life support.

'blue baby' the appearance of an infant born with a congenital heart defect that causes cyanosis, e.g. tetralogy of Fallot or transposition of the great vessels (aorta and pulmonary artery). The appearance, by contrast, of a newborn child suffering from temporary anoxia is described as 'blue asphyxia'. → asphyxia.

blue-green pus bluish discharge from a wound infected with *Pseudomonas aeruginosa*.

blunted affect decreased range and intensity of emotional responsiveness. A negative symptom associated with mental illness such as schizophrenia. It is characterized by: diminished or absent facial expressiveness during interactions with others; unchanging, monotonous or inexpressive voice tone when conversing, and lack of gestures when conversing.

bluxism *n* teeth clenching; it can cause headache from muscle fatigue.

BMI *abbr* body mass index.

BMR *abbr* basal metabolic rate.

BMT *abbr* bone marrow transplant/transplantation. ⇒ graft. ⇒ leukaemia.

BNF *abbr* British National Formulary. ⇒ formulary.

Bobath concept *n* the concept of treatment of abnormal muscle tone and disorder of movement, seen in children with cerebral palsy and adults following a stroke, developed by Berti Bobath and now widely applied to similar dysfunction caused by multiple sclerosis and other neurological conditions.

body cavities central areas of the body, completely or partially protected by bone; they contain various organs; they are named cranial, thoracic, abdominal and pelvic cavity.

body defence mechanisms in a general sense, the body's ability to defend itself; most commonly used in the context of immunity. Immune defence mechanisms may be: nonspecific (innate), such as the intact skin and mucous membranes and phagocytosis, or specific (adaptive), e.g. cell mediated or humoral immunity. ⇒ antitoxin. ⇒ fight or flight mechanism. ⇒ mental defence mechanisms. ⇒ immunoglobulins. ⇒ lymphocyte. ⇒ lysozyme.

body dysmorphic disorder an abnormal preoccupation with a particular part of the body. The person may imagine a defect or exaggerate a very slight body defect, for which they often seek the advice and reassurance of health professionals.

body image the image in an individual's mind of his own body. Distortions of this occur in anorexia nervosa. ⇒ body dysmorphic disorder. ⇒ disfigurement. ⇒ mutilation.

body language nonverbal symbols that express a person's current physical and mental state. They include body movements, postures, gestures, facial expressions, spatial positions, clothes and other bodily adornments. *body language problems* apart from the individuality involved in expression of personality, problems can arise when a person consistently conveys the wrong message, e.g. a dour look may mask a pleasant personality in familiar circumstances. However, a person may temporarily or permanently lack control of some muscles used in body language, for instance after Bell's palsy, cerebrovascular accident, paraplegia and tetraplegia. Communication has to be achieved in the context of the person's deprivation.

body lice ⇒ Pediculus.

body mass index (BMI) a measurement derived from weight and height: weight in kg divided by height in m². Used with other criteria to determine whether an adult is within a healthy weight range and as part of a nutritional assessment.

body surface area (BSA) calculated from a special nomogram using the child's height and weight. May be used to calculate drug doses in children, especially when the difference between the dose giving a therapeutic effect and the dose causing toxicity is small. ⇒ therapeutic index. ⇒ West nomogram.

body temperature the balance between heat production and heat loss in the human body. Body temperature is maintained around 37°C throughout the 24 h, but is subject to a diurnal variation of between 0.5–1.0°C over that period. Metabolism, voluntary and involuntary muscular activities produce most of the heat, and heat is lost by conduction, convection, and evaporation of sweat from the skin; a small amount is lost at defaecation, urination and expiration. *core body temperature* that which registers in the organs of the central cavities of the body (cranium, thorax and abdomen). For most clinical purposes it can be measured in several ways: (a) under the tongue (close to the sublingual artery); (b) by use of an electronic tympanic thermometer or (c) rectally; however the rectal site is no longer advocated unless an electronic rectal probe is available. *shell body temperature* that which registers outwith the trunk, e.g. in the dried axilla or groin. Shell temperature may vary between 35°C at the forehead and 20°C in the feet.

Boeck's disease a form of sarcoidosis.

Bohn's nodules tiny white nodules on the palate of the newly born.

Bohr effect *n* the effect that hydrogen ion concentration (pH) and carbon dioxide levels have on the affinity of haemoglobin for oxygen. As hydrogen ion concentration increases (pH falls) and carbon dioxide increases, the oxygen dissociation curve shifts to the right. The term Bohr effect is usually applied to the shift to the right caused by increasing hydrogen ion concentration. The effect ensures that oxygen is released more easily to metabolically active tissue.

boil *n* (*syn* furuncle) an acute inflammatory condition, surrounding a hair follicle; caused by *Staphylococcus aureus*. Usually attended by suppuration; it has one opening for drainage in contrast to a carbuncle.

Bolam test *n* the test laid down in the case of Bolam v Friern HMC on the standard of care expected of a professional in cases of alleged negligence.

bolus *n* 1. a soft, pulpy mass of masticated food. 2. a large dose of a drug given at the beginning of a treatment programme to raise the concentration in the blood rapidly to a therapeutic level.

bonding *n* the emotional tie one person forms with another, making an enduring and special emotional relationship. There is a fundamental biological need for this to occur between an infant and its parents. When newborn babies have to be nursed in an intensive care unit, special arrangements have to be made to encourage a relationship to form between the parents and their new baby by encouraging contact and touch, despite possible physical barriers. ⇒ attachment.

bone *n* connective tissue that has been mineralized to produce an extremely hard substance that is capable of stretching (tensile strength) and withstanding considerable compressive forces. Bone consists of an organic matrix (osteoid), bone cells (osteocytes, osteoblasts and osteoclasts) and inorganic mineral salts; hydroxyapatites, mainly calcium phosphate, calcium carbonate, calcium hydroxide, and some magnesium and fluoride. There are two types of bone tissue: hard, dense compact (lamellar) bone, and spongy cancellous bone. There are several bone types: long, short, flat, irregular and sesamoid, that form the 206 separate bones of the skeleton. *bone graft* ⇒ bone graft.

bone graft the transplantation of a piece of bone from one part of the body to another, or from one person to another. Used to repair bone defects or to supply osteogenic tissue.

bone marrow the substance contained within the medullary cavity, and spaces in cancellous bone. At birth the cavities are filled with blood-forming *red marrow* which is gradually replaced by *fatty yellow marrow* during childhood, until in adults red marrow is confined to the skull, sternum, ribs, pelvis, vertebrae and the ends of long bones. *bone marrow puncture* an investigation whereby a sample of red marrow is obtained by aspiration after piercing the sternum or iliac crest. *bone marrow transplant (BMT)* ⇒ graft. ⇒ transplant.

Bonnevie-Ullrich syndrome ⇒ Turner's syndrome.

boot *v* the start-up procedure that a PC follows as it runs some checks and loads the operating system when it is first switched on. ⇒ operating system. ⇒ PC.

borborygmi *n* audible bowel sounds. Rumbling noises caused by the movement of flatus and fluid in the intestines.

Bordetella *n* a genus of Brucellaceae bacteria. *B. pertussis* a small Gram-negative bacterium that causes pertussis (whooping cough).

boredom, prevention of this element of nursing is considered essential in children's nursing but it is also necessary for adults. Information written at the patient's initial assessment about their occupation and hobbies, where they live, etc, helps nurses to achieve patient-focused conversation with the objective of helping patients to prevent boredom. Other strategies for preventing boredom include: reading (large print books are available), radio, including local hospital radio stations, television and hobbies such as jigsaws, knitting or sewing. ⇒ institutionalization.

born before arrival (BBA) describes a birth occurring before arrival at hospital or of the midwife or doctor.

Bornholm disease (*syn* epidemic myalgia) a viral disease due to B group of coxsackie viruses named after the Danish island where it was described by Sylvest in 1934. The incubation time is 2–14 days and symptoms include sudden onset of severe pain in lower chest or abdominal or lumbar muscles. Breathing may be difficult, because of the pain, and fever is common. Treatment is symptomatic only.

Borrelia *n* a genus of spiral (spirochaete) bacteria. *Borrelia burgdorferi* causes Lyme disease, a tick-borne relapsing fever.

botulism *n* a rare type of bacterial food poisoning. An intoxication with the exotoxin produced by *Clostridium botulinum*. Vomiting and ocular, pharyngeal and respiratory paralysis manifest within 24–72 h of eating food contaminated with the spores, which require anaerobic conditions to produce the toxin. It is associated with poorly treated tinned food and home preserving of vegetables and meat. There is a high mortality rate.

bougie *n* a cylindrical, flexible instrument made of gum elastic, metal or other material. Used in varying sizes for dilating strictures, e.g. oesophageal or urethral.

bovine *adj* pertaining to the cow or ox. *bovine tuberculosis* ⇒ tuberculosis. *bovine spongiform encephalopathy (BSE)* infective, fatal neurological disease affecting cattle. ⇒ Creutzfeldt-Jakob disease.

bowel *n* the intestine or gut. ⇒ intestine. *small bowel* has three parts: duodenum, jejunum and ileum. It is concerned with food digestion and the absorption of nutrients. *large bowel* runs from the ileocaecal valve to the anus and consists of the caecum, appendix, colon, rectum and anus. The large bowel absorbs water and some nutrients and drugs, stores food residues and eliminates waste as faeces. ⇒ colon. *bowel movement* a lay term for defaecation. ⇒ faeces. *bowel sounds* sounds heard, by auscultation, as food, fluid and gas are moved down the bowel. Different sounds can be indicative of abnormalities, such as obstruction.

bowleg *n* varum genu.

Bowman's capsule *n* the cup-like part of the renal tubule that encloses the glomerulus.

Boyle's law *n* states that at a given temperature the pressure of a gas varies inversely to the volume.

BPD *abbr* bronchopulmonary dysplasia.

BPH *abbr* benign prostatic hyperplasia. ⇒ prostate.

BPRS *abbr* Brief Psychiatric Rating Scale.

Bq *abbr* becquerel.

brace *n* 1. an orthodontic device used in the realignment of teeth. 2. in orthopaedics, any device used to support a body part in its correct position.

brachial *adj* pertaining to the arm. Applied to vessels in this region and a nerve plexus at the root of the neck. *brachial artery* is used for recording arterial blood pressure. *brachial plexus* the nerve plexus formed from the spinal nerves C5–C8 and T1. It innervates the shoulder, arm and forearm. ⇒ Erb's palsy. ⇒ Klumpke's palsy.

brachiocephalic *adj* pertaining to the arm and head. Applied to the artery and vein. *brachiocephalic artery* large artery arising from the aortic arch which forms the right common carotid and right subclavian arteries. Also called the innominate.

brachium *n* the arm (especially from shoulder to elbow), or any arm-like appendage — **brachial** *adj*.

brachytherapy *n* radiotherapy delivered from a small radioactive source or sources which are implanted in or adjacent to the tumour. The technique may be used to treat cancers of the cervix, tongue, anus, lung, breast and oesophagus.

Braden scale *n* a pressure ulcer risk scale based on the Norton scale used extensively in the United States.

Bradford frame a stretcher type of bed used for: (a) immobilizing spine; (b) resting trunk and back muscles; (c) preventing deformity. It is a tubular steel frame fitted with two canvas slings allowing 100–150 mm gap to facilitate the use of a bedpan.

bradycardia *n* abnormally slow heart rate, usually defined as below 60 beats per minute in an adult. ⇒ arrhythmia.

bradykinesia from 'brady' (slow) and 'kinesia' (movement). The slowness of voluntary movement characteristic of Parkinsonism syndrome that accounts for patients' difficulty in turning over in bed, chewing food, dressing, walking and other activities of daily living.

Braille *n* a printing method which produces a pattern of raised dots representing the letters of the alphabet. Visually impaired individuals are able to read by feeling the dots.

brain *n* the encephalon; the largest part of the central nervous system; it is contained in the cranial cavity and is surrounded by three membranes called meninges. It comprises the cerebral hemispheres, cerebellum, pons varolii, midbrain and medulla oblongata. The cerebrospinal fluid inside the brain contained in the ventricles, and outside in the subarachnoid space, acts as a shock absorber to the delicate nerve tissue. *brain death* ⇒ death. *brain scan* imaging techniques which include: radionuclides, computed tomography (CT), magnetic resonance (MRI) and positron emission tomography (PET).

brainstem lowest part of the brain consisting of the midbrain, pons varolii and medulla oblongata. Controls vital automatic functions, such as respiratory rate etc.

bran *n* the husk of grain. The coarse outer part of cereals, especially wheat, high in nonstarch polysaccharides and the vitamin B complex.

branchial *adj* pertaining to the gills. The fissures or clefts which occur on each side of the neck of the human embryo and which are involved in the development of the nose, ears and mouth. *branchial cyst* a cyst in the neck arising from abnormal development of the branchial clefts.

Braun's frame a metal frame, bandaged for use, and equally useful for drying a lower leg plaster and for applying skeletal traction (Steinmann's pin or Kirschner wire inserted through the calcaneus) to a fractured tibia, after reduction.

break-bone fever ⇒ dengue.

breast *n* 1. the anterior upper part of the thorax. 2. the mammary gland. Milk secreting glands. *breast awareness* where a woman regularly examines her breasts, visually and manually, for signs of change. *breast bone* the sternum. *breast cancer* cancer of the breast. One in 12 women is at risk of developing it, and it is responsible for one in five deaths from malignant disease in women. ⇒ lumpectomy. ⇒ mastectomy. *breast feeding* suckling. Breast milk, providing the mother is able to take an adequate diet, provides balanced nutrition in a form which is ideal for the infant. Other advantages include bonding through intimate skin contact, transfer of antibodies and reduced risk of gastrointestinal infections. It is not always desirable or possible for women to breast feed, for instance HIV positive women in developed countries are advised not to breast feed. *breast pump* a glass or plastic cup which encircles the tissue around the nipple; it is attached to a rubber or plastic bulb from which air is evacuated to provide suction which withdraws milk from the breast. *breast reconstruction* performed after mastecto-

my where the skin and nipple are preserved and an implant inserted in place of breast tissue. Implants are also used in breast augmentation to increase size. *breast reduction* surgery to reduce breast tissue in painfully heavy or pendulous breasts.

breast, self-examination part of breast awareness where familiarity with her breasts enables the woman to detect small changes in the breasts. These changes may include: feelings of heaviness, pain or discomfort, nipple discharge or retraction, skin changes, lumps or thickening in the breast or under the arm. Women are encouraged to examine their breasts on a regular basis; either 7–10 days after the first day of menstruation or at set intervals for post menopausal women. Self examination is primarily aimed at finding breast cancers, but benign conditions, such as cysts, can also be felt. Advice and literature about breast self-examination is available from health professionals, such as practice nurses, breast care nurses etc, and is widely available from magazines, charities and self-help groups. ⇒ breast awareness. ⇒ breast cancer.

breath tests noninvasive tests for a variety of gastrointestinal disorders including malabsorption. Breath is analysed for various substances and examples include: H_2 *(hydrogen) breath test* used to assist in the diagnosis of lactose intolerance due to lactase deficieny. When lactose is ingested and not absorbed the amount of hydrogen in the breath increases. *urea breath test* a test for the presence of *Helicobacter pylori* in the stomach.

breech *n* the buttocks. ⇒ buttock.

breech presentation refers to the position of a baby in the uterus such that the buttocks would be born first; the normal position is head first.

bregma *n* the anterior fontanelle. ⇒ fontanelle.

Brief Psychiatric Rating Scale (BPRS) a measure of general psychiatric symptoms. Originally it contained sixteen items; nine of these are scored on verbal responses (somatic concerns, anxiety, guilt, grandiosity, depressive mood, hostility, suspiciousness, hallucinatory behaviour and unusual thoughts); the other seven are scored on observation at time of interview. Scoring is on a Likert scale from 1 (not present) to 7 (extremely severe).

Bright's disease $\Rightarrow$ glomerulonephritis.

British Sign Language *n* a form of signing used in the UK. $\Rightarrow$ Makaton. $\Rightarrow$ sign language.

BRM *abbr* biological response modifier.

Broadbent's sign visible retraction of the left side and back, in the region of the 11th and 12th ribs, synchronous with each heartbeat and due to adhesions between the pericardium and diaphragm. $\Rightarrow$ pericarditis.

broad ligaments lateral ligaments; double fold of parietal peritoneum which hangs over the uterus and outstretched uterine tubes, forming a lateral partition across the pelvic cavity.

broad thumb syndrome Rubenstein-Taybi syndrome.

Broca's area often described as the motor centre for speech; situated at the third convolution in the precentral gyrus, in the left hemisphere of the cerebrum. Injury to this area can result in expressive aphasia.

Brodie's abscess chronic abscess in bone, often affecting the tibia.

bromidrosis *n* a profuse, fetid perspiration, especially associated with the feet — **bromidrotic** *adj*.

bromism *n* chronic poisoning due to continued or excessive use of bromides (a sedative).

bromosulphthalein clearance test a rarely used test of liver function. Its use is limited to the diagnosis of Dubin-Johnson syndrome.

bronchi *npl* the two large tubes into which the trachea divides at its lower end. Each bronchus enters a lung at its hilum, where further subdivision occurs to conduct air to individual lung lobes and segments — **bronchial** *adj* pertaining to the bronchi. *bronchial tree* the network of bronchi as they subdivide within the lungs.

bronchial asthma $\Rightarrow$ asthma.

bronchial cancer the commonest type of lung tumour, accounting for around 50% of tumours, is the squamous type that arises from the epithelium of the bronchus. Other types include: small cell (oat cell), large cell and adenocarcinoma which involves the mucus-secreting glands. Bronchial cancers spread locally and metastasize to the lymph nodes, brain, liver, bone, skin and adrenal glands. Smoking is the most important factor in its aetiology, but passive smoking, environmental pollution and exposure to other carcinogens, e.g. asbestos, are implicated. Presentation is variable and may be with cough, dyspnoea, enlarged lymph nodes, haemoptysis and pleural pain. Some cancers may only cause symptoms when they have grown large and spread. Treatment depends on the type and staging of the cancer and may involve various combinations of surgery, radiotherapy and chemotherapy. The prognosis remains poor because the disease is often at an advanced stage at presentation. $\Rightarrow$ oat cell carcinoma.

bronchiectasis *n* abnormal dilatation of the bronchi. It may be congenital, such as in cystic fibrosis or ciliary dysfunction syndromes. Acquired bronchiectasis may be caused by pneumonia, primary tuberculosis and inhaled foreign bodies during childhood, and in adults, tumours, pneumonia, pulmonary tuberculosis and ciliary dysfunction syndromes. Associated with profuse, offensive, purulent sputum and sometimes haemoptysis. There are recurrent respiratory infections with a decline in general health characterized by anorexia, weight loss, malaise and digital clubbing. May lead eventually to respiratory failure. Management involves physiotherapy and antimicrobial drugs. Surgical resection of an affected lobe may be possible in some cases — **bronchiectatic** *adj*.

bronchiole *n* one of the minute subdivisions of the bronchi which terminate in the alveoli or air sacs of the lungs — **bronchiolar** *adj*.

bronchiolitis *n* inflammation of the bronchioles, caused in most cases by respiratory syncytial virus (RSV) and most common in children in the 1st year of life, peaking in winter months. The younger the child, the more likely the symptoms are to be severe, often requiring hospitalization — **bronchiolitic** *adj*.

bronchitis *n* inflammation of the bronchi. *acute bronchitis* as an isolated incident is usually a primary viral infection as a complication of the common cold, influenza, whooping cough, measles or rubella. Secondary infection occurs with bacteria, commonly *Haemophilus influenzae* or *Streptococcus pneumoniae*. In *chronic bronchitis* the bronchial mucus-secreting glands are hypertrophied with an increase in goblet cells and loss of ciliated cells due to irritation from tobacco smoke or atmospheric pollutants, and the patient's only complaint is of cough productive of mucoid sputum most days for 3 consecutive months in 2 consecutive years. It belongs to the larger group of chronic obstructive pulmonary disease (COPD). The excess mucus production and reduced mucociliary clearance will eventually lead to serious impairment of gaseous exchange in the lungs and heart failure. ⇒ pulmonary emphysema — **bronchitic** adj.

bronchoconstrictor n any agent which constricts the bronchi.

bronchodilator n any agent which dilates the bronchi, e.g. salbutamol. ⇒ beta (β)-adrenoceptor agonist. ⇒ muscarinic antagonists.

bronchogenic adj arising from one of the bronchi.

bronchography n obsolete radiographic examination of the bronchial tree. — **bronchographically** adv.

bronchomycosis n general term used to cover a variety of fungal infections of the bronchi and lungs, e.g. pulmonary candidiasis, aspergillosis — **bronchomycotic** adj.

bronchopleural fistula pathological communication between the pleural cavity and one of the bronchi.

bronchopneumonia n a term used to describe a form of pneumonia in which areas of consolidation are distributed widely around bronchi and not in a lobar pattern. Often seen at the extremes of age or secondary to an existing condition or debilitated state — **bronchopneumonic** adj.

bronchopulmonary adj pertaining to the bronchi and the lungs — **bronchopulmonic** adj.

bronchopulmonary dysplasia (BPD) a chronic respiratory condition, seen in preterm babies born with immature lungs who had long-term treatment with high concentrations of oxygen and positive pressure ventilation. Those infants who survive may be dependent on oxygen therapy and are high risk for repeated chest infections. Eventually the condition may cause pulmonary hypertension and cardiac failure (right side).

bronchorrhoea n an excessive discharge of mucus from the bronchial mucosa — **bronchorrhoeal** adj.

bronchoscope n a fibreoptic or rigid endoscope used for examining, taking biopsies and microbiological specimens from the interior of the bronchi or removing inhaled foreign bodies — **bronchoscopically** adv.

bronchoscopy endoscopic examination of the bronchi. Commonly utilizes a flexible fibreoptic scope but rigid metal instruments may still be used in some situations.

bronchospasm n sudden, but temporary, constriction of the bronchial smooth muscle resulting in narrowing of the airways. There is dyspnoea, cough and wheezing such as in asthma — **bronchospastic** adj.

bronchostenosis n narrowing of one of the bronchi — **bronchostenotic** adj.

bronchotracheal adj pertaining to the bronchi and trachea.

bronchus ⇒ bronchi.

Broselow paediatric resuscitation system system designed in the US for use during paediatric resuscitation. The Broselow tape measure, with its colour segments, is placed alongside the child. This provides the medical team with accurate information, from the colour segment that corresponds to the length of the child, regarding the correct size of equipment and appropriate drug doses to be used for that child. The equipment is stored in colour coded packaging.

brought in dead (BID) describes a corpse when death has occurred prior to arrival at the hospital.

brow n the forehead; the region above the supraorbital ridge.

brown fat present in infant tissue. Contains enzymes which, in the presence of oxygen, rapidly produce energy and heat – a form of nonshivering thermogenesis. ⇒ fat.

Brucella n a genus of bacteria causing brucellosis. Brucella abortus is the bovine strain causing abortion in cattle and undulant fever in humans. Brucella melitensis the goat strain causes Malta fever in humans. Both strains are transmissible to humans via infected milk.

brucellosis *n* an infection caused by a micro-organism of the *Brucella* group: *B. abortus* in cattle, *B. melitenis* in sheep and goats and *B. suis* in pigs. It is transmitted to humans from farm animals, through contaminated milk or contact with the carcass of an infected animal, and can be an occupational hazard for farmers, veterinary surgeons and abattoir workers. The incubation period is around 21 days. There are recurrent attacks of continuous or undulating fever and mental depression. Other signs and symptoms include headache, aches and pains, and splenomegaly. Some infections are subclinical and the condition may last for months with relapses. The condition is also called 'Malta fever', 'abortus fever' and 'undulant fever'.

Brudzinski's sign immediate flexion of knees and hips on raising head from pillow. Seen in meningeal irritation, such as with meningitis.

bruise *n* (*syn* contusion) a discolouration of the skin due to an extravasation of blood into the underlying tissues; there is no abrasion of the skin. ⇒ ecchymosis.

bruit *n* abnormal sound heard during auscultation of a structure or organ, e.g. blood vessel. ⇒ murmur.

bruxism *n* abnormal grinding of teeth, often producing excessive wear or attrition.

Bryant's 'gallows' traction fixed skin traction applied to the lower limbs, the legs are then suspended vertically (from an overhead beam), so that the buttocks are lifted just clear of the bed. May be used for fractures of the femur in children, (usually under twelve months of age, but depends on the size of the child), it has been largely replaced by hoop traction.

BSA *abbr* body surface area.

BSE *abbr* bovine spongiform encephalopathy.

BSS *abbr* Beck Scale for Suicide Ideation.

bubo *n* inflammation and enlargement of lymphatic nodes, especially in the groin or axilla. A feature of soft sore (chancroid), granuloma inguinale and plague — **bubonic** *adj*.

bubonic plague *n* ⇒ plague.

buccal *adj* pertaining to the cheek or mouth (buccal cavity).

Buchanan bib *n* a cotton mesh, foam bib worn over a tracheostomy. It protects the respiratory tract by warming and moistening inspired air and by removing particles from the air. Especially useful for patients with a permanent tracheostomy.

Budd-Chiari syndrome serious liver condition, with hepatic portal hypertension caused by hepatic venous obstruction.

budget holder the individual designated to authorize expenditure from the budget within certain constraints.

Buerger's disease (*syn* thromboangiitis obliterans) a chronic obliterative vascular disease affecting the leg arteries of young or middle-aged males. It results in progressive ischaemia of the legs with intermittent claudication, skin changes and gangrene. May eventually require amputation. *Buerger's exercises* were designed to treat this condition by increasing blood flow to the legs.

buffer *n* 1. substances which limit pH change by their ability to accept hydrogen ions or donate hydrogen ions as appropriate. In the body they prevent differences in pH that would inhibit cell homeostasis and function. The important buffer systems in the body include: hydrogen carbonate (bicarbonate) system, hydrogen phosphates and proteins such as haemoglobin. 2. anything used to reduce shock or jarring due to contact.

bug *n* a mistake in a computer system or program that causes it to either crash completely or malfunction. ⇒ crash.

bulbar *adj* pertaining to the medulla oblongata. *bulbar palsy or paralysis* paralysis which involves the labioglossopharyngeal (lips, tongue and pharynx) region and results from degeneration of the motor nuclei in the medulla oblongata. The patient is deprived of the safety reflexes and is in danger of choking and aspiration pneumonia. Associated with feeding difficulties in children with some types of profound learning disability.

bulbourethral *adj* pertaining to the bulb of the urethra. *bulbourethral glands* two tiny glands located inferior to the prostate gland with openings into the male urethra. They secrete lubricating mucus into the urethra prior to ejaculation. Also known as Cowper's glands.

bulimia nervosa *n* (*syn* binge-purge syndrome) an eating disorder involving repeated episodes of uncontrolled consumption of large quantities of food in a short time, with self-induced vomiting or misuse of laxatives thereafter. Many people with anorexia nervosa have a history of such episodes. ⇒ eating disorders.

bulla *n* a large watery blister. In dermatology, bulla formation is characteristic of the pemphigus group of dermatoses, but occurs sometimes in other diseases of the skin, such as impetigo and some types of eczema — **bullate, bullous** *adj*.

bundle of His *n* ⇒ atrioventricular bundle.

bunion *n* (*syn* hallux valgus) a deformity on the head of the metatarsal bone at its junction with the great toe. Friction and pressure of shoes at this point cause a bursa to develop. There is inflammation of the bursa, soreness, swelling and lateral displacement of the great toe. ⇒ Keller's operation.

buphthalmos *n* congenital glaucoma.

burden of proof the duty of a party to litigation to establish the facts, or, in criminal proceedings, the duty of the prosecution to establish the facts.

Burkitt's lymphoma a nonHodgkin's lymphoma, principally affecting children in tropical Africa, but it does occur in other areas. It mainly affects the jaw and abdomen and is often seen in people previously infected with the Epstein-Barr (EB) virus.

burn *n* traumatic damage of the tissues due to chemicals, dry heat, electricity, flame, friction or radiation; classified as partial or full thickness according to the depth of skin and other structures destroyed, the latter requiring skin grafts. Priorities of treatment include: fluid replacement and prevention of shock, pain relief, emotional support, preventing infection and later maintaining increased nutritional needs, and minimizing scarring and loss of function. Prognosis depends upon the percentage of body area burnt, age and general condition. ⇒ hypercatabolism. ⇒ Lund and Browder's chart. ⇒ scald. ⇒ Wallace's rule of nine.

burnout describes a state that results from exposure to stressors. The stressors are often chronic and work-related, but burnout may occur following exposure to an acute stressor and may also result from stressful family roles such as caring for a relative, or a combination. Health professionals are at particular risk of burnout because of their prolonged contact with ill people. It has been described as emotional exhaustion, isolation, being hardened towards others and an inability to deal positively with problems. The adverse effects can be divided into physical, emotional, intellectual, social and spiritual, and may include ineffective coping strategies, anxiety, insomnia, inability to make decisions, appetite and weight changes, extreme tiredness, apathy, lack of motivation, relationship difficulties and misuse of alcohol and drugs. ⇒ counselling. ⇒ general adaptation syndrome. ⇒ stress. ⇒ stressor.

burr *n* an attachment for a surgical drill which is used for cutting into tooth or bone.

bursa *n* a fibrous sac lined with synovial membrane and containing synovial fluid. Bursae are found between (a) tendon and bone; (b) skin and bone; (c) muscle and muscle. Their function is to facilitate movement without friction between these surfaces — **bursae** *pl*.

bursitis *n* inflammation of a bursa. *olecranon bursitis* inflammation of the bursa over the point of the elbow. *prepatellar bursitis* (*syn* housemaid's knee) a fluid-filled swelling of the bursa in front of the patella (kneecap). It is frequently associated with excessive kneeling. A blow can result in bleeding into the bursa and there can be infection with pyogenic pathogens.

buttock *n* one of the two projections posterior to the hip joints. Formed mainly of the gluteal muscles.

butyrophenones *npl* a group of neuroleptic (antipsychotic) drugs, e.g. haloperidol. Used in schizophrenia, other psychoses and for the short-term management of severe agitation etc.

byssinosis *n* a form of pneumoconiosis caused by inhalation of cotton or linen dust and seen in the textile industries. It is characterized by acute bronchiolitis with airflow obstruction.

byte *n* a unit of computer data storage capacity. One byte contains eight bits. Larger units include the kilobyte (Kb) containing 1024 bytes and the megabyte (Mb) which has 1048576 bytes. ⇒ binary. ⇒ bit.

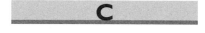

C *n* a complex but powerful computer language. ⇒ computer language.

Ca-125 a substance that can be detected in the serum and can act as a tumour marker for ovarian cancers.

CABG *abbr* coronary artery bypass graft.

cachexia *n* a state characterized by extreme emaciation and debility with anaemia, muscle weakness and malnutrition. Often seen as a feature of advanced cancer — **cachectic** *adj*.

cadaver *n* a dead body. If the dead person had an infectious disease, including blood-borne viruses, such as hepatitis B, AIDS and HIV-antibody positive, the body is put in a cadaver bag bearing a biohazard label.

cadmium (Cd) *n* a poisonous metallic element present in zinc ores and used in several industrial processes, e.g. engraving, welding and electroplating. *cadmium poisoning* food can be contaminated, e.g. by contact with cadmium-containing industrial waste or from storage containers. Inhalation of fumes over time can cause chronic lung disease: bronchitis and emphysema.

caecostomy *n* a surgically established fistula between the caecum and anterior abdominal wall, usually to achieve drainage and/or decompression of the caecum. It is usually created by inserting a wide-bore tube into the caecum at operation.

caecum *n* the blind, pouch-like commencement of the colon in the right iliac fossa. To it is attached the vermiform appendix; it is separated from the ileum by the ileocaecal valve — **caecal** *adj*.

caesarean section delivery of the fetus through an abdominal incision. It is said to be named after Caesar, who is supposed to have been born in this way. A low, horizontal 'lower segment caesarian section' is preferable to the 'classical' which involves a vertical incision in the body of the uterus.

caesium-137 (¹³⁷Cs) radioactive isotope of caesium which, when sealed in needles or tubes, can be used for brachytherapy instead of radium.

caffeine *n* an alkaloid present in tea, coffee, 'cola' and other drinks. Used in some analgesic preparations. It is a stimulant and has a diuretic action.

caisson disease (*syn* the bends, decompression sickness) results from sudden reduction in atmospheric pressure, as experienced by divers on return to surface and aircrew ascending to great heights. The sudden decompression causes nitrogen bubbles to form in the blood with variable, but sometimes fatal, consequences. The condition is largely preventable by proper and gradual decompression technique.

calamine *n* zinc carbonate tinted pink with ferric oxide. Widely employed in lotions and creams for its mild astringent action on the skin. *calamine lotion* calamine dissolved in a weak solution of carbolic acid (phenol) for its anaesthetic effect in relieving itch.

calcaneus *n* the heel bone, also known as the os calcis.

calcareous *adj* pertaining to or containing lime or calcium; of a chalky nature.

calciferol *n* ⇒ ergocalciferol.

calcification *n* the hardening of an organic substance by a deposit of calcium salts within it. May be normal, as in bone, or pathological, as in arteries.

calcitonin *n* (*syn* thyrocalcitonin) hormone produced in the thyroid parafollicular or 'C' cells. It has a fine-tuning role in regulating calcium homeostasis. As an antagonist of parathyroid hormone, it reduces serum calcium and phosphate levels by its action on the kidneys and bone. It inhibits calcium reabsorption from bone and stimulates the excretion of calcium and phosphate in the urine. Calcitonin is released when the serum calcium level rises. Synthetic calcitonin is used therapeutically in the management of Paget's disease and metastatic bone disease.

calcitriol *n* 1,25-dehydroxycholecalciferol (or 1,25-dehydroxyvitamin) the active form of vitamin D. It is involved in calcium homeostasis.

calcium (Ca) *n* a metallic element. It is required by the body for neuromuscular action and blood clotting and is an important constituent of bone and teeth. An essential dietary mineral. *calcium carbonate* a salt of calcium used in many antacid preparations. *calcium gluconate* a salt of calcium used to treat calcium deficiencies and disorders such as rickets. ⇒ calcium antagonists (channel blockers).

calcium antagonists (channel blockers) *npl* drugs that inhibit the flow of calcium ions in smooth muscle, e.g. verapamil, nifedipine and diltiazem. Used in the management of angina, some arrhythmias and hypertension. They decrease myocardial contractility and are negatively inotropic. They cause vasodilatation. ⇒ inotropes.

calcium oxalate a calcium salt which forms a major component of urinary calculi in the UK. ⇒ hyperoxaluria.

calculus *n* abnormal deposits composed chiefly of mineral substances and formed in the passages which transmit secretions, or in the cavities which act as reservoirs for them. The stones or concretions found in the urinary tract, gallbladder or salivary gland. *dental calculus* mineralized dental plaque deposited on the tooth surface — **calculous** *adj*.

Caldwell-Luc operation a radical operation previously used in the management of sinusitis. An opening made above the upper canine tooth into the anterior wall of the maxillary antrum increased drainage. ⇒ antrostomy. ➡ functional endoscopic sinus surgery.

Calgary Depression Scale (CDS) a nine-item structured interview scale developed to assess depression in people suffering from schizophrenia.

calibrate *v* to check or correct graduations of an instrument against a known standard.

caliper *n* 1. a two-pronged instrument with sharp points which are inserted into bone, used to fix bones or apply traction in the treatment of fractures. 2. a supportive metal device worn on the leg to facilitate mobility. *Thomas' walking caliper* is similar to the Thomas' splint, but the W-shaped junction at the lower end is replaced by two small iron rods which slot into holes made in the heel of the boot. The ring should fit the groin perfectly, and all weight is then borne by the ischial tuberosity.

calipers *n* instrument used for measuring thickness or distances, e.g. skin-fold thickness.

callosity *n* (*syn* keratoma) a local hardening of the skin caused by pressure or friction. The epidermis becomes hypertrophied. Most commonly seen on the feet and palms of the hands.

callus *n* 1. a callosity; hardened thickened skin on the plantar or palmar surfaces subject to considerable friction. 2. the partly calcified tissue which forms about the ends of a broken bone and ultimately accomplishes repair of the fracture — **callous** *adj*.

calor *n* heat; one of the four classic local signs of inflammation; the others are dolor, rubor, tumor.

caloric test an otological test of vestibular function. Irrigation of the external auditory canals with water at 30 °C and then at 44 °C is used to stimulate the lateral semicircular canals. Each ear is tested separately. Where the vestibular system is intact the test produces nystagmus.

calorie *n* unit of heat. The small calorie (c) is that amount of heat required to raise the temperature of 1 gram (g) of water through 1°Celsius. In clinical nutritional practice the calorie is too small a unit to be useful and the kilocalorie (kcal) is used. One kilocalorie (kcal), sometimes termed a large calorie (C), is that amount of heat required to raise the temperature of 1 kilogram (kg) of water through 1°Celsius. The energy of food and metabolic needs can be measured in kilocalories, e.g. 1 gram (g) of fat releases 9 kcal. See Nutrition Appendix. 1000 calories = 1 kilocalorie. Calories and kilocalories have been replaced by the SI derived unit, for heat, energy and work, the joule (J) or kilojoule (kJ). Approximately 4.2 kilojoules = 1 kilocalorie.

calorific *adj* describes any phenomena which pertain to the production of heat.

calyx *n* a cup-shaped organ or cavity such as the recesses of the renal pelvis — **calyces** *pl*.

Camberwell Assessment of Need (CAN) an assessment used by mental health nurses and others to rate met and unmet service needs.

CAMI *abbr* Carers Assessment of Managing Index.

cAMP *abbr* cyclic adenosine monophosphate.

Campylobacter *n* a genus of Gram-negative motile bacteria of the family Spirillaceae. *Campylobacter jejuni* is a common cause of food poisoning. It is characterized by bloodstained diarrhoea and abdominal pain lasting 10–14 days. Associated with raw meat and poultry, unpasteurized milk and infected pets who excrete the bacteria in faeces, thereby contaminating their hair. Treatment is with antibiotics, e.g. erythromycin or gentamicin.

CAN *acr* Camberwell Assessment of Need.

canaliculus *n* a minute capillary passage. Any small canal, such as the passage leading from the edge of the eyelid to the lacrimal sac or one of the numerous small canals leading from the haversian canals and terminating in the lacunae of bone — **canaliculi** *pl* — **canaliculization** *n*.

cancellous *n* resembling latticework; light and spongy; like a honeycomb. A type of bone tissue. ⇒ bone.

cancer *n* a general lay term which covers any malignant growth in any part of the body. The growth is purposeless, parasitic, and flourishes at the expense of the human host. Characteristics are the tendency to cause local destruction, to invade adjacent tissues and to spread by metastasis. Cancer develops from the loss of normal cellular regulation. Frequently recurs after removal. Carcinoma refers to malignant tumours of epithelial tissue, sarcoma to malignant tumours of connective tissue. *cancer early warning* people are encouraged to observe for the early warning signs for cancer and seek the help of a health professional should they occur. (See Figure 10). ⇒ leukaemia. ⇒ lymphoma — **cancerous** *adj*.

cancer in situ ⇒ carcinoma.

cancer screening ⇒ screening.

Cancer Units *npl* in the UK. Units in District General Hospitals that support the work of the Regional Cancer Centres by managing the treatment and care of patients with common cancers, e.g. lung, colorectal etc.

cancrum oris *n* gangrenous stomatitis of cheek as a result of dental sepsis. Often called 'noma'. Commoner in children from developing countries and mostly associated with malnourishment.

candela (cd) *n* a measurement of luminous intensity. One of the seven base units of the International System of Units (SI).

- A change in normal bladder or bowel habits, such as frequency of micturition or constipation alternating with diarrhoea
- Any unusual bleeding or discharge, such as blood in the urine, faeces or sputum, unusual vaginal bleeding or discharge, or nipple discharge
- Any thickening or a lump, e.g. in a breast, testis or mouth
- A sore on the skin, lips or in the mouth, that does not heal
- Obvious changes such as darkening, increasing in size or bleeding, occurring in a mole or wart
- Loss of appetite, persistent indigestion or difficulty in swallowing
- Persistent cough or hoarseness

Note: contrary to popular opinion, pain and weight loss are usually late symptoms/signs of cancer.

Figure 10   Cancer – early warning.

Candida *n* (*syn* Monilia) a genus of fungi (yeast) which form some filaments. They are widespread in nature. *Candida albicans* causes candidiasis (thrush).

candidiasis *n* (*syn* moniliasis, thrush) disease caused by infection with a species of Candida, usually *Candida albicans*. It can affect various sites: mouth, gastrointestinal tract, lungs, skin, nails and genitourinary tract (vulvovaginitis, balanitis), especially in people who are debilitated, e.g. cancer, diabetes mellitus, or immunosuppressed and following longterm or extensive use of antimicrobial agents, which disturbs the microbial flora, and other drugs, e.g. corticosteroids. Oral infection can be due to poor oral hygiene, including carious teeth and ill-fitting dentures. The management depends on the site, severity and underlying reason, but antifungal drugs can be administered topically, orally or intravenously and include: nystatin, clotrimazole, miconazole, fluconazole and amphotericin. The presence of pulmonary or oesophageal candidiasis is an AIDS defining condition according to the CDC/WHO classification of HIV disease.

canicola fever human disease caused by *Leptosira canicola*, a micro-organism carried by pigs and dogs. ⇒ Leptospira. ⇒ leptospirosis.

canine *adj* of or resembling a dog. *canine teeth* four in all, two in each jaw, situated between the incisors and the premolars. Those in the upper jaw are popularly known as the 'eye teeth'.

cannabinoids *npl* antiemetic drugs derived from cannabis, e.g. nabilone. Used for the nausea associated with cytotoxic drugs.

cannabis indica (*syn* marihuana, hashish etc). A psychoactive drug which is usually smoked, it produces hallucinations and euphoria. In the UK, its supply, possession or cultivation are criminal offences under the provisions of the Misuse of Drugs Act 1971. There is considerable interest in the possibility of medicinal uses, e.g. to relieve the effects of multiple sclerosis, and trials are currently taking place. ⇒ cannabinoids.

cannula *n* a hollow tube of plastic or metal used for the introduction or withdrawal of fluid from the body. In some types, e.g. intravenous, the lumen is fitted with a sharp-pointed trocar to facilitate insertion which is withdrawn when the cannula is in situ — **cannulae** *pl*.

cannulation *n* insertion of a cannula, such as into a vein.

canthus *n* the angle formed by the junction of the eyelids. The inner one is known as the *nasal canthus* and the outer as the *temporal canthus* — **canthi** *pl* — **canthal** *adj*.

CAPD *abbr* continuous ambulatory peritoneal dialysis.

CAPE *acr* Clifton Assessment Procedures for the Elderly.

capillary *n* (literally, hair-like) any tiny thin-walled vessel forming part of a network which facilitates rapid exchange of substances between the contained fluid and the surrounding tissues. *bile capillary* begins in a space in the liver and joins others, eventually forming a bile duct. *blood capillary* unites an arteriole and a venule (see Figure 11). *capillary fragility* an expression of the ease with which blood capillaries may rupture. *lymph capillary* begins in the tissue spaces throughout the body and joins others, eventually forming a lymphatic vessel.

capital budget an allocation of money for the purchase of items, such as equipment, that have a life of more than 12 months, or items with a cost in excess of an agreed level. ⇒ revenue budget.

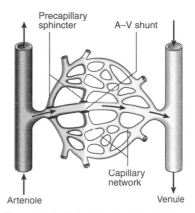

Figure 11　Capillaries. (Reproduced from Brooker 1996 with permission.)

capitalism describes an economic system where the infrastructure for the production of goods and services is privately owned and organized to be profit making within the market. The labour for this production is provided by people who are paid wages/salary.

capitate *n* one of the carpals or wrist bones.

capitation funding a way of allocating money and other resources based on the number of people living in a geographical area. *weighted capitation* the allocation of funds based on the number of people in a geographical area that is adjusted for the age profile or the relative economic and social conditions, e.g. areas with a high level of social deprivation would attract extra funds. Other factors may be the extra costs involved in providing the service in a sparsely populated rural area or in a city.

capping *n* a process by which cell surface molecules are caused to aggregate (usually using antibody) on the cell membrane.

capsaicin *n* a substance present in sweet peppers. It acts on membrane nociceptors and prevents the transmission of pain impulses. Applied topically to relieve pain in postherpetic neuralgia following shingles.

capsule *n* **1.** the outer membranous covering of certain organs, such as the kidney, liver, spleen and adrenal glands. *joint capsule* the fibrous tissue enclosing the joint cavity of a freely movable joint. It is further reinforced by various extracapsular and intracapsular ligaments. **2.** a gelatinous or rice paper container enclosing drugs for swallowing. **3.** the mucus layer forming a protective envelope around certain bacteria. It prevents dessication (drying) in hostile environmental conditions — **capsular** *adj*.

capsulectomy *n* the surgical excision of a capsule. Refers to a joint or lens; less often to the kidney.

capsulitis *n* inflammation of a capsule. Sometimes used as a synonym for frozen shoulder.

capsulotomy *n* incision of a capsule, usually referring to that surrounding the crystalline lens of the eye.

caput the head. *caput medusae* dilated knot of veins around the umbilicus, associated with hepatic portal hypertension. *caput succedaneum* a serous swelling of the infant's soft scalp tissue caused by pressure during labour. It is apparent at or shortly after birth. The swelling is diffuse, not delineated by scalp suture lines and usually disappears rapidly.

carbaminohaemoglobin *n* a compound formed between carbon dioxide and haemoglobin. Part of the carbon dioxide in the blood is carried in this form.

carbapenems *npl* a group of beta (β)-lactam antibiotics that include the broad spectrum imipenem.

carbohydrate *n* an organic compound containing carbon, hydrogen and oxygen. Formed in nature by photosynthesis in plants; they include starches, sugars and cellulose, and are classified in three groups: monosaccharides, disaccharides and polysaccharides. Carbohydrates are the principal energy source in humans. $\Rightarrow$ kilojoule.

carbolic acid $\Rightarrow$ phenol.

carbon *n* a nonmetallic element occurring in all organic molecules and living matter. A huge number of complex molecules can be formed because carbon is able to bond with four other atoms to form many different structures. $\Rightarrow$ valence. *carbon dioxide* a gas; a waste product of many forms of combustion and metabolism, excreted via the lungs. Accumulates in respiratory insufficiency or respiratory failure and carbon dioxide tension in arterial blood ($PaCO_2$) increases above the reference range of 4.4–6.1 kPa. $\Rightarrow$ hypercapnia.

carbon monoxide a poisonous gas present in exhaust fumes and produced from the combustion of other hydrocarbon fuels, such as natural gas. It forms a stable compound with haemoglobin, thus blocking its normal reversible oxygen-carrying function. Hypoxia will occur, but the signs and symptoms may be insidious with prolonged exposure. It is characterized by headache, agitation, dizziness, confusion, convulsions, altered consciousness, increased respiratory rate, flushed or pale skin and cardiac arrhythmias. *carbon tetrachloride* colourless volatile liquid. Used in dry cleaning and in some antifreeze. Exposure may lead to liver damage.

carbonic anhydrase a zinc-containing enzyme which catalyses the reversible conversion of carbon dioxide and water to carbonic acid. It facilitates the transfer of carbon dioxide from tissues to blood and from blood to alveolar air for excretion.

carbonic anhydrase inhibitors *npl* drugs used to reduce intraocular pressure in glaucoma by limiting the production of aqueous humor, rather than as diuretics, e.g. acetazolamide. They also act at the proximal tubule by preventing the reabsorption of hydrogen carbonate, sodium, potassium and water, all of which increases urine production. $\Rightarrow$ carbonic anhydrase.

carboxyhaemoglobin *n* a stable compound formed by haemoglobin and carbon monoxide (CO). Haemoglobin has a high affinity for CO. In this form, haemoglobin is unable to transport oxygen and hypoxia occurs, as in CO poisoning.

carboxyhaemoglobinaemia *n* carboxyhaemoglobin in the blood — **carboxyhaemoglobinaemic** *adj*.

carboxyhaemoglobinuria *n* carboxyhaemoglobin in the urine — **carboxyhaemoglobinuric** *adj*.

carbuncle *n* an acute inflammation, usually caused by a staphylococcal infection. Often on the back of the neck, involving several hair follicles and surrounding subcutaneous tissue, forming an extensive slough with several discharging sinuses.

carcinoembryonic antigen (CEA) *n* a fetal antigen. Elevated levels in the serum of adults can act as a tumour marker for colorectal cancers; however, the test may be positive in other conditions, such as alcoholic cirrhosis.

carcinogen *n* an agent that causes or predisposes to cancer. Examples include: the chemicals in tobacco, viruses (e.g. human papilloma virus and Epstein-Barr virus), sunlight and diet.

carcinogenesis *n* the process of cancer formation — **carcinogenetic** *adj.*

carcinoid syndrome a clinical syndrome which occurs following the development and spread of carcinoid tumours which secrete 5-hydroxytryptamine (5-HT) (also called serotonin) and other substances that cause flushing, bronchospasm and diarrhoea. The tumours usually occur in the gastrointestinal tract, but may metastasize to the liver. Management involves surgical excision and drugs to block the effects of 5-HT or prevent its release, e.g. octreotide.

carcinoma *n* a cancerous growth of epithelial tissue (e.g. mucous membrane). *basal cell carcinoma* a localized, slow-growing tumour, usually occurring on the face. Also known as a rodent ulcer. *carcinoma-in-situ* previously called preinvasive carcinoma or cancer. It is a very early cancer that is asymptomatic and that has not invaded the basement membrane. Well described in uterine cervix and prostate. ⇒ cervical intraepithelial neoplasia. Previously called preinvasive carcinoma. *squamous carcinoma* a malignant tumour arising from squamous epithelium — **carcinomatous** *adj.*

carcinomatosis *n* disseminated malignant disease.

cardia *n* the upper part of the stomach, enclosing the cardiac orifice and adjacent to the gastro oesophageal (cardiac) sphincter. *cardiac* pertaining to the cardia. *cardiac achalasia* food fails to pass normally into the stomach, though there is no obvious obstruction. The oesophagus does not demonstrate normal peristalsis after swallowing; this prevents the normal relaxation of the gastro-oesophageal (cardiac) sphincter. Associated with loss of ganglion cells within muscle layers of at least some areas of the affected oesophagus.

cardiac/cardio- *adj* pertaining to the heart. *cardiac arrest* cessation of an effective output from the heart; asystole, electromechanical dissociation (EMD), ventricular fibrillation (VF) or pulseless ventricular tachycardia (VT). Causes include myocardial ischaemia, electrolyte imbalance and electrocution. *cardiac arrhythmias* an abnormality of heart rhythm. *cardiac bed* one which can be manipulated so that the patient is supported in a sitting position. *cardiac bypass* the circulation of blood through an extracorporeal pump and oxygenator, used to facilitate heart surgery or to support critically ill patients. *cardiac catheterization* ⇒ catheterization. *cardiac cycle* the events occurring in the heart during one heart beat; takes around 0.8 s where the heart rate is approximately 70/min. ⇒ diastole. ⇒ systole. *cardiac enzymes* include aspartate aminotransferase, lactate dehydrogenase and creatine kinase, released by damaged myocardial cells. Elevated levels in the blood are used to confirm the diagnosis of myocardial infarction. *cardiac failure* inability of either the right or left side of the heart to pump effectively. It may occur in one side or both sides may fail. Common causes include coronary heart disease, cardiomyopathy or chronic respiratory disease. It may occur acutely, as in left ventricular failure characterized by dyspnoea and pulmonary oedema, but more usually it is chronic. ⇒ congestive cardiac failure. ⇒ cor pulmonale. *cardiac index* the cardiac output per metre^2 of body surface area. It is calculated by dividing the cardiac output by the body surface area. *cardiac oedema* gravitational oedema. Such patients excrete excessive aldosterone which increases excretion of potassium and conserves sodium and chloride. Aldosterone antagonists are useful, e.g. spironolactone, triamterene. Both act as diuretics. ⇒ oedema. *cardiac output* the amount of blood pumped by the ventricles in one minute. *cardiac pacemaker* an electrical device for maintaining myocardial contraction by stimulating the heart muscle. A pacemaker may be temporary or permanent. Some are fixed rate, whereas others fire on demand when the heart rate falls below a preset rate. ⇒ pacemaker. *cardiac sphincter* ⇒ gastro-oesophageal sphincter. *cardiac tamponade* compression of heart. Can occur in surgery and penetrating wounds or rupture of the heart from haemopericardium. *cardiac transplantation* ⇒ heart transplant. ⇒ transplant.

cardialgia *n* literally, pain in the heart or cardia. Often used to mean heartburn (pyrosis).

cardiogenic *adj* of cardiac origin.

cardiogenic shock *adj* the shock syndrome caused by a failure of the heart to pump sufficient blood around the circulation. The pump failure leads to a low cardiac output and may occur with myocardial infarction, certain arrhythmias, cardiomyopathies, myocarditis and valvular disease. ⇒ shock.

cardiogram the tracing obtained from the use of a cardiograph.

cardiograph *n* an instrument for recording graphically the force and form of the heartbeat. — **cardiographically** *adv.*

cardiologist *n* a medically qualified person who specializes in diagnosing and treating diseases of the heart.

cardiology *n* study of the structure, function and diseases of the heart.

cardiomegaly *n* enlargement of the heart.

cardiomyopathy *n* acute or chronic disease of the myocardium, it may be an inherited condition, secondary to infections and serious systemic disorders, or of unknown aetiology. There are three main types: dilated, restrictive or obliterative, and hypertrophic. Management involves treatment of the cause where possible, treatment of heart failure and, in some cases, heart transplantation — **cardiomyopathic** *adj.*

cardiomyotomy *n* surgical procedure where the muscle at the lower end of the oesophagus is split in an effort to relieve achalasia (cardiospasm) and dysphagia. ⇒ Heller's operation.

cardioplegia *n* the induction of electromechanical cardiac arrest. *cold cardioplegia* cardioplegia combined with hypothermia to reduce the myocardial oxygen requirements during open heart surgery.

cardiopulmonary *adj* pertaining to the heart and lungs *cardiopulmonary bypass* used in open heart surgery. The heart and lungs are excluded from the circulation and replaced by a pump oxygenator. ⇒ cardiac bypass. *cardiopulmonary resuscitation (CPR)* ⇒ cardiopulmonary resuscitation — **cardiopulmonic** *adj.*

cardiopulmonary resuscitation (CPR) means of artificially maintaining respiration and circulation after a cardiopulmonary arrest. It involves maintenance of a clear airway, ventilation of the person's lungs using mouth-mouth, mouth-nose, oxygen with a bag and face mask, or via an endotracheal tube, and maintenance of circulation by external or internal chest compressions.

cardiorenal *adj* pertaining to the heart and kidney.

cardiorespiratory *adj* pertaining to the heart and the respiratory system.

cardiorraphy *n* stitching of the heart wall; usually reserved for traumatic surgery.

cardioscope *n* obsolete instrument for examining the inside of the heart.

cardiothoracic *adj* pertaining to the heart and thoracic cavity. A specialized branch of surgery.

cardiotocograph (CTG) *n* the instrument used in cardiotocography.

cardiotocography *n* a form of fetal monitoring used during labour to detect fetal hypoxia (lack of oxygen); fetal heart rate, fetal movements and uterine contractions are recorded simultaneously. The measurements are fed through a monitor in such a way that extraneous sounds are excluded and recorded on heat-sensitive paper.

cardiotomy syndrome pyrexia, pericarditis and pleural effusion following heart surgery. It may develop weeks or months after the operation and is thought to be an autoimmune reaction.

cardiotoxic *adj* describes any agent which has an injurious effect on the heart.

cardiovascular *adj* pertaining to the heart and blood vessels.

cardioversion *n* use of electrical countershock to convert a cardiac arrhythmia, such as atrial fibrillation, to sinus rhythm.

carditis *n* inflammation of the heart. A word seldom used without the appropriate prefix, e.g. endo-, myo-, pan-, peri-.

care *n* a component of nursing; often used to imply its psychological and social (psychosocial) dimensions, it also covers physical care interventions. Each nurse/patient interaction and nursing activity which involves touching the patient has a psychosocial aspect which can be perceived by the patient as negative, neutral or positive.

care pathway the integrated plan or pathway agreed locally by the multidisciplinary team for specific patient/client groups. The agreed pathway is based on available evidence and guidelines.

care plan the document on which nursing information is recorded. In some instances, it is used as a collective term which includes: information from the initial patient assessment; statement of patient's actual and potential problems with everyday living activities which are amenable to nursing intervention; statement of the goals related to the problems to be achieved by the patient; and the plan of nursing interventions and their implementation, together with information from ongoing assessment and evaluation of whether or not the goals have been, or are being, achieved. ⇒ patient participation.

care programme approach (CPA) developed because of several high profile scandals concerning inadequate continuing care in the community of people with severe learning disabilities and mental health problems. The CPA is designed to ensure that these people do not slip through the net by prescribing and monitoring essential requirements for good practice in their care and supervision. These principles are: (a) assessment of health and social care needs; (b) a written plan of care agreed with the user and carers; (c) a key worker appointed with responsibility for co-ordinating the care programme; (d) regular reviews with multidisciplinary professional and user/carer involvement.

Caregiver Strain Index (CSI) used by mental health nurses and others to assess caregiver strain, using a simple questionnaire. Thirteen predetermined questions answered yes or no by interviewee. Has the benefit of being quick and simple, although crude.

carer *n* someone who takes the responsibility for caring for another (child, sick, disabled or older person). The Association of Carers seeks to restrict the term to cover the 6 million unpaid family, friends and neighbours of vulnerable people in the UK, and not to paid helpers such as care workers, nurses or social workers. They also oppose the term 'informal carer'. ⇒ Caregiver Strain Index. ⇒ Carers Assessment of Managing Index. ⇒ Experience of Caregiving Inventory.

Carers Assessment of Managing Index (CAMI) used by mental health nurses and others to assess coping styles and management of stress by questionnaire.

Carers are given examples of coping strategies, asked if they use these and if they are effective. Important in that it assumes that carers have coping strategies which can be enhanced.

caries *n* **1.** a microbial disease of the calcified tissue of the teeth, characterized by demineralization of the inorganic portion and destruction of the organic substance of the tooth. Potentiated by sugary substances. **2.** inflammatory decay of bone, usually associated with pus formation — **carious** *adj*.

carina *n* a keel-like structure exemplified by the keel-shaped cartilage at the bifurcation of the trachea into two bronchi — **carinal** *adj*.

cariogenic *adj* any agent causing caries, by custom referring to dental caries.

carminative *adj, n* having the power to relieve flatulence and associated colic. The chief carminatives administered orally are aromatics, e.g. cinnamon, cloves, ginger, nutmeg and peppermint.

carneous mole a missed abortion. A fleshy mass in the uterus comprising blood clot and a dead fetus or parts thereof which have not been expelled.

carotenes *npl* naturally occurring yellow or orange carotenoid pigments found in many fruit and vegetables, such as dark green leafy vegetables and carrots. β*carotene* a provitamin converted in the body to retinol. ⇒ vitamin A.

carotenoids *npl* a group of about 100 naturally occurring yellow to red pigments found mostly in plants, some of which are carotenes.

carotid *n* the principal artery on each side of the neck. At the bifurcation of the common carotid into the internal and external carotids there are: (a) the *carotid bodies* a collection of chemoreceptors which monitor blood oxygen levels and pH; (b) the *carotid sinus* a collection of baroreceptors sensitive to pressure changes; increased pressure causes slowing of the heart beat and lowering of blood pressure. *carotid angiogram* the inspection of the carotid arteries after injection of a radiopaque medium.

carpal pertaining to the wrist. *carpal tunnel syndrome* nocturnal pain, numbness and tingling in the area of distribution of the median nerve in the hand. A common condition due to compression as the nerve passes under the fascial band. Often caused by repetitive wrist movements, it may also be a feature of rheumatoid arthritis. Management includes: avoiding a particular movement, splinting or surgical decompression of the carpal tunnel.

carphology *n* involuntary picking at the bedclothes, as seen in exhaustive or febrile delirium.

carpometacarpal *adj* pertaining to the carpal and metacarpal bones, the joints between them and the ligaments joining them.

carpopedal *adj* pertaining to the hands and feet. *carpopedal spasm* painful spasm of hands and feet in tetany due to reduced calcium levels in the blood. ⇒ Chvostek's sign. ⇒ Trousseau's sign.

carpus the wrist. The eight bones of the wrist; capitate, hamate, lunate, pisiform, scaphoid, trapezium, trapezoid and triquetral.

carrier *n* **1.** a person who, without manifesting an infection, harbours the microorganism which can cause the overt infection, and who can transmit infection to others. **2.** a person who is heterozygous for a recessive gene at a specific chromosome location (locus). They do not exhibit the disease or trait (not expressed in heterozygous state) but may pass the gene to their offspring who will exhibit the disease or trait if they inherit the gene from both parents. ⇒ heterozygous. ⇒ homozygous.

carrier molecule *n* a protein molecule present in a cell membrane that facilitates the movement of substances that cannot pass through the lipid cell membrane, such as some ions, nutrients and drugs.

cartilage *n* a dense connective tissue capable of withstanding compressive forces and pressure. Consists of a solid matrix containing chondrocytes (cartilage cells). There are three types which perform different functions: yellow elastic, hyaline and white fibrous. Yellow elastic helps structures, such as the pinna of the ear, to maintain their shape. Hyaline, a smooth tissue, forms the embryonic bones and in adults covers the ends of long bones and forms the cartilage of the larynx, nose, bronchi and costal cartilages. Most of the hyaline cartilage forming embryonic

bones becomes bone tissue during childhood and adolescence. White fibrous is a flexible, but very strong, tissue such as that found as pads between the vertebrae. ⇒ chondrocyte. ⇒ intervertebral disc — **cartilaginous** *adj*.

cascara *n* purgative bark, used as the dry extract in tablets and as liquid extract and elixir for chronic constipation. ⇒ laxatives.

case control study a retrospective study which compares outcomes for a group with a particular condition with those of a control group without the condition.

case manager nurses and member of social services community care team whose role is to assess older or disabled clients living in their own homes, for the amount and type of home care and support they require to live as independently as possible. Each assessment leads to the construction of an individualized 'package of care' for that client, one that may involve intervention by a home carer/care worker, district nurse, occupational therapist and physiotherapist. The case manager's role is that of assessor, coordinator and evaluator of care.

Case Managers Rating Scale (CMRS) used in the assessment of substance misuse. It contains a five point scale, with each point operationally defined in terms of levels of substance misuse and their biopsychosocial consequences.

case study research study that examines data from one case, or a small group of cases.

caseation *n* a form of tissue necrosis characterized by the formation of a soft, cheese-like mass, as occurs in tuberculosis — **caseous** *adj* pertaining to caseation.

casein *n* a protein formed by the action of rennin on caseinogen in milk.

caseinogen *n* the principal protein in milk. The proportion to lactalbumin is much higher than in cow's milk than in human milk. In the presence of rennin it is converted into insoluble casein.

cast *n* **1.** fibrous material and exudate which has been moulded to the form of the cavity or tube in which it has collected; this can be identified under the microscope. **2.** a rigid casing made with plaster of Paris, fibreglass or plastics and applied to a part of the body.

caste in Hinduism practised on the Indian subcontinent, the system of social division and stratification which determines the social position of individuals at birth.

castor oil a vegetable oil which has a purgative action when taken orally. Also used with zinc ointment to protect the skin from excoriation.

castration *n* surgical removal of the testes in the male, or of the ovaries in the female. Castration can be part of the treatment for a hormone-dependent cancer — **castrate** *n, vt.*

CAT *acr* computed axial tomography.

cat cry syndrome ⇒ 'cri du chat' syndrome.

cat scratch fever a viral infection resulting from a cat scratch or bite. There is fever and lymph node swelling about a week after the incident. Recovery is usually complete, although there may be abscess formation.

catabolism *n* the series of chemical reactions in the body in which complex molecules are broken down into simpler ones to release energy. ⇒ anabolism. ⇒ metabolism — **catabolic** *adj* pertaining to catabolism. A feature of the postabsorptive (or fasted state) where fuel molecules are in short supply and body processes are geared to energy release through catabolic reactions. *catabolic state* produced when protein turnover in the body increases during severe illness or injury, such as trauma, sepsis and major surgery. Dietary protein intake is insufficient for the increased amino acid breakdown and the individual is said to be in negative nitrogen balance. ⇒ hypercatabolism. ⇒ nitrogen balance.

catalase *n* an enzyme present in most human cells to catalyse the breakdown of hydrogen peroxide.

catalysis *n* an increase in the rate at which a chemical action proceeds to equilibrium through the medium of a catalyst or catalyser. If there is retardation it is negative catalysis — **catalytic** *adj.*

catalyst *n* a substance that controls or speeds up the rate of a chemical reaction without itself being permanently altered.

cataplexy *n* a condition of sudden muscular rigidity induced by severe mental shock or fear. The patient remains conscious — **cataplectic** *adj.*

cataract *n* an opacity of the crystalline lens or its capsule. It may be congenital, associated with aging, traumatic or due to metabolic defects, in particular diabetes mellitus. *hard cataract* contains a hard nucleus, tends to be dark in colour and occurs in older people. *soft cataract* one without a hard nucleus, occurs at any age, but particularly in the young. Cataract usually develops slowly and when mature is called a *ripe cataract*. Treatment is by removal or destruction of the lens and replacement of focusing ability with an intraocular lens implant, contact lens or spectacles — **cataractous** *adj.*

catarrh *n* chronic inflammation of a mucous membrane with constant flow of a thick sticky mucus. Usually applied to the upper respiratory tract — **catarrhal** *adj.*

catatonia state characterized by immobility or impulsive motor activity. Seen in some types of schizophrenia.

catatonic schizophrenia ⇒ schizophrenia.

catchment area a geographical area which is serviced by e.g. a health centre, a district general hospital, a specialist service such as an oncology unit.

catecholamines *npl* a group of important physiological amines, such as adrenaline (epinephrine), noradrenaline (norepinephrine) and dopamine. They are produced in the body from the amino acid tyrosine and act as neurotransmitters and hormones. They have effects on blood pressure, heart rate, respiratory rate and blood sugar. They have a short half-life and their metabolites are excreted in the urine. Abnormally high levels are secreted by adrenal and other tumours and can be detected in the urine. ⇒ adrenergic. ⇒ phaeochromocytoma.

categorical data data that can be put in categories, e.g. eye colour. ⇒ nominal data. ⇒ ordinal data.

catgut *n* a form of suture material prepared from sheep's intestines.

catharsis *n* 1. in psychology, it describes the purging of emotion through experiencing it deeply. 2. purging or cleansing — **cathartic** *adj.*

catheter *n* a hollow tube of variable length and bore, usually having one fluted end and a tip of varying size and shape according to function. Catheters are made of many substances including soft and hard rubber, gum elastic, glass, silver, other metals and many synthetic materials with a variety of coatings, which may be radiopaque. They have many uses including: introduction of contrast medium in angiography, cardiac catheterization, insufflation of hollow tubes, the introduction of nutrients, administration of drugs, such as cancer chemotherapy, via an arterial catheter and withdrawal/drainage of fluid from body cavities, e.g. urinary bladder. ⇒ arterial cannula. ⇒ catheterization. ⇒ central venous catheter/line. ⇒ Foley catheter. ⇒ self-retaining catheter. ⇒ suprapubic catheter. ⇒ ureteric catheter. ⇒ urinary catheter.

catheterization *n* insertion of a catheter, most usually into the urinary bladder. *cardiac catheterization* a long plastic catheter or tubing is inserted into a vein or artery and manipulated under radiographic guidance into the heart. A catheter passed into the femoral or brachial vein can be passed into the right atrium, ventricle and pulmonary artery, and catheters passed into an artery can be used to access the left side of the heart. Cardiac catheterization can be used for: (a) recording pressures in the heart and measuring cardiac output. ⇒ pulmonary artery flotation catheter. ⇒ pulmonary artery wedge pressure; (b) introducing contrast medium prior to angiography; (c) treatments, such as stent insertion and ablation techniques. ⇒ catheter — **catheterize** *vt*.

cation *n* an ion with a positive electrical charge, such as sodium (Na$^+$). During electrolysis it is attracted to the negative electrode (cathode). ⇒ anion. ⇒ ion.

CATS points *acr* Credit Accumulation and Transfer System. See Box – APEL, APL and CATS.

cauda *n* a tail or tail-like appendage — **caudal, caudate** *adj*.

caudal anaesthetic an anaesthetic administered by means of an approach to the epidural space through the caudal canal in the sacrum.

caul *n* the amnion, instead of rupturing as is usual to allow the baby through, persists and covers the baby's head at birth.

causalgia *n* excruciating neuralgic pain, resulting from physical trauma to a cutaneous nerve.

caustic *adj, n* a substance, usually a strong acid or alkali, that destroys cells and can cause chemical burns. Corrosive or destructive to organic tissue. Used to destroy excess granulation tissue, warts or polypi, e.g. silver nitrate.

cauterize *vt* to cause the destruction of tissue by applying a heated instrument, a cautery — **cauterization** *n*.

cautery *n* an agent or device, e.g. electricity, chemicals or extremes of temperature, which destroys cells and tissues. May be used to destroy diseased tissue or to arrest haemorrhage during surgery.

cavernous *adj* having hollow spaces. *cavernous sinuses* bilateral channels for venous blood, between the sphenoid bone and the dura mater. They drain venous blood from the brain and the orbit. Sepsis in these areas can cause cavernous sinus thrombosis.

cavitation *n* the formation of a cavity, as in pulmonary tuberculosis.

Cavitron *n* proprietary name for an ultrasonic surgical aspirator.

cavity *n* an enclosed area of the body. ⇒ body cavities.

CBA *abbr* cost-benefit analysis.

CCK *abbr* cholecystokinin.

CCPNS *abbr* cell cycle phase nonspecific.

CCPS *abbr* cell cycle phase specific.

CCU *abbr* coronary care unit. ⇒ high dependency unit. ⇒ intensive therapy unit.

CD *abbr* controlled drug.

CDC *abbr* Centres (Centers) for Disease Control and Prevention.

CDH *abbr* congenital dislocation of the hip. ⇒ developmental dysplasia of the hip (DDH).

CD-ROM *abbr* for Compact Disk Read-Only Memory. Used as a storage and distribution device for data and programs that can be read by a PC.

CDS *abbr* Calgary Depression scale.

CEA *abbr* carcinoembryonic antigen.

cell *n* the basic structural unit of living organisms. A mass of protoplasm (cytoplasm) and usually a nucleus within a plasma or cell membrane (see Figure 12A). Some cells, e.g. the erythrocytes, are non-nucleated whereas others, such as voluntary muscle, may be multinucleated. The cytoplasm contains various subcellular organelles – mitochondria, ribosomes and endoplasmic reticulum – that per-

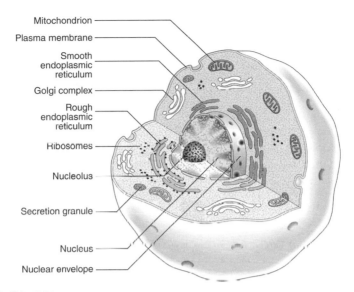

Mitochondrion

Plasma membrane

Smooth endoplasmic reticulum

Golgi complex

Rough endoplasmic reticulum

Ribosomes

Nucleolus

Secretion granule

Nucleus

Nuclear envelope

Figure 12A Cell.

form the metabolic processes of the cell. *cell cycle* the sequence of events occurring within a cell from one mitotic division to the next: interphase, mitosis and cyto-kinesis (see Figure 12B) — **cellular** *adj*.

cell cycle phase nonspecific describes a cytotoxic drug that is active at any time in the cell cycle.

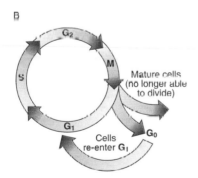

B

G₂

S

M

G₁

G₀

Mature cells (no longer able to divide)

Cells re-enter G₁

Figure 12B Cell cycle. G_1 (gap 1) A variable length period between mitosis and the synthetic phase. S (synthetic) A period of DNA replication and growth. G_2 (gap 2) Preparation for complete separation, growth and maturation. M (mitotic) Period when mitosis and cytokinesis occur. G_0 (quiescent) A 'resting' phase where no division occurs but some cells can rejoin the cell cycle when extra cells are needed, e.g. liver cells after surgical resection. (Adapted from Westwood 1999 with permission.)

cell cycle phase specific describes a cyto-toxic drug that only acts during a specific part of the cell cycle.

cell mediated immunity part of the immune response involving the action of specific T-lymphocytes that destroy abnormal/foreign cells and the release of regulatory chemicals. ⇒ immunity.

cellulitis *n* a diffuse inflammation of the skin and connective tissue, especially the loose subcutaneous tissue. When it occurs in the floor of the mouth it is called Ludwig's angina.

cellulose *n* a polysaccharide found in plant cell walls. It is not digested by humans and provides the nonstarch polysac-charide (NSP dietary fibre) required to increase faecal mass, stimulate peristalsis and reduce transit time.

Celsius the derived SI unit (International System of Units) for temperature. ⇒ centi-grade.

cementum *n* connective tissue that covers the root of a tooth and helps to support it within the socket. ⇒ gomphosis.

censor *n* term employed by Freud to define the resistance which prevents repressed material from readily re-entering the conscious mind from the subconscious (unconscious) mind.

centigrade *n* having one hundred divisions or degrees. Usually applied to the thermometric scale in which the freezing point of water is fixed at 0° and the boiling point at 100°. The centigrade thermometer was first constructed by Celsius (1701–1744). Usually known as Celsius in science and medicine.

centimetre (cm) *n* a unit of length. One hundredth part of a metre.

central cyanosis ⇒ cyanosis.

central limit theorem in research. Sampling distribution becomes more normal as more samples are taken.

central nervous system (CNS) the brain and spinal cord. ⇒ peripheral nervous system.

central processing unit *n* the chip which ultimately controls PC function. ⇒ chip.

Central Sterile Supplies Department (CSSD) an area in which packets are prepared containing the equipment and/or swabs and dressings necessary to carry out particular activities requiring aseptic technique. ⇒ Hospital Sterilization and Disinfection Unit (HSDU).

central tendency statistic averages. In statistics, the tendency for observations to centre around a specific value rather than across the complete range. ⇒ mean. ⇒ median. ⇒ mode.

central venous catheter/line a special catheter inserted into a large central vein via a peripheral vein or by using a skin tunnel. Used in critical care situations for measuring pressures, administering drugs and for infusing hypertonic fluids. It also allows long term vascular access for the administration of nutritional support, drugs (chemotherapy, analgesics and antibiotics) and blood products.

central venous pressure (CVP) *n* measures pressure of blood in the right atrium and can reflect fluid status (see Figure 13). See Box – Central venous pressure.

Centres (Centers) for Disease Control and Prevention (CDC) a federal agency of the United States of America. Sited in Atlanta, it provides services and facilities to investigate, identify, prevent and control disease. Originally only communicable diseases were studied, but it now deals with many other areas, e.g. smoking and disease.

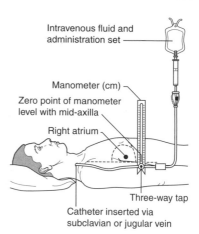

Intravenous fluid and administration set

Manometer (cm)

Zero point of manometer level with mid-axilla

Right atrium

Three-way tap

Catheter inserted via subclavian or jugular vein

Figure 13 Central venous pressure. (Reproduced from Brooker 1998 with permission.)

centrifugal *adj* efferent. Having a tendency to move outwards from the centre, such as nerve impulses from the brain to peripheral structures.

centriole *n* a cell organelle involved in spindle formation during nuclear division. ⇒ mitosis.

centripetal *adj* afferent. Having a tendency to move towards the centre, as the rash in chickenpox.

centromeres *npl* structures that join the double chromosome (2 chromatids) and eventually become arranged along the equator of the spindle during nuclear division. ⇒ mitosis.

centrosome *n* an area near the cell nucleus that contains the centrioles.

cephalalgia *n* pain in the head; headache.

cephalhaematoma *n* a subperiosteal haemorrhage on the head of the infant, usually due to pressure during a long labour. It is delineated by suture lines and is gradually absorbed.

cephalic *adj* pertaining to the head; near the head. *cephalic version* ⇒ version.

cephalocele *n* hernia of the brain; protrusion of part of the brain through the skull.

cephalohaematoma cephalhaematoma.

cephalometry *n* measurement of the living human head.

cephalopelvic pertaining to the size of fetal head and maternal pelvis. *cephalopelvic disproportion* where the fetal head is too

---

Central venous pressure

Central venous pressure (CVP) is used in the clinical setting to reflect fluid status. A central venous catheter (central line) is inserted into a large vein such as the subclavian or internal jugular and progressed until the catheter tip is in or very near the right atrium of the heart. This is an aseptic procedure and a chest X-ray is performed after insertion to check: (a) the correct position of the catheter and (b) that during the procedure the pleura had not been accidentally punctured causing a pneumothorax.

The CVP can be measured using a water manometer or a pressure transducer attached to a monitor. The normal values are 5–12 cm H_2O and 3–9 mm Hg respectively. There are a number of factors in addition to fluid status that can affect the CVP including pulmonary hypertension, right ventricular failure and peripheral vasodilatation. Therefore, CVP should only be interpreted in conjunction with other observations such as heart rate and blood pressure. In addition, the trend in CVP is more meaningful than a single, isolated reading.

---

large or the maternal pelvis is too small to facilitate a vaginal delivery, a caesarian section is needed.

cephalosporins *npl* beta (β)-lactam antibiotics, e.g. cefaclor, ceftazidime etc. They are closely related to the penicillins. Bacterial resistance is a problem and hypersensitivity reactions may occur. Some have a narrow spectrum, but later drugs are wider spectrum.

cerebellar gait ⇒ gait.

cerebellum *n* that part of the brain which lies behind and below the cerebrum. Its chief functions are the coordination of fine voluntary movements and the control of posture — **cerebellar** *adj*.

cerebral *adj* pertaining to the cerebrum. *cerebral compression* arises from any space-occupying intracranial lesion. ⇒ intracranial pressure. *cerebral cortex* thin outer layer of grey matter (cells) *cerebral embolus* blood clot, or rarely air or fat, becomes lodged in the cerebral blood vessels. *cerebral haemorrhage* bleeding into the brain from a ruptured vessel. It results in tissue damage. *cerebral hemisphere* one half of the cerebrum. *cerebral lateralization* in the main the functional areas are duplicated in both hemispheres but others, such as speech, appear on one side only. There is lateralization of other functions. *cerebral palsy* nonprogressive brain damage before the completion of brain development, resulting in mainly motor conditions ranging from clumsiness to severe spasticity. Speech, hearing and vision may be affected. Causes include: hypoxia and birth injury. *cerebral thrombosis* formation of a thrombus within the cerebral circulation. ⇒ cerebrovascular accident.

cerebral perfusion pressure (CPP) *n* an indirect measure of the amount of blood reaching the brain. It is the mean systolic arterial blood pressure minus the intracranial pressure.

cerebrospinal *adj* pertaining to the brain and spinal cord. *cerebrospinal fluid (CSF)* the clear fluid produced by specialized capillaries of the choroid plexus. It circulates in the ventricles of the brain, central canal of the spinal cord and in the subarachnoid space of the cranial and spinal meninges. It protects the brain and facilitates the exchange of substances.

cerebrovascular *adj* pertaining to the blood vessels of the brain. *cerebrovascular accident (CVA)* interference with the cerebral blood flow due to embolism, haemorrhage or thrombosis. Signs and symptoms vary according to the duration, extent and site of tissue damage; there may only be a passing, even momentary, inability to move a hand or foot; weakness or tingling in a limb; stertorous breathing, incontinence of urine and faeces, coma; paralysis of a limb or limbs and speech deficiency (aphasia). ⇒ transient ischaemic attacks.

cerebrum *n* the largest and uppermost part of the brain. The longitudinal fissure divides it into two hemispheres, each containing a lateral ventricle. The internal substance is white matter (fibres), the outer convoluted cortex is grey matter (cells). It contains major sensory and motor areas and is involved with the higher functions of the brain — **cerebral** *adj*.

ceruloplasmin *n* a plasma protein that transports copper around the body.

cerumen *n* ear wax. Sticky yellow-brown substance that helps to trap dust and foreign bodies entering the ear — **ceruminous** *adj* pertaining to cerumen. *ceruminous glands* modified sweat glands, that produce cerumen, sited in the external auditory canal.

cervical *adj* **1.** pertaining to the neck. *cervical collar* a device used to immobilize the neck where cervical spine injury is a possibility, or to maintain position and give support for neck injuries. *cervical rib* (*syn* thoracic inlet syndrome) a supernumerary rib in the cervical region, which may be asymptomatic or it may press on nerves of the brachial plexus. *cervical vertebrae* the seven vertebrae of the neck. ⇒ atlas. ⇒ axis. **2.** pertaining to the cervix (neck) of an organ. Usually of the uterus *cervical amnioscopy* ⇒ amnioscopy. *cervical canal* the lumen of the cervix uteri, from the internal to the external os. *cervical cap* ⇒ diaphragm. *cervical smear* ⇒ Papanicolaou test.

cervical intraepithelial neoplasia (CIN) staging of cellular changes in the cervix uteri that occur prior to the development of carcinoma-in-situ and invasive cancer. Abnormal cells are detected by a smear test and the diagnosis is confirmed by colposcopy and biopsy. CIN1 – mild dysplasia. CIN2 – moderate dysplasia. CIN3 – severe dysplasia, carcinoma-in-situ. ⇒ cone biopsy.

cervicectomy *n* excision of the uterine cervix, usually for cancer. Rarely performed.

cervicitis *n* inflammation of the uterine cervix.

cervix *n* a neck. *cervix uteri, uterine cervix* the neck of the uterus.

cestode *n* tapeworm. ⇒ Taenia.

CF *abbr* cystic fibrosis.

CFT *abbr* complement fixation test.

CFTR gene *abbr* cystic fibrosis transmembrane regulator gene.

Chaga's disease ⇒ trypanosomiasis.

chaining see Box – Chaining.

chalazion *n* Meibomian cyst. A small retention cyst in the eyelid, caused by a blockage of the secretion of the Meibomian glands.

challenging behaviour *n* behaviour which, by the nature of its character, frequency or severity, may seriously threaten the safety of the individual or other people, or behaviour that hinders the integration of the individual into the community by preventing his or her access to various facilities and activities, such as mainstream education. It may be a feature of some forms of learning disability.

chalone *n* a polypeptide hormone-like substance that inhibits rather than stimulates.

chancre *n* the primary syphilitic ulcer, associated with swelling of local lymph nodes. The presence of the chancre with regional adenitis constitutes 'primary syphilis'. The chancre is painless, indurated, solitary and highly infectious.

chancroid *n* (*syn* soft sore) a type of highly contagious, sexually transmitted infection prevalent in warmer climates. Causes multiple, painful, ragged ulcers on the penis and vulva, often associated with bubo formation. Infection is by the bacillus *Haemophilus ducreyi*.

change management see Box – Change management.

Chaining

Chaining is a technique that may be used when helping people with learning disabilities to master complex sequences of behaviour. The idea is to reward each stage of the process so that it sets up a positive link in a whole chain of actions. There are two forms of chaining, forward and backward. Forward chaining means analysing a behaviour such as eating a meal by starting with sitting at an appropriate place, then picking up one utensil, then another etc. On successful accomplishment of each stage the individual receives a reward, praise in the early stages, enjoyment of the food later on. In contrast, backward chaining starts at the end of a complex chain of behaviour and uses rewards to create links with the stage before. So when teaching dressing, one might begin by encouraging the individual to perform only the final step, putting on the second shoe and then rewarding with praise and an admiring glance in a mirror to see the process completed. Next time the encouragement is to put on the first shoe and then the second with the same reward at the end of the chain. The advantage of this approach is that the overall goal is usually a strong reward and is seen as achievable from beginning to end.

Change management
We all experience change in every aspect of our lives – it is a normal phenomenon. The principles of change management originate from the discipline of psychology, and can be applied to either the individual, or to an organization. Over the past years, the pace and level of change within healthcare contexts have been unprecedented. Whilst this is going on, the service has to be maintained and also new initiatives introduced.

Effective change management is an important part of the role of both managers and clinical professionals. Change management is more than 'just getting something done differently'. It requires that the individuals involved take a different approach to doing something – i.e. it requires a change in their attitudes towards the initiative.

Managing change effectively requires skills of effective communication, active listening, negotiation, planning and the ability to be open, flexible and to be able to consider the 'what if' scenario. This means to think through 'what if x happened. . . .' etc. It is important also to consider the effect of the change you are managing on other people – the stakeholders. Including any stakeholders in your early thoughts and plans for the change is a positive step, which often saves time at a later stage.

---

character *n* **1.** a numeral, letter or any other mark that can be seen on the computer screen or printed. **2.** the sum total of the known and predictable mental characteristics of an individual. *character change* denotes change in the form of conduct to one foreign to the patient's natural disposition, e.g. indecent behaviour in a hitherto respectable person. Common in the psychoses.

charcoal *n* the residue after burning organic substances at a high temperature in an enclosed vessel. Used in medicine for its adsorptive and deodorant properties. Activated charcoal pads may be used for preventing odour from malodorous discharging wounds. ⇒ deodorants.

Charcot's joint neuropathic joint disease. Characterized by destructive joint changes associated with less pain than would be expected. It is seen in syringomyelia or tabes dorsalis (locomotor ataxia). *Charcot's triad* manifestation of nystagmus, intention tremor and staccato speech in multiple sclerosis.

Charles' law a gas law stating that at a constant pressure the volume of a specific mass of gas is directly proportional to the temperature. Also called Gay-Lussac's law.

charts *npl* documents on which diverse data, such as TPR (temperature, pulse and respiration), blood pressure, intake and output, central venous pressure, haemoglobin oxygen saturation, relief of pressure, and medications, are recorded; accepted as part of nursing documentation.

CHC *abbr* Community Health Council.

CHD *abbr* coronary heart disease. ⇒ ischaemic heart disease.

cheilitis *n* inflammation of the lip. *angular cheilitis* the term used when the inflammation is confined to the two angles of the lips.

cheiloplasty *n* plastic surgery repair of a defect to the lip.

cheilorrhaphy *n* operation to repair a cleft lip or a lacerated lip.

cheilosis *n* maceration at the angles of the mouth; fissures occur later. May be due to vitamin B deficiency.

cheiropompholyx *n* symmetrical eruption of skin of hands (especially fingers) characterized by the formation of tiny vesicles and associated with itching or burning. On the feet the condition is called podopompholyx. → eczema. → pompholyx

chelating agents soluble organic compounds that combine with certain metallic ions to form complexes that can be safely eliminated from the body by the kidneys. Used as treatment for poisoning or overload, e.g. desferrioxamine for iron and penicillamine for copper. ⇒ haemochromatosis. ⇒ thalassaemia. ⇒ Wilson's disease.

chemonucleolysis *n* injection of an enzyme, usually into an invertebral disc, for dissolution of same — **chemonucleolytic** *adj*.

chemopallidectomy *n* the destruction of a predetermined section of globus pallidus by chemicals.

chemoprophylaxis use of drugs to prevent infection, e.g. antimalarial drugs, antibiotics for certain surgical procedures and for people who have been in contact with meningitis.

chemoreceptor *n* a cell or specialized sensory nerve ending able to respond to chemical stimuli, such as pH and oxygen levels in the blood, taste and smell.

chemoreceptor trigger zone (CTZ) *n* an area in the brain involved in the vomiting reflex. It responds to chemical stimuli, e.g. morphine, cytotoxic drugs and endogenous toxins such as produced with uraemia. ⇒ vomiting.

chemosis *n* an oedema or swelling of the bulbar (occular) conjunctiva — **chemotic** *adj.*

chemotaxis *n* movements of a cell (e.g. leucocyte) or an organism in response to chemical stimuli; attraction towards a chemical is *positive chemotaxis*, repulsion is *negative chemotaxis* — **chemotactic** *adj.*

chemotherapy *n* use of a specific chemical agent to arrest the progress of, or eradicate, disease in the body without causing irreversible injury to healthy tissues. Chemotherapeutic agents are administered mainly by oral, intramuscular and intravenous routes, and are distributed usually by the bloodstream. The term is used mainly in relation to the treatment of cancer with cytotoxic chemotherapy. Some of these agents may also be given via the intra-arterial route or directly into a body structure, e.g. the bladder. ⇒ alkylating agents. ⇒ antimetabolites. ⇒ antitumour antibiotics. ⇒ cytotoxic. ⇒ vinca alkaloids. See Box – Chemotherapy (cytotoxic).

chenodeoxycholic acid ⇒ bile acids. Used to disperse certain types of gallstones.

Cheyne-Stokes respiration abnormal breathing pattern in which breathing waxes and wanes. It is characterized by repeated cycles where depth of breathing increases followed by decreasing depth and a period of apnoea. It is usually a feature of serious disruption to the respiratory centres, such as may occur where blood chemistry is altered.

CHF *abbr* congestive heart failure.

chi one of several terms used in complementary medicine to describe the individual's innate energy. ⇒ Qi energy.

CHI *abbr* Commission for Health Improvement.

chi-square statistic (χ^2) statistical technique that analyses the relationship between expected frequency and the actual frequency of data obtained. A test of statistical significance used to assess the probability of results occurring by chance. ⇒ nonparametric tests.

chiasma *n* an X-shaped crossing or decussation. *optic chiasma* ⇒ optic — **chiasmata** *pl.*

chickenpox *n* (*syn* varicella) an infection with the varicella/zoster virus (VZV), primarily affecting children. The incubation period is 12–21 days. There is mild pyrexia and a skin rash. Successive crops of vesicles appear first on the trunk and develop through various stages to pustules that scab and usually heal without leaving scars, but scarring is possible.

chief cells *npl* stomach cells that secrete pepsinogen; the proteolytic enzyme precursor. Also known as zymogen cells.

Chemotherapy (cytotoxic)

Cytotoxic chemotherapy refers to the use of drugs to kill cancer cells. Chemotherapy is increasingly used to shrink a tumour prior to surgery or radiotherapy or to mop up microscopic cancer cells afterwards. It may be used to achieve cure or remission, or to alleviate the symptoms of advanced disease within a palliative care context. There are five groups of chemotherapy drugs that all have slightly different effects but ultimately serve to disrupt DNA synthesis preventing cellular replication. Chemotherapy has a non-discriminatory affect on healthy and cancer tissue so it relies on combination treatment, scheduling and timing of therapy to maximize the response, without causing life-threatening toxicity. As the tumour develops and cells are exposed to chemotherapy they may develop resistance so that alterations in treatment are required (Peterson and Goodman 1997). The patient's response to chemotherapy is determined by the type of cancer cell involved, the size of the tumour at presentation, developing drug resistance, dose reduction and treatment delays as a result of treatment related toxicity. The nursing role is to provide information to the patient and their family, monitoring, proactive management of potential toxicity and support.

References
Peterson J, Goodman M 1997 Principles of chemotherapy. In: Gates R A, Fink R M (eds) Oncology Nursing Secrets. Hanley and Belfus, Philadelphia, pp 39–55

chikungunya *n* a mosquito-borne viral haemorrhagic fever. Occurs in Africa.

chilblain *n* (*syn* erythema pernio) congestion, inflammation and swelling attended with severe itching and burning sensation in reaction to cold. Usually affects the toes, fingers or ears.

child abuse ⇒ abuse.

childbirth *n* the act of giving birth. *natural childbirth* giving birth without medical intervention.

child mishandling ⇒ abuse.

Child protection officer/co-ordinator a suitably qualified and experienced individual (with a nursing, health visiting or social work background) employed by social services to oversee/co-ordinate the interagency child protection activities in a particular location. In addition, many NHS trusts employ a designated nurse with a child protection role. ⇒ child protection register. ⇒ emergency protection order.

child protection register in the UK, a register of children deemed to be at risk of neglect, abuse etc. The register is administered by social services but is used in interagency child protection work. ⇒ child protection officer/co-ordinator.

Children Act 1989 an Act of Parliament (became law in 1991) which clearly defines the rights of children, their protection, welfare and care.

Children's Charter introduced by the UK Government in 1996 it aimed to ensure that children and their parents had a better understanding of their rights in terms of health care, such as having treatment and care explained, and certain expectations, e.g. being on a ward specifically for children and young people.

chip *n* an integrated circuit where electronic components are formed from a single silicon wafer. They control a range of functions from simple tasks to extremely complex procedures. ⇒ central processing unit.

chiropodist *n* an obsolete term for podiatrist.

chiropody *n* ⇒ podiatry.

chiropractic *n* a technique of manipulation of the spine, based on the principle that problems with the vertebral alignment may result in muscular, organic, neural or sensory problems caused by aberrations in the functioning of the nervous system.

chiropractor *n* a person who uses chiropractic. The practitioner aims to identify areas of the spine affecting normal movement and, if manipulation is appropriate, to attempt to restore normal movement. The underlying principle is that mechanical function or dysfunction is directly related to biological function and thus health and illness.

Chlamydia *n* micro-organisms of the genus Chlamydia. They are intracellular parasites and have features common to both bacteria and viruses. Chlamydial infections are treated with antibiotic drugs, e.g. tetracyclines and erythromycin. *Chlamydia psittaci* infects birds and causes psittacosis in humans. ⇒ ornithosis. *Chlamydia trachomatis* causes trachoma. The organism commonly infects the genitourinary tracts of both sexes. In men it causes nonspecific urethritis, epididymitis and prostatitis. Infected women may be asymptomatic, but infection can lead to salpingitis, pelvic inflammatory disease (PID) and infertility. Infants infected during birth can develop serious eye infections and pneumonia. ⇒ lymphogranuloma venereum. ⇒ ophthalmia neonatorum.

chloasma *n* pigmentation of the skin, especially the face. *chloasma gravidarum* brown pigmentation during pregnancy. It may also be associated with the use of some oral contraceptives.

chlorhexidine *n* a bactericidal solution used as a disinfectant on human tissues. Its main uses are for preoperative skin preparation and for hand decontamination, in an alcoholic handrub, as part of infection control. ⇒ handwashing.

chloride *n* a salt of hydrochloric acid. A major extracellular anion. *chloride shift* a chemical reaction whereby chloride ions enter the red blood cell, to restore electrical balance, as hydrogen carbonate (bicarbonate) ions move into the blood as part of carbon dioxide transport.

chlorine *n* a greenish-yellow, irritating gaseous element. Powerful disinfectant, bleaching and deodorizing agent in the presence of moisture, when nascent oxygen is liberated. Used chiefly as hypochlorites or other compounds which slowly liberate active chlorine.

chloroform *n* a heavy liquid, previously used as a general anaesthetic. Much used in the form of chloroform water as a flavouring and preservative in aqueous mixtures.

choanae *npl* funnel-shaped openings. ⇒ nares — **choanal** *adj*.

choanal atresia congenital abnormality where there is no communication between the nose and the nasopharynx. Bilateral atresia presents as a respiratory emergency at birth.

chocolate cyst an endometrial cyst containing altered blood. The ovaries are the most usual site.

choked disc ⇒ papilloedema.

cholaemia *n* the presence of bile in the blood — **cholaemic** *adj*.

cholangiography *n* the radiographic examination of the biliary ducts (hepatic, cystic and common bile ducts). Can be performed: (a) after oral or intravenous administration of contrast medium; (b) by direct injection at operation to detect any further stones in the ducts; (c) during or after operation by way of a T-tube in the common bile duct; (d) by means of an injection via the skin on the anterior abdominal wall and the liver, when it is called percutaneous transhepatic cholangiography. ⇒ endoscopic retrograde cholangiopancreatography — **cholangiographically** *adv*.

cholangiohepatitis *n* inflammation of the liver and bile ducts.

cholangitis *n* inflammation of the bile ducts.

cholecalciferol *n* vitamin D_3. It is essential as a precursor for the active forms of vitamin D responsible for calcium homeostasis. Deficiency causes rickets in children and osteomalacia in adults.

cholecystectomy *n* surgical removal of the gallbladder. Usually advised for gallstones, inflammation and occasionally for growths. *laparoscopic cholecystectomy* surgical removal of the gallbladder via the minimally invasive transperitoneal approach, using specially designed instruments, diathermy and laser, usually under video control.

cholecystenterostomy *n* literally, the establishment of an artificial opening (anastomosis) between the gallbladder and the small intestine.

cholecystitis *n* inflammation of the gallbladder.

cholecystoduodenal *adj* pertaining to the gallbladder and duodenum as an anastomosis between them.

cholecystoduodenostomy *n* the establishment of an anastomosis between the gallbladder and the duodenum.

cholecystography *n* radiographic examination of the gallbladder after administration of contrast medium — **cholecystographically** *adv*.

cholecystojejunostomy *n* an anastomosis between the gallbladder and the jejunum. Performed for obstructive jaundice due to growth in head of pancreas.

cholecystokinin (CCK) *n* a regulatory peptide hormone secreted by the duodenal mucosa. It stimulates gallbladder contraction and relaxation of the sphincter of Oddi with the release of bile into the duodenum and the secretion of pancreatic enzymes. Cholecystokinin also inhibits gastric secretion and motility.

cholecystolithiasis *n* the presence of stone or stones in the gallbladder.

cholecystostomy *n* a surgically established fistula between the gallbladder and the abdominal surface; used to provide drainage, in empyema of the gallbladder or occasionally after the removal of stones.

cholecystotomy *n* incision into the gallbladder.

choledochoduodenal *adj* pertaining to the bile ducts and duodenum, e.g. *choledochoduodenal fistula*.

choledochoduodenostomy *n* an anastomosis between the common bile duct and the duodenum.

choledochography *n* cholangiography.

choledocholithiasis *n* the presence of a stone or stones in the bile ducts.

choledocholithotomy *n* surgical removal of a gallstone from the common bile duct.

choledochostomy *n* drainage of the common bile duct using a T-tube, usually after exploration for a gallstone.

choledochotomy *n* incision into the common bile duct.

cholelithiasis *n* the presence of stones in the gallbladder or bile ducts.

cholera *n* acute enteritis caused by the bacterium *Vibrio cholerae*. Endemic and epidemic in Asia and Africa where it is associated with faecal contamination of water, overcrowding and poor hygiene conditions. It is characterized by severe diarrhoea (rice-water stools) accompanied by agonizing cramp and vomiting which lead to dehydration, electrolyte imbalance and severe collapse. Mortality rates are high where patients do not have access to adequate fluid and electrolyte replacement.

choleric temperament *n* one of the four classical types of temperament, hasty and prone to emotional outbursts.

cholestasis *n* obstruction to the free flow of bile. It is characterized by severe jaundice, pruritus, metallic taste in the mouth, dark urine and pale (clay-coloured) stools. *intrahepatic cholestasis* where the small bile ducts within the liver are obstructed, for example in hepatitis, cirrhosis or metastatic cancer. *extrahepatic cholestasis* when a larger duct, such as the common bile duct, is blocked by a gallstone or a cancer in the pancreas — **cholestatic** *adj*.

cholesteatoma *n* collection of abnormally sited squamous epithelium in the middle ear. *acquired cholesteatoma* usually seen in a chronically diseased ear. If untreated, erodes bone and may lead to intracranial complications, such as cerebral abscess or facial nerve palsy. *congenital cholesteatoma* squamous epithelial cysts that can arise anywhere within the temporal bone. Aetiologically this has no relationship with acquired cholesteatoma — **cholesteatomatous** *adj*.

cholesterol *n* a sterol found in many tissues. It is an important constituent of cell membranes and is the precursor of many biological molecules, such as steroid hormone, vitamin D and bile salts. High levels in the blood have, however, been linked with the formation of some types of gallstones and arterial disease. ⇒ hypercholesterolaemia.

cholesterosis *n* abnormal deposition of cholesterol.

cholic acid ⇒ bile acids.

choline *n* organic base found as a constituent of many important biological molecules, such as phosphoglycerides and acetylcholine. Important in lipid metabolism and in the formation of plasma (cell) membranes. Rich dietary sources include: offal and egg yolk.

cholinergic *adj* applied to nerves which use acetylcholine as their neurotransmitter. Includes nerves which cause voluntary skeletal muscle to contract, all parasympathetic nerves and a few postganglionic sympathetic nerves. ⇒ adrenergic *ant*. *cholinergic crisis* severe muscle weakness and respiratory failure resulting from overtreatment with anticholinesterase drugs. *cholinergic receptors* receptors sites on the effector structures innervated by parasympathetic and voluntary motor nerves. The receptors are termed nicotinic or muscarinic according to how they respond to acetylcholine. They may be excitory or inhibitory depending on their location. Both muscarinic and nicotinic receptors are further subdivided, e.g. muscarinic: M1, M2 and M3.

cholinesterase *n* an enzyme which hydrolyses and inactivates the neurotransmitter acetylcholine into choline and acetic acid at nerve endings.

choluria *n* biliuria — **choluric** *adj*.

chondritis *n* inflammation of cartilage.

chondroblast *n* immature blast cell that forms cartilage. ⇒ fibroblast. ⇒ haemocytoblast. ⇒ osteoblast.

chondrocostal *adj* pertaining to the costal cartilages and ribs.

chondrocyte *n* a cartilage cell.

chondrodynia *n* pain in a cartilage. Also called chondralgia.

chondrolysis *n* dissolution of cartilage — **chondrolytic** *adj*.

chondroma *n* a benign, slow-growing tumour of cartilage; tends to recur after removal.

chondromalacia *n* softening of cartilage.

chondrosarcoma *n* malignant growth of cartilage — **chondrosarcomatous** *adj*.

chondrosternal *adj* pertaining to the rib cartilages and sternum.

chorda tympani a branch of the facial nerve supplying anterior two-thirds of the tongue, which may be damaged during middle ear surgery.

chordae tendineae *n* the thin cords which stabilize the atrioventricular valves by attaching them to the papillary muscle of the heart.

chordee *n* 1. a congenital structural defect of the penis. 2. painful penile erection associated with urethritis.

chorditis *n* inflammation of the spermatic or vocal cords.

chordotomy ⇒ cordotomy.

chorea *n* describes irregular and jerky movements, beyond the patient's control. Chorea may follow childhood rheumatic fever *Sydenham's chorea*, but usually results from a disorder or drug affecting the basal nuclei. In adults, chorea is a feature of the inherited condition Huntington's disease and the administration of drugs that include the phenothiazines and L-dopa used in parkinsonism — **choreal, choreic** *adj*.

choreiform *n* resembling chorea.

choriocarcinoma *n* (*syn* chorionepithelioma) a malignant tumour of chorionic cells which may develop following abortion or evacuation of a hydatidiform mole or rarely following a normal pregnancy. Metastatic spread, e.g. to lung or brain, is common, but treatment with cytotoxic drugs offers a very high cure rate. ⇒ human chorionic gonadotrophin.

chorion *n* forms from the trophoblast; it develops into the placenta and the tough outer membrane forming the embryonic or fetal sac. *chorion biopsy* ⇒ chorionic villus sampling — **chorial, chorionic** *adj chorionic gonadotrophin (hCG)* a hormone produced by the trophoblast cells and later the chorion. It maintains the corpus luteum until placental hormone secretion is sufficiently advanced. The presence of hCG in blood or urine is used to confirm pregnancy. High levels may indicate choriocarcinoma (chorionepithelioma). *chorionic villi* projections from the chorion from which the fetal part of the placenta is formed. Through the chorionic villi, diffusion of gases, nutrients and waste products, from the maternal to the fetal blood and vice versa, occurs.

chorionepithelioma ⇒ choriocarcinoma.

chorionic villus sampling (CVS) *n* also known as chorion or chorionic villus biopsy. A prenatal screening test for chromosomal and other inherited disorders. Samples of fetal tissue are obtained via the cervix for the detection of genetic abnormalities during early pregnancy (around 11 weeks). Although the test can be done at an earlier stage and provides a rapid diagnosis, research has shown it to be less safe than amniocentesis, and decreased accuracy means that retesting may be required. If CVS is performed too early in pregnancy there is a risk that the developing limbs will be malformed.

chorioretinitis *n* (*syn* choroidoretinitis) inflammation of the choroid and retina.

choroid *n* the middle pigmented, vascular coat of the posterior five-sixths of the eyeball, continuous with the iris in front. It lies between the sclera and the retina, and prevents the passage of light rays — **choroidal** *adj*.

choroid plexus *n* the specialized capillaries derived from pia mater and covered by ependymal cells, which line the ventricles of the brain. They produce cerebrospinal fluid.

choroiditis *n* inflammation of the choroid. *Tay's choroiditis* degenerative change affecting the retina around the macula lutea.

choroidocyclitis *n* inflammation of the choroid and ciliary body.

choroidoretinal *adj* pertaining to the choroid and the retina.

choroidoretinitis *n* ⇒ chorioretinitis.

Christmas disease an inherited defect of blood coagulation, where blood clotting factor IX is deficient. Also called haemophilia B.

Christmas factor *n* factor IX in coagulation. Also known as antihaemophilic factor B.

chromatid *n* one of the strands resulting from the duplication of chromosomes during nuclear division. ⇒ mitosis.

chromatin *n* the thread-like nuclear material that forms the chromosomes. It consists of DNA and proteins. *sex chromatin* in females one of the X chromosomes becomes inactivated and appears in a somatic cell nucleus as a mass known as the Barr body.

chromatography analytical techniques. Consists of several methods of separating different gaseous or dissolved substances which include: gel filtration chromatography, ion exchange chromatography and gas chromatography.

chromosomes *npl* the genetic material present in the nucleus of the cell. They appear as microscopic threads within the cell nucleus as the cell prepares to divide. Chromosomes consist of strands of DNA molecules known as genes. Humans have 23 pairs (46) in each somatic cell: 22 pairs of autosomes and 1 pair of sex chromosomes (females have XX and males have XY). The exception are the mature gametes (oocytes and spermatozoa) with half the usual number (haploid number) as a result of reduction division. This means that the set of 23 unpaired chromosomes inherited from each parent results in an individual with 46 chromosomes (diploid number). The male gamete determines genetic sex of the embryo by whether it contributes a Y chromosome (genetic male) or an X chromosome (genetic female). Genetic material is not exclusive to the nucleus. It is present in some organelles, such as the mitochondria, where it codes for metabolic processes and can be reponsible for the inheritance of conditions, such as optic nerve atrophy. ⇒ meiosis. ⇒ mitosis — **chromosomal** adj.

chronic adj lingering, lasting, opposed to acute. The word does not imply anything about the severity of the condition. chronic fatigue syndrome ⇒ myalgic encephalmyelitis. chronic heart failure ⇒ congestive heart failure. chronic leukaemias ⇒ leukaemia. ⇒ chronic obstructive pulmonary disease.

chronic obstructive pulmonary disease (COPD) n group of respiratory diseases where airway resistance is increased with impaired airflow, e.g. chronic bronchitis and pulmonary emphysema. It is characterized by dyspnoea, expiratory problems, wheeze, cough and poor gaseous exchange. Often linked to smoking tobacco and atmospheric pollution. Complications include: pneumothorax, respiratory failure or cor pulmonale. Those affected may be severely disabled and require oxygen therapy for many hours a day. ⇒ asthma.

chronic wounds npl wounds such as pressure ulcers and leg ulcers. They often have delayed healing and more complex aetiology than acute wounds. ⇒ wound healing.

chronological age a person's actual age in years.

chronotherapy n administration of treatment, such as drugs or radiotherapy, at the most efficacious time.

chunking in psychology, it describes the organization and coding of chunks of information that allows us to increase the effective capacity of short term memory, which can only store around seven items of information.

Chvostek's sign excessive twitching of the face on tapping the facial nerve: a sign of tetany.

chyle n milky (containing fats) fluid formed from chylomicrons within the lymphatic lacteals of the intestinal villi — **chylous** adj.

chylomicron n tiny particles formed from triacylglycerols (triglycerides), cholesterol and lipoproteins within the cells of the intestinal mucosa following the absorption of digested fat. They enter the lymphatic lacteal to form chyle. ⇒ lipoprotein.

chylothorax n leakage of chyle from the thoracic duct into the pleural cavity.

chyluria n chyle in the urine — **chyluric** adj.

chyme n acidic liquid formed from partially digested food in the stomach. Its acidity controls the pylorus so that chyme is ejected at frequent intervals, thus ensuring that the duodenum is not deluged. ⇒ enterogastric reflex — **chymous** adj.

chymotrypsinogen n an inactive precursor of a proteolytic enzyme secreted by the pancreas; it is activated by trypsin. Used therapeutically to reduce soft tissue inflammation.

cicatrix n ⇒ scar.

cilia npl 1. the eyelashes. 2. microscopic hair-like projections from certain epithelial cells. Membranes containing such cells, e.g. those lining the respiratory tract and uterine tubes, are known as ciliated membranes — **ciliary, ciliated, cilial** adj.

ciliary adj hair-like. ciliary body a specialized structure in the eye connecting the anterior part of the choroid to the iris; it is composed of the ciliary muscles and processes. ciliary muscles fine hair-like muscle fibres that control accommodation. ciliary processes are projections on the undersurface of the choroid which are attached to the ciliary muscles. Contain blood vessels which produce aqueous humor. ⇒ Schlemm's canal.

ciliary dysfunction syndromes *npl* characterized by a reduction in ciliary action and hence mucociliary clearance from the bronchi. May be congenital or acquired. ⇒ bronchiectasis. ⇒ Kartagener's syndrome. ⇒ Young's syndrome.

ciliary dyskinesia abnormal movement of the cilia, particularly in the respiratory tract. ⇒ Kartagener's syndrome.

Cimex *n* a genus of insects of the family Cimicidae. *Cimex lectularius* is the common bedbug, parasitic to man and bloodsucking.

CIN *abbr* cervical intraepithelial neoplasia.

CINAHL *abbr* Cumulative Index to Nursing and Allied Health Literature.

circadian rhythm rhythm with a periodicity of approximately 24 h. May refer to hormone secretion, urine production, etc.

circinata *n* ⇒ tinea.

circinate *adj* in the form of a circle or segment of a circle, e.g. the skin eruptions of late syphilis, ringworm, etc.

circle of Willis circular anastomosis of arteries supplying the brain. Located at the base of the brain and formed from the internal carotid, vertebral and basilar arteries.

circulation *n* passage in a circle. Usually means circulation of the blood, i.e. the passage of blood from heart to arteries to capillaries to veins and back to heart. *circulation of bile* ⇒ enterohepatic circulation. *circulation of cerebrospinal fluid (CSF)* takes place from the ventricles of the brain, where it circulates to the cisterna magna, central canal of the spinal cord and in the subarachnoid space of the cranial and spinal meninges. It is absorbed into the blood in the cerebral venous sinuses. *collateral circulation* ⇒ collateral. *coronary circulation* the system of vessels which supply oxygenated blood to the myocardium and return venous blood to the heart. ⇒ coronary arteries. ⇒ coronary sinus. *extracorporeal circulation* ⇒ extracorporeal. *fetal circulation* ⇒ fetal. *hepatic portal circulation* venous blood from the digestive tract, pancreas and spleen, which is rich in nutrients and hormones, passes through the liver, via the hepatic portal vein, prior to its return to the systemic circulation. *lymph circulation* lymph is collected from the tissue spaces and transported in the lymphatic capillaries, vessels and through lymph nodes to the two main ducts (right lymphatic duct and thoracic duct) that return lymph to the venous system via connections with the great veins in the neck. *pulmonary circulation* deoxygenated blood leaves the right ventricle via the pulmonary artery which branches to each lung. The artery branches again within the lung to eventually form capillary networks around the alveoli. Gaseous exchange occurs: oxygen into the blood and carbon dioxide into the alveoli, and oxygenated blood returns to the left atrium via the pulmonary veins. *systemic circulation* oxygenated blood returned to the left atrium passes into the left ventricle and is pumped out to the body via the aorta. It moves through smaller arteries to the capillary networks where nutrients, oxygen and waste diffuse between the blood and cells. The blood, with high levels of waste, returns via veins eventually forming the venae cavae which empty into the right atrium — **circulate** *vi, vt*.

circumcision *n* excision of the prepuce or foreskin of the penis, usually for religious or cultural reasons. The operation is sometimes required for phimosis or paraphimosis. *female circumcision* excision of the clitoris, labia minora and labia majora. The extent of cutting varies from country to country. The simplest form is clitoridectomy; the next form entails excision of the prepuce, clitoris and all or part of the labia minora. The most extensive form, infibulation, involves excision of clitoris, labia minora and labia majora. The vulval lips are sutured together but total obliteration of the vaginal introitus is prevented by inserting a piece of wood or reed to preserve a small passage for urine and menstrual fluid. These procedures are illegal in many countries.

circumcorneal *adj* around the cornea.

circumoral *adj* surrounding the mouth. *circumoral pallor* a pale appearance of the skin around the mouth, in contrast to the flushed cheeks. A characteristic of scarlet fever — **circumorally** *adv*.

circumvallate *adj* surrounded by a raised ring, as the large circumvallate papillae at the base of the tongue.

cirrhosis *n* hardening of an organ. There are diffuse degenerative changes in the tissues. *cirrhosis of liver* fibrosis and structural damage leads to loss of liver cells (hepatocytes) and obstruction to the hepatic portal circulation. The causes include: viral hepatitis, alcohol misuse, drugs and metabolic disorders. It is characterized by hepatomegaly, jaundice, ascites, splenomegaly, oesophageal varices, hepatic encephalopathy, endocrine problems, circulatory changes, digital clubbing and a tendency to bleed and bruise — **cirrhotic** adj.

cirsoid adj resembling a tortuous, dilated vein (varix). *cirsoid aneurysm* a tangled mass of pulsating blood vessels appearing as a subcutaneous tumour, usually on the scalp.

cisterna n any closed space serving as a reservoir for a body fluid. *cisterna chyli* dilated portion of the thoracic duct which collects lymph. *cisterna magna* is a subarachnoid space in the cleft between the cerebellum and medulla oblongata — **cisternal** adj.

cisternal puncture ⇒ puncture.

citizen advocacy n ⇒ advocacy.

citric acid n an organic acid present in citrus and soft fruit. *citric acid cycle* ⇒ Krebs'cycle.

citrus fruit includes lemons, limes, oranges and grapefruit. An important source of vitamin C in the prevention of scurvy.

civil law n law relating to noncriminal matters. ⇒ litigation. *civil action* proceedings brought in the civil courts. *civil wrong* act or omission which can be pursued in the civil courts by the person who has suffered the wrong. ⇒ tort.

CJD abbr Creutzfeldt-Jakob disease.

claim form n the commencement of a civil action. Previously called a writ.

claimant n person who brings legal action to obtain compensation or other redress for an alleged civil wrong. Previously known as the plaintiff.

class a sociological term that describes the socioeconomic variations between groups that account for differences in the level of affluence and influence. ⇒ social class.

claudication n limping caused by interference with the blood supply to the legs. The cause may be spasm or disease of the vessels themselves. In *intermittent claudication* the patient experiences severe pain in the calves when walking but is able to continue after a short rest. A symptom of arterial insufficiency.

claustrophobia n a form of mental disturbance in which there is an irrational fear of enclosed spaces — **claustrophobic** adj.

clavicle n the collar-bone. Articulates with the sternum and scapula. Acts as an anterior brace for the shoulder — **clavicular** adj.

clavus n a corn.

claw-foot adj, n (syn pes cavus) a deformity where the longitudinal arch of the foot is increased in height and associated with clawing of the toes. It may be acquired or congenital in origin.

claw-hand n claw-shaped deformity due to flexor spasm followed by contraction of the muscles flexing the fingers; often due to ulnar nerve damage.

cleanser n, adj (describes) a cleansing agent. Term often applied to drugs of the cetrimide type, which have both antiseptic and cleaning properties, and so are valuable in removing grease, dirt, etc from skin and wounds, and scabs and crusts from skin lesions.

clearance the ability of the kidney to clear the blood of a particular substance. *renal clearance* measurement of glomerular filtration rate and kidney function by calculating the volume of blood cleared of a substance, e.g. creatinine, in a given time, usually one minute.

cleft lip a congenital defect where the top lip fails to fuse in the midline, resulting in a fissure extending from the margin of the lip to the nostril; may be single or double, and is often associated with cleft palate.

cleft palate congenital defect where the developing palate fails to fuse in the midline. The cleft may vary, but, when complete, extends through both soft and hard palates into the nasal cavity. Often associated with cleft lip.

cleidocranial dysostosis n rare hereditary condition inherited as an autosomal dominant trait. It is characterized by a failure of ossification in the cranial bones and a partial or total absence of clavicles.

client n the person to whom a (nursing) service is supplied. Community nurses, including mental health nurses in particular, prefer this word, as it does not have the illness connotation of the word 'patient'.

Clifton Assessment Procedures for the Elderly a series of tests which measure cognitive function as well as behaviour.

climacteric *n* in the female, describes a period of time during which ovarian activity declines and eventually ceases. It generally occurs between the mid forties to mid fifties. The cessation of menstruation is a distinct event during the climacteric. ⇒ menopause.

clinical *adj* pertaining to a clinic or the observation, nursing and treatment of patients. *clinical equipment* used in the treatment or nursing of patients. ⇒ clinical nurse specialist (CNS). ⇒ clinical thermometer.

clinical audit part of quality assurance. A critical and systematic analysis of the quality of clinical care and treatment. It includes diagnostic procedures, treatment, resource use and outputs including quality of life for the individual concerned.

clinical effectiveness ⇒ effectiveness.

clinical governance see Box – Clinical governance.

clinical guidelines *npl* systematically developed statements which assist the clinical practitioner and patient in making decisions about a specific aspect of care. ⇒ effectiveness. ⇒ evidence-based practice.

clinical nurse specialist (CNS) a nurse who develops skills in relation to a particular group of patients, e.g. those with a stoma or with diabetes, or a particular area of nursing, e.g. infection control or intravenous therapy. ⇒ higher level practice. ⇒ specialist nursing practice.

clinical risk management ⇒ risk management. See Box – Risk management.

clinical supervision see Box – Clinical supervision.

clinical thermometer traditionally, glass and mercury thermometers of various types were used. These have mostly been replaced by safer alternatives, such as electronic probes and single-use thermometers. ⇒ body temperature. ⇒ clinical thermometry. ⇒ temperature.

Clinical Governance

A term for the framework introduced following the English White Paper *The New NHS: Modern, Dependable* (Department of Health 1997) within which all NHS organizations are accountable for their services, and are required to have in place an active programme of continuous quality improvement within an overall, coherent framework of cost effective service delivery. It embraces the process of clinical audit as a quality improvement tool. Clinical governance requires that good practice is identified and built upon; that there is in place in all NHS organizations a programme to manage risk; that mistakes are learnt from, free from a culture of blame; and that lifelong learning is encouraged in order that professionals may be supported and developed in their role of delivering quality care.

Clinical supervision

Clinical supervision is defined as "a method of assuring the delivery of high quality health care" (UKCC 1996). The process of clinical supervision is aimed to assist practitioners to develop skills, knowledge and professional values throughout their careers, and implies the need to reflect and measure risk.

The United Kingdom Central Council (UKCC) prefers no single method of supervision, and they suggest developing a model of clinical supervision by selecting and using elements of recognized models to suit local and individual requirements. The ultimate aim of clinical supervision is to enable individuals to develop a deeper understanding of what it is to be an accountable practitioner. Currently, clinical supervision is not a statutory requirement for nurses and health visitors, though of course, continuing professional development through PREP is a requirement.

The benefits of clinical supervision encompass the practitioner, patients/clients, and the overall contexts and environments in which care is delivered, and the NHS Executive (1995) set out six medium term priorities, one of which is "develop NHS organizations as good employers with particular reference to workforce planning, education and training, employment policy and practice, the development of team work, reward systems, staff utilization and staff welfare".

References
NHS Executive 1995 Priorities and Planning Guidance for the NHS: 1996/97. Department of Health, London
UKCC 1996 Position Statement on Clinical Supervision for Nursing and Health Visiting. UKCC, London

clinical thermometry traditionally, measuring the body temperature was accomplished by using a clinical thermometer (glass/mercury); research supports an oral placement time of 2–3 minutes. Increasingly, glass/mecury thermometers are being replaced by electronic thermometers which use a probe in the same way as a clinical thermometer; many of them register in as short a time as 3 seconds, without sacrificing accuracy. Electronic thermometers are available for routine oral, rectal and tympanic membrane measurement of temperature. Chemical crystals, made into a band, can be applied to the skin of the forehead, and change colour as they register the temperature. These are especially useful for babies, children and older people. A type of chemical dot thermometer is also available for oral use. Placed in the sublingual socket, it takes only seconds to register. The flexibility of the stem can help with efficient sublingual placing, even in the presence of dentures. Since it is a single-use item it cannot contribute to hospital-acquired infection. ⇒ body temperature.

clinician *n* in a nursing/midwifery/health visiting context, the word is used to designate those individuals who work with patients/clients as opposed to those who indirectly serve patients, e.g. managers and educators. Also used to describe all those involved directly with patient care, such as chiropodists, dentists, dieticians, doctors, medical laboratory scientific officers, optists, physiotherapists, radiographers and speech and language therapists. ⇒ practitioners.

clitoridectomy *n* the surgical removal of the clitoris. ⇒ female circumcision.

clitoriditis *n* inflammation of the clitoris.

clitoris *n* a small erectile organ situated just below the mons veneris at the junction anteriorly of the labia minora, homologous to the penis. It contains abundant nervous tissue, is very sensitive and involved in the female sexual response.

cloaca *n* in osteomyelitis, the opening through the involucrum which discharges pus — **cloacal** *adj*.

clonic *adj* ⇒ clonus.

clonus *n* a series of intermittent muscular contractions and relaxations. A feature of some types of epilepsy. ⇒ tonic — **clonicity** *n*.

closed urinary drainage system a means of draining urine via a self-retaining catheter into a drainage bag, which has a nonreturn valve at the inlet and may have a drainage tap as an outlet. The capacity of the bag may be 2 litres, for those patients who are in bed and/or are prescribed bladder irrigation. There are also a variety of body-worn bags with a capacity of 350–750 mL to which a 2 litre bag may be attached at night 'piggy back'. The 2 litre bag is discarded in the morning. The leg bag may be worn for up to 7 days without disconnection from the catheter.

Clostridium *n* a genus of spore-forming Gram-positive anaerobic bacilli found as commensals of the gut of animals and man and as saprophytes in the soil. Many species are pathogenic because of the exotoxins produced, e.g. *Clostridium tetani* (tetanus), *C. botulinum* (botulism), *C. perfringens* (gas gangrene), *C. difficile* (pseudomembranous colitis) — **clostridial** *adj*.

clothing, modification of may be required by people with a physical or learning disability, frail and older people and those who are incontinent, in order to promote independent living. The Disabled Living Foundation's Clothing Advisory Service will answer enquiries about clothing and dressing.

club-foot *n* ⇒ talipes.

clubbing enlargement of the terminal phalanges of the fingers and sometimes the toes. It is usually associated with chronic cardiovascular and respiratory conditions, but may also be a feature of liver cirrhosis, thyrotoxicosis and inflammatory bowel disease.

clumping *n* agglutination.

Clutton's joints joints which show symmetrical swelling, usually painless. The knees are often involved. Associated with congenital syphilis.

CMRS *abbr* Case Managers Rating Scale.

CMV *abbr* 1. cytomegalovirus. 2. controlled mandatory ventilation.

CNS *abbr* 1. central nervous system. 2. clinical nurse specialist.

coagulase *n* an enzyme produced by some bacteria of the genus Staphylococcus: it coagulates plasma. It can be used to classify staphylococci as coagulase-negative or coagulase-positive.

coagulation one of four overlapping processes involved in haemostasis. Coagulation (clotting) involves a series of complex reactions that use enzyme cascade amplification to initiate the formation of a fibrin clot to arrest bleeding. There are two pathways/systems: intrinsic (initiated by the exposure of factor XII and platelets to collagen and platelet breakdown) and extrinsic (dependent on tissue damage and thromboplastin release), which converge to follow a common final pathway. Coagulation is initiated when platelets break down, tissue is damaged and thromboplastins are released. Various factors are involved in coagulation: I – Fibrinogen, II – Prothrombin, III – Tissue thromboplastin, IV – Calcium ions, V – Labile factor (proaccelerin), VII – Stable factor (proconvertin), VIII – Antihaemophilic factor (AHF), IX – Christmas factor, X – Stuart-Prower factor, XI – Plasma thromboplastin antecedent, XII – Hageman factor and XIII – Fibrin-stabilizing factor. The final common pathway involves the conversion of inactive prothrombin to thrombin, the active enzyme. Thrombin reacts with the soluble protein fibrinogen to form insoluble fibrin, which forms a network of strands in which blood cells are trapped to form the clot. (See Figure 14). ⇒ fibrinolysis. ⇒ haemostasis. ⇒ platelet plug.

coal tar the black substance obtained by the distillation of coal. It is used in various topical preparations for psoriasis and eczema.

coalesce *vi* to grow together; to unite into a mass. Often used to describe the development of a skin eruption, when discrete areas of affected skin coalesce to form large areas of a similar appearance — **coalescent** *adj.*

coarctation *n* contraction, compression, stricture, narrowing; applied to a vessel or canal. *coarctation of the aorta* a congenital narrowing of the aorta in the region of the ductus arteriosus (a structure of the fetal circulation).

coarse tremor violent trembling.

cobalamins *npl* molecules containing a cobalt atom and four pyrrole units. A constituent of substances having vitamin B_{12} activity. ⇒ cyanocobalamin.

cobalt (Co) *n* an essential trace element, utilized as a constituent of vitamin B_{12} (cobalamin). Required for healthy red

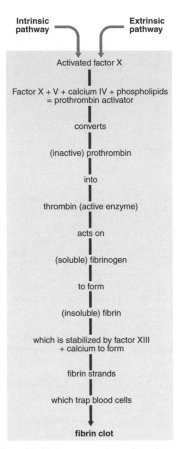

Figure 14 Final common pathway of coagulation. (Reproduced from Brooker 1998 with permission.)

blood cell production and proper neurological function.

cocaine *n* a powerful local anaesthetic obtained from the leaves of the coca plant. Controlled drug under the Misuse of Drugs Act (1971) and Misuse of Drugs Regulations (1985). It is addictive and subject to considerable criminal misuse. *crack cocaine* a highly potent and addictive form.

cocainism *n* mental and physical degeneracy caused by a morbid craving for, and excessive use of, cocaine. ⇒ addiction. ⇒ drug dependence. ⇒ dependence.

coccidiodomycosis *n* infection caused by the spores of the fungus *Coccidioides immitis*. Seen in the southern United

States and Central and South America. It has similarities with tuberculosis and is treated with antifungal drugs, e.g. amphotericin.

coccus *n* a spherical or nearly spherical bacterium — **coccal, coccoid** *adj.*

coccyalgia *n* pain in the region of the coccyx.

coccygectomy *n* surgical removal of the coccyx.

coccyx *n* the last part of the vertebral column formed from four or five fused vestigial tail bones. It is triangular in shape and curved slightly forward. It is cartilaginous at birth, ossification being completed at about the 30th year — **coccygeal** *adj* pertaining to the coccyx. *coccygeal injuries* commonly occur following slipping on a step, and result in pain and difficulties with sitting. Recovery may take months, and injections of local anaesthetic and corticosteroids or surgical removal may be necessary. *coccygeal plexus* formed from part of the 4th sacral, the 5th sacral and coccygeal spinal nerves. It innervates the pelvic floor and the skin over the coccyx.

cochlea *n* a spiral fluid-filled canal resembling a snail shell, in the anterior part of the bony labyrinth of the ear. It contains the organ of Corti and the nerve endings of the vestibulocochlear nerve — **cochlear** *adj.*

code of practice *n* guidelines setting out how a healthcare professional should fulfil their role, duties, obligations and responsibilities, such as those produced by the statutory bodies set up to regulate the registration and work of healthcare professionals.

codon *n* in genetics, the three complementary bases carried by messenger RNA (mRNA) concerned with the transcription stage of protein synthesis.

coeliac *adj* relating to the abdominal cavity; applied to arteries, veins, nerves and a plexus. *coeliac disease* (*syn* gluten-induced enteropathy) due to intolerance to the protein gluten in barley, wheat, oats and rye, it being gliadin (part of gluten) that is the harmful substance. Sensitivity occurs in the villi of the small intestine, and produces the malabsorption syndrome. It presents in infants under two years of age and usually within six months of weaning with cereal foods. Affected infants are irritable and unhappy. They pass high volume pale stools due to undigested fat and have abdominal distention. Eventually there is failure to thrive and anaemia. The condition may present during adult life for the first time and is characterized by diarrhoea, weight loss and anaemia. The management includes a gluten-free diet and supplementation with minerals and vitamins.

coenzyme *n* an enzyme activator, such as those derived from the B vitamins, e.g. nicotinamide adenine dinucleotide (NAD), involved in many oxidation-reduction reactions.

coffee ground vomit vomit containing blood, which, in its partially digested state, resembles coffee grounds. Indicative of upper gastrointestinal bleeding. ⇒ haematemesis.

cognition *n* a general term used to describe all the psychological processes by which people become aware of and gain knowledge about the world in which they live. ⇒ affection. ⇒ conation — **cognitive** *adj* pertaining to cognition. ⇒ cognitive behaviour therapy. ⇒ cognitive therapy.

cognitive behaviour therapy an approach to the psychological treatment of many mental health problems. It uses techniques from both the cognitive and behavioural view of therapy. The emphasis is on a meditational model and makes use of both classical and operant conditioning to assist clients to deal with their problems.

cognitive therapy an approach to the psychological treatment of depression, anxiety and anxiety-related disorders, eating disorders and schizophrenia. It focuses on, and is effective through, correcting the patient's cognitive dysfunctions, such as errors in thinking and poor problem-solving.

cohabitation when a couple live together in a close relationship without marriage.

cohort *n* a group of people who have some common characteristic, e.g. age. ⇒ cohorting.

cohort study a research study that investigates a population that shares a common feature, such as year of birth.

cohorting an infection control measure whereby people in hospital with the same infection are grouped together.

coitus *n* insertion of the erect penis into the vagina; the act of sexual intercourse or copulation. *coitus interruptus* removal from the vagina of the penis before ejaculation of semen as a means of contraception. The method is considered unsatisfactory as it is not only unreliable but can lead to sexual problems — **coital** *adj.*

cold abscess ⇒ abscess.

cold sore oral herpes.

colectomy *n* excision of part or the whole of the colon.

colic *n* severe pain resulting from periodic spasm in an abdominal organ. *biliary colic* ⇒ biliary. *intestinal colic* abnormal peristaltic movement of an irritated gut. *painter's (lead) colic* spasm of intestine and constriction of mesenteric vessels, resulting from lead poisoning. *renal colic* ⇒ renal. *uterine colic* ⇒ dysmenorrhoea — **colicky** *adj.*

coliform *adj* a word used to describe any of the enterobacteria, such as *Escherichia coli.*

colitis *n* inflammation of the colon. May be acute or chronic, and may be accompanied by ulcerative lesions. *ulcerative colitis* ⇒ inflammatory bowel disease.

collagen *n* the main protein constituent of white fibrous tissue. ⇒ elastin. The *collagen diseases* are characterized by inflammation of unknown aetiology affecting collagen and small blood vessels. They involve autoimmune responses and include dermatomyositis, systemic lupus erythematosus (SLE), polyarteritis nodosa, rheumatoid arthritis and scleroderma — **collagenic, collagenous** *adj.*

collapse *n* **1.** the 'falling in' of a hollow organ or vessel, e.g. collapse of lung from change of air pressure inside or outside the organ. **2.** physical or nervous prostration.

collapsing pulse Corrigan's pulse. The water-hammer pulse of aortic regurgitation characterized by a surge of arterial distension followed by sudden emptying and absence of force.

collar-bone *n* the clavicle.

collateral *adj* accessory or secondary. *collateral circulation* an alternative route provided for the blood by secondary blood vessels when a primary vessel is blocked.

Colles' fracture fracture at the lower end of the radius following a fall on the outstretched hand. The backward displacement of the hand produces the typical 'dinner fork' deformity. A common fracture of older women with osteoporosis.

collodion *n* an inflammable liquid that forms a clear flexible film when applied to the skin. Previously used as a protective dressing.

colloid *n* a glue-like noncrystalline substance; diffusible but not soluble in water; unable to pass through an animal membrane. Therapeutic uses include colloid solutions used intravenously to increase extracellular volume. Some drugs can be prepared in their colloidal form, such as gold. *colloid degeneration* mucoid degeneration of tumours. *colloid goitre* abnormal enlargement of the thyroid gland, due to the accumulation in it of viscid, iodine-containing colloid.

colloidal gold test also known as the Lange test. Carried out on cerebrospinal fluid to assist the diagnosis of neurosyphilis.

coloboma *n* a congenital fissure or gap in the eyeball or one of its parts, particularly the uvea — **colobomata** *pl.*

colon *n* the large bowel, extending from the caecum to the rectum. In its various parts it has appropriate names: ascending, transverse, descending and sigmoid colon. ⇒ flexure. *spasmodic colon* ⇒ megacolon — **colonic** *adj.*

colonization *n* the establishment of micro-organisms in a specific environment, such as a body site with minimal or no response. There is no disease or symptoms, but colonization leads to the creation of a reservoir of micro-organisms that may cause infection — **colonize** *vt.*

colonoscopy *n* use of a flexible fibreoptic colonoscope to view the colonic mucosa. A short colonoscope is used to examine the sigmoid and the left-hand side of the colon, whereas a long colonoscope is required to examine the entire colon. During colonoscopy it is possible to take biopsy specimens and remove polyps — **colonoscopically** *adv.*

colony *n* a mass of bacteria which is the result of multiplication of one or more organisms. A colony may contain many millions of individual organisms and may become macroscopic; its physical features are often characteristic of the species.

colony stimulating factors (CSF) *npl* growth factors that stimulate blood stem cells to produce a particular cell line; for example, granulocyte CSF (G-CSF) promotes the production of neutrophils.

colorectal *adj* pertaining to the colon and the rectum.

colostomy *n* a surgically established fistula between the colon and the surface of the abdomen; this acts as an artificial anus.

colostrum *n* the fluid secreted by the breasts in late pregnancy and during the first 3 days after parturition, before the formation of true milk is established. A source of maternal antibodies, more protein, vitamins and minerals, but less fat and lactose than true milk.

colotomy *n* incision into the colon.

colour blindness applies to various conditions in which certain colours are confused with one another. Inability to distinguish between reds and greens is called daltonism.

colpectomy *n* excision of the vagina.

colpitis *n* inflammation of the vagina.

colpocele *n* protrusion of prolapse of either the bladder or rectum so that it presses on the vaginal wall.

colpocentesis *n* withdrawal of fluid from the vagina, as in haematocolpos.

colpohysterectomy *n* removal of the uterus through the vagina. More commonly called vaginal hysterectomy.

colpoperineorrhaphy *n* the surgical repair of an injured vagina and deficient perineum.

colpophotography *n* a photograph of the cervix taken in women who have had an abnormal smear result. ⇒ colposcopy.

colporrhaphy *n* surgical repair of the vagina. An anterior colporrhaphy repairs a cystocele and a posterior colporrhaphy repairs a rectocele.

colposcope *n* an endoscopic instrument that utilizes low-powered magnification to examine the cells of the vagina and cervix by direct observation — **colposcopically** *adv*.

colposcopy *n* an examinatiom of the vagina and cervix using a colposcope to detect abnormal cells and give laser treatment. The cervix may be painted with acetic acid and iodine to highlight abnormal cells. ⇒ cervical intraepithelial neoplasia.

colposuspension operation the vagina is suspended from the ileopectineal ligament. Carried out for severe stress incontinence of urine.

colpotomy *n* incision of the vaginal wall. A posterior colpotomy drains an abscess in the rectouterine pouch through the vagina.

coma *n* a state of altered consciousness where the individual is insensible and does not respond to painful stimuli. Causes include: brain pathology, trauma, drugs, alcohol and metabolic disturbances. ⇒ Glasgow coma scale.

comatose *adj* in a state of coma.

comedone, comedo *n* caused by accumulations of sebum and cell debris blocking the outlet of a hair follicle in the skin; a feature of acne vulgaris. Comedones may be closed (whiteheads) or open (blackheads), which have a black colour because of pigmentation.

commensals *npl* parasitic micro-organisms adapted to grow on the skin and mucous surfaces of the host, forming part of the normal flora. Commensals cause no harm in their correct location and may have beneficial effects. They are potentially pathogenic in other locations, such as the bowel commensal *Escherichia coli* which causes wound and urinary tract infection.

Commission for Health Improvement *n* a body appointed by the Secretary of State for Health with statutory powers to inspect and support the implementation of clinical governance arrangements in Health Authorities and NHS trusts. Their remit also includes targeted support when requested by organizations with a specific problem, and in more serious situations they may intervene by direction of the Secretary of State or at the request of Health Authorities, NHS Trusts or Primary Care Groups/Trusts.

commissioning see Box – Commissioning.

commissure *n* 1. connecting structure, such as a bundle of nerves connecting different sides of the brain or spinal cord. 2. the point at which two structures meet, such as the corner of the lips, eyelids or labia.

> **Commissioning**
> Commissioning is a multi-faceted process – the aim of which is to ensure that a given population has an appropriate level of service provision. The first stage is to make an assessment of the needs of the given population, then from that assessment, priorities are drawn up, taking into account the overall national policy guidance from government. When this process is completed, an appropriate range of services are purchased from relevant providers. The final stage in the commissioning process is that of evaluation. Organizations/bodies responsible for commissioning have the responsibility of not only evaluating the clinical outcomes of the services, but also of evaluating the outcomes in relation to value for money (VFM). Normally, where available, it is expected that only evidence-based interventions should be purchased. Commissioning organizations are also responsible for ensuring resources are used effectively by all users – be they the public or the clinicians.

Committee on Safety of Medicines the body that monitors drug safety and advises the UK licensing authority about quality, efficacy and safety of medicines. ⇒ yellow card reporting.

common law *n* that derived from decisions made by judges, case law, judge made law.

communicable disease *n* a microbial disease that is transmissible directly or indirectly from one person or animal to another.

communicating *v* the exchange of information between at least two people. It is usually accomplished by using language: verbal, which can be spoken, written, word processed/typed, printed or displayed on a screen; or nonverbal, which transmits attitudes, values and beliefs relevant to the information exchanged. When two people do not speak the same language, miming can be used to exchange information, or an interpreter may be required. Some profoundly deaf people and those with learning disability communicate by sign language. ⇒ British sign language. ⇒ Makaton. ⇒ sign language. People with a partial hearing loss are usually helped to continue communicating by the use of a hearing aid and lip reading. After e.g. a stroke or head injury, the person may have language difficulties. ⇒ aphasia. ⇒ body language. ⇒ dysarthria.

community a social group determined by geographical boundaries and/or common values and interests. Community has also come to imply shared relationships, lifestyles, and a greater frequency and intimacy of contact among those who live in a community. For example, the Chinese community in China town and the East End community in London, where the common interests, values and bonds maintain cohesive networks. *community care* term applied to the care of people in the community (outside hospital). Such care is delivered by health and social care professionals and unpaid carers such as family and friends. The community concept hence circumscribes the idea of primary health care and nursing practice. The community or primary care setting is increasingly being recognized to be at the forefront of health services development and delivery. ⇒ community nurse. ⇒ Health Action Zone. ⇒ Health Improvement Programme. ⇒ inequalities in health. ⇒ primary healthcare team. ⇒ social exclusion unit. ⇒ specialist community practitioner.

community development whole-community initiatives that enable individual communities to assess their needs, such as for health, and decide on what action should be taken by the community. *community development health worker* a person appointed locally to facilitate the process of community development by assisting individuals to acquire the skills needed to take an action plan forward.

Community Health Council (CHC) a statutory and independent body comprising lay members of the community who monitored local health services and represented the views of local consumers to the relevant health authorities. Replacement of Community Health Councils by statutory patient forums, patient advocacy liaison service in NHS and primary care trusts, and the relevant local government authority is planned for 2002 depending on the necessary legislation.

community nurse generic term which describes those nurses based in the community and concerned with the health, well-being and care of people in their homes and other community settings. Their role also includes health promotion, health education and the prevention of illness and disability. Community nurses may be e.g. health visitors, public health nurses, district nurses, community psychiatric nurse (CPN) or learning disability nurses, community children's nurses, practice nurses, family planning nurses or school nurses. ⇒ specialist community practitioner.

community occupational therapist *n* one employed by a social services department to work in the community, typically providing services to clients in their own homes and other community settings.

comparative study a study that compares two populations.

compartment syndrome compromise of circulation and function of tissue within a closed space (usually a muscle compartment) due to increased pressure, leading to muscle necrosis. ⇒ Volkmann's ischaemic contracture.

compatibility *n* suitability; congruity. The power of a substance to mix with another without unfavourable results, such as blood crossmatched prior to transfusion, tissue for transplant or two medicines. ⇒ blood groups — **compatible** *adj*.

compensation *n* 1. a mental mechanism, employed by a person to cover up a weakness, by exaggerating a more socially acceptable quality. 2. the state of counterbalancing a functional or structural defect, e.g. cardiac compensation, where the heart enlarges by hypertrophy to maintain an adequate cardiac output when heart disease is present.

compensatory techniques *npl* used by occupational therapists to compensate for physical or cognitive deficits, such as teaching different ways of completing tasks or by adapting the environment or equipment, e.g. the use of velcro fastening instead of shoe laces.

competence/competencies see Box – Competence/competencies.

complaints management the procedures and protocols in place to manage complaints that arise from any aspect of care or treatment. ⇒ ombudsman.

Competence/competencies

It has arguably been taken for granted that nursing and midwifery are professions which encompass competence within the workforces. However, currently the issue of competence is a major topic, and is being debated and decided upon through a number of initiatives that include: the UKCC Commission for Education (1999) *Fitness for Practice*; the NHS Executive (1999) *Agenda for Change*; and the Department of Health (1999) *Making a Difference*.

All of these documents discuss and promote the development of nursing competencies, spanning pre-registration nursing and midwifery programmes, and practitioners who work at higher levels (see Higher level practice). Reference is also made to the uses of National and Scottish Vocational Qualifications (S/NVQs) for non-professional carers.

The available literature demonstrates that there are a number of definitions for the word 'competence', (WHO 1998, Hogston 1993), but the UKCC Commission for Education (1999) uses the term competence, in the context of preregistration programmes, to "describe the skills and ability to practice safely and effectively without the need for direct supervision".

On the whole, the notion is that an individual, a health care assistant, a nursing student, a qualified practitioner working at higher level, demonstrates competence to an assessor through normal working practices and the compilation and presentation of a portfolio of evidence (see personal professional profile).

The theme of competence is not restricted to the UK, and members of the European Community are debating similar issues, striving to define the term, and to define competencies for nursing which are acceptable to all members of the European Union.

References
Commission for Education 1999 Fitness for Practice. UKCC, London
Department of Health 1999 Making a Difference. The Stationery Office, London
Hogston R 1993 From competent novice to competent expert: a discussion of competence in the light of postregistration education and practice project (PREPP). Nurse Education Today 13(3):341–344
NHS Executive 1999 Agenda for Change. NHSE, Leeds
World Health Organization 1998 Learning to Work Together for Health. Report of a WHO study group on multiprofessional education for health personnel; a team approach. WHO, Geneva

complement a group of more than twenty proteins present in the plasma, which, when activated, enhance the immune response, inflammation and bacteriolysis. They act through a cascade where one substance activates the next in the sequence and so on. (See Figure 15). *complement fixation test (CFT)* serological test where the fixation of complement is used to detect the presence of specific antigen-antibody complexes.

complemental air the extra air that can be drawn into the lungs by deep inspiration.

complementary feed a bottle feed given to an infant to complement breast milk, if this is an insufficient amount. Now generally accepted to interfere with the establishment of lactation.

complementary medicine see Box – Complementary medicine. ⇒ integrated medicine.

complete abortion ⇒ abortion.

complex *n* a series of emotionally charged ideas, repressed because they conflict with ideas acceptable to the individual, e.g. Oedipus complex, Electra complex.

compliance ⇒ patient compliance.

complication *n* in medicine, an accident or second disease arising in the course of a primary disease.

compos mentis of sound mind. Having mental capacity, i.e. mentally competent, is the preferred term.

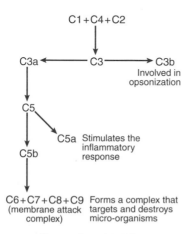

$$C1 + C4 + C2$$

C3a ← C3 → C3b
Involved in opsonization

C5

C5a Stimulates the inflammatory response

C5b

C6+C7+C8+C9 Forms a complex that (membrane attack targets and destroys complex) micro-organisms

C = complement protein

Figure 15 Complement cascade (simplified). (Adapted from Hinchliff et al 1996 with permission.)

compound *n* a substance composed of two or more elements, chemically combined in a definitive proportion to form a new substance with new properties. *compound fracture* ⇒ fracture.

comprehension *n* the understanding of ideas and their meaning and the relationships between them.

compress *n* usually refers to a folded pad of gauze or other material used to stop bleeding or apply pressure, medication, heat, cold or moisture. Used to reduce inflammation, swelling or pain, such as a cold compress on the forehead may relieve headache.

compression *n* the state of being compressed. The act of pressing or squeezing together. ⇒ intermittent pneumatic compression. *compression bandage/therapy* used in the management of venous leg ulcers to increase venous return and reduce venous hypertension. Compression stockings are used to prevent venous leg ulcers occurring where there is venous insufficiency, or to reduce the risk of deep vein thrombosis following surgery or immobility. ⇒ antiembolic hose. *compression fracture* ⇒ fracture.

compromise *n* in psychiatry, a mental mechanism whereby a conflict is evaded by disguising the repressed wish to make it acceptable in consciousness.

compulsion *n* in psychiatry, an urge to carry out an act recognized to be irrational. Resisting the urge leads to increasing tension which is only relieved by carrying out the act.

computed axial tomography (CAT) ⇒ computed tomography.

computed tomography (CT) computer-constructed imaging technique of a thin horizontal slice through the body, derived from X-ray absorption data collected during a circular scanning motion. See Box – Computed tomography.

computer language the form in which computer programs are written. ⇒ BASIC. ⇒ C. ⇒ Java. ⇒ Pascal.

computer memory the electronic storage areas which store the data that the computer is processing and the program which is running. PC's have two types of memory. ⇒ RAM. ⇒ ROM. Powerful computers with considerable memory can use complex programs and handle data

Complementary medicine

Complementary medicine refers to a range of therapeutic modalities currently perceived as adjuncts to conventional medicine. These include: acupuncture, homeopathy, yoga, osteopathy or aromatherapy. More recently the term *integrated medicine* has been promoted implying a fusion between allopathic and complementary systems of health care. This is not to subsume one form of medicine within another but proffers a new form of health care embodying the best of two differing world views in order to promulgate health and well-being.

Such therapies present a multidimensional perception of health and well-being. This is broadly based upon a premise that health represents a harmonious state of being, involving a conscious awareness and balanced interaction between an individual's mind, body, emotional well-being, spirit and the environment in which they live. Care of a person is tailored to meet specific individual needs by recognizing the interaction and impact of each of those dimensions upon health and well-being. Complementary medicine also affords value to the healing potential of the therapeutic relationship between client and therapist (Rankin-Box 1995, 2001).

Complementary therapies are rooted in a world view that integrates one with another by suggesting that time and energy are intrinsically related as various aspects of the same phenomena. Many therapies share a perception of some form of universal energy that is present in all forms of life. This energy may manifest at a submolecular and molecular level to subtly influence cellular, emotional, spiritual and environmental energy. Thus therapies may be referred to as energy medicine or energetic treatments (Graham 1999).

Imbalances in one or more dimensions of an individual's existence may result in an energy imbalance or illhealth at some level. Complementary therapies aim to rebalance or reharmonize differing energy dimensions in the human body by stimulating the body's own innate predisposition towards health and well-being. It is also postulated that some form of reciprocal energy exchange may occur between client and therapist, which may facilitate the healing process.

References

Graham H 1999 Complementary Therapies in Context: The psychology of healing. Jessica Kingsley Publishers, London

Rankin-Box D (ed) 1995 The Nurses' Handbook of Complementary Therapies. Churchill Livingstone Edinburgh

Rankin-Box D (ed) 2001 The Nurse's Handbook of Complementary Therapies, 2nd edn. Baillière Tindall, Edinburgh

Computed tomography

Computed tomography (CT or CAT) imaging was developed in 1972 by Godfrey Hounsfield. Unlike plain X-ray films the CT tube rotates around the patient, scanning in multiple directions. Opposite arrays of radiation detectors then measure the extent of absorption. Computer processing the reconstruction produces a series of 'slices' through the body, depicting bone and soft-tissue structures. CT has the advantages of improved sensitivity, excellent definition of structures and organs, and also has the ability to display slices of anatomy without superimposition.

In recent years spiral CT has been introduced which is capable of imaging a volume in a single breath-hold, thus reducing breathing artifacts and examination times. CT is fast and readily available and is often the first line investigation for stroke (cerebrovascular accident) and head and spinal trauma. It is also useful for imaging the chest, abdomen and pelvis, musculoskeletal, central nervous and vascular systems.

Patient preparation is dependent on the area under investigation, and patients may need to be fasted, or require administration of contrast media (which improves the delineation of structures within the body). Therefore it is important that the CT department is informed beforehand if the patient has a history of diabetes, asthma, or allergies, as these may be contraindications to the administration of contrast media.

Further reading

Romans L E 1995 Introduction to computerized tomography. Williams and Wilkins, Baltimore

Sutton D 1998 Radiology and imaging for medical students. 7th edn. Churchill Livingstone, Edinburgh.

very quickly. Work must still be saved onto a disk before the computer is switched off as RAM memory only holds data whilst the computer is working.

computer virus *n* a program installed maliciously. Viruses copy automatically and generally destroy or disrupt data, but some are harmless.

conation *n* part of the mental processes – the will, desire and volition. The conscious tendency to action. One of the three aspects of mind, the others being cognition and affection.

concentric having a common centre or point. *concentric muscle work* shortening of a muscle to draw its attachments closer together and produce movement at a joint. The quadriceps group of muscles work concentrically to straighten the knee. ⇒ eccentric muscle work.

concept *n* the abstract idea or image of the properties of a class of objects.

conception *n* the creation of a state of pregnancy: impregnation of the oocyte by a spermatozoon. *assisted conception* ⇒ assisted fertility/conception — **conceptive** *adj*.

conceptual framework for nursing a group of concepts which are defined and organised in such a way that they describe the author's interpretation of the highly complex activity called nursing. The framework provides the matrix in which the selected concepts are related to each other, thus providing a way of 'thinking about nursing'.

conceptualizing *n* the mental processes involved in developing and continually refining a concept.

concretion *n* a deposit of hard material; a calculus.

concurrent audit open chart audit. A type of nursing audit where care in progress is assessed and evaluated by examination of charts and nursing records. ⇒ audit.

concussion *n* a violent jarring or shaking, e.g. from a blow; the term is usually applied to the brain. It interferes with brain function and may cause: altered consciousness, headache, dizziness, pallor, vomiting and visual problems. ⇒ Glasgow coma scale. ⇒ neurological assessment.

conditioned reflex a reflex in which the response occurs, not to the sensory stimulus which caused it originally, but to another stimulus which the subject has learned to associate with the original stimulus; it can be acquired by training and repetition. In Pavlov's classic experiments, dogs learned to associate the sound of a bell with the sight and smell of food; even when food was not presented, salivation occurred at the sound of a bell.

conditioning *n* the encouragement of new (desirable) behaviour by modifying the stimulus/response associations. *classical conditioning* where the conditioned reflex occurs in response to a neutral stimulus. ⇒ conditioned reflex. *operant conditioning* the term used when there is a programme to reward a response (or withold a reward) each time it occurs, so that, given time, it occurs more (or less) frequently. ⇒ counterconditioning. ⇒ deconditioning.

condom *n* a thin latex sheath worn over the penis that prevents conception and reduces the spread of sexually transmitted infections (STIs). *female condom* a polyurethane tube that fits inside the vagina to provide contraception and protection against STIs.

condom urinary drainage used for males suffering urinary incontinence. It comprises application to the penis of a modified condom which has a tube attached to its base, via which urine escapes into a body-worn drainage bag which has a clamped outlet at its base to facilitate emptying. ⇒ closed urinary drainage system.

conduction *n* 1. the passage of heat, light, or sound waves through suitable media. 2. the transmission of electrical impulses within the body, such as nerve impulses.

conductor *n* a substance or medium which transmits heat, light, sound, electric current, etc. The words bad, good or non-conductor designate the degree of conductivity.

condyle *n* round projection at the end of some bones, e.g. tibia.

condyloma *n* wart-like or papillomatous growth. *condylomata acuminata* acuminate (pointed) viral warts found on the genitalia and/or on the skin of the perianal region. *condylomata lata* highly infectious, moist, flat papules found in moist areas of the body (vulva, anus, axilla, etc) as a manifestation of secondary syphilis — **condylomatous** *adj*.

cone biopsy *n* excision of a cone-shaped part of the cervix. Used in the treatment of certain stages of CIN. Also known as a conization.

cones *npl* photoreceptors found in the retina. They function in bright light to give high definition colour vision. ⇒ rod.

confabulation *n* a symptom common in confusional states when there is impairment of memory for recent events. The gaps in the patient's memory are filled in with fabrications of his own invention, which nevertheless he appears to accept as fact. Occurs in senile and toxic confusional states, cerebral trauma and Korsakoff's psychosis/syndrome.

confidence interval in statistics, a level, e.g. 95%, that indicates the level of confidence that the test result, e.g. sample mean, will fall within a specified range.

confidentiality *n* a legal and professional requirement to protect all confidential information concerning patients and clients obtained in the course of professional practice, and make disclosures only with consent, where required by the order of a court, or by the law, or where [they] can justify disclosure in the wider public interest.

conflict *n* in psychiatry, presence of two incompatible and contrasting wishes or emotions. When the conflict becomes intolerable, repression of the wishes may occur. Mental conflict and repression form the basic causes of many neuroses.

confluence *n* becoming merged; flowing together; a uniting, as of neighbouring pustules.

conformity a tendency to change views and/or behaviour to better fit the prevailing social norms in response to social pressure.

confounding factors outside factors, apart from the variables already taken into account, that distort the results of research.

confusion *n* a mental state which is out of touch with reality and associated with a clouding of consciousness, disorientation and loss of decision-making ability. Can occur in many illnesses but particularly associated with postepileptic fits, cerebral arteriosclerosis, dementia, infection, trauma and severe toxaemia. *acute confusional state (ACS)* sudden and acute onset of confusion which, when seen in older people, may be mistaken for dementia. It usually has an acute medical cause, such as anaemia, cerebral vascular accident or chest or urinary tract infection, but may be due to incorrect medication or recent bereavement or loss. ⇒ polypharmacy.

chronic confusional state has a slow onset and may be due to a chronic, unnoticed condition such as hypothyroidism.

congenital *adj* of abnormal conditions, present at birth, often genetically determined. ⇒ genetic. Existing before or at birth, usually associated with a defect or disease, e.g. developmental dysplasia of the hip (DDH) (previously known as congenital dislocation of the hip), congenital heart disease.

congestion *n* hyperaemia. Accumulation of blood in a part of the body. May be active, which involves dilatation of arterioles and capillaries, or passive, which is due to venous stasis, as in the lower limbs or the lungs — **congest** *vi, vt*.

congestive cardiac failure (CCF) a chronic inability of the heart to maintain an adequate output from one or both ventricles. It is characterized by congestion in organs and veins that leads to systemic and pulmonary oedema and poor tissue oxygenation.

conization *n* ⇒ cone biopsy

conjugate *n* a measurement of the bony pelvis used to assess its adequacy for childbirth.

conjugation *n* 1. joining together of substances. Important in biochemical processes, especially in the liver, whereby toxic substances are rendered less harmful prior to being excreted. An example is the conjugation of bilirubin with glucuronic acid. 2. a method by which bacteria use sex pili to transfer genetic material during sexual reproduction. Allows genes for drug resistance to pass between bacterial strains. ⇒ plasmid. ⇒ transduction. ⇒ transformation.

conjunctiva *n* the delicate transparent vascular membrane which lines the eyelids (palpebral conjunctiva) and reflects over the front of the eyeball (bulbar or ocular conjunctiva) — **conjunctival** *adj*.

conjunctivitis *n* inflammation of the conjunctiva. ⇒ pink-eye. ⇒ trachoma inclusion conjunctivitis.

connective tissue *n* diverse group of tissues situated throughout the body which include: areolar, adipose, reticular, fibrous, elastic, cartilage, bone and blood/blood-forming tissue. They are characterized by a matrix containing cells and fibres. *connective tissue massage* stretching manipulations of the superficial and deep connective tissue to stimulate the circulation.

Conn's syndrome a primary oversecretion of aldosterone from the adrenal cortex, such as occurs in hyperplasia or adenoma. Results in hypertension, hypokalaemia and muscular weakness. ⇒ hyperaldosteronism.

consanguinity *n* blood relationship. This varies in degree from close (as between siblings) to less close (as between cousins etc) — **consanguineous** *adj*.

conscientious objection recognition in law that an individual is not bound to take part in a specific activity, e.g. termination of pregnancy. May also refer to a strongly held belief which is not recognized by law.

consciousness *n* a complex concept which implies that a person is consciously perceiving the environment via the five senses, and responding to the perceptions. ⇒ anaesthesia. ⇒ sleep.

consent patients are legally required to consent to treatment, surgery and any intervention that requires touching the patient. Consent may be given in writing, by word of mouth or be implied, i.e. nonverbal communication. However, where there are likely to be risks or disputes, written consent is advisable. It is the responsibility of the professional carrying out the treatment to explain to the patient in advance of treatment or surgery what the procedure will involve and any additional measures that may be required and to obtain written consent. This is usually the doctor concerned, but increasingly other health professionals are undertaking treatments. If the patient is a minor, or incapable of giving informed consent, the next-of-kin must sign the consent form. See Box – Consent. ⇒ informed consent.

conservative treatment aims at preventing a condition from becoming worse without using radical measures, i.e. preservation or repair. Examples include breast conservation by lumpectomy rather than mastectomy.

consolidation *n* becoming solid, as, for instance, the state of the lung due to exudation and organization in lobar pneumonia.

constipation *n* an implied chronic condition of infrequent, incomplete and often difficult evacuation of hard faeces. Causes include: insufficient intake of nonstarch polysaccharides (NSPs), dehydration, ignoring or being unable to respond to the urge to defaecate, immobility and lack of exercise, medication, hypokalaemia, hormonal, e.g. pregnancy, depressive illness, systemic disease, e.g. hypothyroidism, colorectal cancer (alternating with diarrhoea) and anorectal conditions causing pain on defaecation. Leakage of liquid faeces around an impacted mass of hard constipated faeces may be mistaken for diarrhoea. Acute constipation may indicate obstruction or paralysis of the gut of sudden onset. ⇒ laxatives. ⇒ spurious diarrhoea.

consumer protection laws giving rights to the consumer if there are defects in any products.

consumption *n* **1.** act of consuming or using up. **2.** a once popular term for pulmonary tuberculosis (which 'consumed' the body) — **consumptive** *adj*.

contact *n* **1.** direct or indirect exposure to infection. **2.** a person who has been so exposed. *contact lens* of glass or plastic, worn under the eyelids in direct contact with conjunctiva (in place of spectacles) for therapeutic or cosmetic purposes. *contact tracer* a person, often a nurse, who works from a chest clinic tracing contacts of people with tuberculosis, or a genitourinary clinic tracing the sexual contacts of people diagnosed with sexually transmitted infections (STIs), to encourage them to attend the clinic in an attempt to prevent the spread of STIs.

contagious *adj* capable of transmitting infection or of being transmitted.

containment isolation separation of a patient with, or suspected of having, a communicable disease to prevent spread of the condition to others. ⇒ protective isolation.

contingency fund an amount of money built into the costings of a project that would be used for some unplanned or unpredictable expense.

Continuing Professional Development (CPD) also referred to as Continuing Education (CE), and it can be thought of as lifelong learning, which embraces the acceptance of education occurring at all points in the lifespan. This implies, of course, that the teaching methods appropriate to adult learners must be used,

Consent

Consent or other lawful justification is required to prevent treatment constituting the actionable wrong of trespass to the person. A trespass to the person is one of a group of civil wrongs known as 'torts' which are actionable in the civil courts. The claimant must establish on a balance of probabilities that there has been a direct interference with his person. A trespass to the person is actionable per se, i.e. in its own right, without the need to establish that harm has occurred. This contrasts with an action for negligence, where harm must be established.

To be valid as a defence to an action for trespass, the consent must be given voluntarily by a mentally competent adult (a person over 18 years – for children see below) with no fraud or coercion. Consent can be given by non-verbal communication (implied consent), by word of mouth or in writing. For evidential purposes the latter is preferable. The capacity of the individual must be commensurate with the nature of the decision to be made. To be defined as having the necessary capacity a person must be able to comprehend and retain treatment information; to believe it and to weigh it in the balance to arrive at a choice. (Re C (Adult: Refusal of Medical Treatment) [1994] 1 WLR 290) If a person has the necessary capacity then he or she can refuse treatment for a good reason, a bad reason or for no reason at all. (Re MB (Medical Treatment) [1997] 2 FLR 426)

Consent given by a mentally competent person in broad terms to what is proposed will prevent an action for trespass to the person succeeding.

However, where a person has consented to treatment but has not been informed of the significant risks of substantial harm, then legal action lies not in an action for trespass to the person, but in an action for negligence (qv) alleging breach of the duty of care to inform. In this situation, the standard of information giving to the patient is determined according to the Bolam Test of the reasonable practitioner following approved practice. (Sidaway v. Bethlem RHG [1985] 1 All ER 643 where the House of Lords stated that informed consent was not a doctrine recognized in the English Courts) The claimant would have to prove that had he or she been informed of the risks of the harm which has occurred he or she would not have given consent to the treatment.

Where an adult is mentally incapacitated, then no-one at present has the right in law to give consent on his behalf. However, the House of Lords has recognized the right at common law to act in the best interests of a mentally incapacitated adult following the reasonable standard of care. (Re F. (Mental Patient: Sterilization) [1990] 2 AC 1) The Government has prepared proposals for statutory provision for decision making on behalf of a mentally incapacitated adult (Making Decisions Lord Chancellor's Office 1999, The Stationery Office)

Children become adults at 18 years. They have a statutory right to give consent to treatment at 16 or 17 years under the Family Law Reform Act 1969, but cannot refuse to give consent to life saving, necessary treatment in their best interests until they are 18 years. (Re W. (A Minor)(Medical Treatment) [1992] 4 All ER 627) The House of Lords recognized in the Gillick case (Gillick v. West Norfolk and Wisbech Area Health Authority [1986] 1 AC 112) that a competent child could give a valid consent to treatment if he or she had the mental capacity commensurate with the decision that was to be made. Parents also have the right to give consent on behalf of their children until 18 years.

focusing on learning derived from experience, using a student-centred, needs-based approach. This approach allows the learner to set her or his own agenda and assess its success. It stresses active, rather than passive, learning, frequently using peers as a source for knowledge. It also embraces the linkage of education and work – the application of learning to practice and the notion that practice itself is not static. Alongside this is the acceptance that theory not only informs practice, but also that knowledge can be embedded in, and emerge from, practice. Dynamic, changing practice is underpinned by education that is work-focused.

The nature of work changes rapidly these days. The education that fits a practitioner for practice now will not be relevant in 5 years, let alone for a whole working life. Practitioners need to be able to access knowledge and skills, and to develop attitudes to upgrade, consciously, systematically and continuously, their existing repertoire. CPD is a way of meeting this need for education 'on the job', and practitioners should be encouraged and supported to undertake professional development additional to the statutory 5 days of study every 3 years currently required for re-registration as a nurse in the UK. ⇒ PREP.

continuous ambulatory peritoneal dialysis (CAPD) a type of dialysis carried out each day by patients, with renal failure, at home. ⇒ dialysis.

continuous positive airways pressure (CPAP) the administration of a constant pressure of humidified gas to the airway during spontaneous inspiration. It prevents alveolar collapse at the end of expiration and can be used as ventilatory support to prevent the need for mechanical ventilation, to treat respiratory failure, to wean patients from ventilators and long term nocturnal use for sleep apnoea.

continuous quality improvement for continuous improvement to occur, it is necessary to: know the 'customer' and link this knowledge to the activities of the organization; have leaders that create an organizational culture that encourages pride, co-operation and scientific thought; work to reduce variations in processes and outcomes.

continuous service the length of service required before an employee is entitled to certain statutory and contractual rights.

continuous subcutaneous insulin infusion (CSII) the use of a pump to deliver a continuous controlled dose of insulin subcutaneously to achieve almost physiological control of diabetes mellitus.

contraceptive *n, adj* describes an agent used to prevent conception, e.g. male or female condom, spermicidal vaginal pessary or cream, sponge, rubber cervical cap or diaphragm, intrauterine device or emergency contraceptive. ⇒ coitus. ⇒ oral contraceptive. ⇒ postcoital — **contraception** *n*.

contract *v* 1. draw together; shorten; decrease in size. 2. acquire by contagion or infection.

contract *n* an agreement enforceable in law. *contract for services* agreement whereby one party provides services, not being employment, in return for payment or other consideration from the other. *contract of service* a contract for employment.

contractile *adj* possessing the ability to shorten, usually when stimulated; special property of muscle tissue — **contractility** *n*.

contraction *n* shortening, especially applied to muscle fibres.

contracture *n* shortening of muscle or scar tissue, producing deformity. ⇒ Dupuytren's contracture. ⇒ Volkmann's ischaemic contracture.

contraindication *n* a sign or symptom suggesting that a certain line of treatment (usually used for that disease) should be discontinued or avoided.

contralateral *adj* on the opposite side — **contralaterally** *adv*.

contrecoup *n* injury or damage through transmission of the force of a blow, remote from the original point of contact, such as damage to the brain as it hits the inside of the skull on the opposite side to the blow.

control group in research, the group that is not exposed to the independent variable, such as a particular nursing intervention. ⇒ experimental group. ⇒ variables.

control of infection the policies and measures taken to control infection in hospital and the community. It involves patient care, hygiene, use of aseptic technique, isolation etc. The most important contribution is the use of effective handwashing techniques by all healthcare staff. Policies and procedures that include policies for cleaning, disinfection and restricting the use of antibiotics. Public health measures such as immunization programmes, disease notification and environmental health. ⇒ containment isolation. ⇒ Infection Control Committee. ⇒ Infection Control Nurse. ⇒ protective isolation. ⇒ source isolation.

control of substances hazardous to health (COSHH) regulations requiring risk assessment and action to be taken, such as with the use of glutaraldehyde.

controlled cord traction withdrawal of the placenta and membranes after birth by holding back the contracted uterus while applying traction to the umbilical cord. Forms part of the active management of the third stage of labour. May lead to acute uterine inversion if improperly performed.

controlled drugs (CD) drugs that are subject to statutory control. In the UK they are defined and controlled by the Misuse of Drugs Act (1971), the Misuse of Drugs (Notification of and supply to Addicts) Regulations (1973) and the Misuse of

Drugs Regulations (1985). Examples include: cocaine, diamorphine (heroin), morphine, methadone, barbiturates etc.

controlled mandatory ventilation (CMV) ⇒ mechanical ventilation.

contusion *n* ⇒ bruise — **contuse** *vt*.

convalescence *n* the period after an illness before achievement of previous health status, or coping with a changed health status. ⇒ rehabilitation.

conversion *n* a mental defence mechanism. A psychological conflict manifesting as a physical symptom.

conversion disorder a psychological disorder in which conflict is converted into physical symptoms, e.g. loss of sensation or blindness.

convolutions *npl* folds, twists or coils as found in the intestine, renal tubules and the surface of the brain — **convoluted** *adj*.

convulsions *npl* involuntary contractions of muscles resulting from abnormal cerebral stimulation; there are many causes, e.g. epilepsy, head injury. They occur with or without loss of consciousness. *clonic convulsion* associated with muscle contraction and relaxation with violent jerky movements of the face and limbs, incontinence of urine and tongue biting. *febrile convulsions* → febrile. *tonic-clonic convulsions*, also called grand mal convulsions or seizures. The person becomes rigid (tonic) falls to the ground and jerks all over (clonic). *tonic convulsions* sudden contraction of muscles leading to sustained rigidity. The person may be cyanosed with loss of consciousness — **convulsive** *adj*.

convulsive therapy ⇒ electroconvulsive therapy.

Cooley's anaemia β thalassaemia major.

Coombs' test a highly sensitive test designed to detect antibodies to red blood cells: the 'direct' method detects those bound to the red cells; the 'indirect' method detects those circulating unbound in the serum. The 'direct' method is especially useful in the diagnosis of haemolytic syndromes.

coordination *n* moving in harmony. *muscular coordination* is the harmonious action of muscles, permitting free, smooth and efficient movements under perfect control.

COPD *abbr* chronic obstructive pulmonary disease.

coping the way in which a person deals with a circumstance which can be either negative or positive. The coping response can be negative, e.g. foregoing social activities because of increased frequency of micturition; or it can be positive, e.g. increasing one's level of physical exercise although confined to a wheelchair.

copper (Cu) *n* essential trace element in all animal tissues. Needed for the synthesis of catecholamines, enkephalins, certain proteins and enzymes, e.g. superoxide dismutase. Required for healthy blood cell formation.

coprolalia *n* filthy or obscene speech. Occurs as a symptom most commonly in cerebral deterioration or trauma affecting frontal lobes of the brain. ⇒ Tourette's syndrome.

coprolith *n* faecalith.

coproporphyrin *n* naturally occurring porphyrin in the faeces, formed in the intestine from bilirubin.

copropraxia *n* rude or obscene gestures. → Tourette's syndrome.

copulation *n* coitus.

cord *n* a thread-like structure. *spermatic cord* that which suspends the testes in the scrotum. Runs in the inguinal canal where it encloses nerves, blood vessels and the vas deferens. *spinal cord* a cord-like structure which runs inside the vertebral column, reaching from the foramen magnum to the first or second lumbar vertebra. It is part of the central nervous system. *umbilical cord* the cord attaching the fetus to the placenta. It contains two arteries and a vein. *vocal cord* the membranous bands in the larynx, vibrations of which produce the voice.

cordectomy *n* surgical excision of a cord, usually reserved for a vocal cord.

cordotomy *n* (*syn* chordotomy) division of the anterolateral nerve tracts in the spinal cord to relieve intractable pain in the pelvis or lower limbs.

core *n* central portion, usually applied to the slough in the centre of a boil.

Cori cycle *n* a biochemical reaction whereby lactic acid is converted to glucose for cell use. It occurs in the liver but only when oxygen is available (i.e. aerobically).

Cori's disease *n* a glycogen storage disease.

corn *n* a painful, cone-shaped overgrowth and hardening of the epidermis, with the point of the cone in the deeper layers; it is produced by friction or pressure. A *hard corn* usually occurs over a toe joint; a *soft corn* occurs between the toes.

cornea *n* the outwardly convex transparent membrane forming part of the anterior outer coat of the eye. It is avascular and allows light to enter the eye — **corneal** *adj*.

corneal graft (*syn* corneoplasty, keratoplasty) a corneal opacity is excised and replaced by healthy, transparent, human cornea from a donor.

corneoplasty *n* corneal graft.

corneoscleral *adj* pertaining to the cornea and sclera, as the circular junction of these structures.

cornu *n* horn-like structure. Describes one of two structures at the apex of the sacrum. Or the projections where the uterine tubes enter either side of the upper part of the uterus.

coronary *adj* crown-like; encircling, as of a vessel or nerve. *coronary arteries* those supplying the heart muscle, the first pair to be given off by the aorta as it leaves the left ventricle. Spasm, narrowing or blockage of these vessels causes angina pectoris or myocardial infarction. Diseased vessels may be cleared by lasers, balloon angioplasty or replaced with veins taken from the legs. ⇒ angioplasty. *coronary sinus* channel receiving venous blood from some of the cardiac veins and opening into the right atrium. *coronary thrombosis* occlusion of a coronary artery by a thrombus. The area deprived of blood becomes necrotic and is called an infarct. ⇒ ischaemic heart disease. ⇒ myocardial infarction.

coronary artery bypass graft (CABG) *n* surgical procedure by which diseased coronary arteries are bypassed using a vein graft (usually the saphenous vein).

coronary care unit (CCU) *n* a unit that provides specialist care for acutely ill patients with cardiac conditions, such as myocardial infarction, arrhythmias and unstable angina.

coronary heart disease (CHD) *n* another name for ischaemic heart disease. ⇒ angina pectoris. ⇒ coronary thrombosis. ⇒ myocardial infarction.

coronaviruses *npl* a group of viruses that can cause acute respiratory illnesses.

coroner *n* in England and Wales, an officer of the Crown, usually a solicitor, barrister or doctor, who presides over the Coroner's Court responsible for determining the cause of unexpected or suspicious death. When doubt exists, a doctor is advised to consult the coroner and act on his/her advice. The coroner must be notified if a patient is admitted to hospital and dies within 24 h. Likewise, all theatre/anaesthetic deaths must be reported to the coroner. Any death where the deceased has not consulted a doctor recently means that a coroner's postmortem may be ordered at the discretion of the coroner. In Scotland, reports about such deaths are submitted to the Procurator Fiscal but a postmortem is normally only ordered if foul play is suspected. The Scottish equivalent of the Coroner's Inquest is the Fatal Accident Enquiry, presided over by the Sheriff.

corporate governance the term used to describe the accountability of NHS organizations for standards in corporate dealings such as statutory financial obligations.

cor pulmonale right heart failure resulting from chronic respiratory disease, such as COPD or pulmonary fibrosis.

corpus *n* a body. *corpus albicans* white body. Scar on the ovary resulting from the degeneration of the corpus luteum. *corpus callosum* white matter (fibres) joining the two cerebral hemispheres. *corpus cavernosa* two lateral columns of erectile tissue in the penis. *corpus luteum* yellow body which forms in the ovary after rupture of a Graafian follicle. It secretes hormones which maintain pregnancy if fertilization occurs, until placental hormone secretion takes over. In the absence of fertilization it degenerates and menstruation commences. *corpus spongiosum* a single ventral column of erectile tissue in the penis. *corpus striatum* part of the basal nuclei — **corpora** *pl*.

corpuscle *n* a microscopic mass of protoplasm. Outdated term for blood cells — **corpuscular** *adj*.

corrective *adj, n* (something) which changes, counteracts or modifies something harmful.

Corrigan's pulse ⇒ collapsing pulse.

cortex *n* the outer layer of an organ beneath its capsule or membrane, as in the kidney or adrenal glands. ⇒ adrenal. ⇒ cerebral cortex. *renal cortex* the outer tissue of the kidney, underneath the renal capsule — **cortical** *adj*.

corticospinal *adj* pertaining to the cerebral cortex and the spinal cord. *corticospinal tracts* main voluntary motor pathways in the brain and spinal cord. Also called pyramidal tracts.

corticosteroids *npl* 1. steroid hormones produced by the adrenal cortex. There are three groups: glucocorticoids, e.g. cortisol, mineralocorticoids, e.g. aldosterone, and sex hormones, e.g. androgens. ⇒ glucocorticoids. ⇒ mineralocorticoids. 2. synthetic corticosteroids, such as prednisolone and dexamethasone, are used for their anti-inflammatory and immunosuppressive properties, e.g. in asthma, inflammatory bowel disease, rheumatoid arthritis, some skin conditions or following transplant surgery. The benefits of therapy must always be weighed against the risk of serious side-effects associated with high doses and/or sustained use (see Figure 16).

corticotrophin *n* ⇒ adrenocorticotrophic hormone (ACTH). *corticotrophin releasing factor (CRF)* hypothalamic factor that stimulates the anterior pituitary gland to secrete adrenocorticotrophic hormone.

cortisol *n* hydrocortisone, one of the principal steroid hormones of the adrenal cortex. It is increased in Cushing's disease and syndrome, and decreased in Addison's disease. It is essential to life.

cortisone *n* one of the steroid hormones of the adrenal gland. It is converted into cortisol before use by the body. It is given as physiological replacement treatment in Addison's disease and hypopituitarism. *cortisone suppression test* differentiates primary from secondary hypercalcaemia.

Corynebacterium *n* a genus of Gram-positive, rod-shaped (bacilli) bacteria. Many strains are commensals colonizing the upper respiratory tract and some are pathogenic, e.g. *Corynebacterium diphtheriae*, which causes diphtheria and produces a powerful exotoxin.

coryza *n* the common cold. An acute upper respiratory infection of short duration; highly contagious; causative viruses include rhinoviruses, coronaviruses and

Adverse effects usually occur with high doses or the sustained use of corticosteroid drugs and may include:

- Sodium and water retention leading to hypertension and oedema; muscle weakness due to potassium loss
- Changes in fat and protein metabolism leading to typical 'moon' face, fat redistribution to the abdomen and back ('buffalo hump') and muscle wastage in the limbs
- Weight gain
- Hyperglycaemia, due to excessive gluconeogenesis, leading to diabetes mellitus
- The suppression of inflammatory response which delays wound healing and masks signs of infection
- Reactivation of tuberculosis
- The skin becomes thin, fragile and easily damaged; striae and excessive bruising
- Hirsutism and acne
- Menstrual cycle disturbance
- Osteoporosis and spontaneous fractures, especially vertebral collapse as calcium is lost
- Peptic ulcer development linked to an increase in gastric acid secretion
- Cataracts
- Mood changes and serious mental illness—paranoia, euphoria and depression

Figure 16 Adverse effects of corticosteroid therapy.

adenoviruses. Antibiotics are not effective and they should not be prescribed.

COSHH *abbr* control of substances hazardous to health.

cosmetic *adj, n* (that which is) done to improve the appearance or prevent disfigurement.

cost-benefit analysis (CBA) a complex method of analysing the costs (as opportunity costs) of the provision and the benefits of a particular health intervention in terms of money. The cost of each benefit (cost-benefit ratio) is calculated, with difficulty because of the subjectivity of judging quality of life measures, which allows comparisions to be made between different interventions.

cost centre a department, e.g. pharmacy or catering, for which a budget covering staff and other resources has been set.

cost-effectiveness analysis an assessment of efficiency. The comparison of measurable health gains (outcomes) with the net cost of the healthcare intervention (input). ⇒ clinical audit. ⇒ efficiency. ⇒ Performance Indicators. ⇒ quality assurance.

costal *adj* pertaining to the ribs. *costal cartilages* those which attach the ribs to the sternum.

costive *adj* lay term for constipated. ⇒ constipation — **costiveness** *n*.

costochondral *adj* pertaining to a rib and its cartilage.

costochondritis *n* inflammation of the costochondral cartilage. ⇒ Tietze syndrome.

costoclavicular *adj* pertaining to the ribs and the clavicle.

cot death ⇒ sudden infant death syndrome.

cotyledon *n* one of the subdivisions of the maternal surface of the placenta.

cough *n* explosive expulsion of air from the lungs as a voluntary or protective reflex action to expel a foreign body such as a crumb, mucus or sputum. Coughing is associated with numerous respiratory and cardiac conditions. A cough which achieves expulsion of sputum is said to be moist/productive. Patients who are at risk of chest infection postoperatively are taught to cough productively while supporting an abdominal wound with the palms of both hands. ⇒ postural drainage.

counselling *n* a professional helping relationship with a client who is experiencing psychological problems. The counsellor listens actively and helps the client to identify and clarify the problems, and supports them as they make a positive attempt to overcome them.

counterconditioning a behavioural technique that seeks to replace a learned response with one that is more acceptable.

countercurrent *n* a change in the direction of fluid flow. *countercurrent heat exchanger* the heat exhange system in the blood vessels of the legs where cold venous blood is warmed by arterial blood before returning to the body core. *countercurrent multiplication theory* a hypothesis which can be used to explain osmolarity gradients, within the interstitial fluid surrounding the renal tubule, required for the production of urine of different concentrations.

counterirritant *n* an agent which, when applied to the skin, produces a mild inflammatory reaction (hyperaemia) and relief of pain and congestion associated with a more deep-seated inflammatory process — **counterirritation** *n*.

countertraction *n* a force that counters the pull of traction, often the body weight of the person.

couvade syndrome *n* a custom in some cultures whereby a father exhibits the symptoms of his partner's pregnancy and childbirth.

covalent bond *n* a chemical bond where electrons are shared between the atoms to form molecules or compounds, such as the formation of a molecule of hydrogen (H_2). Carbon forms covalent bonds with hydrogen, oxygen and nitrogen to form the important organic molecules used by the body. ⇒ hydrogen bond. ⇒ ionic bond.

Cowper's glands ⇒ bulbourethral glands.

coxa *n* the hip joint. *coxa valga* an increase in the normal angle between neck and shaft of femur. *coxa vara* a decrease in the normal angle plus torsion of the neck, e.g. slipped femoral epiphysis — **coxae** *pl*.

coxalgia *n* pain in the hip.

Coxiella *n* a genus closely related to *Rickettsia*, including *Coxiella burneti* which causes Q fever.

coxitis *n* inflammation of the hip joint.

coxsackie viruses first isolated at Coxsackie, NY. One of the three groups included in the family of enteroviruses. Divided into groups A and B. They cause diseases that include: aseptic meningitis, herpangina, Bornholm disease, pericarditis, myocarditis, hand, foot and mouth disease, gastroenteritis and infections in neonates.

CPA *abbr* care programme approach.

CPAP *abbr* continuous positive airways pressure.

CPD *abbr* Continuing Professional Development.

CPK *abbr* creatine phosphokinase. ⇒ creatine kinase.

CPN *abbr* Community Psychiatric Nurse. ⇒ specialist community practitioner.

CPR *abbr* cardiopulmonary resuscitation.

CPU *abbr* central processing unit.

crab louse Pediculus pubis.

cradle cap thick, yellow scaling of the scalp of infants; seborrhoeic eczema (dermatitis).

cramp *n* sudden tonic contraction of a muscle or group of muscles; involuntary and painful; may result from fatigue. *occupational cramp* is such as occurs amongst certain groups of workers, e.g. miners.

cranial *adj* pertaining to the cranium. *cranial cavity* skull cavity containing and protecting the brain. *cranial nerves* twelve pairs of peripheral nerves that originate in the brain. Known by names and Roman numerals, e.g. the facial or VIIth nerve.

craniofacial *adj* pertaining to the cranium and the face. *craniofacial resection* a procedure which can be used in all age groups for the removal of paranasal sinus tumours, particularly those inaccessible through a usual nasal approach. It avoids the need for a total neurosurgical approach.

craniometry *n* the science which deals with the measurement of skulls.

craniopharyngioma *n* a pituitary tumour seen in children. It develops from cells of Rathke's pouch, an embryonic structure that forms in the roof of the mouth and develops into the anterior lobe of the pituitary gland.

cranioplasty *n* operative repair of a skull defect — **cranioplastic** *adj*.

craniosacral *adj* pertaining to the skull and sacrum. *craniosacral outflow* applied to the parasympathetic nerves which leave the central nervous system with the cranial nerves and from the sacral region of the spinal cord.

craniostenosis *n* a condition in infancy in which the skull sutures fuse too early and the fontanelles close. It may cause raised intracranial pressure requiring surgery.

craniotabes *n* condition in which parts of the vault of the skull are unusually soft and can be indented. May be found in newborn (usually preterm) infants, caused by delayed calcification; also associated with rickets. Infants are otherwise normal — **craniotabetic** *adj*.

craniotomy *n* a surgical opening of the skull in order to remove a growth, relieve pressure, evacuate blood clot or arrest haemorrhage.

cranium *n* the part of the skull enclosing the brain. It is composed of eight bones: the occipital, two parietals, frontal, two temporals, sphenoid and ethmoid — **cranial** *adj*.

crash sudden and serious malfunction or complete loss of program. ⇒ bug.

c-reactive protein test (CRP) an acute phase protein. Elevated amounts are present in the plasma in response to tissue damage and inflammation. It is a very sensitive indicator of the progress of many inflammatory conditions, such as infective endocarditis.

creatinase *n* ⇒ creatine kinase.

creatine *n* a nitrogenous compound synthesized in vitro. *phosphorylated creatine* is an important storage form of high-energy phosphate in muscle tissue. *creatine kinase (CK)* (syn ATP: creatine phosphokinase) occurs as three isoenzymes, each having two components labelled M and B; the form in brain tissue is BB, in skeletal muscle and serum MM, and in heart muscle both MM and MB. *creatine kinase test* the MB isoenzyme is raised in serum in acute myocardial infarction.

creatinine *n* a waste product of protein and nucleic acid metabolism found in muscle and blood and excreted in normal urine. *creatinine clearance test* ⇒ clearance.

creatinuria *n* an excess of the nitrogenous compound creatine in the urine. Occurs in conditions in which muscle protein is rapidly broken down, e.g. acute fevers, starvation.

creatorrhoea *n* the presence of excessive nitrogen in the faeces. It occurs particularly in pancreatic dysfunction.

Credit Accumulation and Transfer System (CATS) see Box – APEL, APL and CATS.

crenation the shrinkage of red blood cells placed in a hypertonic solution.

crepitation *n* 1. (crepitus) grating of bone ends in fracture. 2. crackling sound in joints, e.g. in osteoarthritis. 3. crackling sound heard via stethoscope. 4. crackling sound elicited by pressure on tissue containing air (surgical emphysema).

crepitus *n* ⇒ crepitation.

cresol *n* a phenolic disinfectant derived from coal tar. Present in a wide range of general disinfectants.

Creutzfeldt-Jakob disease (CJD) form of progressive dementia transmissible through prion protein. New variant CJD, found in young adults, is possibly linked with bovine prion of spongiform encephalopathy. It runs a rapid degenerative course and is usually fatal.

CRF *abbr* chronic renal failure. ⇒ renal.

cribriform *adj* perforated, like a sieve. *cribriform plate* that portion of the ethmoid bone allowing passage of fibres of olfactory nerve.

cricoid *adj* ring-shaped. Applied to the cartilage forming the inferior posterior part of larynx. *cricoid pressure* pressure applied to the cartilage to prevent aspiration of stomach contents during the induction of general anaesthesia.

cricothyroid ligament *adj* relating to the cricoid and thyroid cartilages of the larynx. *cricothyroid ligament* fibro-elastic membrane that attaches the cricoid cartilage to the thyroid cartilage.

'cri du chat' syndrome congenital condition caused by an anomaly of chromosome 5. It is characterized by a high-pitched cry like that of a kitten, micrognathia, low set ears and severe learning disability.

criminal abortion ⇒ abortion.

criminal law *n* law creating offences heard in the criminal courts. *criminal wrong* an act or omission which can be pursued in the criminal courts.

crisis *n* **1.** a critical turning point in an acute illness, such as the point of defervescence in a fever. ⇒ lysis *ant*. **2.** sudden severe pain or other form of deterioration associated with certain conditions, such as *Dietl's crisis* severe kidney pain (nephralgia) caused by obstruction of the ureter. **3.** *crisis intervention* in psychiatry, when the therapeutic team intervenes to assist in solving an immediate crisis and its associated problems.

critical appraisal a technique for making an objective judgement regarding a research study in terms of research design, methodology, analysis, interpretation of results and how appropriate the study findings are to a particular area of practice.

critical path analysis a project management technique used where operations, tasks and actions are deemed to be interdependent. The timing of each action or stage is crucial to the overall success of the project, medical treatment or nursing intervention, because some actions or stages must be completed before others can be started. The technique has many applications in the identification of the key components of patient care and assuring high quality outcomes.

Crohn's disease also called regional ileitis. ⇒ inflammatory bowel disease.

Crosby capsule a special tube which is passed through the mouth to the small intestine; manoeuvre of the tube selects tissue for biopsy. Endoscopic biopsy is often used in preference to this time-consuming investigation.

cross infection ⇒ infection.

cross-over studies a research study where participants experience both the experimental agent and the placebo one after another.

croup *n* laryngeal obstruction. Croupy breathing in a child is often called 'stridulous', meaning noisy or harsh-sounding. Narrowing of the airway, which gives rise to the typical attack with crowing inspiration, may be the result of oedema or spasm, or both.

crown the portion of a tooth above the gum.

CRP *abbr* ⇒ c-reactive protein test.

cruciate *adj* shaped like a cross. *cruciate ligaments* the ligaments giving stability to the knee joint.

'crush' syndrome traumatic uraemia. Occurs following extensive crush trauma to muscle tissue. Shock and myoglobin release into the circulation causes changes to renal perfusion with tubular necrosis and eventual failure. Management includes renal replacement therapy. ⇒ haemodiafiltration. ⇒ haemodialysis. ⇒ haemofiltration.

crutch palsy paralysis of extensor muscles of wrist, fingers and thumb from repeated pressure of a crutch upon the radial nerve in the axilla.

cryaesthesia *n* **1.** the sensation of coldness. **2.** exceptional sensitivity to a low temperature.

cryoanalgesia *n* relief of pain achieved by use of a cryosurgical probe to block peripheral nerve function. Ice packs can also be used to relieve pain. ⇒ cryoprobe. ⇒ cryosurgery.

cryoextractor *n* a type of cryoprobe used for extraction of the lens in cataract surgery.

cryogenic *adj, n* (anything) produced by low temperature. Also used to describe any means or apparatus involved in the production of low temperature.

cryoglobulins *npl* cold antibodies. Immunoglobulins which precipitate at low temperatures and are associated with diseases, such as systemic lupus erythematosus.

cryopexy *n* surgical fixation by freezing, as replacement of a detached retina.

cryoprecipitate therapy use of factor VIII to prevent or treat bleeding in haemophilia, and the use of fibrinogen enriched factor VIII for DIC. The term refers to the preparation of factor VIII for injection. Subarctic temperatures make it separate from plasma. ⇒ coagulation.

cryoprobe *n* freezing probe. Can be used for biopsy. A flexible metal tube attached to liquid nitrogen equipment. The cryoprobe has tips of various sizes which can be cooled to a temperature of -180°C. Causes less tissue trauma and 'seeding' of malignant cells.

cryosurgery *n* the use of intense, controlled cold to remove or destroy diseased tissue. Instead of a knife or guillotine, a cryoprobe is used.

cryothalamectomy *n* freezing applied to destroy groups of neurons within the thalamus in the treatment of Parkinson's disease and other hyperkinetic conditions.

cryotherapy *n* the use of cold for the treatment of disease.

cryptococcosis *n* the disease resulting from infection with the yeast *Cryptococcus neoformans*, which occurs in soil and pigeon excreta. It affects the lungs, skin, bones and meninges. Meningitis is the most frequent manifestation. Patients who are immunocompromised, such as those with AIDS, are at increased risk. It is an AIDS defining condition according to CDC/WHO.

Cryptococcus *n* a genus of fungi. *Cryptococcus neoformans* is an occasional cause of disease in humans. ⇒ yeast.

cryptogenic *adj* of unknown or obscure cause.

cryptomenorrhoea *n* hidden menstruation. Apparent amenorrhoea with retention of the menses due to a congenital obstruction, such as an imperforate hymen or atresia of the vagina. ⇒ haematocolpos.

cryptorchism *n* undescended testes. A developmental defect whereby the testes do not descend into the scrotum; they are retained within the abdomen or inguinal canal. Untreated, it may impair fertility, lead to emotional distress and is associated with an increased risk of testicular cancer. Treatment is surgical. ⇒ orchidopexy. ⇒ testis — **cryptorchid, cryptorchis** *n*.

cryptosporidiosis *n* disease caused by cryptosporidium species (protozoa). The protozoa are present in the faeces of domestic and farm animals, and transmission to humans occurs through contamination of water and food. Infection may result in profuse watery diarrhoea but patients may be asymptomatic. Patients with AIDS and other conditions that cause immunodeficiency may be seriously affected with abdominal pain, anorexia, weight loss and fever.

cryptosporidium ⇒ cryptosporidiosis.

crystal violet *n* (*syn* gentian violet) a brilliant, violet-coloured, antiseptic aniline dye, used as 0.5% solution for ulcers and skin infections. It must only be applied to intact skin because it is carcinogenic.

crystalline *adj* like a crystal; transparent. Applied to various structures. *crystalline lens* a biconvex body, oval in shape, which is suspended just behind the iris of the eye, and separates the aqueous from the vitreous humor. It is slightly less convex on its anterior surface and it refracts the light rays so that they focus directly on to the retina.

crystallins *npl* protein constituents of the lens of the eye.

crystalloids *npl* substances in solution that will diffuse through a selectively permeable membrane. Crystalloid solutions are administered intravenously to maintain fluid and electrolyte balance. May be used in conjunction with colloids in severely ill patients.

crystalluria *n* excretion of crystals in the urine.

CSF *abbr* 1. cerebrospinal fluid. 2. colony stimulating factors.

CSI *abbr* Caregiver Strain Index.

CSII *abbr* continuous subcutaneous insulin infusion.

CSM *abbr* Committee on Safety of Medicines.

CSSD *abbr* Central Sterile Supplies Department.

CSSU *abbr* central sterile supply unit. ⇒ Central Sterile Supplies Department. ⇒ Hospital Sterilization and Disinfection Unit.

CT *abbr* computed tomography.

CTG *abbr* cardiotocograph.

CTZ *abbr* chemoreceptor trigger zone.

cubital tunnel external compression syndrome ulnar paralysis resulting from compression of the ulnar nerve within the cubital tunnel situated on the inner and posterior aspects of the elbow, sometimes referred to as the 'funny bone'.

cubitus *n* the forearm; elbow — **cubital** *adj.*

cue *n* in the context of communicating, a verbal or nonverbal signal from another person which is perceived by the observer to warrant sensitive exploration (by prompting or reflection) as to its meaning for the person exhibiting it.

culdocentesis *n* aspiration of the rectouterine pouch via the posterior vaginal wall.

culdoscope *n* an endoscope used for pelvic examination via the vaginal route.

culdoscopy *n* passage of an endoscope through the posterior vaginal fornix, behind the uterus to enter the peritoneal cavity, for viewing of the rectouterine pouch — **culdoscopically** *adv.*

cultural capital the degree to which an individual absorbs the dominant culture. It has implications for success in education, where those with a high degree of social capital are more successful.

culture *n* 1. the growth of micro-organisms on artificial media under ideal conditions. 2. the attitudes, beliefs, ideas, knowledge, practices and values which members of different groups hold about themselves, and which inform the total behaviour of a group. See Box – Culture.

cumulative action if the dose of a slowly excreted drug is repeated too frequently, an increasing action is obtained. This can be dangerous as, if the drug accumulates in the system, toxic symptoms may occur, e.g. with digoxin.

Cumulative Index to Nursing and Allied Health Literature *n* computerized database of literature relevant to nursing and allied health.

cupping *n* a method of counter-irritation. A small bell-shaped glass (in which the air is expanded by heating, or exhausted by

---

Culture

The conceptual framework of culture encompasses dimensions such as human behaviour and the influences of knowledge and inheritance: the acquisition of ideas, values, customs, codes, rituals, taboos, language, ceremonies and other related cultural forces, such as spirituality and religion. The evolution of culture is contingent upon man's innate potential to gain knowledge and to transfer his experiential learning to succeeding generations.

Although culture is often defined as a sociological concept, its role in behavioral science is recognized. For example, how a person communicates is influenced not only by social backgrounds and sociocultural beliefs (Béphage 2000), but these influences will also determine the expression of psychological needs.

Psychological distress and/or the experience of pain for example differ from one ethnic group to another. In addition, some authors (e.g. Loveman and Gaie 2000) have drawn attention to oppressive practice, when professionals fail to assess the ethnic client's pain experience accurately. In this context, one can argue that a professional's cultural background can affect his/her perception of clients' pain phenomena.

A prerequisite to good healthcare practice is considered to be able to recognize and being sensitive to clients' diverse sociocultural beliefs and practices. Interventions used should also involve clients to recognize how sociocultural factors can influence pain in addition to biopsychological factors (Kwekkeboom 1999).

References
Béphage G 2000 Social and Behavioural Sciences for Nurses: An integrated approach. Churchill Livingstone, Edinburgh
Loveman E, Gale A 2000 Factors influencing nurses' inferences about patient pain. British Journal of Nursing 9(6):334–337
Kwekkeboom K L 1999 A model for cognitive behavioural interventions in cancer pain management. Image: Journal of Nursing Scholarship 31(2):151–156

compression of an attached rubber bulb) is applied to the skin, resultant suction producing hyperaemia.

curettage *n* the scraping of unhealthy or exuberant tissue from a cavity. This may be as treatment or to establish a diagnosis through laboratory analysis of the scrapings.

curette *n* a spoon-shaped instrument or a metal loop which may have sharp and/or blunt edges for scraping out (curetting) cavities.

curettings *npl* the material obtained by scraping or curetting and usually sent for examination in the pathology department.

curie *n* old unit of radioactivity, now replaced by the SI unit the becquerel (Bq).

Curling's ulcer acute peptic ulceration which occurs either in the stomach or duodenum as a response to the physiological stress of extensive burns or scalds.

curriculum vitae literally 'the course of one's life'. A summary of personal details, education, professional qualifications and attainment and employment experience.

CUSA *abbr* Cavitron ultrasonic surgical aspirator.

Cuscoe's speculum *n* → speculum.

cushingoid *adj* used to describe the moon face and central obesity common in people with elevated levels of plasma corticosteroid from whatever cause.

Cushing's disease a rare disorder, mainly affecting females, characterized principally by functional obesity with fat accumulations on the back, chest and face ('moon face'), muscle wastage and weakness, bruising, purpura, striae, acne, hirsutism, osteoporosis, hyperglycaemia, glycosuria, hypertension, increased infection, poor wound healing and psychotic disturbances. Due to excessive corticosteroid production by hyperplastic adrenal glands as a result of increased ACTH (corticotrophin) secretion by a tumour or hyperplasia of the anterior pituitary gland.

Cushing's reflex a rise in blood pressure and a fall in pulse rate; occurs in cerebral space-occupying lesions.

Cushing's syndrome a disorder clinically similar to Cushing's disease and also due to elevated levels of plasma corticos-teroids, but where the primary pathology is not in the pituitary gland. It can be due to adenoma or carcinoma of the adrenal cortex and to the secretion of ACTH by nonendocrine tumours such as bronchial carcinoma. It can also be iatrogenic due to prolonged or excessive administration of corticosteroids.

cusp *n* a projecting point, such as the edge of a tooth or the segment of a heart valve. The cardiac tricuspid valve has three, the bicuspid (mitral) valve two cusps.

cutaneous *adj* relating to the skin.

cuticle *n* 1. the thickened area situated at the base of a nail. Also called the eponychium. 2. the epidermis — **cuticular** *adj*.

CV *abbr* curriculum vitae.

CVA *abbr* cerebrovascular accident.

CVP *abbr* central venous pressure.

CVS *abbr* 1. chorionic villus sampling. 2. cardiovascular system.

CVVH *abbr* continuous venous venous haemofiltration. ⇒ haemofiltration.

CVVHD *abbr* continuous venous-venous haemodiafiltration. ⇒ haemodiafiltration.

cyanocobalamin *n* a commercially produced substance with vitamin B_{12} activity. → cobalamins. ⇒ hydroxocobalamin.

cyanosis *n* a bluish or purple colouration of the skin and mucous membranes due to poor oxygenation of the blood. It may be observed centrally or in peripheral structures, such as the digits — **cyanosed, cyanotic** *adj*.

cyclic adenosine monophosphate (cAMP) *n* an important metabolic molecule that acts as the 'second messenger' in the action of several hormones, e.g. adrenocorticotrophic hormone.

cyclical syndrome a term used to describe the diverse effects seen in the premenstrual phase of the menstrual cycle. Some people prefer this term to that of premenstrual syndrome.

cyclical vomiting periodic attacks of vomiting in children, usually associated with ketosis and usually with no demonstrable pathological cause. Occurs mainly in highly-strung children. Recovery is usually spontaneous; in some cases, dehydration can occur.

cyclitis *n* inflammation of the ciliary body of the eye, shown by deposition of small collections of white cells on the posterior cornea called 'keratitic precipitates' (KP). Often coexistent with inflammation of the iris. ⇒ iridocyclitis.

cyclodialysis *n* operation to improve drainage from the anterior chamber of the eye which aims to reduce intraocular pressure in glaucoma.

cyclodiathermy *n* use of diathermy to destroy part of the ciliary body as a treatment for glaucoma.

cycloplegia *n* paralysis of the ciliary muscle of the eye — **cycloplegic** *adj.*

cycloplegics *npl* drugs which cause paralysis of the ciliary muscle, e.g. atropine, homatropine and cyclopentolate. ⇒ mydriatics.

cyclothymia *n* a tendency to alternating, but relatively mild, mood swings between elation and depression — **cyclothymic** *adj.*

cyclotron *n* an apparatus in which radioactive isotopes can be prepared. These isotopes may be used in imaging, or used to treat various cancers with proton or neutron beams.

cyesis *n* pregnancy. ⇒ pseudocyesis.

cyst *n* a sac with membranous wall, enclosing fluid or semisolid matter — **cystic** *adj.*

cystadenoma *n* a benign cystic growth of glandular epithelium. Liable to occur in the female breast or ovary.

cystathioninuria *n* inherited disorder of cystathionine metabolism marked by excessive excretion of cystathionine in the urine, an intermediate product in conversion of methionine to cysteine. Associated with learning disabilities, Marfan-like syndrome and thrombotic episodes.

cystectomy *n* usually refers to the removal of part or the whole of the urinary bladder as a treatment for bladder cancer. This may necessitate urinary diversion, such as implanting the ureters into an isolated ileal segment (ileal conduit). ⇒ ileoureterostomy.

cysteine *n* a sulphur-containing amino acid. Easily oxidized to cystine.

cystic fibrosis (CF) (*syn* fibrocystic disease of the pancreas, mucoviscidosis) an autosomal recessive disorder caused by the mutated CFTR gene that affects the exocrine glands (especially those in the gastrointestinal tract, pancreas, goblet cells in the respiratory mucosa and sweat glands). The condition is particularly common in Caucasian populations, where it has a frequency of around 1 in 2500 live births; diagnosis may be confirmed by high levels of sodium in sweat. Meconium ileus, causing intestinal obstruction in newborns, may be an early physical effect. The affected glands have faulty cell membrane ion (chloride and sodium) transport, and produce viscous mucus which leads to blocked dilated ducts, stasis, infection and fibrosis. The lungs and pancreas are primarily affected, giving rise to repeated chest infections, respiratory problems and cardiac failure and digestive problems leading to malabsorption. Current management centres upon physiotherapy, antimicrobial drugs and replacement of pancreatic enzymes, but advances in management include: recent identification of the defective mutated gene, gene therapy, heart/lung transplants, antenatal testing and genetic counselling. ⇒ iontophoresis. ⇒ sweat test.

cystic fibrosis transmembrane regulator (CFTR) a gene located on chromosome 7. It is concerned with the movement of chloride ions through the cell membrane. Mutations may occur which disrupt the movement of chloride and sodium ions through the cell membrane. ⇒ cystic fibrosis.

cysticercosis *n* infection of humans with cysticercus, the larval stage of *Taenia solium* (pork tapeworm). After ingestion, the ova do not develop beyond this form, but form 'cysts' in subcutaneous tissues, skeletal muscles and the brain, where they provoke epilepsy. Treatment is with anthelmintics: praziquantel, albendazole.

cysticercus *n* the larval form of *Taenia solium*. ⇒ cysticerosis.

cystine *n* a sulphur-containing amino acid. It is readily reduced to two molecules of cysteine.

cystinosis *n* a recessively inherited metabolic disorder in which crystalline cystine is deposited in the body. Cystine and other amino acids are excreted in the urine. ⇒ Fanconi syndrome.

cystinuria *n* excretion of cystine and other amino acids in the urine associated with an inborn error of metabolism, where basic amino acids are not reabsorbed by the renal tubules. Stones containing cystine form in the kidneys. ⇒ cystinosis. ⇒ Fanconi syndrome — **cystinuric** *adj.*

cystitis *n* inflammation of the urinary bladder. The cause is usually bacterial, but other causes include: tumour or calculi. ⇒ urinary tract infection.

cystocele *n* prolapse of the posterior wall of the urinary bladder into the anterior vaginal wall. ⇒ colporrhaphy.

cystodiathermy *n* the application of a cauterizing electrical current to the walls of the urinary bladder through a cystoscope, or by open operation.

cystography *n* radiographic examination of the urinary bladder, after it has been filled with a contrast medium. ⇒ micturating cystogram — **cystographically** *adv.*

cystolithiasis *n* the presence of a stone or stones in the urinary bladder.

cystometrogram *n* a record of the changes in pressure within the urinary bladder under various conditions; used in the study of bladder dysfunction.

cystometry *n* the study of pressure changes and capacities within the urinary bladder. Results recorded graphically as a cystometrogram — **cystometric** *adj.*

cystoplasty *n* surgical repair of the urinary bladder — **cystoplastic** *adj.*

cystoscope *n* an endoscope used in diagnosis and treatment of bladder, ureter and kidney conditions — **cystoscopically** *adv.*

cystoscopy *n* use of a cystoscope to view the inside of the urinary bladder. It can also incorporate a biopsy or fulguration of a bladder tumour.

cystostomy *n* (*syn* vesicostomy) an operation whereby a fistulous opening is made into the urinary bladder via the abdominal wall.

cystotomy *n* incision into the urinary bladder via the abdominal wall; often done to remove a large stone or tumour or occasionally to gain access to the prostate gland in the operation of transvesical prostatectomy.

cystourethritis *n* inflammation of the urinary bladder and urethra.

cystourethrography *n* radiographic examination of the urinary bladder and urethra, after the introduction of a contrast medium — **cystourethrographically** *adv.*

cystourethropexy *n* forward fixation of the urinary bladder and upper urethra in an attempt to combat incontinence of urine.

cytochromes *npl* a series of iron or copper containing proteins with a similar structure to haemoglobin. They are involved in the mitochondrial oxidation-reduction reactions of the electron transport chain which generate energy as ATP. *cytochrome* P_{450} a liver enzyme involved in the oxidation and clearance of lipid soluble drugs.

cytodiagnosis *n* diagnosis by the microscopic study of cells — **cytodiagnostic** *adj.*

cytogenetics *n* the study of cells with a particular emphasis upon chromosomes, genes and their behaviour. Chromosomes can be studied by culture techniques, using either lymphocytes or a piece of tissue such as skin, or cells such as those of the amniotic fluid (fetal cells). Chromosome abnormalities of either number or make-up (structure) can be associated with physical and mental disorder or with spontaneous abortion or stillbirth — **cytogenesis** *n.*

cytokines *npl* a general term for the signalling molecules produced by immune cells, e.g. macrophages and lymphocytes. They include interleukins, interferons and tumour necrosis factors, and are responsible for controlling the immune system. Cytokines produced by lymphocytes are also known as lymphokines.

cytokinesis *n* cell (cytoplasmic) division; the process by which a cell divides into two following nuclear division. ⇒ mitosis.

cytology *n* the microscopic study of cells. ⇒ exfoliative cytology — **cytological** *adj.*

cytolysis *n* the degeneration, destruction, disintegration or dissolution of cells — **cytolytic** *adj.*

cytomegalovirus (CMV) *n* a herpesvirus. Can cause latent and symptomless infection. Virus particles are excreted in urine and saliva. Commonly transmitted to the fetus in utero, where it may cause abortion, stillbirth or serious neonatal disease characterized by hepatosplenomagaly, purpura, encephalitis and microcephaly with learning disability and delay in motor development or neonatal death. In adults it causes an illness similar to infectious mononucleosis and respiratory problems. The virus is a serious threat to immunocompromised individuals, such as those with AIDS, where it may cause serious pneumonitis, retinitis and systemic infection. The antiviral drug ganciclovir is used to treat serious infections.

cytometer *n* device for counting cells, such as blood cells.

cytopathic *adj* pertaining to abnormality of the living cell.

cytopheresis *n* the separation and removal of specific cellular components of blood. It may be used therapeutically to collect components needed by patients, or to remove abnormal components. ⇒ apheresis.

cytoplasm *n* the protoplasm of a cell excluding that surrounding the nucleus. The fluid part that contains the subcellular organelles is termed the cytosol — **cytoplasmic** *adj*.

cytosine *n* nitrogenous base derived from pyrimidine. A component of nucleic acids (DNA, RNA).

cytosol ⇒ cytoplasm.

cytostasis *n* arrest or hindrance of cell development — **cytostatic** *adj*.

cytotoxic *adj* any substance which is toxic to cells. *cytotoxic drugs* the drugs used mainly for the treatment of malignant conditions, but sometimes for other conditions. They work in different ways, but they all eventually cause cancer cell death by either disrupting DNA or causing apoptosis. Some are cell cycle phase specific and others work at any point in the cell cycle. They also harm some normal cells and some have longer term side-effects. The handling of cytotoxic drugs is a health and safety issue and all health-care workers should follow local policies regarding handling, protection and incident reporting. ⇒ chemotherapy. ⇒ toxicity. They belong to five groups: (a) alkylating agents that disrupt DNA, e.g. busulfan (busulphan), cyclophosphamide; (b) antimetabolites that disrupt DNA by

blocking enzymes required for its synthesis, e.g 5-fluorouracil; (c) antitumour antibiotics that disrupt DNA and the cell membrane, e.g. bleomycin; (d) vinca alkaloids and other plant extracts disrupt microtubules during cell division, e.g. vincristine; (e) miscellaneous group that work in a variety of ways, e.g. asparaginase.

cytotoxins *npl* antibodies which are toxic to cells.

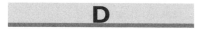

D

D and C *abbr* dilatation and curettage.

D₂-receptor antagonists *npl* antiemetic drugs that block the dopamine receptors, e.g. prochlorperazine which belongs to the phenothiazine group, and metoclopramide. These drugs are used for vomiting associated with cytotoxic drugs, radiation, toxins and gastrointestinal disorders.

Da Costa syndrome cardiac neurosis. An anxiety state in which palpitations and left-sided chest pain are the most prominent symptoms in the absence of cardiac disease.

dacry(o)adenitis *n* inflammation of a lacrimal gland.

dacryocyst *n* an old term for the lacrimal sac (tear sac). The word is still used in its compound forms.

dacryocystectomy *n* excision of any part of the lacrimal sac.

dacryocystitis *n* inflammation of the lacrimal sac, which usually results in abscess formation and obliteration of the tear duct, giving rise to epiphora.

dacryocystography *n* radiographic examination of the tear drainage apparatus after it has been rendered radiopaque — **dacryocystographically** *adv*.

dacryocystorhinostomy *n* an operation to establish drainage from the lacrimal sac into the nose when there is obstruction of the nasolacrimal duct.

dacryocystotomy *n* incision into the lacrimal sac.

dacryolith *n* a concretion in the lacrimal passages.

dactyl *n* a digit, finger or toe — **dactylar, dactylate** *adj*.

dactylitis *n* inflammation of finger or toe. The digit becomes swollen due to periostitis.

dactylology *n* finger spelling. A form of communication used with people with hearing impairment. Can be used in conjunction with British Sign Language. ⇒ Makaton. ⇒ sign language.

DADL *abbr* Domestic Activities of Daily Living. ⇒ Activities of Daily Living.

daltonism *n* red/green colour blindness.

Dalton's law *n* a gas law. States that the pressure of a mixture of gases is a sum of the partial pressures that each gas would exert if it completely filled the space.

damages sum of money awarded by a court as compensation for a tort or breach of contract.

dandruff *n* (*syn* scurf) the common scaly condition of the scalp. It consists of dead keratinized epidermal cells. May be associated with skin diseases, such as seborrhoeic eczema (dermatitis). Fungal infections may be a factor in the aetiology.

dandy fever dengue.

Dane particle *n* the term used to describe the entire hepatitis B virus particle.

dark adaptation adjustments required by the eye to facilitate vision in poor light or darkness. The pupils dilate, the cones stop working, rhodopsin is formed and the activity of the rods increases.

data *npl* pieces of information, usually collected for a specific purpose. In clinical nursing, data which are requested on the patient assessment form are collected at an initial interview with the patient. Other data are collected by ongoing assessment and evaluation — **datum** *sing*.

data analysis data collected at the initial interview are analysed, with the patient when possible, to identify the patient problems (actual or potential) which are being experienced in everyday living that are amenable to nursing intervention. The cause may or may not be the medical diagnosis. Also describes statistical analyses on data. ⇒ data processing.

database a computer file or files, which stores information, e.g. a mailing list, where each record contains a number of fields. The stored information can be accessed and sorted as required.

data collection data can be collected by interviewing, during which a structured form, such as a patient assessment form, may be used. In some circumstances an unstructured interview might be appropriate. The data are referred to as subjective or soft data. The nurse, as a skilled interviewer, prompts and reflects so that the patient describes his/her condition as factually as possible. The nurse records the information as factually as possible to decrease bias. Other data are the result of measurement, e.g. the amount of urine passed in 24 h, and yet others are the result of testing, e.g. urine, and these are called objective or hard data. ⇒ confidentiality. ⇒ data. ⇒ database. ⇒ data analysis. ⇒ data protection.

data processing storage, sorting and analysis of data, usually electronically by computers.

data protection rules relating to security and access to information held about individuals, as in Data Protection Act 1998.

data set the collection of data relating to a specific group.

dawn phenomenon early morning hyperglycaemia; it does not result from the waning of subcutaneously injected insulin and has been found in nondiabetic subjects, as well as those with type 1 (insulin dependent) diabetes mellitus and type II (noninsulin dependent) diabetes mellitus. Large surges of growth hormone (GH) secretion have been implicated in the pathogenesis of the phenomenon. ⇒ Somogyi phenomenon.

day case surgery patients are admitted for surgery but discharged home the same day. The practice is increasingly common, especially with children. Ideally, patients are admitted to a specialized day surgery unit but some day admissions are cared for on a general ward. Also known as ambulatory surgery.

day centre a centre which people attend for 1, 2 or more days weekly. Recreational and occupational therapy and physiotherapy, or other services as appropriate, are provided. Greatest use is for people with mental health problems and for older people.

DDH *abbr* developmental dysplasia of the hip.

deafness *n* a partial or complete loss of hearing. *conductive deafness* is due to an obstruction which prevents the conduction of sound waves from the atmosphere to the inner ear, such as excess ear wax. *mixed deafness* combination of both conductive and sensorineural deafness. *sensorineural* or *nerve deafness* is due to damage to hearing receptors, the nerve or the auditory cortex in the brain, such as damage by the rubella virus during early pregnancy, or exposure to loud noise. ⇒ body language. ⇒ finger spelling. ⇒ Rinne's test. ⇒ sign language. ⇒ Weber's test.

deamination *n* removal of an amino group (NH$_2$) from organic compounds such as amino acids. The liver is able to deaminate excess amino acids and use the amino group to synthesize nonessential amino acids and urea.

death *n* irreversible cessation of the body's vital functions, usually assessed by the absence of a pulse and breathing. Death may be immediate and unexpected as when a child is killed in an accident; it can be sudden and unexpected, e.g. a person collapses and within 24 hours is dead; death can be expected because of the medical diagnosis, but in the end it can occur suddenly; or a person can be terminally ill for a period varying from a few days to several weeks or months. Nowadays, life-support systems, such as mechanical ventilation, can maintain vital functions despite brainstem damage; consequently stringent tests may be necessary to diagnose death in some situations. ⇒ coroner. *biological death* death of tissues. ⇒ gangrene. ⇒ necrosis. *brain death* a state characterized by a complete lack of brainstem activity due to irreversible damage requiring life support mechanisms if life is to be maintained. It can be ascertained by testing certain reflexes, e.g. gag and pupillary. Different countries have different criteria to diagnose brain death. The diagnosis can only be made in the absence of factors that could depress brainstem activity. Brain death is confirmed when there is no evidence of cerebral or brainstem activity, according to strict criteria. It is distinguishable from irreversible coma, when the brainstem and cerebellum remain functional so vital functions continue and patients are maintained with nursing care, feeding and fluids. *death certificate* official document issued, by the registrar of deaths, to relatives or authorized person which allows for the disposal of the body. It is issued after a notification of probable cause of death is completed by the medical officer in attendance upon the deceased or the appropriate documentation from the coroner. *death rate* ⇒ mortality.

debility *n* a condition of weakness with lack of muscle tone.

debridement *n* the removal of foreign matter and injured or infected tissue from a wound to expose healthy viable tissue. *chemical/medical debridement* is accomplished by the external application of a substance to the wound. ⇒ alginates. ⇒ enzymatic agents. ⇒ hydrocolloid dressings. ⇒ hydrogel dressings. *surgical debridement* is accomplished by removing the affected tissue using sterile instruments and aseptic technique.

decalcification *n* the removal of calcium and other salts, as from teeth in dental caries, or bone in disorders of calcium metabolism.

decannulation *n* the removal of a cannula.

decapsulation *n* the surgical removal of a capsule.

decay in psychology, the term used to describe the loss of information from the memory thar occurs spontaneously over time.

decerebrate *adj* without cerebral function; a state of deep unconsciousness. *decerebrate posture* a condition of the unconscious patient in which all four limbs are spastic and which indicates severe damage to the cerebrum.

decibel (dB) *n* a unit of sound intensity (loudness).

decidua *n* the endometrial lining of the uterus thickened and altered for the reception of the fertilized ovum. It is shed when pregnancy ends. *decidua basalis* that part which lies under the embedded ovum and forms the maternal part of the placenta. *decidua capsularis* that part that lies over the developing ovum. *decidua vera* the decidua lining the rest of the uterus — **decidual** *adj.*

deciduous *adj* by custom refers to the primary (or milk) teeth which, on shedding, are normally replaced by permanent teeth.

decision-making *n* in nursing, decision-making by both nurses and patients is becoming increasingly overt as patient participation in care and care planning is actively encouraged. The concept of informed consent acknowledges the patient's right to make decisions. ⇒ consent. ⇒ informed consent.

decompensation *n* a failure of compensation, usually referring to heart disease.

decompression *n* removal of pressure or a compressing force. *decompression of brain* achieved by trephining the skull. ⇒ trephine. *decompression of bladder* in cases of chronic urinary retention, by continuous or intermittent drainage via catheter inserted per urethra. *decompression chamber* used when returning deep sea divers to the surface. *decompression sickness* ⇒ caisson disease.

deconditioning eliminating an unwanted particular response to a particular stimulus. ⇒ aversion therapy. ⇒ conditioning.

decongestants *npl* agents which reduce or eliminate congestion, usually referring to nasal congestion. They can be taken by mouth, or they can be applied locally as drops or sprays, e.g. ephedrine.

decongestion *n* relief of congestion — **decongestive** *adj*.

decortication *n* surgical removal of cortex or outer covering of an organ, such as the kidney or the lung.

decubitus *n* the recumbent position; lying down. *decubitus ulcer* ⇒ pressure ulcer — **decubital** *adj*.

decussation *n* intersection; crossing of nerve fibres at a point beyond their origin, as in the optic and pyramidal tracts.

deep vein thrombosis (DVT) phlebothrombosis. A thrombosis occurring mainly in the deep veins of the legs and pelvis, but they can form in the axillary vein in the upper limb. Associated with venous stasis caused by immobility or heart failure, injury to vessel walls, and where blood coagulation has been altered, e.g. oral contraceptive. Material may become detached from the thrombus to form an embolus which travels through the heart to the lung. ⇒ antiembolic. ⇒ intermittent pneumatic compression. ⇒ pulmonary.

defaecation *n* voluntary intermittent voiding per anus of faeces previously stored in the rectum.

defence mechanisms ⇒ body defence mechanisms. ⇒ mental defence mechanisms.

defervescence *n* the time during which a fever is declining.

defibrillation *n* the conversion of certain cardiac arrhythmias (atrial and ventricular fibrillation and some tachycardias) to sinus rhythm. A defibrillator is used to deliver an electric shock to the heart that may be delivered externally through the chest wall or internally. ⇒ arrhythmia. ⇒ cardiac arrest — **defibrillate** *vt*.

defibrillator *n* a device used to convert certain cardiac arrhythmias to sinus rhythm.

defibrinated *adj* rendered free from fibrin. A necessary process in the preparation of serum from whole blood. ⇒ blood **defibrinate** *v*.

deficiency disease disease resulting from dietary deficiency of any substance essential for good health, especially the vitamins.

degeneration *n* deterioration in quality or function. Regression from more specialized to less specialized type of tissue. When the structural changes are marked, descriptive changes are sometimes used, e.g. colloid, fatty, hyaline etc — **degenerate** *vi*.

deglutition *n* the process of swallowing, partly voluntary, partly involuntary.

dehiscence *n* the process of splitting or bursting open, as of a wound.

dehydration *n* water depletion. Occurs when excess fluid is lost or intake is inadequate. It is often accompanied by varying degrees of electrolyte imbalance. In the body this condition arises when the fluid intake fails to replace fluid loss. This is liable to occur when there is vomiting, diarrhoea, excessive gastrointestinal drainage, e.g. after surgery, excessive exudation from a raw area, e.g. a burn, excessive sweating, haemorrhage, polyuria caused by disease such as diabetes mellitus or diuretic drugs. Presentation includes: a dry flushed skin, dry mouth with sticky saliva and furred tongue, thirst, oliguria and dark concentrated urine, constipation and, if severe, the person can develop hypovolaemic shock. If suitable fluid and electrolyte replacement cannot be achieved orally then fluid may be administered subcutaneously, rectally, via the intraosseous route and intravenously. ⇒ oral rehydration solution — **dehydrate** *vt, vi.*

7-dehydrocholesterol *n* a sterol present in the skin, converted to vitamin D by the action of sunlight.

deindividuation feeling that personal identity has been lost with an anonymous joining with a group.

déjà vu phenomenon an intense feeling of familiarity as if everything had happened before. It may occur in epilepsy involving temporal lobes of the brain and in certain epileptic dream states.

Delhi boil ⇒ oriental sore.

deliberate self-harm (DSH) ⇒ parasuicide.

delirium *n* abnormal mental condition based on hallucinations or illusion. May occur in high fever, in mental health problems, or be toxic in origin. *delirium tremens* results from alcoholic intoxication and is represented by a picture of confusion, terror, restlessness and hallucinations — **delirious** *adj.*

Delphi technique a research method where a consensus of expert opinion is obtained by a seven-step process with the chosen group of contributors, who are asked to rate a number of items, e.g. areas for research, in order of importance.

delta (δ) *n* fourth letter of the Greek alphabet. *delta cells* ⇒ islets of Langerhans. *delta wave (rhythm)* high amplitude brain waves with a frequency of less than 4 Hz. Recorded during deep sleep and when the reticular activating system is inhibited.

delta virus old term for hepatis D virus. It is an incomplete RNA virus that causes hepatitis D, but only in the presence of the active hepatitis B virus infection. Transmission is the same as for hepatitis B.

deltoid *adj* triangular. *deltoid muscle* covers the shoulder joint and is inserted into the mid-humerus. Acts at the shoulder, with other muscles, to facilitate a wide range of movements.

delusion *n* a false belief, inconsistent with the individual's culture, use and level of intelligence, which cannot be altered by argument or reasoning. Found as a psychotic symptom in several types of mental illness, notably schizophrenia, paraphrenia, paranoia, senile psychoses, mania and depressive states. ⇒ Delusions Rating Scale. ⇒ Insight Scale.

Delusions Rating Scale (DRS) unpublished scale that uses a structured interview designed to elicit details regarding different delusional beliefs. It consists of six items that range from the amount of preoccupation to intensity of distress and disruption.

demarcation *n* an outlining of the junction of diseased and healthy tissue, often used when referring to gangrene.

dementia *n* (*syn* organic brain syndrome, OBS) the irreversible deterioration of mental functioning resulting from organic brain disease. It is increasingly known as brain failure. The causes include: Alzheimer's disease, arteriosclerosis, multiple infarcts, toxins, trauma, infective agents and age-related atrophy occurring in old age. It affects memory, personality, intellect, judgement, and the ability to self-care. *presenile dementia* signs and symptoms of dementia occurring in people between 40 and 60 years of age, due to early degeneration of both the medium and small cerebral blood vessels. ⇒ Alzheimer's disease. ⇒ Creutzfeldt-Jakob disease. ⇒ Huntington's disease. ⇒ Pick's disease. See Box – Dementia.

demography *n* the study of population — **demographic** *adj* pertaining to demography. *demographic indices* such as age distribution, birth and mortality rates, occupation and geographical distribution, are used to provide a profile of a given population and to plan services.

demulcent *n* a slippery, mucilaginous fluid which allays irritation and soothes inflammation, especially of mucous membranes.

demyelination *n* demyelinization. Degenerative process by which the myelin sheath surrounding some nerve fibres is lost; occurs in multiple sclerosis and other demyelinating diseases.

dendrite *n* (*syn* dendron) one of many branched processes which are given off from the nerve cell body. That part of a neuron that receives impulses from other neurons and transmits them to the nerve cell body — **dendritic** *adj.*

Dementia

Dementia, the outcome of a variety of disease processes, leads to a decline in cognitive function. One of the leading causes of dementia is Alzheimer's disease but other causes are Creutzfeldt-Jakob disease (a transmissible dementia) and cerebrovascular disease. The prevalence of dementia rises markedly with age. The development of dementia can be described in three stages. In the early stages of dementia severe memory loss in the sufferers may be noticed along with subtle personality changes which family and friends are likely to notice. In the middle stages of dementia, when cognitive decline is severe, behavioural changes in the sufferer may become a problem and these include wandering, aggression and eating inappropriate substances and over eating. Incontinence of urine and faeces may also be a problem and while many families are able to care for sufferers at home for a considerable period it is also the case that the development of problems such as incontinence lead the family to seek help with care. As a result people with dementia may be admitted to nursing homes, continuing care wards, psychogeriatric wards and residential homes. The final stage of dementia is one where the sufferer becomes uncommunicative, unwilling to eat and eventually dies.

dendritic cells *npl* antigen presenting cells found in the spleen, lymph nodes and the blood. ⇒ Langerhans' cells.

dendritic ulcer a linear corneal ulcer that sends out tree like branches. Caused by the herpes simplex virus. Treated with idoxuridine. Also called dendritic keratitis, it can cause permanent corneal scarring with impaired vision.

dendron *n* ⇒ dendrite.

denervation *n* the means by which a nerve supply is cut off. Usually refers to incision, excision or blocking of a nerve.

dengue *n* (*syn* 'break-bone fever') one of the mosquito-borne viral haemorrhagic fevers, a disease of the tropics. It varies in severity and is characterized by limb pains, fever, headache, vomiting and a rash etc. The haemorrhagic form has a high mortality from disseminated intravascular coagulation and acute circulatory collapse.

denial *n* a complex unconscious mental defence mechanism in which difficult situations, or unacceptable or painful facts, are not acknowledged, in order to avoid distress, anxiety and emotional conflict. It may occur in response to changed circumstances, e.g. sudden incapacitating illness, impending loss of part of the body, or terminal illness. Psychological support provided by nurses can help the patient gradually to bear the reality in consciousness, and begin planning to cope. Recognized as one of the phases of the grieving process.

Denis Browne splints splints used to correct congenital talipes equinovarus (clubfoot). The splints are of metal padded with felt, with a joining bar to which the baby's feet are strapped. ⇒ club-foot. ⇒ talipes.

dens *n* a tooth.

dental *adj* pertaining to the teeth.

dental alveolus *n* a tooth socket in the jaw bone. ⇒ gomphosis.

dental amalgam ⇒ amalgam.

dental calculus *n* ⇒ calculus.

dental hygienist *n* a person with specialist training who is able to provide dental hygiene services under the supervision of a dentist. They are primarily concerned with dental hygiene, such as scaling, and the promotion of dental health.

dental plaque *n* noncalcified deposit on the surface of a tooth, composed of a soft mass of bacteria and cellular debris which accumulates rapidly in the absence of effective oral hygiene.

dental pulp *n* the connective tissue located within the pulp chamber/cavity inside a tooth. It contain nerves, blood vessels and lymph vessels.

dentalgia toothache.

dentate *adj* having own teeth present.

dentine *n* the very hard, calcified tissue forming the body of the tooth beneath the enamel and cementum, enclosing the pulp chamber and root canals.

dentition *n* refers to the teeth or their development and eruption (teething). ⇒ teeth.

denture *n* a removable dental prosthesis containing one or several teeth, or may be a complete upper or lower denture.

deodorants *npl* substances used to deal with odours at an environmemtal level or used for personal hygiene. In a nursing context, substances used to reduce malodour in infected wounds: describes diverse substances such as charcoal dressings; topical use of the antibiotic metronidazole etc.

deontological ethical theory that supports the view that there is a duty to act within certain universal rules of morality. This approach is associated with the work of Immanuel Kant. ⇒ utilitarianism.

deoxygenation *n* the removal of oxygen — deoxygenated *adj*.

deoxyribonucleic acid (DNA) a nucleic acid molecule found in the chromosomes of all organisms (except some viruses). See Box – Deoxyribonucleic acid and Figure 17. ⇒ chromosomes. ⇒ gene. ⇒ ribonucleic acid.

dependence *n* 1. the level of reliance a person has on others for activities of daily living. ⇒ dependency. 2. on a drug or chemical substance. Characterized by a compulsion to continue taking the substance, and often the presence of specific symptoms if the drug is withdrawn.

dependency *n* a measure of the level of nursing care a patient will require. May be used to calculate how many nursing staff will be required for a particular group of patients.

dependency culture in sociology, describes the view that unlimited State welfare provision may reduce the ability of individuals to be assertive and support themselves.

depersonalization *n* a subjective feeling of having lost one's personality, sometimes

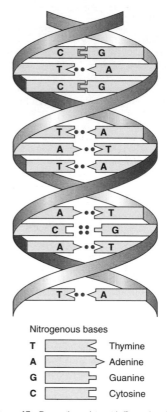

Nitrogenous bases

T	Thymine
A	Adenine
G	Guanine
C	Cytosine

Figure 17 Deoxyribonucleic acid. (Reproduced from Brooker 1996 with permission.)

that one no longer exists. Occurs in schizophrenia and, more rarely, in depressive states.

depilate *vt* to remove hair from — depilation *n*.

Deoxyribonucleic acid

Deoxyribonucleic acid (DNA) is the chemical which comprises the genes. It is a polymer consisting of nucleotides which, in turn, are molecules consisting of either a purine or pyrimidine ring (the bases of DNA: adenine (A), thymine (T), guanine (G) and cytosine (C)), a deoxyribose sugar (a pentose or 5 carbon sugar) and phosphate. The nucleotide units are bound covalently into long strands which form a double helix with the two strands held together by hydrogen bonds between specific bases: the adenine of one strand always lies opposite the thymine of the other and the same for guanine and cytosine.

The double strands of DNA confer its ability to replicate and conserve the genetic code. DNA replicates by unwinding and forming two new strands in which the genetic code is conserved by the base pairing between strands. The genetic code consists of triplets of bases called codons each of which codes for the incorporation of a specific amino acid into a protein molecule. The genetic code in DNA is transcribed into ribonucleic acid (RNA) which is a template for the translation, by incorporation of specific amino acids, into protein molecules. The processes of replication, transcription and translation are known as the *central dogma of genetics*.

depilatories *npl* substances used to remove superfluous hair on a temporary basis. May be used preoperatively to remove hair from the operation site. Being nonabrasive, they do not cause skin damage that could lead to infection. ⇒ epilation.

depolarization the inside of a membrane becomes electrically positive in respect to the outside in excitable cells. Occurs during nerve transmission. ⇒ polarized.

depot *n* a body area in which a substance, usually a drug, can be deposited or stored, and from which it can be distributed, such as contraceptives or hormone replacement therapy. *depot injections* preparations given by deep intramuscular injection, usually of a psychotrophic drug, used when clients fail to take their medications regularly.

depression *n* **1.** a hollow place or indentation. **2.** diminution of power or activity. **3.** a common psychiatric disorder. It may be described as *reactive*, usually occurring in response to loss or some other stressful event, or *endogenous*, which is more severe and occurs without apparent cause. See Box – Depression. *bipolar (BP) depression* (manic depression) coexists with episodes of hypomania, possibly accompanied by hostility, irritability and, in extreme cases, delusions and hallucinations. The main methods of management of depression are with drugs (⇒ antidepressants) and, in severe cases, electroconvulsive therapy. *unipolar (UP) depression* is characterized only by feelings of depression. ⇒ Beck Depression Inventory. ⇒ Calgary Depression Scale. ⇒ seasonal affective disorder (SAD).

deprivation indices *npl* a set of census variables and weightings used to assess levels of deprivation within a population. They include: levels of unemployment, overcrowded households, single-parent households, pensioners living alone and households without a car etc.

Derbyshire neck goitre.

Depression

"I am so depressed" is a term commonly used in everyday language by lay people to describe feeling down or low. The majority of people have a tendency to feel low at some time or another, however, these feelings are usually sporadic and go away without affecting daily living activities or functioning.

The medical definition of depression is somewhat different. A person's low mood is not alleviated by circumstances and it persists over time. There is both physical and psychological deterioration. Sleep, appetite and concentration are affected, the person often feels guilty, worthless and loses interests in all activities, sees little point to the future, expresses the desire to die and contemplates suicide (Craig 2000).

The ICD-10 classifies depression based on symptom patterns and the longtitudinal occurrence of the disorder.

Core symptoms

(a) depressed mood;
(b) loss of interest and enjoyment;
(c) decreased energy;
(d) reduced concentration and attention;
(e) reduced self-esteem;
(f) ideas of guilt and unworthiness;
(g) bleak and pessimistic view of the future;
(h) ideas or acts of self-harm or suicide;

(i) sleep disturbance;
(j) change in appetite and corresponding weight change.

Severity classification

Symptoms must persist for at least two weeks.

* Core symptoms: mild depression at least two of (a) to (c) plus at least one from (d) to (j); moderate depression at least two of (a) to (c) plus at least three from (d) to (j); severe depression all three from (a) to (c) plus at least four from (d) to (j).
* Somatic syndrome, at least four of: marked loss of interest/pleasure; lack of emotional reactions to events; waking in the morning two or more hours before usual time; depression worse in the morning; marked psychomotor retardation or agitation; weight loss of 5% or more in the previous month; loss of libido.
* Psychotic symptoms: mood congruent delusions and hallucinations.

References

Craig T K J 2000 Severe mental illness: symptoms, signs and diagnosis. In: Gamble C, Brennan G (eds) Working with Serious Mental Illness: A manual for clinical practice. Baillière Tindall, Edinburgh
World Health Organization 1992 ICD-10 Classification of Mental and Behavioural Disorders. WHO, Geneva

derealization *n* feelings that people, events or surroundings have changed and are unreal. Similar sensations may occur in normal people during dreams. May sometimes be found in schizophrenia and depressive states.

dereistic *adj* of thinking, not adapted to reality. Describes autistic thinking.

dermabrasion *n* ⇒ abrasion.

dermatitis *n* inflammation of the skin. A term used synonymously with eczema. *atopic dermatitis* ⇒ atopic eczema. *contact dermatitis* an exogenous dermatitis (eczema) that may be irritant or allergic in aetiology. Irritant substances, such as detergents, solvents and abrasives, may be encountered occupationally or at home. Napkin dermatitis is another form of irritant contact dermatitis caused by ammonia (in urine) and faeces; less common since the development of disposable nappies. Allergic dermatitis (eczema) results from a delayed hypersensitivity reaction to substances that include: nickel, latex, cosmetics and sticking plaster. *dermatitis herpetiformis* a bullous skin disease that responds to dapsone, sulphapyidine and a gluten-free diet. ⇒ pemphigus. *seborrhoeic dermatitis* ⇒ seborrhoeic eczema.

dermatoglyphics *n* study of the ridge patterns of the skin of the fingertips, palms and soles to discover developmental anomalies.

dermatographia *n* ⇒ dermographia.

dermatologist *n* a physician who studies skin diseases and is skilled in their treatment. A skin specialist.

dermatology *n* the study of the skin, its structure, functions, diseases and their treatment — **dermatologically** *adv*.

dermatome *n* **1.** an instrument for cutting slices of skin of varying thickness, usually for grafting. **2.** an area on the body surface or a segment of skin that receives sensory innervation from the cutaneous branches of a particular spinal nerve.

dermatomycosis *n* a fungal infection of the skin — **dermatomycotic** *adj*.

dermatomyositis *n* a rare connective tissue disease, more common in females. It is characterized by muscle weakness and pain, inflammation of the skin with a rash and scaling and periorbital oedema.

dermatophytes *npl* the three genera of fungi that cause superficial infections of skin, nails and hair, e.g. athlete's foot.

dermatophytosis *n* infection of the skin with dermatophyte species.

dermatosis *n* generic term for skin disease — **dermatoses** *pl*.

dermis *n* the true skin; the layer below the epidermis — **dermal** *adj*.

dermographia *n* (*syn* dermatographia) a condition in which weals occur on the skin after a blunt instrument or fingernail has been lightly drawn over it. Seen in vasomotor instability and urticaria — **dermographic** *adj*.

dermoid *adj* pertaining to or resembling skin. *dermoid cyst* a tumour derived from embryonic tissue. It is a benign cystic teratoma, usually of the ovary. It contains a variety of tissues: hair, nail, skin, teeth, bone and fatty tissue.

Descemet's membrane *n* posterior membrane of the cornea.

descriptive statistics that which describes or summarizes the observations of a sample. ⇒ inferential statistics.

desensitization *n* **1.** technique used to increase resistance to a particular allergen (antigen) by repeated exposure to small doses. Injected allergens are given to diminish or cancel out hypersensitivity to insect venoms, drugs, pollen and other causes of acute hypersensitivity reactions. **2.** a behavioural therapy used to help phobic patients overcome their irrational fear of specific objects or situations. The person is exposed to the irrational fear through imagining the objects, looking at pictures or by confronting the real object or situation — **desensitize** *vt*.

desiccation *n* drying out.

desloughing the process of removing slough from a wound. ⇒ proteolytic enzymes.

desmosome *n* a type of junction between cells formed from an adaptation of the plasma membrane. They hold cells together, especially where the tissue is subjected to mechanical stresses, such as in the skin. ⇒ gap junction. ⇒ tight junction.

desquamation *n* shedding; peeling off; casting off — **desquamate** *vi*, *vt*.

detached retina separation of the neuroretina (containing the nervous tissue) from the pigment epithelium. ⇒ retina.

detained patient *n* a person suffering from a mental disorder who has been detained under the Mental Health Act.

deterioration *n* progressive impairment of function; worsening of the patient's condition.

determinant, of health those factors that impact on the health of individuals and populations, such as economic conditions, social class, culture, access to health services, working conditions, unemployment, living conditions, level of education, community networks, personal lifestyle, age, gender and genetic inheritance.

detoxication *n* the process of removing the harmful property of a substance — **detoxicate** *vt*.

detritus *n* waste matter from disintegration.

detrusor *n* expelling muscle. See Box – Detrusor. *detrusor instability* failure to inhibit a reflex contraction of the detrusor. ⇒ detrusor/sphincter dyssynergia. ⇒ incontinence.

detrusor/sphincter dyssynergia a loss of the normal balance between detrusor contraction and sphincter relaxation to allow normal micturition to occur. The sphincter remains contracted although the detrusor contracts, and the result is incomplete voiding and an increase in the residual volume of urine.

detumescence *n* subsidence of a swelling.

developmental dysplasia of the hip (DDH) *n* also known as congenital dislocation of the hip. However, the term DDH is more useful as it covers the varying degrees and causes of the disorder.

There is usually poor development of the acetabulum allowing femoral head dislocation. It is essential to recognize the condition as soon as possible after birth and commence early treatment, usually involving various types of splinting, or possibly surgical intervention. ⇒ Barlow's sign/test. ⇒ frog plaster. ⇒ Ortolani's sign/test.

deviance *n* a variation from normal. In sociology, a departure from the accepted social norm, such as behaviour that does not fit the current norm.

devitalized *n* without life or vitality. Describes dead tissue. ⇒ necrosis.

dextran *n* a colloid solution obtained by the action of a specific bacterium on sugar solutions. Previously used for replacing fluids in hypovolaemia.

dextrin *n* a soluble polysaccharide formed during the hydrolysis of starch.

dextrocardia *n* transposition of the heart to the right side of the thorax — **dextrocardial** *adj*.

dextrose *n* (*syn* glucose) a soluble carbohydrate (monosaccharide) widely used in intravenous infusion solutions. Also given orally as a readily absorbed sugar in rehydration fluids for fluid and electrolyte replacement, for hypoglycaemia and other nutritional disturbances.

dextroxylase test xylose test.

dhobie itch *n* tinea cruris.

DI *abbr* donor insemination.

diabetes *n* a disease characterized by polyuria. Used without qualification it means diabetes mellitus. ⇒ diabetes insipidus. ⇒ diabetes mellitus.

Detrusor

The detrusor is the smooth muscle of the urinary bladder which stores urine until it is convenient for the urine to be expelled by micturition. The smooth muscle of the bladder is capable of stretching due to its convoluted structure and changes from pear shaped when empty to spherical when the bladder is partly full of urine. When there are about 200 mL of urine in the bladder, stretch receptors in the smooth muscle detect this but we are able to suppress the desire to micturate until it is socially convenient to do so or the bladder is extremely distended. Once we are prepared to micturate there is co-operation between the involuntary internal sphincter, which is formed from the detrusor, and the external sphincter which is voluntary and formed from the skeletal muscle of the pelvic floor. The sphincters relax together and urine is expelled from the bladder via the urethra. Disorders of the detrusor due to injury or infection may lead to an inability to sense the filling of the bladder (this may also occur due to damage to the nervous system) and incontinence of urine may arise as a result.

diabetes insipidus *n* there is polyuria with the excretion of large volumes (5–20 L/day) of dilute urine and excessive polydipsia (thirst). It may be: *cranial diabetes insipidus* caused by deficiency of ADH. Usually due to trauma or tumour involving posterior pituitary, but may be idiopathic. Treated with desmopressin, a long-acting analogue of vasopressin. *nephrogenic diabetes insipidus* where the renal tubules are insensitive to ADH. Treatment is with thiazide diuretics, such as bendroflumethiazide (bendrofluazide).

diabetes mellitus *n* a common syndrome caused by an absolute or relative deficiency of insulin. There is hyperglycaemia leading to glycosuria, which in turn causes polyuria (high specific gravity urine) and polydipsia. Impaired utilization of carbohydrate is associated with increased secretion of antistorage hormones such as glucagon, cortisol and growth hormone in an attempt to provide alternative metabolic substrate. Glycogenolysis, gluconeogenesis and lipolysis are all increased. The latter results in excessive formation of ketone bodies which in turn leads to acidosis. If untreated, this will eventually cause coma (ketoacidotic diabetic coma) and death. Diabetes mellitus may be: *insulin dependent diabetes mellitus (IDDM) or Type I* usually diagnosed in people aged under 40 years and requiring insulin and dietary control, or *noninsulin dependent diabetes mellitus (NIDDM) or Type II* which occurs mainly in people over 50 years, but can occur at an earlier age. It is generally controlled with oral hypoglycaemic drugs and dietary control, but insulin may be required in some circumstances. *potential diabetics* have a normal glucose tolerance test but are at increased risk of developing diabetes for genetic reasons. *latent diabetics* have a normal glucose tolerance test but are known to have had an abnormal test under conditions imposing a burden on the pancreatic beta cells, e.g. during infection or pregnancy. In the latter instance, the term *gestational diabetes* is commonly used. Gestational diabetes can only be accurately diagnosed in retrospect, as pregnancy onset diabetes can clear up or develop into the disease. ⇒ glucose tolerance test. ⇒ hyperosmolar diabetic coma. ⇒ hypoglycaemia. ⇒ ketoacidosis. ⇒ lactic acidosis — **diabetic** *adj, n*.

diabetogenic *adj* causing diabetes.

diagnosis *n* the identification of the disease or condition. *clinical diagnosis* one based on examination and consideration of the signs and symptoms. *differential diagnosis* made after comparing the features of two or more similar diseases. *laboratory diagnosis* one based on the result of laboratory tests. *nursing diagnosis* a statement of actual or potential health problems requiring nurse-initiated interventions that the nurse is qualified and compentent to deliver.

diagnostic *adj* **1.** pertaining to diagnosis. **2.** serving as evidence in diagnosis — **diagnostician** *n*.

dialysate *n* the fluid used in dialysis.

dialyser *n* used for dialysis. Contains two compartments, one for blood and the other for dialysate; these are separated by a semipermeable membrane. ⇒ haemodialysis.

dialysis *n* separation in solution of small molecular weight substances such as electrolytes, from a mixture containing colloids, using a semipermeable membrane. A technique employed to remove waste products from the blood in renal failure and reduce high levels of toxic substances such as drugs. It takes advantage of their differing diffusability through a semipermeable membrane, as in the artificial kidney. ⇒ haemodialysis. ⇒ haemodiafiltration. ⇒ haemofiltration. *peritoneal dialysis* the peritoneum is used as the semipermeable membrane in achieving dialysis for the removal of urea and other waste products. Dialysing fluid (dialysate) is run into the peritoneal cavity via the abdominal wall, waste moves from the blood vessels in the peritoneum into the dialysate, which is then drained out of the abdomen. Peritoneal dialysis can be used intermittently or continuously. ⇒ continuous ambulatory peritoneal dialysis (CAPD) — **dialyse** *vt*.

diapedesis *n* the passage of cells, e.g. leucocytes in inflammation, from within blood vessels through spaces in the vessel walls into the tissues — **diapedetic** *adj*.

diaphoresis *n* perspiration.

diaphragm *n* **1.** the dome-shaped muscular partition between the thorax above and the abdomen below. **2.** any partitioning membrane or septum. **3.** vaginal diaphragm. A rubber cap which covers the cervix to prevent conception. Reliable when used properly with a spermicidal chemical — **diaphragmatic** adj.

diaphragmatic hernia ⇒ hernia.

diaphysis n the shaft of a long bone. ⇒ epiphysis — **diaphyseal** adj.

diarrhoea n frequent loose stools that may, if prolonged or excessive, lead to dehydration, perianal soreness, hypokalaemia, acidosis (metabolic) and malabsorption. Causes include: infection, dietary change or indiscretion, food sensitivity, drugs such as antibiotics, laxative misuse, anxiety, irritable bowel syndrome, inflammatory bowel disease, colorectal cancer (alternating with constipation) and systemic diseases, e.g. hyperthyroidism. ⇒ spurious diarrhoea.

diarthrosis n a synovial, freely movable joint — **diarthrodial** adj.

diastasis n a separation of bones without fracture; dislocation.

diastole n the relaxation period of the cardiac cycle when the heart fills with blood. ⇒ systole — **diastolic** adj pertaining to diastole. ⇒ blood pressure.

diastolic murmur an abnormal sound heard during diastole; occurs in valvular diseases of the heart.

diathermy n the passage of a high frequency electric current through the tissues, whereby heat is produced. When both electrodes are large, the heat is diffused over a wide area according to the electrical resistance of the tissues. In this form it is widely used in the treatment of inflammation, especially when deeply seated (e.g. sinusitis, pelvic cellulitis). When one electrode is very small, the heat is concentrated in this area and becomes great enough to destroy tissue. In this form (surgical diathermy) it is used to stop bleeding at operation by coagulation of blood, or to cut through tissue in operation for malignant disease.

dibenzodiazepines a group of neurolepic drugs, e.g. clozapine.

DIC abbr disseminated intravascular coagulation.

dicephalous adj two-headed.

dicrotic adj, n (pertaining to, or having,) a double beat, as indicated by a second expansion of the artery during diastole. *dicrotic wave* the second rise in the tracing of a dicrotic pulse.

diencephalon n part of the brain between mesencephalon and telencephalon; contains the thalamus, hypothalamus, epithalamus and the third ventricle.

dietary fibre ⇒ nonstarch polysaccharides.

dietary reference values (DRV) n values that provide a range of intakes for most nutrients (macronutrients and micronutrients). ⇒ EAR. ⇒ LRNI. ⇒ RNI. See Box – Dietary reference values (nutritional requirement).

Dietary reference values (nutritional requirement)
Nutritional requirement is the amount of a specific nutrient required by an individual to reduce the risk of diet-related disease and maintain health. These differ for different individuals depending on age, gender, activity and physiological status. In the UK nutritional requirements have been estimated for different groups of the population and have been published as Tables of Dietary Reference Values (DRV) (DoH 1991).

Three different values are usually given. These are for populations of healthy individuals with no metabolic abnormalities.

Estimated average requirement
Estimated average requirement (EAR) is an estimate of the average requirement of a group of people. This means that 50% of the group will actually require more and 50% will actually require less. The EAR is usually used to estimate energy requirement.

Reference nutrient intake
Reference nutrient intake (RNI) is the amount of the nutrient that is required to ensure that the needs of most of the group (97.5%) are met. RNI is commonly used as an estimate of the micronutrient requirement of a population.

Lower reference nutrient intake
Lower reference nutrient intake (LRNI) is the amount of the nutrient that is sufficient for that small group of the population (2.5%) who have a low requirement.

When referring to these values it is important to ensure they are applied to the correct population group. The use of these values replaces the recommended daily allowances (RDAs).

Reference
Department of Health 1991 Report on Health and Social Subjects 41. Dietary Reference Values for food energy and nutrients for the United Kingdom. HMSO, London

dietetics *n* the study, interpretation and application of the scientific principles of nutrition to maintaining health and managing illness.

dietitian *n* a person qualified in the principles of nutrition and dietetics. They work in a variety of settings that include: the community, hospitals, schools, institutions such as residential homes, retail food outlets such as shops, restaurants and hotels, with large employers, e.g. local authorities, and in the food processing industry.

Dietl's crisis ⇒ crisis.

differential blood count ⇒ blood count.

differential diagnosis ⇒ diagnosis.

differentiation the process by which cells and tissues develop the ability to perform specialized functions that distinguish them from other cell types. Cancer cells are graded by their degree of differentiation: well differentiated cancer cells resemble their tissue of origin whereas poorly differentiated cancer cells are more primitive. ⇒ grading. ⇒ staging. ⇒ TNM.

diffusion *n* the process whereby gases and liquids of different concentrations intermingle when brought into contact, until their concentration is equal throughout (see Figure 18). ⇒ dialysis.

digestion *n* the mechanical and chemical processes by which food is converted to simple substances that can be absorbed into the blood or lymph — **digest** *vt*.

digit *n* a finger or toe — **digital** *adj*.

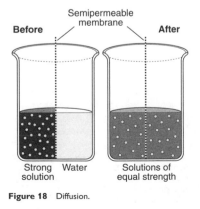

Figure 18 Diffusion.

digital compression pressure applied by the fingers, usually to an artery to stop bleeding.

digitalis *n* leaf of the common foxglove containing glycosides, such as digoxin. ⇒ glycosides.

1,25-dihydroxycholecalciferol *n* active form of vitamin D produced by the kidneys. Also known as calcitriol.

dilatation *n* stretching or enlargement. May occur physiologically, pathologically or be induced artificially. *dilatation and curettage* by custom refers to artificial stretching of the cervical os to procure endometrial curettings. ⇒ hysteroscopy.

dimercaprol (BAL) *n* an organic compound used as an antidote for heavy metal poisoning, e.g gold. It acts by binding to the heavy metal to form a stable compound that can then be rapidly excreted in the urine.

Diogenes syndrome gross self-neglect, usually an older person living in the most appalling conditions of squalor, often with many companion animals. The person concerned strenuously resists any attempts to change their environment.

dioptre *n* a unit of measurement in refraction. A lens of one dioptre has a focal length of 1 metre.

dioxide *n* oxide with two atoms of oxygen in each molecule, such as carbon dioxide (CO_2).

dipeptidases *npl* intestinal enzymes able to split dipeptides into individual amino acids.

dipeptide *n* a pair of linked amino acids.

diphenylbutylpiperazines a group of neuroleptic drugs, e.g pimozide.

2,3-diphosphoglycerate (2,3-DPG) *n* substance present in erythrocytes that decreases the affinity of haemoglobin for oxygen, thus ensuring that oxygen is released to the tissues. Production of 2,3-DPG by erythrocytes increases at high altitudes and in chronic lung disease.

diphtheria *n* a serious, notifiable infectious disease caused by *Corynebacterium diphtheriae*. Characterized by a grey, adherent, false membrane growing on a mucous surface, usually that of the upper respiratory tract. Locally there is pain, swelling and airway obstruction. The production of exotoxins cause serious systemic effects which include damage to heart muscle and nerves. Patients are isolated and close contacts are offered immunization and antibiotic prophylaxis. Immunization is available as part of the routine programme offered to babies and children — **diphtheritic** *adj*.

diphtheroid *adj* any bacterium morphologically and culturally resembling *Corynebacterium diphtheriae.*

diplegia *n* symmetrical paralysis of legs, usually associated with cerebral damage — **diplegic** *adj*.

diplococcus *n* a coccal bacterium characteristically occurring in pairs. Diplococcus may be used in a binomial to describe a characteristically paired coccus, e.g. *Diplococcus pneumoniae (Pneumococcus or Streptococcus pneumoniae).*

diploid (2n) *adj* refers to a cell with a full set of paired chromosomes; seen in all cells apart from the gametes. In humans the diploid number is 46 arranged in 23 pairs (2n). There are 44 autosomes and 2 sex chromosomes. → haploid.

diplopia *n* the word used alone implies the seeing of two objects when only one exists (double vision). May be due to a disorder of the extraocular muscles or of their nerve supply. Also known as ambiopia.

dipsomania *n* alcoholism in which heavy drinking occurs in bouts, often with long periods of sobriety between — **dipsomaniac** *adj, n*.

direct cost a cost that can be directly attributed to the budget of a specific department, e.g. catering costs in a given department.

disability *n* any restriction or lack of ability (resulting from an impairment) to perform an activity in the manner or within the range considered normal for age. Disability is likely to result in social disadvantage, in a society geared towards the majority, with impairment, e.g. when a person in a wheelchair is faced with an unramped flight of steps or a deaf person is interviewed by a nurse unable to use sign language.

disaccharide *n* a carbohydrate (sugar) formed from two monosaccharide units that join together by dehydration to form a glycosidic linkage. They include: lactose (glucose plus galactose), maltose (glucose plus glucose) and sucrose (glucose plus fructose). Chemical digestion breaks the glycosidic linkage between the two monosaccharides by adding water (hydrolysis) to produce two simple sugar units for use by the cells.

disarticulation *n* amputation at a joint.

discectomy *n* surgical removal of a disc, usually an intervertebral disc.

discharge *n* 1. used to designate a person's exit from treatment in the health service, e.g. from a community nursing service, health centre, outpatients' clinic, ward, or special unit. 2. the exudate from an infected wound. 3. excessive secretion from a mucous membrane (usually inflamed), e.g. vaginal and urethral.

disciplinary action the action taken by an employer, e.g. NHS trust, that follows the agreed disiplinary procedure, when a member of staff has made a serious error, acted unprofessionally or negligently or been convicted of a criminal offence ⇒ professional disciplinary process.

disclosing tablet *n* contains a substance that, when chewed, identifies dental plaque by staining it red.

discogenic *adj* arising in or produced by a disc, usually an intervertebral disc.

discrete *adj* distinct, separate, not merging.

discrimination *n* 1. attitude to, and treatment of, a person solely on the grounds of prejudice towards a characteristic of the group to which the person belongs, v.g. gender, religious beliefs, age, sexual preference or skin colour. 2. ability to distinguish between certain characteristics, e.g. sounds.

disease *n* any deviation from or interruption of the normal structure and function of any part of the body. It is manifested by a characteristic set of signs and symptoms and in most instances the aetiology, pathology and prognosis are known. It can be of an acute or chronic nature.

disease prevention see Box – Disease prevention.

disengagement theory *n* one of the psychosocial theories of ageing. It describes a process whereby people gradually disengage from life (physical activities and social contacts) as they become older. ⇒ activity theory.

Disease Prevention
Reducing the risk of disease, premature death, illness or disability is part of work to improve the population's health. Traditionally, prevention is classified into primary prevention (seeking to prevent the onset of a disease or condition), secondary prevention (aiming to halt progression of a disease once it is established), tertiary prevention (concerned with the rehabilitation of people with an established disease and prevent further complications). Strategies for prevention include immunization and vaccination programmes to reduce or eliminate infectious diseases, health education to encourage changes in behaviour and screening to detect early indications of the presence of disease so that treatment can be started.

disfigurement *n* disfigurement occurs after, e.g. removal of any part of the body, or formation of a scar with consequent disruption of body image. It usually takes longer to come to terms with visible disfigurement but all need to go through a psychological process of incorporating the change into the body image.

disimpaction *n* separation of the broken ends of a bone which have been driven into each other during the impact which caused the fracture. Traction may then be applied to maintain the bone ends separate and in good alignment.

disinfectants *npl* a word usually reserved for chemicals that destroy micro-organisms. They are too corrosive or toxic to be applied to tissues, but are suitable for application to inanimate objects. Their effectiveness may be seriously impaired by the presence of organic material.

disinfection *n* the removal or destruction of harmful microbes but not usually bacterial spores. It is commonly achieved by using heat or chemicals.

disinfestation *n* extermination of infesting agents, especially lice (delousing).

disk *n* a general term describing various types of storage medium which permanently store computer data files. Most work by recording data by magnetic means, but some, such as CD-ROM, operate optically. *floppy disk* so called because it uses flexible magnetic material. It is removable from the computer which allows the physical transfer of data (maximum around 2 megabytes Mb) to another location. *hard disk* so called because it uses several metal platters. It is usually a fixed device in the computer and is capable of storing very large amounts of data. Often referred to as drive C. ⇒ byte. ⇒ CD-ROM. ⇒ drive.

dislocation *n* a displacement of organs or articular surfaces, so that all apposition between them is lost. It may be congenital, spontaneous, traumatic, or recurrent. ⇒ subluxation — **dislocate** *vt*.

disobliteration *n* rebore. Removal of that which blocks a vessel, most often intimal plaques in an artery, when it is called endarterectomy.

disorientation *n* loss of orientation. An inability to place oneself in terms of person, time and place. Occurs in toxic states, trauma and many mental health problems.

displacement *n* **1.** an unconscious mental defence mechanism whereby a distressing emotion is transferred to a substitute person or object. **2.** the loss of items of information from short term memory as new information is added. ⇒ chunking.

dissection *n* separation of tissues by cutting.

disseminated *adj* widely spread or scattered. ⇒ disseminated intravascular coagulation (DIC).

disseminated intravascular coagulation (DIC) a pathological overstimulation of the coagulation processes characterized by a rapid consumption of clotting factors which leads to microvascular thrombi and bleeding. It occurs in situations where there is inadequate organ perfusion, such as hypovolaemia and or sepsis. ⇒ multiple organ dysfunction syndrome. ⇒ systemic inflammatory response syndrome.

dissociation *n* **1.** separation of complex substances into their components. **2.** ionization; when ionic compounds dissolve in water they dissociate or ionize into their ions. **3.** in psychiatry, an abnormal mental process by which the mind achieves non-recognition and isolation of certain unpalatable facts. This involves the actual splitting off from consciousness of all the unpalatable ideas so that the individual is no longer aware of them. It is seen in its most exaggerated form in delusional psychoses, e.g. a woman who, being deluded, believes she is the head of state, cheerfully scrubbing the ward floor. Her elevated status and her actions are completely separated or dissociated in her mind and she does not recognize the incongruity.

dissociative state conflict converted into psychological symptoms, e.g. amnesia.

distal *adj* farthest from the head or source. *distal convoluted tubule* ⇒ nephron. ⇒ proximal — **distally** *adv.*

distichiasis *n* an extra row of eyelashes at the inner lid border, which is turned inward against the eye.

distractibility *n* in psychiatry, a disorder of the power of attention, which can only be applied momentarily.

distraction therapy a term preferred by some nurses for diversional therapy.

distress negative stress. ⇒ stress.

district nurses registered nurses holding a specialist qualification who are employed to provide skilled nursing for patients in the community. They are qualified and accountable for assessing, prescribing and evaluating the nursing plan for such patients. ⇒ nurse prescribing. ⇒ specialist community practitioner.

diuresis *n* increased secretion of urine. ⇒ diuretics.

diuretics *npl* substances that increase the production of urine by the kidney. ⇒ caffeine. ⇒ carbonic anhydrase inhibitors. ⇒ loop diuretics. ⇒ osmotic diuretics. ⇒ potassium sparing diuretics. ⇒ thiazide diuretics.

divalent bivalent, having a valence of two, such as oxygen which combines with two atoms of hydrogen to form water.

divarication separation of two points on a straight line.

diversional therapy distraction therapy. The conscious use of diverting the focus of attention from one activity, object or person to another. It can be used to prevent boredom, institutionalization and in minimizing pain. Especially useful in children.

diver's paralysis caisson disease.

diverticulitis *n* inflammation of a diverticulum. Specially applied to those diverticula occurring in the colon.

diverticulosis *n* a condition in which there are many diverticula, especially in the colon.

diverticulum *n* a pouch or sac protruding from the wall of a tube or hollow organ, most commonly the colon, but also occur in the urinary bladder, small intestine and oesophagus. May be congenital or acquired. ⇒ diverticulitis. ⇒ diverticulosis. ⇒ Meckel's diverticulum — **diverticula** *pl* — **diverticular** *adj* pertaining to diverticula. *diverticular disease* term describing diverticulitis and diverticulosis.

dizygotic pertaining to two zygotes. Describes twins arising from two zygotes. Nonidentical twins who are genetically no more alike than siblings born at separate times. ⇒ monozygotic.

DNA *abbr* deoxyribonucleic acid.

DNA viruses *npl* several families of viruses that contain DNA as their nucleic acid, e.g. herpesvirus, hepadnavirus etc.

documentation of nursing documentation usually reflects the phases of the process of nursing – assessing, planning, implementing and evaluating. Nursing records and documentation are required for day-to-day communication and may be needed for the investigation of complaints, disciplinary or professional conduct proceedings, an inquiry, litigation for damages or a criminal prosecution.

Döderlein's bacillus a nonpathogenic Gram-positive rod which is normally part of the vaginal flora in women of reproductive age. It contributes to the protective acidic environment by the production of lactic acid. ⇒ Lactobacillus

doll's eye reflex a reflex present in the newborn where the eyes remain still when the head is moved from side to side. Normally disappears as development occurs.

dolor *n* pain; usually used in the context of being one of the four classical signs of inflammation – the others being calor, rubor, tumor.

dominant *adj* describes a gene with the capacity to overpower other recessive genes. Dominant genes are expressed in both the homozygous state (inherited from one parent) and the heterozygous state (inherited from both parents). Examples of dominant characteristics and diseases include: freckles, normal skin and hair pigmentation and Huntington's disease. ⇒ Mendel's law. ⇒ recessive.

dominant hemisphere on the opposite side of the brain to that of the preferred hand. The dominant hemisphere for language is the left in 90% of right-handed and 30% of left-handed people.

donor *n* 'to give a gift', such as blood for transfusion, semen or oocytes for fertility treatment, or an organ for transplantation.

donor insemination (DI) insemination of a female with donor sperm, either by direct insertion into the cervical canal or combined with IVF techniques. The donor undergoes screening for various conditions, including HIV infection.

Donovan bodies Leishman-Donovan bodies.

dopa *n* dihydroxyphenylalanine. An important compound formed in the intermediate stage in the synthesis of catecholamines from tyrosine.

dopamine *n* a monoamine neurotransmitter found in the central nervous system, especially the basal nuclei where its lack is linked to the development of parkinsonism. Used intravenously to increase cardiac output and renal blood flow in the treatment of shock.

Doppler technique used to measure the velocity of blood flow through a vessel to determine the degree of occlusion or stenosis. *Doppler ultrasound technique* in critical care the technique is used to calculate cardiac output and stroke volume by measuring blood flow in the aorta via a probe passed into the oesophagus. Used to monitor haemodynamic status and response to treatment. *Doppler scanning* combines ultrasonography with pulse echo.

Dornier lithotriptor a piece of equipment which can destroy certain types of kidney stones by shock waves, thereby rendering invasive surgery unnecessary. The technique is called extracorporeal shock-wave lithotripsy (ESWL).

dorsal *adj* pertaining to the back, or the posterior part of an organ.

dorsiflexion *n* bending backwards. In the case of the great toe, upwards. ⇒ Babinski's reflex.

dorsolumbar *adj* pertaining to the lumbar region of the back.

dorsum the posterior or upper surface of a body structure, e.g. foot, or the back of the body.

dosimeter, dosemeter *n* a device worn by personnel or placed within equipment to measure incident X-rays or gamma rays. Thermoluminescent dosimeters, using lithium fluoride powder impregnated into plastic discs, are used in personnel monitoring. Previously, photographic film in a special filter holder was used.

double vision ⇒ diplopia.

douche *n* a stream of fluid directed against the body externally or into a body cavity.

down regulation process, used in assisted conception, of temporarily 'switching off' the pituitary gland, preventing ovulation and therefore making easier the management of superovulation.

Down's syndrome a chromosomal abnormality, usually of chromosome 21 which fails to separate during meiosis, resulting in an individual with 47 chromosomes (trisomy 21). It may also be due to a problem between chromosomes of groups 13–15 and 21–22. ⇒ trisomy. See Box – Down's syndrome.

Down's syndrome

Down's syndrome is named after James Langdon Down who gave a detailed description of the condition in 1866. It is caused by chromosomal abnormality, either a third chromosome or trisomy involving chromosome 21 or in about 5% of cases a fused chromosome. The latter is inherited from a carrier parent whereas the risk of trisomy rises with maternal age from 1 in 800 at age 30 to as high as 1 in 50 when the mother is age 44 years or older. Both types of chromosomal abnormality produce multisystem disorders. These include generalized disturbance of growth, leading to characteristic facial features such as an upward slant of the eyes and a fold around the angle of the eyelids; muscle tone is poor in babies with Down's syndrome; the central nervous system is affected with the overall average weight of the brain decreased by 10–20%; intellectual disability shows as a delay in the achievement of developmental milestones although there is considerable variability in overall intellectual attainment. Other problems associated with the syndrome are congenital heart disease, upper respiratory tract infections, ear infections which may lead to conductive deafness, thyroid disease and acute lymphatic leukaemia.

dracontiasis *n* infestation with *Dracunculus medinensis* the Guinea worm. Found in parts of Africa, Asia and the Middle East, it is spread through contaminated drinking water. The female worm migrates from the intestine to emerge through the skin surface to deposit her larvae. There is inflammation and a cord-like thickening which ulcerates. Treatment is with anthelmintic drugs, e.g. praziquantel, mebendazole.

Dracunculus medinensis (*syn* Guinea worm) a tissue dwelling nematode parasite which infests humans. ⇒ dracontiasis.

drain *n* ⇒ wound drains.

drama therapy the promotion of personal growth by using games and improvisation to encourage spontaneity and positive ways of relating to self and others by means of verbal and nonverbal techniques. Incorporates many of the ideas of psychodrama but is more of an art therapy than a psychotherapy.

dreaming altered state of consciousness where fantasies and remembered events are confused with reality

dressings *npl* ⇒ wound dressings.

Dressler's syndrome *n* post-myocardial infarction syndrome characterized by pyrexia, pericarditis, pleurisy and effusion.

drive *n* that part of a computer that writes to and reads from a disk. ⇒ disk.

drop attacks periodic falling with vertigo due to transient interruption of cerebral blood flow. May be associated with cervical spondylosis. ⇒ vertebrobasilar insufficiency.

droplet infection transmission of pathogens via moisture droplets produced by sneezing, coughing, talking etc.

dropsy *n* ⇒ oedema — **dropsical** *adj.*

DRS *abbr* Delusions Rating Scale.

drug *n* the common name for any substance used for symptom control, or the prevention, diagnosis and treatment of disease. The word medicine is usually preferred for therapeutic drugs to distinguish them from the addictive drugs which are used illegally. For alleviating unpleasant symptoms of self-limiting illnesses, any remedy which does not require a prescription is termed an 'over-the-counter' (OTC) medicine. ⇒ general sales list (GSL). ⇒ pharmacy only (P). *drug clearance* ⇒ clearance. *drug dependence* a state of physical or psychological dependence on a particular drug arising from repeated administration of a drug on a periodic or continuous basis. Also called drug addiction. *drug error* see Box – Drug errors. *drug interaction* occurs when the pharmacological action of one drug is affected by another drug, food or beverage taken previously or simultaneously, e.g. monoamine oxidase inhibitors. *drug misuse* the term used by many lay and professional people for the illegal use of drugs. The term 'substance abuse' includes other substances, such as alcohol and solvents, as well as drugs. *drug*

Drug errors

Drug errors are preventable prescribing, dispensing or administration mistakes, and in UK hospitals around one in twenty doses is given incorrectly (Taxis et al 1998). As human error is inevitable, no matter how knowledgeable and careful healthcare workers are, a technique developed in industry known as 'failure mode and effects analysis' should be used to reduce errors (Cohen et al 1994). This involves identifying mistakes that will happen before they happen, and determining whether the consequences of those mistakes would be tolerable or intolerable. Where potential effects are unacceptable actions are taken to eliminate the possibility of error, trap error before it reaches a patient or minimize the consequences of the error when potential errors cannot be eliminated. For example, potassium chloride for injection in vials of 20 mmol per 20 ml, has been involved in more fatal medication errors than any other drug (Davis, 1995). Failure mode and effects analysis identifies the answer to this problem as removal of the possibility of error, i.e. remove potassium chloride for injection concentrate from ward environments and stock minibags of potassium chloride injection 20 mmol per 100 mL instead.

References

Cohen M R, Senders J, Davis N M 1994 Failure mode and effects analysis: a novel approach to avoiding dangerous medication errors and accidents. Hospital Pharmacy 29(4):319–330

Davis N 1995 Potassium perils. American Journal Nursing 95(3):14

Taxis K, Dean B S, Barber N D 1998 Hospital drug distribution systems in the UK and Germany — a study of medication errors. Pharmacy World and Science 21(1):25–31 *reaction* an adverse or unexpected effect associated with the administration of a drug, e.g. a rash. ⇒ adverse drug reactions. *drug resistance* the ability of various micro-organisms, e.g. methicillin resistant *Staphylococcus aureus*, to develop resistance to antibiotics. *drug tolerance* where the therapeutic effects of a drug reduce over time, requiring an increased dose.

drug trials *npl* the stages of testing that occur during the development of a new drug. (a) phase I trials involve a small number (20–80) of healthy vounteers, usually male. Only small doses are given and volunteers are monitored for adverse reactions. Blood samples are taken to ascertain drug distribution and excretion. (b) phase II trials involve patients (100–300) and the efficiency of the new drug is compared with other therapies. (c) phase III trials involve large scale multicentre studies prior to the drug being approved and licensed by the appropriate bodies, e.g. Committee on Safety of Medicines/Medicines Control Agency in the UK. (d) phase IV trials occur after the drug is in clinical use. Idiosyncratic reactions and adverse reactions not seen in earlier phase trials are monitored and reported. ⇒ Medicines Control Agency.

DRV *abbr* dietary reference values.

dry eye syndrome ⇒ Sjögren syndrome.

DSA *abbr* digital subtraction angiography.

DSH *abbr* deliberate self-harm ⇒ parasuicide.

DTPer *abbr* diphtheria, tetanus and pertussis vaccine. An injectable vaccine offered to infants at 2, 3 and 4 months; the triple vaccine.

dualism in psychology, a view that mind and body are distinct.

Dubin-Johnson syndrome *n* rare genetic condition where bile transport is abnormal. Leads to conjugated hyperbilirubinaemia and mild jaundice.

Dubowitz score assesses gestational age in low birth weight infants.

Duchenne muscular dystrophy a degenerative myopathy inherited as a sex-linked recessive disorder where a female carrier passes the abnormal gene on the X chromosome to her male offspring. The disorder usually begins to show between 3 and 5 years, and is characterized by progressive muscle weakness and loss of locomotor skills. Death usually occurs during the teens or early twenties from respiratory or cardiac failure.

Ducrey's bacillus *Haemophilus ducreyi*.

duct *n* a tube or duct carrying glandular secretions or excretions.

ductless glands *npl* ⇒ endocrine glands.

ductus a duct or small canal. *ductus arteriosus* a blood vessel connecting the left pulmonary artery to the aorta, to bypass the lungs in the fetal circulation. At birth the duct closes, but occasionally it remains patent. ⇒ patent ductus arteriosus. *ductus venosus* blood vessel which bypasses the fetal liver by shunting blood from the umbilical vein to the inferior vena cava. After birth it empties and becomes fibrous tissue.

dumbness *n* ⇒ mutism.

'dumping syndrome' the name given to the symptoms which sometimes follow a partial gastrectomy – epigastric fullness, dizziness, faintness, nausea and sweating soon after a meal. It results from the rapid movement of hypertonic stomach contents into the duodenum where fluid moves from the blood to the lumen of the intestine. ⇒ epigastrium.

duodenal *adj* pertaining to the duodenum. *duodenal intubation* ⇒ intubation. *duodenal ulcer* a type of peptic ulcer occurring in the duodenal mucosa. The aetiology includes a genetic predisposition and the vast majority are associated with the presence of the bacterium *Helicobacter pylori* in the upper gastrointestinal tract. Epigastric pain occurs some time after meals (hunger pains) and the person may wake during the night. The pain is relieved by food, antacids and vomiting. The ulcer can bleed, leading to haematemesis and/or melaena, or it can perforate, constituting an abdominal emergency. Severe scarring following chronic ulceration may produce pyloric stenosis and gastric outlet obstruction. Management includes: (a) general measures; smoking cessation, avoiding foods that cause pain, avoiding aspirin and NSAIDs; (b) drugs to irradicate *H. pylori*; specific anti-ulcer drugs, including H_2 receptor antagonists, e.g. ranitidine and the proton pump inhibitor, omeprazole, and antacids based on calcium, magnesium or aluminium salts; (c) surgical treatment may be required where medical treatment fails, in an emergency, such as perforation, or to improve gastric drainage. ⇒ vagotomy.

duodenectomy *n* partial or total excision of the duodenum.

duodenitis *n* inflammation of the duodenum.

duodenoenterostomy *n* operation to establish an anastomosis between the duodenum and another part of the small intestine.

duodenojejunal *adj* pertaining to the duodenum and jejunum.

duodenopancreatectomy *n* surgical excision of the duodenum and part of the pancreas, carried out for cancer of the head of pancreas. ⇒ Whipples operation.

duodenoscope *n* a side-viewing flexible fibreoptic endoscope — **duodenoscopy** *n*.

duodenostomy *n* a surgically made fistula between the duodenum and another cavity, e.g. cholecystoduodenostomy, a fistula between the gallbladder and duodenum made to relieve jaundice in inoperable cancer of the head of the pancreas.

duodenum *n* horseshoe shaped first portion of the small intestine, connecting the stomach above to the jejunum below. Secretes digestive enzymes, contains the openings of the bile and pancreatic ducts and is concerned with absorption — **duodenal** *adj*.

Dupuytren's contracture painless, chronic flexion of the digits of the hand, especially the third and fourth, towards the palm. The aetiology is uncertain but some cases are associated with hepatic cirrhosis. Management includes: exercises, or fasciotomy.

dura mater *n* fibrous outer meningeal membrane. ⇒ falx cerebri. ⇒ meninges. ⇒ tentorium cerebelli.

duty of care the legal obligation in the law of negligence that a person must take reasonable care to avoid causing harm.

DVT *abbr* deep vein thrombosis.

dwarf *n* person of stunted growth. May be due to growth hormone deficiency. Also occurs in untreated congenital hypothyroidism and juvenile hypothyroidism, achondroplasia and other conditions.

dwarfism *n* arrested growth and development, as occurs in hypothyroidism and in some chronic diseases, such as intestinal malabsorption, renal failure and rickets.

dynamic psychology a psychological approach which stresses the importance of (typically unconscious) energy or motives, as in Freudian or psychoanalytic theory.

dynamometer *n* apparatus to test the strength of grip.

dysaesthesia *n* impairment of touch sensation.

dysarthria *n* a speech disorder resulting from disturbance in muscular control of the speech mechanism due to damage to the central and/or peripheral nervous system. The loss of muscular control may involve weakness, slowness and/or incoordination. Disturbance may involve respiration, phonation, articulation, resonance and prosody — **dysarthric** *adj*.

dyscalculia *n* impairment of numeral ability.

dyschesia *n* difficult or painful defaecation.

dyschondroplasia *n* inherited developmental problem, where cartilage is deposited within bones or on the cortical surface. Also called enchondromatosis.

dysentery *n* inflammation of the bowel with evacuation of blood and mucus, accompanied by tenesmus and colic. *amoebic dysentery* is caused by the protozoon *Entamoeba histolytica*. → amoebiasis. *bacillary dysentery* is caused by *Shigella boydii*, *S. dysenteriae*, *S. flexneri* or *S. sonnei*. Disease results from poor sanitation, and the house-fly carries the infection from faeces to food. ⇒ Shigella — **dysenteric** *adj*.

dysfunction *n* 1. a temporary or permanent inability to perform the normal activities (roles, occupations and relationships) expected for a person of that age, culture and gender. 2. abnormal functioning of any organ or part.

dysfunctional uterine bleeding *n* heavy periods or intermenstrual bleeding in the absence of demonstrable pelvic pathology. There are, however, histological changes in the endometrium and it is linked to an imbalance between levels of oestrogen and progesterone during the luteal phase. All cases of abnormal uterine bleeding should be fully investigated to exclude serious pathology.

dysgammaglobulinaemia *n* an inherited immunodeficiency due to a failure to produce certain classes of immunoglobulins. It results in repeated infection. ⇒ globulins.

dysgenesis *n* abnormal development — **dysgenetically** *adv.*

dysgerminoma *n* a rare tumour of the ovary. It arises from undifferentiated germ cells of the embryonic gonad and is histologically identical to a seminoma.

dysgraphia *n* an acquired disorder of written language due to brain injury. The ability to spell familiar and/or unfamiliar words is affected in one or many modalities (handwriting, wordprocessing, etc). A number of different types of dysgraphia are recognized — **dysgraphic** *adj.*

dyshidrosis *n* an abnormality of sweating — **dyshidrotic** *adj* relating to dyshidrosis. *dyshidrotic eczema* ⇒ eczema.

dyskaryosis *n* abnormal cellular change. ⇒ dysplasia.

dyskinesia *n* (clumsy child syndrome) a long recognized but only recently diagnosed condition. There is inability to coordinate and programme voluntary movement, so that the child appears to be clumsy, writes badly, cannot tie shoelaces and so on. Responds to a special system of behavioural training — **dyskinetic** *adj.*

dyslexia *n* a disorder of reading. A number of different types of dyslexia are recognized, e.g. deep dyslexia and surface dyslexia. Many patients with dyslexia may also present with dysgraphia — **dyslexic** *adj.*

dysmaturity *n* signs and symptoms of growth retardation at birth. ⇒ low birthweight.

dysmelia *n* malformation in the development of the limbs.

dysmenorrhoea *n* painful menstruation, which in some women responds to simple analgesia, an oral antiprostaglandin and in others to an oral contraceptive. *spasmodic or primary dysmenorrhoea* most often affects young women once ovulatory cycles have become established. It comes on during the first day of a period, often within an hour or two of the start of bleeding. It comes in spasms of acute colicky pain in the lower part of the abdomen, and sometimes in the back and inner parts of the thighs. The spasms can be bad enough to cause fainting and vomiting. *congestive or secondary dysmenorrhoea* usually affects women in their late twenties and may be associated with pelvic pathology, such as fibroids or endometriosis. Women know several days in advance that their period is coming, because they have a dull aching pain in the lower abdomen, increasing heaviness, perhaps constipation, nausea and lack of appetite. There may also be breast tenderness, headache and backache.

dysmorphogenic *adj* ⇒ teratogen.

dysostosis *n* abnormal bone formation.

dyspareunia *n* painful or difficult coitus. ⇒ vaginismus.

dyspepsia *n* indigestion — **dyspeptic** *adj.*

dysphagia *n* difficulty in swallowing. See Box – Dysphagia — **dysphagic** *adj.*

dysphasia *n* ⇒ aphasia. See Box – Dysphasia.

dysphonia *n* a disorder of voice due to organic, neurological, behavioural or psychogenic causes — **dysphonic** *adj.*

Dysphagia

Dysphagia is a disorder of swallowing. Difficulty in swallowing can occur in many different medical conditions including cerebral palsy, motor neurone disease, stroke (cerebrovascular accident), dementia, head and neck cancer and so forth. A person can experience difficulty swallowing fluids and/or foods and the degree of difficulty can range from a mild to a severe difficulty. Assessment and management of dysphagia is best conducted by a multidisciplinary team that may include a speech and language therapist. The composition of the team will be determined by the needs of the patient, the medical condition underlying the swallowing problem and the clin-

ical setting. The signs and symptoms which may be indicative of a swallowing problem include:

- Excessive coughing;
- Chest infections;
- Weight loss;
- Failure to thrive;
- Aversion to eating;
- Oral sensitivity and drooling;
- Prolonged time to eat a meal;
- Avoidance of certain types of foods.

Further reading
Logemann J A 1989. Evaluation and treatment of swallowing disorders. 2nd Edn. Austin, Texas: Pro-Ed.

Dysphasia

Dysphasia, sometimes called aphasia, is a disorder of language and is not a disorder of intellect. It occurs most commonly following a left-sided stroke (cerebrovascular accident), but can occur after a head injury or neurosurgery. Dysphasia can affect a person's ability to understand language and also to use language to express themselves. People with dysphasia vary greatly in their profiles of skills and difficulties and it is important that detailed, individual consideration is given to their difficulties. Understanding language includes both understanding what is said and what is written. Likewise, expressing oneself includes both verbal expression and written expression. A discrepancy between the level of understanding and expression of language is common. Most often, individuals with dysphasia have impairments both in comprehension and in expression although the degree of impairment in each may vary. Assessment and treatment of dysphasia requires a detailed understanding of language and the breakdown of language. Speech and language therapists can provide therapy to assist individuals and their carers to improve their communication. Rehabilitation may take many months. Dysphasia has a considerable impact on many aspects of life such as work and leisure activities and also on relationships. People with dysphasia can become very withdrawn and isolated if they do not receive sufficient support.

dysphoria restless mood with depression and anguish.

dysplasia *n* changes in epithelial cell size and shape; results from chronic irritation or inflammation. Commonly affects the skin, cervix and oesophagus. They are serious changes that can progress to the development of cancer — **dysplastic** *adj*.

dyspnoea *n* difficulty in, or laboured, breathing; can be mainly of an inspiratory nature as in choking, or expiratory as in asthma — **dysponoeic** *adj*.

dyspraxia *n* lack of voluntary control over muscles, particularly the orofacial ones. A range of different dyspraxias can occur, e.g. limb dyspraxia, dressing dyspraxia and ideometer dyspraxia. Articulatory dyspraxia affects the ability to control the positioning of speech muscles and the sequencing of speech movements. Developmental dyspraxias may be found in children. ⇒ apraxia — **dyspraxic** *adj*.

dysreflexia *n* ⇒ autonomic dysreflexia.

dysrhythmia *n* disordered rhythm, usually of heart. ⇒ arrhythmia — **dysrhythmic** *adj*.

dystaxia *n* difficulty in controlling voluntary movements. ⇒ ataxia — **dystaxic** *adj*.

dystocia *n* difficult or slow labour.

dystrophy *n* defective nutrition of an organ or tissue, usually muscle. ⇒ Duchenne muscular dystrophy. ⇒ muscular dystrophies.

dysuria *n* painful micturition — **dysuric** *adj*.

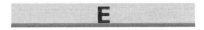

EAB *abbr* ⇒ extra-anatomic bypass.

ear *n* the sensory organ for hearing and balance. Consists of the outer (external), middle (tympanic cavity) and inner (internal) ear. The outer ear comprises the pinna (auricle) and the external auditory canal along which sound waves pass to vibrate the tympanic membrane which separates it from the middle ear. The middle ear is an air-filled cavity and contains three tiny bones or ossicles: malleus, incus and stapes. The sound waves are transmitted by the ossicles to the inner ear via the oval window. The middle ear communicates with the nasopharynx via the pharyngotympanic tube (also known as the eustachian tube). The fluid-filled inner ear comprises the organ of hearing; the cochlea and the semicircular canals which are concerned with balance. The cochlea and semicircular canals contain the nerve endings of the cochlear and vestibular branches of the vestibulocochlear or auditory nerve (VIIIth cranial). (See Figure 19). ⇒ cerumen. ⇒ cochlea. ⇒ organ of Corti.

EAR *acr* estimated average requirement.

eardrum *n* the tympanic membrane at the end of the external auditory canal. To its inner surface is attached the first of the auditory ossicles. ⇒ ear.

Early Signs Scale (ESS) an assessment scale used to predict relapse in people with schizophrenia. It describes the

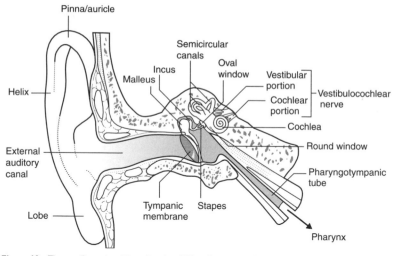

Figure 19 The ear. (Reproduced from Brooker 1996 with permission.)

problems and complaints that people sometimes have prior to relapse. There are thirty four items that describe feelings and behaviours which can occur prior to relapse. Each item is rated on a 0 (not a problem) to 3 (marked problem) scale.

early warning signs various signs, such as behaviour changes, that indicate the imminent worsening of a mental health problem. Indications of potential deterioration, through the use of specialized assessment tools, allow mental health nurses to plan early interventions aimed at preventing serious effects. ⇒ cancer early warning. ⇒ Early Signs Scale.

eating disorders *npl* a group of disorders that include anorexia nervosa, bulimia nervosa and binge eating. See Box – Eating disorders.

EB *abbr* epidermolysis bullosa.

EBM *abbr* **1.** expressed breast milk. **2.** Evidence-based medicine. See Box – Evidence-based practice.

Ebola *n* one of the viral haemorrhagic fevers occuring as epidemics and sporadically in Africa. Mortality is very high and management consists of supportive measures only. ⇒ filoviruses.

EBP *abbr* Evidence-based Practice.

Eating disorders

Eating disorders may be divided into three categories (see below). All three categories are psychological illnesses in which anxiety and distress are expressed in disordered eating behaviours such as binge eating, restriction of food intake or the alternation of severe dietary restriction with binge eating. Eating disorders are more prevalent amongst females than males.

Anorexia nervosa

In anorexia nervosa the distorted body image of the individual means that they have a fear of fatness and gaining weight and find it impossible to believe that they are a normal weight. People with anorexia nervosa show the signs and symptoms of severe malnutrition including muscle wasting, osteoporosis and amenorrhoea in females.

Bulimia nervosa

Bulimia nervosa is a condition in which the sufferer eats an enormous amount of food in a short period of time and then attempts to prevent weight gain by one or more of the following: taking laxatives; excessive exercising; and fasting. Individuals may be spending a large proportion of their income on food to maintain the high levels of food intake.

Binge eating disorder

Binge eating disorder is a less well documented disorder in which periods of binge eating are interspersed with periods of strict dieting which result in large fluctuations in body weight. It has been estimated that 20–30% of people who are obese suffer from binge eating disorder.

EBV *abbr* Epstein-Barr virus.

ecbolic *adj* describes any agent which stimulates contraction of the gravid uterus and hastens expulsion of its contents, e.g. ergometrine. ⇒ oxytocic.

eccentric not positioned centrally. *eccentric muscle work* paying out of a muscle, allowing attachments to be drawn further apart. Walking down stairs, the hamstring group of muscles work eccentrically to control straightening of the knee. ⇒ concentric muscle work.

ecchondroma *n* a benign tumour composed of cartilage which protrudes from the surface of the bone in which it arises — **ecchondromata** *pl*.

ecchymosis *n* an extravasation of blood under the skin. ⇒ bruise — **ecchymoses** *pl*.

eccrine *n* the most abundant type of sweat gland. They play a major role in temperature homeostasis; wherein the evaporation of sweat from the skin surface results in heat loss. ⇒ apocrine.

ECF *abbr* extracellular fluid.

ECG *abbr* electrocardiogram. → electrocardiograph. Also electrocorticography.

Echinococcus *n* a genus of cestodes, tapeworms, e.g. *Echinococcus granulosa* that infects dogs and other canines as the primary host. Its larval stage can infect humans through handling affected dogs or drinking water contaminated with eggs. The encysted larvae cause hydatid disease in human and other animals, e.g. sheep and cattle who act as a secondary host. ⇒ hydatid cyst.

echocardiography *n* a noninvasive cardiac investigation that uses ultrasound as a diagnostic tool for studying blood flow, the heart structure and the movement of heart valves and the myocardium.

echoencephalography *n* passage of ultrasound waves across the head. Can detect abscess, blood clot, injury or tumour within brain.

echolalia *n* repetition, almost automatically, of words or phrases heard. Occurs most commonly in schizophrenia and dementia; sometimes in toxic delirious states. A normal characteristic of all infants' speech — **echolalic** *adj*.

echopraxia *n* involuntary mimicking of another's movements.

echoviruses *npl* a group of enteroviruses. The various strains (around 40) cause conditions that include: meningitis, encephalitis, rashes, respiratory infection and gastroenteritis. The name derives from Enteric Cytopathic Human Orphan.

ECI *abbr* Experience of Caregiving Inventory.

eclampsia *n* **1.** a severe manifestation of pregnancy-induced hypertension, associated with fits and coma. ⇒ pre-eclampsia. **2.** a sudden convulsive attack — **eclamptic** *adj*.

ecmnesia *n* impaired memory for recent events with normal memory of remote ones. Common in old age and in early cerebral deterioration.

ECMO *abbr* extracorporeal membrane oxygenation.

ecological study a research study where a group of people, e.g. colleges, towns etc, are the observation unit.

economy spending or using as little as possible and still maintain quality.

Ecstasy *n* colloquial name for an amfetamine (amphetamine) derivative (methylenedioxymethamphetamine) that causes euphoria and hallucinations. Its illegal misuse is widespread at 'raves' and clubs. Many users consider it to be safe, but there may be serious effects from extreme physical acitivity and dehydration which leads to hyperpyrexia and possibly death. ⇒ MDMA.

ECT *abbr* electroconvulsive therapy.

ectasia dilatation of a hollow structure, such as a duct.

ecthyma *n* a type of impetigo characterized by pustule formation with crusts and ulceration. It most frequently affects the skin of the legs.

ectoderm *n* the outer of the three primary germ layers of the early embryo. From it are developed some epithelial and nervous tissue. Surface ectoderm gives rise to skin structures (epidermis, nails, hair and sebaceous glands), lens of the eye, inner ear, enamel on teeth, the mammary glands and the anterior pituitary glands. Neuroectoderm forms the central nervous system, cranial, spinal and autonomic nerves, adrenal medulla, posterior pituitary gland, pineal body (gland) and the retina of the eye. ⇒ endoderm. ⇒ mesoderm — **ectodermal** *adj*.

ectodermosis *n* disease of any organ or tissue derived from the ectoderm.

ectogenesis *n* the growth of the embryo outside the uterus (in vitro fertilization).

ectogenous *adj* originating outside an organism. ⇒ endogenous *ant.*

ectoparasite *n* a parasite that lives on the exterior surface of its host, such as a flea — **ectoparasitic** *adj.*

ectopia *n* malposition of an organ or structure, usually congenital. *ectopia vesicae* an abnormally placed urinary bladder which protrudes through or opens on to the abdominal wall — **ectopic** *adj.*

ectopic outside the normal place or time. *ectopic beat* ⇒ extrasystole. *ectopic pregnancy* ⇒ ectopic pregnancy.

ectopic pregnancy (*syn* tubal pregnancy) extrauterine gestation, the uterine tube being the most common site, but rarely the embryo implants in the peritoneal cavity. An ectopic pregnancy may result in: rupture of the tube with varying degrees of haemorrhage and shock, or the formation of a tubal mole (mass of tissue etc) when the embryo dies; this mole may be absorbed or cause a tubal abortion or rupture.

ectozoa *npl* external parasites.

ectrodactyly, ectrodactylia *n* congenital absence of one or more fingers or toes or parts of them.

ectropion *n* an eversion or turning outward, especially of the lower eyelid or of the pupil margin – *ectropion uveae.*

ECV *abbr* external cephalic version.

eczema *n* an inflammatory skin condition accompanied by intense itching of the affected area. The eczema skin reaction begins with erythema, then vesicles appear. These rupture, forming crusts or leaving pits which ooze serum. This is the exudative or weeping stage. In the process of healing, the area becomes scaly. Some authorities limit the word eczema to the cases with internal (endogenous) causes, while those caused by external (exogenous) contact factors are called dermatitis or eczematous dermatitis; however, the terms eczema and dermatitis are used synonomously. The lesions may be colonized or infected with hospital strains of *Staphylococcus aureus*. Due to the exfoliative nature of eczema, modification of patient management is required to protect others from infection. ⇒ dermatitis. The endogenous eczemas include: *asteatotic eczema* dry scaly skin associated with reduced sebaceous gland activity. It is exacerbated by frequent use of alkaline soap, dehydration and central heating. A particular problem for older adults. *atopic eczema* there is a genetic predisposition to react inappropriately to a variety of antigens leading to the development of eczema, along with diseases that include hay fever, asthma and other allergies. ⇒ atopy. *dyshidrotic eczema* a type of eczema that may be precipitated by stress and heat. Those affected may develop bullae and vesicles on the hands and feet. Also known as pompholyx. *eczema herpeticum* a vesiculopustular skin eruption caused by a herpes simplex infection in an existing rash, such as atopic eczema. It requires urgent referral to a specialist. Also called Kaposi's varicelliform eruption. *seborrhoeic eczema* a chronic skin condition characterized by scales and crusts that may be dry or wet. Fungal infections may be a factor in the aetiology. It takes three forms: (a) scalp, eyebrows and face. ⇒ dandruff; (b) skin folds or flexures, e.g. axillae, groin and under the breasts; (c) the chest and back. *varicose (gravitational stasis) eczema* occurs on the lower leg and is associated with signs of venous insufficiency and leg ulcers — **eczematous** *adj.*

EDD *abbr* expected date of delivery.

edentulous *adj* without natural teeth.

edrophonium test a diagnostic test for myasthenia gravis. An intravenous injection of edrophonium chloride (a short-acting anticholinesterase) will improve muscle power almost immediately, albeit temporarily, in patients with myasthenia gravis.

education consortia groups consisting of representatives from organizations who provide health care, e.g. NHS Trusts, Health Authorities, private sector etc, who are responsible for allocating resources to NMET for pre and postregistration education and training for all groups other than doctors and dentists. Plans to phase them out are in progress.

Edward's syndrome trisomy 18 or trisomy E. An abnormality affecting chromosomes in group E; 17–18; the individual has a third chromosome 18 which results in them having 47 chromosomes. It is characterized by micrognathia, low-set malformed ears, overlapping fingers, 'rocker bottom' feet, multiple congenital anomalies, such as heart defects, and severe learning disability. Few babies survive more than a few months. ⇒ trisomy.

EEG *abbr* electroencephalogram. ⇒ electroencephalograph.

EFAs *abbr* ⇒ essential fatty acids.

effective dose *n* the amount of a drug that can be expected to cause a specific intensity of effect in the individuals receiving the drug.

effectiveness using resources to achieve the required outcomes.

effector *n* a motor or secretory nerve ending in a muscle, gland or organ.

efferent *adj* carrying, conveying, conducting away from a centre. ⇒ afferent *ant*.

efficiency using the minimum resources to achieve the maximum outcomes.

effleurage *n* a massage manipulation using long, whole-hand strokes in the direction of venous and lymphatic drainage, with the aim of assisting venous return to the heart and reduction of oedema. Deep effleurage causes dilatation of the arterioles by stimulating the axon reflex.

effort syndrome a form of anxiety neurosis, manifesting itself in a variety of cardiac symptoms including precordial pain, for which no pathological explanation can be discovered.

effusion *n* extravasation of fluid into body tissues or cavities. ⇒ pleural effusion.

ego *n* refers to the conscious self, the 'I' which, according to Freud, deals with reality, is influenced by social forces and controls unconscious instinctual urges (the id).

egocentric self-centred.

EHEC *abbr* enterohaemorrhagic *Escherichia coli*.

EIA *abbr* exercise induced asthma. ⇒ asthma.

EIEC *abbr* enterovasive *Escherichia coli*.

ejaculation *n* the sudden emission of semen from the erect penis at the moment of male orgasm. *retrograde ejaculation* occurs when semen is transported backwards into the bladder. May be a complication of diabetic autonomic neuropathy or prostate surgery.

elastin *n* a protein found in elastic fibres of some connective tissues and in the extracellular matrix holding cells together. ⇒ collagen.

elder abuse ⇒ abuse.

Electra complex excessive emotional attachment of daughter to father. The name is derived from Greek mythology.

electroacupuncture *n* originated in Europe but widely used in China. A mild electric current is applied to inserted acupuncture needles in order to intensify the sensory stimulation and stimulate the therapeutic effect.

electrocardiogram (ECG) *n* a recording of the electrical activity of the heart muscle during the cardiac cycle on a moving paper strip, made by an electrocardiograph. The normal heart produces a typical waveform, sinus rhythm, which consists of five deflection waves, known universally as PQRST. ⇒ PQRST complex. *ambulatory ECG (Holter monitoring)* method of recording heart rhythm and rate over a 24 hour period to detect transient ischaemia or arrhythmias. The person continues with their normal activities and keeps a log of times and activities. *exercise (stress) ECG* performed during increasing levels of exertion, such as on a treadmill, to detect arrhythmias or ischaemic changes caused by physical stress.

electrocardiograph *n* a device which records the electrical activity of the heart muscle from electrodes on the limbs and chest (see Figure 20) — **electrocardiographically** *adv*.

electrocardiography technique used to diagnose myocardial ischaemia and infarction, conduction problems and arrhythmias. Also provides information regarding drug toxicity and changes in body chemistry that affect heart rhythm.

electrocoagulation *n* technique of surgical diathermy. Coagulation, especially of bleeding points, by means of electrodes.

electrocochleography (ECoG) *n* direct recording of the action potential generated following stimulation of the cochlear nerve. ⇒ vestibulocochlear nerve.

electroconvulsive therapy (ECT) a form of physical treatment used by psychiatrists, mainly in the treatment of severe

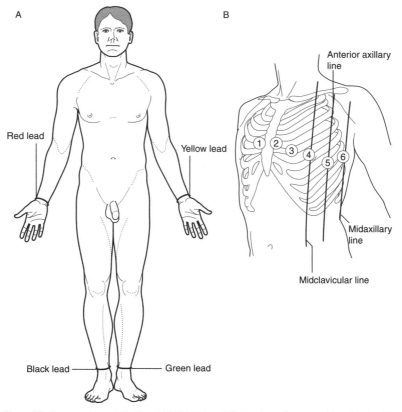

A

B

Anterior axillary
line

Red lead

Yellow lead

① ② ③ ④ ⑤ ⑥

Midaxillary
line

Midclavicular line

Black lead —— —— Green lead

Figure 20 Electrocardiograph. Position of (A) limb leads and (B) chest leads. (Reproduced from Nicol et al 2000 with permission.)

depression. A device is used which delivers a definite electrical voltage for a precise fraction of a second to electrodes placed on the head, producing a convulsion. The convulsion is modified by use of an intravenous anaesthetic and a muscle relaxant prior to treatment. *unilateral ECT* avoids the sequela of amnesia for recent events. The mechanism for memory of recent events is probably in the dominant cerebral hemisphere which is the left in practically all people. ECT is therefore applied to the right hemisphere to minimize memory disturbance.

electrocorticography *n* direct recording from the cerebral cortex during operation — **electrocorticographically** *adv*.

electrode *n* in medicine, a conductor in the form of a pad or plate, whereby electricity enters or leaves the body.

electrodesiccation *n* a technique of surgical diathermy. There is drying and subsequent removal of tissue, e.g. papillomata.

electroencephalogram (EEG) *n* a recording of the electrical activity of the brain on a moving paper strip, made by an electroencephalograph.

electroencephalograph *n* a device which records the electrical impulses derived from the brain. These can be amplified and recorded on paper — **electroencephalographically** *adv*.

electroencephalography technique that records the electrical activity of the brain by use of an electroencephalograph connected to electrodes placed on the scalp. Used in the diagnosis of conditions, such as epilepsy.

electrolaryngography an investigation used for voice analysis. It involves recording the electrical currents produced by the laryngeal muscles during speech.

electrolysis *n* 1. term used for the destruction of individual hairs (epilation), eradication of moles, naevi, etc using electricity. 2. chemical decomposition by electricity, with migration of ions shown by changes at the electrodes.

electrolyte *n* a liquid or solution of a substance, such as sodium chloride, which dissociates into electrically charged ions that conduct electricity. ⇒ anion. ⇒ cation. In medical usage it refers to the ion itself, e.g. sodium, chloride and potassium ions in the body. *electrolyte balance* the balance of relative amounts of electrolytes, such as sodium, potassium, calcium, magnesium, chloride, bicarbonate (hydrogen carbonate) and phosphate in blood fluids and tissues. The balance between positively and negatively charged ions ensures overall electrical neutrality within the fluid compartments of the body. Various conditions and diseases can cause electrolyte imbalance which is often associated with loss of fluid and pH homeostasis — **electrolytic** *adj.*

electromagnetic waves the spectrum of electric and magnetic radiation energy that includes the short wavelength gamma rays up to the long wavelength radio waves. ⇒ infrared rays. ⇒ ultraviolet rays. ⇒ X-rays.

electromechanical dissociation (EMD) a form of cardiac arrest characterized by an ineffective cardiac output where electrical activity is normal or nearly so. ⇒ cardiac arrest.

electromotive force (EMF) a measurement of the force needed for an electric current to flow between two points. The volt (V), a derived SI unit(International System of Units), is used.

electromyography (EMG) *n* the use of an instrument which records electric currents generated in active muscle — **electromyographically** *adv.*

electron *n* a subatomic particle with a negative charge. *electron microscope* uses a beam of electrons to visualize minute objects, such as virus particles. *electron transfer chain* a series of oxidation-reduction reactions occurring in the mitochondria that generate energy as ATP.

electro-oculography *n* the use of an instrument which records eye position and movement, and potential difference between front and back of the eyeball using electrodes placed on skin near socket. Can be used as a diagnostic test — **electro-oculographically** *adv.*

electrophoresis an analytical technique. Charged particles are separated in a liquid medium by their characteristic speed and direction of migration in an electrical field. It is commonly used for measuring serum proteins.

electroretinogram (ERG) *n* graphic record of electrical currents generated in the retina in response to exposure to light.

electroretinography *n* technique that records the electrical responses of the retina. Used in the diagnosis of eye problems.

element *n* a primary part. In chemistry, elements are the primary substances which in pure form, or combined into compounds, constitute all matter. They cannot be broken down by ordinary chemical processes.

elephantiasis *n* the swelling of a limb, usually a leg, as a result of lymphatic obstruction caused by filarial infestation. The skin and subcutaneous tissues are thickened (pachydermia), coarsened and fissured. ⇒ filaria. ⇒ filariasis. ⇒ lymphoedema.

elimination *n* the passage of waste from the body, usually reserved for urine and faeces — **eliminate** *vt.*

ELISA *abbr* enzyme linked immunosorbent assay.

elixir *n* a sweetened, aromatic solution of a drug, often containing an appreciable amount of alcohol.

elliptocytosis *n* elliptical red blood cells. Seen in autosomal dominant disorder hereditary elliptocytosis, a congenital haemolytic anaemia. May be found in small numbers in other types of anaemia, e.g. megaloblastic.

emaciation *n* excessive leanness, or wasting of body tissue — **emaciate** *vt.*

E-mail *abbr* electronic mail. A system of communication where messages are stored centrally prior to being dispatched via networks or modem to other computers.

emasculation *n* castration in the male.

embolectomy *n* surgical removal of an embolus.

embolic *adj* pertaining to an embolism or an embolus.

embolism *n* the condition in which there is obstruction of a blood vessel by a body of undissolved material. Most commonly due to thrombus, but other causes include: fat, malignant cells, amniotic fluid, gases, bacteria and parasites. Rarer emboli, such as fat, may follow long bone fractures, air may enter the circulation via a penetrating chest wound or during surgery, and amniotic fluid during labour. *arterial embolism* arising from the left side of the heart or a diseased artery, may travel to various sites including brain, bowel or limb; the effects depend on the size of vessel occluded and location, e.g. gangrene of a limb. ⇒ cerebrovascular accident. *pulmonary embolism* ⇒ pulmonary embolism. ⇒ deep vein thrombosis.

embologenic *adj* capable of producing an embolus.

embolus *n* solid body or gas bubble transported in the circulation. ⇒ embolism — **emboli** *pl*.

embrocation *n* a liquid which is applied topically by rubbing.

embryo *n* the early developmental stage starting two weeks after fertilization of the oocyte until the end of week eight of gestation. ⇒ gastrulation — **embryonic** *adj*.

embryology *n* study of the development of an embryo — **embryologically** *adv*.

embryoma *n* ⇒ teratoma.

embryopathy *n* disease or abnormality in the embryo — **embryopathically** *adv*.

embryotomy *n* describes an obsolete procedure that involved the destruction of the fetus to facilitate delivery.

EMD *abbr* electromechanical dissociation.

emergency protection order (EPO) replaces a place of safety order. An order issued by the court when they believe that a child may suffer significant harm. It transfers parental responsibility rights and allows for the child's removal to a safe place.

emesis *n* vomiting.

emetic *n* any agent used to produce vomiting, e.g. ipecacuanha. ⇒ antiemetic *ant*.

emetogenic describes substances that causes vomiting or have the potential to do so, e.g. cytotoxic drugs.

emission *n* an ejaculation or sending forth, especially an involuntary ejaculation of semen.

EMLA *abbr* eutectic mixture of local anaesthetics.

emmetropia *n* normal or perfect vision — **emmetropic** *adj*.

emollient *adj, n* (an agent) which softens, moisturizes and soothes skin or mucous membrane. Used to reduce scaly skin and water loss from the skin.

emotion *n* the tone of feeling recognized in ourselves by certain bodily changes, and in others by tendencies to certain characteristic behaviour. Aroused usually by ideas or concepts. See Box – Emotions.

emotional *adj* characteristic of or caused by emotion. *emotional bias* tendency of emotional attitude to affect logical judgement. *emotional lability* rapid change in mood. *emotional state* effect of emotions on normal mood, e.g. agitation.

empathy *n* identifying with another person or the actions of another person. See Box – Empathy — **empathic** *adj*.

emphysema *n* gaseous distension of the tissues. ⇒ crepitation. ⇒ pulmonary emphysema. ⇒ surgical emphysema — **emphysematous** *adj*.

empirical *adj* based on observation and experience and not on scientific reasoning.

employment law the law, common law and statute, relating to the relationship of employer and employee.

empowerment *n* the enabling process by which individuals gain power and control over decisions that affect their lives. For example, it may occur when individuals with learning disabilities acquire the ability to live independently in the community, or when a group of professionals who share the same goals are able to take collective control or responsibility for the decisions which affect their practice. The concept of empowerment and enabling activities can be applied to any situation.

empyema *n* a collection of pus in a cavity, hollow organ or space.

emulsion *n* fluid that contains two immiscible fluids; the particles of one are suspended in the other, such as milk which is a uniform suspension of fat particles in an aqueous continuous phase.

Emotions

Psychologists view the concept of emotion as consisting of two states: a cognitive mechanism and a state of arousal. The former determines what emotions the individual will experience. An appraisal of the emotion-generating stimuli, based on experience, will, therefore, cause the person to respond accordingly. Sometimes the individual may be aroused physiologically and subsequently searches for an explanation (cognitively aroused) for the feelings (e.g. fear, anxiety, depression) experienced.

In nursing practice, attending to clients and their families may alleviate their anxiety and fears (Gelling 1999). Further, using strategies (e.g. catharsis, counselling, biofeedback) to help the person reassess and evaluate the situation that is causing the emotional reactions can improve personal control over subjective experiences, and develop understanding.

In the field of mental health and psychiatric practice, it is argued that emotional dysfunc-tion is often attributed to biological problems – a common feature in psychopathy (Butler 2000). Furthermore, in chronically depressed individuals, psychosurgical interventions (which involve the destruction of specific fibres in the frontal lobes of the brain matter), have been known to improve emotional functioning, with a 50–60% recovery rate from depression (Butler 2000). Intense sufferings caused by some illnesses and diseases can elicit intense emotions. The need to talk to others, as a consequence, is accentuated (Davison et al 2000).

References
Butler G 2000 Emotion and the brain. The Psychologist 13(3):131–132
Davison K, Pennbaker J W, Dickerson J 2000 Who talks; the social psychology of illness support groups. American Psychologist 55(2):205–217
Gelling L 1999 The role of hope for relatives of critically ill patients: a review of the literature. Nursing Standard 14(1):33 38

Empathy

Empathy is related to a demonstration of insightful awareness of another person's biopsychosocial experiences. In contrast with sympathy, the empathetic person shows objectivity during interpersonal communication. Some researchers have described the latter as 'empathic concern' (being concerned for patients); and the former (sympathy) as 'emotional contagion' (sharing the emotions of patients) (Omdahl & O'Donnell 1999). Emotional contagion is hence regarded as detrimental as it encourages nurses professionals to become emotionally exhausted.

Empathy is considered to be one of the key variables in nurse-client interpersonal relationship (Yegdich 1999). The empathetic person is, however, not detached from all emotions, but is able to recognize when personal feelings are aroused in the process, which could block the therapeutic encounter.

The skilled practitioner can show empathy by listening and reflecting the sufferer's cathartic response; using silence appropriately while being a supportive presence, and tactfully guiding and directing the client to manage his/her emotions effectively.

References
Omdahl B L, O'Donnell C 1999 Emotional contagion, empathic concern and communicative responsiveness as variables affecting nurses stress and occupational commitment. Journal of Advanced Nursing 29(6):1351–1359
Yegdich T 1999 On the phenomenology of empathy in nursing: empathy or sympathy? Journal of Advanced Nursing 30(1):83–93

---

enamel *n* extremely hard substance covering the crown of a tooth.

encapsulation *n* enclosure within a capsule.

encephalins *npl* ⇒ enkephalins.

encephalitis *n* inflammation of the brain, due to viral or bacterial infection. *encephalitis lethargica* occurred in the 1920s possibly due to a virus. May lead to parkinsonism.

encephalocele *n* protrusion of brain substance through the skull. Often associated with hydrocephalus, when the protrusion occurs at a suture line.

encephalography a technique to examine the brain, to produce a printed or visible record of the investigation findings. ⇒ echoencephalography. ⇒ electroencephalography. ⇒ pneumoencephalography — **encephalogram** *n*.

encephalomalacia *n* softening of the brain.

encephalomyelitis *n* inflammation of the brain and spinal cord.

encephalomyelopathy *n* disease affecting both brain and spinal cord — **encephalomyelopathic** *adj*.

encephalon *n* the brain.

encephalopathy *n* any disease of the brain. Generally applied to those of toxic, nutritional or metabolic aetiology — **encephalopathic** *adj*.

enchondroma *n* a tumour of cartilage growing within a bone. ⇒ chondroma — **enchondromata** *pl*.

encopresis *n* involuntary passage of faeces at an age by which faecal continence is normally achieved. May be associated with mental health problems — **encopretic** *adj, n*.

encounter group a form of psychotherapy. Members of a small group focus on becoming aware of their feelings and developing the ability to express them openly, honestly and clearly. The objective is to increase self-awareness, promote personal growth and improve interpersonal communication.

Endamoeba ⇒ Entamoeba.

endarterectomy *n* the surgical removal of the intimal lining and atheromatous core from an artery, sometimes called disobliteration or 'rebore'. ⇒ atheroma. *gas endarterectomy* carbon dioxide gas can be used to separate the tunica intima and tunica media.

endarteritis *n* inflammation of the intima or inner lining coat of an artery. *endarteritis obliterans* the new intimal connective tissue obliterates the lumen.

endaural *adj* incision of external meatus, extending in front of the ear, used in ear surgery.

end-diastolic volume (EDV) *n* the volume of blood in the ventricles at the end of diastole. ⇒ stroke volume.

endemic *adj* recurring in an area. Applied to a disease that is always present in an area, such as a particular communicable disease. ⇒ epidemic *ant*.

endemiology *n* the special study of endemic diseases.

endocardial mapping the recording of electrical potentials from various sites in the heart to determine the site of origin of cardiac arrhythmia. It is performed via a wire inserted into the heart via the femoral vein. Where an abnormal pathway producing arrhythmias is discovered, it can be destroyed by transvenous catheter radiofrequency ablation.

endocarditis *n* inflammation of the endothelial lining of the heart (endocardium), and particularly of the valves. It may complicate rheumatic fever, leading to valve damage. *infective endocarditis* is caused by micro-organisms: *Streptococcus viridans*, *Streptococcus pneumoniae*, *Staphylococcus aureus*, and, less commonly, rickettsiae, chlamydiae and fungi such as Candida. It may be acute or subacute and occasionally occurs following heart valve surgery. Vegetations, consisting of micro-organisms, platelets and fibrin, which form on the valves, may break off in to the circulation to form emboli. There may be permanent valve damage. Treatment is with the appropriate antimicrobial drug. Both normal and abnormal hearts and all ages may be affected. Prophylactic antimicrobial drugs are used to cover dental treatment and surgical procedures, where micro-organisms may enter the blood, to protect people with existing heart lesions.

endocardium *n* smooth endothelium tissue that lines the heart and covers the valves.

endocervical *adj* pertaining to the inside of the cervix uteri.

endocervicitis *n* inflammation of the mucous membrane lining the cervix uteri.

endocrine *adj* secreting internally. Describes ductless glands that discharge their hormone secretions directly into the blood or lymph. *endocrine glands* include the hypothalamus, pituitary, thyroid, parathyroids, adrenals, pancreas, gonads, pineal body (gland) and thymus. Other structures that secrete hormones include: the gastrointestinal tract, heart, kidneys and the placenta. ⇒ exocrine *ant*. ⇒ hormone — **endocrinal** *adj*.

endocrinology *n* the study of the endocrine glands and their internal secretions.

endocrinopathy *n* abnormality of one or more of the endocrine glands or their secretions.

endocytosis *n* the general term for the bulk transport processes by which large molecules enter the cell (*ant* exocytosis). ⇒ phagocytosis. ⇒ pinocytosis.

endoderm *n* innermost layer of the three primary germ layers of the early embryo. From it are derived the epithelium of the pharynx, tonsil, thyroid and parathyroid glands, middle ear, respiratory tract, gastrointestinal tract, pancreas and bladder. ⇒ ectoderm. ⇒ mesoderm.

endogenous *adj* originating within the organism. ⇒ ectogenous. ⇒ exogenous *ant*.

endolymph *n* the fluid contained in the membranous labyrinth of the internal ear.

endolymphatic sac decompression a surgical technique used to reduce the distension of the endolymphatic system of the inner ear. Used in the management of Menière's disease.

endometrioma *n* a tumour of misplaced endometrium. ⇒ chocolate cyst.

endometriosis *n* the presence of functional endometrium in ectopic sites, e.g. myometrium, uterine tubes, ovary, peritoneum, bladder or bowel. The clinical presentation depends on the site, but includes pain before menstruation, dyspareunia and infertility. ⇒ chocolate cyst.

endometritis *n* inflammation of the endometrium lining of the uterus.

endometrium *n* the specialized lining mucosa of the uterus — **endometrial** *adj* pertaining to the endometrium. *endometrial destruction* newer surgical techniques where the basal layer of the endometrium is destroyed by laser ablation, resection or destruction using heat. These are performed by the transcervical route and provide a safer and more acceptable alternative to hysterectomy, as a treatment for menorrhagia.

endomyocardium *n* relating to the endocardium and myocardium — **endomyocardial** *adj*.

endomysium *n* thin layer of connective tissue around individual muscle fibres.

endoneurium *n* the delicate, inner connective tissue surrounding the nerve fibres.

endoparasite *n* any parasite living within its host — **endoparasitic** *adj*.

endophthalmitis *n* internal infection of the eye, usually bacterial.

endoplasmic reticulum (ER) *n* a subcellular organelle that consists of a network of channels and membranes. They are concerned with the synthesis and movement of substances within the cell, e.g. proteins and lipids. The rough endoplasmic reticulum found in secretory cells has ribosomes on its surface, whereas the smooth variety has no ribosomes.

endorphins *n* a group of opioid-like neuropeptides activated by the pituitary gland, which have an analgesic effect. Involved in both central and peripheral nervous functions, their role is to modulate pain interpretation and to induce a euphoric aftereffect. → enkephalins.

endoscope *n* a lighted instrument used to visualize body cavities or organs. Most are now fibreoptic endoscopes, where light is transmitted by means of very fine glass fibres along a flexible tube, e.g. bronchoscope or colonoscope. It can permit examination, photography, biopsy and surgery of the cavities or organs, with or without a general anaesthetic. Rigid metal endoscopes are used in some situations, e.g. sigmoidoscope — **endoscopy** *n*.

endoscopic retrograde cholangiopancreatography introduction of a contrast medium into the pancreatic and bile ducts via a catheter from an endoscope located in the duodenum.

endospore *n* a bacterial spore which has a purely vegetative function. It is formed in response to adverse environmental conditions, such as loss of water. Metabolism is minimal and allows the organism to resist heat, desiccation and disinfectants. They may remain dormant for long periods and can germinate when environmental conditions become favourable. The only genera which include pathogenic species that form spores are Bacillus and Clostridium.

endosteoma *n* tumour arising in the medullary cavity of a bone.

endothelioid *adj* resembling endothelium.

endothelioma *n* a malignant tumour derived from endothelial cells.

endothelium *n* the lining membrane of serous cavities, heart, blood and lymph vessels — **endothelial** *adj*.

endotoxin *n* an intracellular toxin found in the cell wall of some Gram-negative bacteria, e.g. *Salmonella typhi* and *Neiserria meningitidis*. It is released on destruction of the cell wall and causes physical effects, e.g. fever. ⇒ exotoxin *ant* — **endotoxic** *adj*.

endotracheal *adj* within the trachea. *endotracheal anaesthesia* the administration of an anaesthetic through an endotracheal tube passed into the trachea. *endotracheal tube* a tube passed into the trachea to establish or maintain an airway or to facilitate ventilation.

end-systolic volume (ESV) *n* the volume of blood remaining in the ventricles following systole. ⇒ stroke volume.

end-tidal CO_2 a noninvasive method of measuring expired carbon dioxide (CO_2) levels which can approximate to $PaCO_2$.

enema *n* the introduction of a liquid into the bowel via the rectum, to be returned or retained. The word is usually preceded by the name of the liquid used. It can be further designated according to the function of the fluid. The evacuant enemas are usually prepared commercially in small bulk as a disposable enema: the chemicals attract water into the bowel, promoting cleansing and peristaltic contractions of the lower bowel. The enemas to be retained are usually drugs, the most common being corticosteroids. ⇒ barium enema. ⇒ laxatives — **enemas, enemata** *pl*.

energy conservation an occupational therapy technique where clients are helped to make maximum use of a limited potential for energy expenditure, such as a person with multiple sclerosis or a chronic cardiac condition.

enkephalins *npl* peptide neurotransmitters found in the central nervous system, pituitary gland and gastrointestinal tract. They have opioid-like effects and act as natural painkillers. Also known as encephalins. ⇒ endorphins.

enophthalmos *n* abnormal retraction of an eyeball within its orbit.

ensiform *adj* sword-shaped; xiphoid.

ENT *abbr* ear, nose and throat.

Entamoeba *n* (*syn* Endamoeba) a genus of protozoon parasites, three species infesting man: *Entamoeba coli*, nonpathogenic, infesting intestinal tract; *E. gingivalis*, nonpathogenic, infesting mouth; *E. hystolytica*, pathogenic causing amoebic dysentery. ⇒ amoebiasis.

enteral *adj* within the gastrointestinal tract. *enteral diets* those which are taken by mouth or through a nasogastric tube; low residue enteral diets can be whole protein/polymeric, or amino acid/peptide. *enteral feeding* method of providing nutrition when the gastrointestinal tract is not functioning. Includes via nasogastric and nasoduodenal tubes or via gastrostomy or jejunostomy tubes. Enteral feeding can be administered by bolus, gravity or pump controlled methods. ⇒ parenteral feeding. ⇒ percutaneous endoscopic gastrostomy (PEG).

enteric *adj* pertaining to the small intestine. *enteric coating* a coating applied to a pill that prevents drug release until it reaches the intestine. *enteric fevers* includes typhoid and paratyphoid fever.

enteritis *n* inflammation of the small intestine.

enteroanastomosis *n* intestinal anastomosis.

Enterobacter *n* a genus of aerobic, nonspore-bearing, Gram-negative bacilli of the family Enterobacteriaceae, e.g. *Enterobacter cloacae* found in faeces (human and animal), soil, water and some foods.

Enterobacteriaceae *n* a family of Gram-negative bacteria found in the human gut that include the genera: Escherichia, Klebsiella, Proteus, Salmonella and Shigella.

enterobiasis *n* infestation with the threadworm *Enterobius vermicularis*. It infests the small and large intestine. There is an autoinfective life-cycle with human as the only host. The eggs are swallowed, they hatch in the small intestine and move to the large bowel and later the rectum. The females emerge at night and deposit their eggs on the skin around the anus. Reinfestation occurs when the person scratches the perianal area and the eggs contaminate the hands. The cycle is completed as the eggs are transferred to the mouth. Treatment aims at complete elimination and all members of the household are given an anthelmintic, mebendazole or less often piperazine citrate, and hygiene measures are also necessary to prevent reinfestation during treatment.

Enterobius a genus of nematode worm, e.g. *Enterobius vermicularis* (threadworm). ⇒ enterobiasis.

enterocele *n* prolapse of intestine through the wall of the vagina.

Enterococcus *n* a genus of Gram-positive cocci commensal in the bowel, e.g. *Enterococcus faecalis* and *Enterococcus faecium*. They cause wound infection and urinary tract infection and occasionally neonatal meningitis. Increasingly common as a cause of hospital-acquired infection, and many strains are developing antibiotic resistance. ⇒ vancomycin-resistant enterococci.

enterocolitis *n* inflammation of the small intestine and colon. ⇒ necrotizing enterocolitis.

enterocyte intestinal cell.

enterogastric reflex *n* a series of neural and hormonal (duodenal) events that inhibit gastric secretion and emptying as acidic chyme enters the duodenum. This limits the rate at which chyme is released and allows time for duodenal processing and prevents damage from a deluge of acidic fluid. The local hormones, (known collectively as enterogastrones), include secretin, gastric inhibitory peptide, cholecystokinin and vasoactive inhibitory peptide.

enterohepatic circulation *n* a recycling process, whereby bile salts and other substances including drugs that are secreted into bile, are absorbed from the intestine and returned to the liver via the hepatic portal vein. Returning bile salts stimulate further bile and bile acid production, but recycled drugs, such as digoxin and morphine, form a reservoir of active drug that prolongs activity and can lead to toxicity.

enterokinase *n* (*syn* enteropeptidase) a proteolytic enzyme secreted by the duodenal mucosa that converts the inactive pancreatic enzyme trypsinogen into active trypsin.

enterolith *n* an intestinal concretion.

enterolithiasis *n* the presence of intestinal concretions.

enteron *n* the gut.

enteropathy disease of the small intestine.

enteropeptidase *n* ⇒ enterokinase.

enterostomy *n* an opening into the small intestine. It may be to connect it to another structure, e.g. gastroenterostomy, or some other surface as in an ileostomy. ⇒ jejunostomy — **enterostomal** *adj*.

enterotomy *n* an incision into the small intestine.

enterotoxin *n* a toxin which has its effect on the gastrointestinal tract, causing vomiting, diarrhoea and abdominal pain.

enterotribe *n* a metal clamp which causes necrosis of the spur of a double-barrelled colostomy, as a preliminary to its closure.

enteroviruses *npl* a group of picornaviruses that enter the body by the alimentary canal/tract. They include the polioviruses, coxsackieviruses and echoviruses.

enterozoa *npl* any animal parasites infesting the intestines — **enterozoon** *sing*.

entropion *n* inversion of an eyelid so that the lashes are in contact with the globe of the eye.

enucleation *n* the removal of an organ or tumour in its entirety, as of an eyeball from its socket.

E-number *n* an identification serial number given to various food additives, e.g. E500 (sodium bicarbonate), E102 (tartrazine).

enuresis *n* incontinence of urine, especially bedwetting. *nocturnal enuresis* incontinence during sleep.

environment *n* external surroundings. The outside physical conditions that surround and influence all living organisms — **environmental** *adj*.

enzymatic agent used for the debridement of wounds, they include streptodornase and streptokinase. → proteolytic enzymes.

enzyme *n* a protein that acts as a biological catalyst (a catalyst controls or speeds up the rate of a reaction without itself being permanently altered). Enzymes are produced by living cells where they catalyse specific biochemical reactions involving specific substrates. Many reactions in biological systems would proceed too slowly without an enzyme, e.g. carbon dioxide would not be cleared from the tissues without the enzyme carbonic anhydrase. The names of enzymes often reflect their function, e.g. aminotransferases catalyse the transfer of amine groups (NH_2) between amino acids — **enzymatic** *adj*.

enzyme cascade amplification *n* the process by which complex physiological processes can proceed rapidly. Amplification occurs as the product of one reaction triggers the next reaction and so on, such as blood coagulation.

enzyme induction the property of substances, such as some environment chemicals, alcohol and some drugs, e.g. rifampicin and barbiturates, to increase the production of liver (microsomal) enzymes. ⇒ cytochromes. This can either have the effect of increasing the rate at which the 'inducer' and sometimes other drugs are metabolized and excreted with loss of drug effects, e.g. rifampicin causes inactivation of oral contraceptives, or sometimes increasing drug effects, such as the toxic metabolites produced in paracetamol overdose.

enzyme inhibitors *npl* agents, including many drugs that act by inhibiting a specific enzyme either reversibly or irreversibly. Some drugs are substrate analogues (very similar to the usual substrate of the enzyme) and act as competitive inhibitors, e.g. the cytotoxic drug methotrexate inhibits the enzyme (dihydrofolate reductase) needed for folic acid use by cancer cells. Some drugs inhibit liver (microsomal) enzymes and increase the effects of other drugs, e.g. aspirin can prevent the metabolism of oral anticoagulants, such as warfarin, which leads to an increased anticoagulant effect. ⇒ false substrate.

enzyme-linked immunosorbent assay (ELISA) enzyme-labelled antibodies are used to test for the presence of other antibodies, including HIV, and antigens. The test is not highly specific for HIV. If positive, it is usually followed by a second ELISA test and then by the more specific Western blot test before HIV infection is confirmed.

enzymology *n* the science dealing with the structure and function of enzymes — **enzymological** *adj*.

eosin *n* a red staining agent used in histology and laboratory diagnostic procedures. ⇒ eosinophil.

eosinophil *n* cells having an affinity for acidic dyes, such as eosin. A polymorphonuclear leucocyte (white blood cell) that contains granules. It is concerned with immune responses involving immunoglobulin (IgE) and allergics. ⇒ granulocyte — **eosinophilic** *adj*.

eosinophilia *n* increased eosinophils in the blood. Often seen in parasitic and allergic disorders, e.g. asthma.

EPEC *abbr* enteropathic *Escherichia coli*.

ependymal cell *n* a type of neuroglial cell (supporting cells) found lining the fluid-filled cavities of the central nervous system. Some cover the choroid plexus and others have cilia that circulate the cerebrospinal fluid. ⇒ neuroglial.

ependymoma *n* tumour arising from ependymal cells in the lining of the cerebral ventricles or central canal of spinal cord. Can occur in all age groups.

ephelides *npl* freckles, an increase in pigment granules with a normal number of pigment cells. ⇒ lentigo — **ephelis** *sing*.

epicanthus *n* a fold of skin obscuring the inner canthus of the eye. It is characteristic of certain groups of people, such as Chinese. Some individuals with Down's syndrome also have epicanthal folds — **epicanthal** *adj*.

epicardium *n* the visceral layer of the pericardium — **epicardial** *adj*.

epicondyle *n* an eminence on a bone, such as the femoral epicondyles.

epicritic *adj* describes the somatic sensations of fine touch, vibration, two-point discrimination and proprioception. ⇒ protopathic.

epidemic *n* a particular disease, such as influenza, simultaneously affecting many people (more than normally expected) in an area. ⇒ endemic *ant*.

epidemic myalgia ⇒ Bornholm disease.

epidemiology *n* the scientific study of the distribution of diseases in populations. See Box – Epidemiology — **epidemiologically** *adv*.

epidermis *n* the external nonvascular layer of the skin; the cuticle — **epidermal** *adj*.

epidermolysis bullosa (EB) rare inherited skin conditions characterized by extreme fragility of the skin, which blisters with minimal contact.

Epidermophyton *n* a genus of fungi which affects the skin and nails.

epidermophytosis *n* infection of the skin or nails with fungi of the genus *Epidermophyton*, e.g. ringworm.

epididymectomy *n* surgical removal of the epididymis.

epididymis *n* a small oblong body attached to the posterior surface of each testis. It consists of the seminiferous tubules which convey the spermatozoa from the testes to the vas deferens.

Epidemiology

Epidemiology deals with the incidence, distribution and control of disease. The elements of epidemiology are statistical in nature, as diagnosis, treatment and prognosis are uncertain in individual cases, and it is only by looking at larger samples that data can be interpreted more meaningfully. Epidemiology is a quantitative discipline, it considers health outcomes such as death or disease, and attempts to establish relationships between these outcomes and other factors.

Samples of subjects from a population are analysed with respect to the occurrence of the outcome, and the presence of various purported risk factors. A classic case of epidemiological work is the link between smoking and lung cancer. An individual who smokes may or may not develop lung cancer, and non-smokers also can develop lung cancer. However, the incidence of lung cancer is far higher among smokers than non-smokers.

epididymitis *n* inflammation of the epididymis.

epididymo-orchitis *n* inflammation of the epididymis and the testis.

epidural *adj* upon or external to the dura, ⇒ dura mater. *epidural block* single injection or intermittent injection through a catheter of local anaesthetic for maternal analgesia during labour or for surgical operations. *epidural space* the region through which spinal nerves leave the spinal cord. It can be approached at any level of the spine, but the administering of anaesthetic is commonly done at the lumbar level or through the sacral cornua for caudal epidural block.

epigastrium *n* the abdominal region lying directly over the stomach. ⇒ abdominal regions — **epigastric** *adj.*

epiglottis *n* the thin, leaf-shaped flap of cartilage behind the tongue which, during the act of swallowing, protects the opening leading into the larynx.

epiglottitis *n* inflammation of the epiglottis.

epilation *n* extraction or destruction of hair roots, e.g. by coagulation necrosis, electrolysis or forceps. ⇒ depilation — **epilate** *vt.*

epilatory *adj, n* (describes) an agent which produces epilation.

epilepsy *n* correctly called the epilepsies, a group of conditions resulting from disordered electrical activity of the brain and manifesting as epileptic seizures or 'fits'. The seizure is caused by an abnormal electrical discharge that disturbs cerebration and results in a generalized or partial seizure, depending on the area of the brain in which the discharge originates. (a) *Generalized seizures* may be: *tonic-clonic (grand mal)* the commonest type of epileptic seizure with loss of consciousness and generalized convulsions. *absences (petit mal)* where there is a brief alteration in consciousness; (b) *Partial seizures* occur when the electrical disturbance is limited to a particular focus of the brain and are manifested in a variety of ways, including motor problems characterized by limb twitching that may spread, known as Jacksonian epilepsy. In other types there may be paraesthesia, visual hallucinations, such as coloured patterns, and psychomotor seizures where there are changes to mood, perception and memory with more complex hallucinations and physical manifestations, such as nausea. *Secondary generalized seizures* occur when partial seizure activity spreads to involve other areas of the brain and awareness is lost. ⇒ status epilepticus.

epileptic 1. *adj* pertaining to epilepsy. **2.** *n* a person with epilepsy. *epileptic aura* premonitory subjective phenomena (tingling in the hand or visual, olfactory or auditory sensations) which precede a generalized tonic-clonic epileptic seizure. ⇒ aura. *epileptic cry* the sound heard as the person expels air due to respiratory muscle spasm during the tonic phase of the seizure.

epileptiform *adj* resembling epilepsy.

epileptogenic *adj* capable of causing epilepsy.

epiloia *n* ⇒ tuberous sclerosis.

epimenorrhoea *n* reduction of the length of the menstrual cycle, resulting in more frequent menstruation.

epimysium *n* fibrous connective tissue enclosing an entire muscle.

epinephrine *n* ⇒ adrenaline.

epineurium *n* outer fibrous coat enclosing a nerve trunk.

epiphora *n* pathological overflow of tears onto the cheek.

epiphysis *n* the end of a growing bone. Separated from the shaft by a plate of cartilage (epiphyseal plate) which disappears due to ossification when growth ceases. ⇒ diaphysis — **epiphyseal** *adj*.

epiphysitis *n* inflammation of an epiphysis.

episclera *n* loose connective tissue between the sclera and conjunctiva — **episcleral** *adj*.

episcleritis *n* inflammation of the episclera.

episiorrhaphy *n* surgical repair of a lacerated perineum.

episiotomy *n* an incision of the perineum made during the second stage of labour to prevent perineal laceration or to facilitate delivery, e.g. forceps delivery.

episodic memory the part of long term memory that stores personal experiences. It is organized with respect to when and where the experience happened, e.g. an episode from your last job interview.

epispadias *n* a congenital opening of the urethra on the dorsum (upper side) of the penis, often associated with ectopia vesicae. ⇒ hypospadias.

epispastic *n* a blistering agent.

epistaxis *n* bleeding from the nose — **epistaxes** *pl*.

epistemology discussion and debate about knowledge and 'truth' and how it varies between different disciplines.

epithalamus *n* part of the brain that lies above and behind the thalamus. It forms part of the third ventricle and contains the pineal body (gland).

epithelialization *n* the migration of epithelial cells over the raw area of a wound; occurs during the proliferative phase of wound healing.

epithelioma *n* a malignant growth arising from epithelial tissue.

epithelium *n* one of four basic body tissues. It covers the body, forms glands and lines cavities. It is classified according to the arrangement and shape of the cells it contains: simple, single layer of squamous, columnar or cuboidal, and stratified with several layers, such as transitional or stratified squamous — **epithelial** *adj*.

epitope *n* ⇒ antigenic determinant.

EPO *abbr* emergency protection order.

eponychium ⇒ cuticle.

Epstein-Barr virus (EBV) a herpesvirus, the causative agent of infectious mononucleosis. Also linked with the formation of some malignant tumours, including Burkitt's lymphoma and nasopharyngeal cancer.

epulis *n* a tumour growing on or from the gums.

equality being equal. *equality of opportunity* having equal access to opportunities for health care, decent housing, employment, redress in the courts etc, regardless of class, age, race or gender. ⇒ equity. ⇒ inequalities in health. ⇒ social exclusion.

equinus describes the condition where the toes point down and the person walks on tiptoe. ⇒ talipes.

equity fairness of the distribution of resources. ⇒ justice. Access to resources according to need and ability to benefit.

Erb's palsy paralysis involving the shoulder and arm muscles from a lesion of the fifth and sixth cervical nerve roots. The arm hangs loosely at the side with the forearm pronated ('waiter's tip position'). Most commonly a birth injury.

ERCP *abbr* endoscopic retrograde cholangiopancreatography.

erectile *adj* upright; capable of being elevated. *erectile dysfunction* an inability to achieve or maintain erection of the penis. *erectile tissue* highly vascular tissue, which, under stimulus, becomes rigid and erect from hyperaemia.

erection *n* the state achieved when erectile tissue is hyperaemic. The enlarged state of the penis and clitoris during sexual arousal and coitus.

erector *n* a muscle which achieves erection of a part, as in the muscles which lift the hairs on the skin. ⇒ arrectores pilorum.

ERG *abbr* electroretinogram.

ergocalciferol *n* vitamin D_2 obtained from the diet. Formed from the plant sterol ergosterol.

ergometry *n* measurement of work done by muscles — **ergometric** *adj*.

ergonomics *n* the scientific study of human working environments and efficient use of energy.

ergosterol *n* a sterol provitamin found in plants and fungi. It is converted to ergocalciferol (vitamin D_2) by U-V light.

ergot *n* a fungus, *Claviceps purpurea*, which infects rye. There are two important medicinal derivatives: (a) ergometrine, used to contract the uterus and prevent or minimize postpartum haemorrhage, and (b) ergotamine, that is used in the management of migraine.

eroticism *n* arousal of sexual desire or instinct through suggestive or symbolic means, or as foreplay before the act of sexual intercourse.

eructation *n* belching: the act of noisily bringing up gas from the stomach and expelling it orally.

eruption *n* the process by which a tooth emerges through the alveolar bone or gingiva. *skin eruption* furuncle or skin rash.

ERV *abbr* expiratory reserve volume.

erysipelas *n* an acute, specific infectious disease, in which there is a spreading, streptococcal inflammation of the skin and subcutaneous tissues, accompanied by fever and constitutional disturbances.

erysipeloid *n* a skin condition resembling erysipelas. It occurs in butchers, fishmongers or cooks. The infecting organism is the *Erysipelothrix* of swine erysipelas.

erythema *n* reddening of the skin due to vascular congestion. *erythema induratum* Bazin's disease. *erythema multiforme* a form of toxic, infective or allergic skin eruption which breaks out suddenly and lasts for days; the lesions are in the form of violet pink papules or plaques. It is associated with allergies, viral and bacterial infection, cancer and radiotherapy and drug sensitivities. Severe form called Stevens-Johnson syndrome. *erythema nodosum* an eruption of painful red nodules on the front of the legs. It is generally accompanied by pyrexia, malaise and joint pains. It may be a symptom of many diseases including: infections, e.g. tuberculosis, drug sensitivities, e.g. sulphonamides, and systemic illnesses, such as sarcoidosis and inflammatory bowel disease. *erythema pernio* ⇒ chilblain. ⇒ perniosis — **erythematous** *adj*.

erythroblast *n* a nucleated precursor cell found in the red bone marrow from which the erythrocytes develop — **erythroblastic** *adj*.

erythroblastosis fetalis ⇒ haemolytic disease of the newborn.

erythrocytes *npl* the non-nucleated red cells of the circulating blood. Erythrocytes carry oxygen and some carbon dioxide, and buffer pH changes in the blood. *erythrocyte sedimentation rate (ESR)* the rate at which erythrocytes fall to the bottom of a narrow tube to leave a column of clear serum above. The ESR, which varies with age and gender, is measured at the end of an hour and reported in millimetres. Tissue destruction and inflammatory conditions cause an increase in the ESR. See Box — Erythrocyte — **erythrocytic** *adj*.

erythrocythaemia *n* overproduction of red cells that may be: (a) a physiological response to hypoxia, such as that experienced at high altitude, in lung disease or due to some congenital heart diseases; (b) inappropriate erythropoietin production from tumours, e.g. kidney and liver cancers. ⇒ erythrocytosis. ⇒ myeloproliferative disorder. ⇒ polycythaemia.

Erythrocyte

The erythrocyte is highly specialized for its purpose of transporting oxygen from the lungs to the peripheral tissues. It has no nucleus and becomes packed with haemoglobin. The erythrocyte lacks mitochondria (and other organelles) and relies only on anaerobic glycolysis for the production of adenosine triphosphate (ATP) meaning that it does not consume the oxygen which it transports. The erythrocyte is a biconcave disc approximately 8 μm (microns) in diameter and 2 μm (microns) thick which gives it an optimal surface area to volume ratio facilitating the transport of oxygen and carbon dioxide into and out of the cell. Erythrocytes stack up alongside one another to travel through peripheral capillaries. In the erythrocyte haemoglobin binds oxygen at high oxygen levels, such as in the lungs, and releases it at relatively low levels of oxygen such as in the peripheral tissues. The surface of the erythrocyte carries antigens which are genetically determined and the common antigens are those which confer the A, B or O blood types.

erythrocytopenia *n* deficiency in the number of red blood cells — **erythrocytopenic** *adj*.

erythrocytosis *n* an abnormal increase in the number of red blood cells. ⇒ erythrocythaemia.

erythroderma *n* excessive redness of the skin caused by desquamation.

erythrogenic *adj* 1. producing or causing a rash. 2. producing red blood cells.

erythropoiesis *n* the production of red blood cells in the red bone marrow as a result of stimulation by the growth factor erythropoietin. Other hormones, such as androgens and thyroid hormones, also stimulate the bone marrow. (See Figure 21). ⇒ haemopoiesis.

erythropoietin *n* a glycoprotein hormone secreted by certain cells in the kidney in response to hypoxia. Active erythropoietin is formed from the renal erythropoietic factor and some is also produced in the liver. It acts on the bone marrow, stimulating erythropoiesis. A synthetic preparation is used therapeutically to manage the anaemia associated with chronic renal failure and dialysis and with some types of chemotherapy. ⇒ anaemia.

eschar *n* a dry scab or crust, as results from a burn, application of caustics, diathermy, etc — **escharotic** *adj* pertaining to an eschar or any agent capable of producing one.

Escherichia *n* a genus of motile, Gram-negative bacilli belonging to the family Enterobacteriaceae. *Escherichia coli* is part of normal bowel flora. Some strains are pathogenic to humans, causing urinary tract infection, gastroenteritis, meningitis, peritonitis and wound infections. The serotypes that cause gastroenteritis are classified into four groups; (a) enterohaemorrhagic *Escherichia coli* (EHEC), e.g *E. coli* 0157. A virulent organism that produces a toxin (verocytotoxin) and causes a range of disease from mild diarrhoea to severe haemorrhagic bowel inflammation. Some of those affected may develop life-threatening haemolytic uraemic syndrome. Outbreaks of infection have been associated with eating meat and meat products, such as undercooked burgers, unpasteurized milk and vegetables washed in water contaminated with faeces; (b) enteropathic *Escherichia coli* (EPEC), causes serious diarrhoea in babies, especially in developing countries. Infection occurs through food handlers or faecal contamination of water supplies; (c) enterotoxigenic *Escherichia coli* (ETEC), affects people travelling to areas where hygiene standards are poor and causes outbreaks of gastroenteritis in developing countries. It results in watery diarrhoea which can cause fluid and electrolyte imbalance; (d) enterovasive *Escherichia coli* (EIEC), infection is usually via food handlers or water contaminated with faeces. It causes bloodstained diarrhoea.

Esmarch's bandage a rubber roller bandage used to procure a bloodless operative field in the limbs.

ESP *abbr* extrasensory perception.

ESPs *abbr* extended scope physiotherapy practitioners.

espundia ⇒ leishmaniasis.

ESR *abbr* erythrocyte sedimentation rate.

ESRD *abbr* end stage renal disease. ⇒ renal.

ESS *abbr* Early Signs Scale.

essential amino acids also known as indispensable. ⇒ amino acids.

essential fatty acids (EFAs) linoleic and linolenic acids. Polyunsaturated fatty acids (PUFA) which cannot be synthesized

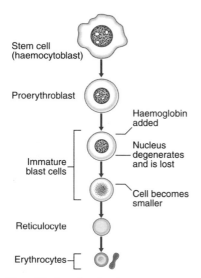

Figure 21 Formation of erythrocytes.
(Reproduced from Brooker 1998 with permission.)

in the body. Arachidonic acid, which can be formed from linoleic acid, becomes essential if linoleic acid is deficient. They have diverse functions, that include being the precursors for many regulatory lipids, e.g. prostaglandins; they fulfil an important role in fat metabolism and form part of the plasma membrane. They are present in natural vegetable seed oils. Various other polyunsaturated fatty acids, such as γlinoleic acid (GLA) are found in fish oils as well as plants.

essential oil *n* the undiluted oil extracted from plants, commonly diluted in a carrier oil prior to use by aromatherapists. ⇒ aromatherapy.

establishment used in the context of planned staffing levels in a particular area. Usually described as the number of WTEs.

ester *n* an organic compound formed from an alcohol and organic acid.

estimated average requirement (EAR) *n* a dietary reference value. See Box – Dietary reference values.

estradiol *n* ⇒ oestradiol.

estrogens *npl* ⇒ oestrogens.

ESWL *abbr* extracorporeal shock-wave lithotripsy. ⇒ Dornier lithotriptor. ⇒ lithotriptor.

ETEC *abbr* enterotoxigenic *Escherichia coli*.

ethanol *n* ethyl alcohol. The alcohol present in intoxicating beverages.

ether *n* an inflammable liquid; previously used as a general anaesthetic.

ethics *n* the study of the code of moral principles derived from a system of values and beliefs and concerned with rights and obli-

gations. The study of nursing ethics as a discipline distinct from bioethics and medical ethics, has developed strongly in recent years. The many areas in health care that involve ethical issues include: abortion, confidentiality, consent, euthanasia, research etc. *ethics committees* bodies set up by Health authorities, NHS trusts and universities etc. to consider proposals for research projects. Funding bodies usually require the approval of the relevant ethics committee prior to the award of a grant. See Box – Ethics and research.

ethmoid *n* a complex cranial bone forming part of the orbital and nasal cavities. It contains many paranasal sinuses, making the bone very spongy and light. ⇒ sinus.

ethmoidectomy *n* surgical removal of a part of the ethmoid bone, usually that forming the lateral nasal walls.

ethnic *adj* pertaining to a social group who share customs and culture.

ethnicity the feeling of belonging to a particular group who share common cultural customs and traditions. See Box – Ethnicity. *ethnicity and health inequality* ⇒ inequalities in health. ⇒ race.

ethnocentrism the belief that one's own ethnic group or life-style is superior to others. An inability to appreciate the validity of other cultures.

ethnography a study of people in their usual surroundings. Used in qualitative research to describe customs, culture and social life through informal interviews, observation etc.

ethnology *n* a branch of anthropology which has implications for health care; it studies mainly the cultural differences between groups, particularly the

---

Ethics and research

When conducting research on humans, a strong ethical approach is needed. In particular there should be voluntary consent by the subject, and the research should be expected to bear fruitful results, and be based on prior knowledge. No experiments where death or disabling injury occurs (unless experimenter is the subject) should be countenanced, and risk should not exceed the importance of the problem. Preparations and facilities to protect from injury should be in place, and the study should be performed by suitably qualified personnel.

The experimenter has the duty to end an experiment if injury is likely. Subjects can withdraw at any time, with no prejudice to treatment. Risks to subjects should be minimized by sound research procedures. Institutional review boards should be in place.

Informed consent needs to be obtained and documented. There is a right to privacy and dignity, and to anonymity. Explanation of the study, and of risks, and of potential benefits should be given, and any questions posed by the subject should be answered honestly.

Ethnicity

Sociologists and psychologists often link the term 'ethnicity' with the study of race. Although the two concepts are interconnected, their meanings are markedly different. Race applies to biological characteristics, e.g. skin colour, height, hair types, facial features, etc. whereas, ethnicity denotes cultural lifestyles based on values, beliefs and practices shared by the ethnic groups.

Ethnicity may be recognized by the language used, religion, dress, dietary habits for example and spiritual practices. Ethnic groups however, may still represent racial groups and their identities.

The role of ethnicity and race in the development and definition of the self (Harris 1995) should be acknowledged. Hence race and ethnicity are two of the many variables that help create individuality.

In clinical practice healthcare practitioners must respond positively to ethnic groups' differing health needs. Research findings (Hanson 1999) for example, indicate that specific beliefs distinguish between smokers and non-smokers, while some beliefs differ by ethnicity. Other studies have established a correlation between ethnicity and the higher level of psychological stress experienced by minority groups when facing adversity (Ritsner et al 2000). In addition, ethnicity is linked with the under utilization of healthcare services, and the misinterpretation of ethnic clients' psychiatric illness (Bhugra et al 1999).

Implications for transcultural healthcare practice are numerous. For example, recognizing that present behaviour is influenced by sociocultural factors can direct professionals to refine their strategies.

References

Bhugra D, Lippett R, Cole E 1999 Pathways into care: an explanation of the factors that may affect minority ethnic groups. In: Bhugra D, Bahl (eds) Ethnicity: An Agenda for Mental Health. Gaskell, London, p 32

Hanson M S 1999 Cross cultural study of beliefs about smoking among teenaged females. Western Journal of Nursing Research 21(5):635–651

Harris H W 1995 A conceptual overview of race, ethnicity and identity. In: Harris H W, Blue H C, Griffith E Z (eds) Racial and Ethnic Identity. Routledge, New York

Ritsner M, Ponizovsky A, Kurs R, Modai I 2000 Somatization in an immigrant population in Israel: a community survey of prevalence, risk factors and help seeking behavior. American Journal of Psychiatry 157(3):385–392

---

attitudes, values and beliefs relating to such life events as birth, contraception, abortion, marriage, diet, health care and death — **ethnologically** *adv*.

ethnomethodology technique used to study the methods applied by different groups to make sense of social living and enable social interaction.

ethology study of the behaviour of animals within the natural environment.

ethyl pyrophosphate (TEPP) organophosphorus compound used as an insecticide in agriculture. Powerful and irreversible anticholinesterase action.

ethylene oxide *n* gas used in specialist units to sterilize delicate equipment that would be damaged by high temperatures.

EU nursing directives since 1979 attempts have been made via EU nursing directives to ensure that nurses in the different European countries have been exposed to a similar education programme to facilitate free movement of nursing personnel throughout the countries.

EUA *abbr* examination (of the uterus) under anaesthetic.

eugenics *n* the study of genetic characteristics aimed at improving the qualities of future generations — **eugenic** *adj*.

eukaryote *n* a cell that has the genetic material contained in a nuclear membrane. Found in all higher organisms, such as animals, and in some microorganisms. It has a true nucleus. ⇒ prokaryote.

eunuch *n* a human male from whom the testes have been removed; a castrated male — **eunuchoid** *adj*.

eupepsia *n* normal digestion.

euphoria *n* in psychiatry, an exaggerated sense of well-being — **euphoric** *adj*.

eustachian tube ⇒ pharyngotympanic tube.

eustress positive stress. ⇒ stress.

eutectic mixture of local anaesthetics a cream for anaesthetizing skin by applying it to the site 1 hour before, e.g. venepuncture of a child.

euthanasia *n* literally an 'easy death'. The act of causing a painless and planned death, such as relieving a person's extreme suffering from an incurable disease, e.g. with an overdose of opioid (opiate) drugs. Presently illegal in UK and opposed by many professional groups, it is practised in some European countries, including the Netherlands. ⇒ homicide.

euthyroid state denoting normal thyroid function.

eutocia *n* a natural and normal labour and childbirth without any complications.

evacuant *n* an agent which causes an evacuation, particularly of the bowel. ⇒ enema.

evacuation *n* the act of emptying a cavity; generally refers to the discharge of faecal matter from the rectum. ⇒ manual evacuation of bowel.

evacuator *n* an instrument for procuring evacuation, e.g. the removal from the bladder of a stone, crushed by a lithotrite.

evaluating *v* commonly accepted as the fourth phase of the nursing process. Care is evaluated to assess whether the stated patient/client goals have been or are being achieved. Although it is the final step in the nursing process, it should occur continuously from the first assessment to the patient's discharge from the healthcare system — **evaluation** *n*.

evaporate *vt, vi* to convert from the liquid to the gaseous state by means of heat.

evaporating lotion one which, applied as a compress, absorbs heat in order to evaporate and so cools the skin.

evening primrose oil *n* a plant oil containing γlinoleic acid. It is used by some women to relieve the effects of the premenstrual syndrome.

eversion *n* a turning outwards, as of the upper eyelid to expose the conjunctival sac.

evidence-based practice (EBP) see Box – Evidence-based practice. ⇒ effectiveness. ⇒ clinical guidelines. ⇒ randomized controlled trial.

evisceration *n* 1. removal of internal organs. 2. protrusion of viscera through a wound or surgical incision.

evulsion *n* forcible tearing away of a structure.

Ewing's tumour a malignant tumour of bone (sarcoma) occurring in children and young adults.

ex gratia as a matter of favour, e.g. without admission of liability, of payment offered to a claimant.

exacerbation *n* increased severity, as of symptoms.

exanthema *n* a skin eruption — **exanthematous** *adj*.

Evidence-based practice

Evidence-based practice describes the delivery of healthcare interventions based on systematic analysis of information available about their effectiveness in relation to cost-effective health outcomes. At present, systematic research-based evidence is not available for all areas of health care, and some types of care do not lend themselves to scientific research methods. Thus some of the evidence-based protocols may be developed from the collection of best expert practice in the field.

Categories of causal evidence are shown below. It should be noted that the strength of the recommendation reflects the robustness of the methodological processes, not the value of the findings to practice.

Categories of evidence for causal relationships and treatment

Ia – Evidence from meta-analysis of randomized controlled trials (RCTs)

Ib – Evidence from at least one RCT

IIa – Evidence from at least one controlled study without randomization

IIb – Evidence from at least one other type of quasi-experimental study

III – Evidence from non-experimental descriptive studies and case-control studies

IV – Evidence from expert committee reports or opinions and/or clinical experience of respected authorities.

Strength of recommendation

A – Directly based on category I evidence

B – Directly based on category II evidence or extrapolated recommendation from category I evidence

C – Directly based on category III evidence or extrapolated recommendation from category I or II evidence

D – Directly based on category IV evidence or extrapolated recommendation from category I, II or III evidence.

Adapted from Shekelle P G, Woolf S H, Eccles M, Grimshaw J 1999 BMJ. 318: 593–596.

excision *n* removal of a part by cutting — **excise** *vt*.

excitability *n* rapid response to stimuli; a state of being easily irritated — **excitable** *adj* **excitable cells** cells that are able to produce an action potential by reversibly altering the potential difference across their membrane, such as nerve and muscle cells.

excitation *n* the act of stimulating an organ or tissue.

exclusion isolation ⇒ protective isolation.

excoriation *n* ⇒ abrasion.

excrement *n* faeces.

excresence *n* an abnormal protuberance or growth of the tissues.

excreta *n* the waste matter which is normally discharged from the body, particularly urine and faeces.

excretion *n* the elimination of waste material from the body, and also the matter so discharged — **excrete** *vt*.

exenteration *n* removal of the viscera from its containing cavity, e.g. the eye from its socket, the pelvic organs from the pelvis.

exfoliation *n* 1. the shedding of the primary (deciduous) teeth. 2. the scaling off of tissue in layers, such as the outer layers of the skin — **exfoliative** *adj*.

exfoliative cytology *n* the study of cells that have been shed, or exfoliated, from the surface of an organ or lesion. Used in screening for malignant conditions, such as cervical cytology. ⇒ cytology. ⇒ smear.

exhibitionism *n* 1. any kind of 'showing off'; extravagant behaviour to attract attention. 2. a psychosexual disorder confined to males and consisting of repeated exposure of the genitals to a stranger. No further contact is sought with the victim, who is usually a female adult or a child — **exhibitionist** *n*.

Eximer laser laser used to perform photorefractive keratectomy (PRK).

exocrine *adj* describes glands from which the secretion or excretion passes via a duct; secreting externally, e.g. sweat gland, salivary gland and exocrine pancreas. ⇒ endocrine *ant* — **exocrinal** *adj*.

exocytosis *n* process by which some molecules leave the cell, such as mucus and some hormones (*ant* endocytosis).

exogenous *adj* of external origin. ⇒ endogenous *ant*.

exomphalos *n* a condition present at birth and due to failure of the gut to return to the abdominal cavity during fetal development. The intestines protrude through a gap in the abdominal wall, still enclosed in peritoneum.

exophthalmos *n* protrusion of the eyeball. ⇒ Graves' disease. ⇒ hyperthyroidism — **exophthalmic** *adj*.

exostosis *n* an overgrowth of bone tissue forming a benign tumour.

exotoxin *n* a toxin released through the cell walls of living Gram-positive bacteria, e.g *Clostridium tetani*. Exotoxins have widespread systemic effects, such as muscle spasm and peripheral neuropathy. Exotoxins are antigenic proteins and can thus be neutralized by antibodies produced during the immune response. ⇒ endotoxin *ant* — **exotoxic** *adj*.

expanded role of the nurse nurses are increasingly taking on additional roles and responsibilities, traditionally regarded as belonging to doctors and other professionals. These include specific skills, such as intravenous cannulation and venepuncture, and roles, such as nurse-led clinics. The UKCC has set out the professional framework in which such practice may develop in its document 'The Scope of Professional Practice'.

expected date of delivery (EDD) usually calculated from the first day of the last normal menstrual period.

expectorant *n* a drug which may promote expectoration. They are of doubtful value.

expectoration *n* 1. the elimination of secretion from the respiratory tract by coughing. 2. sputum — **expectorate** *vt*.

Experience of Caregiving Inventory (ECI) used by mental health nurses and others to assess both burden and coping. Sixty six questions which cover ten areas. Eight areas described as 'negative'; two areas described as 'positive'. Negative areas: difficult behaviours; negative symptoms; stigma; problems with services; effects on family; need to backup; dependency and loss. Positive areas: positive personal experiences; good relationships with patients.

experimental group in a research study, the group exposed to the independent variable (the experimental agent or intervention). ⇒ control group. ⇒ variables.

experimental method ⇒ research methods.

expert witness *n* evidence given by a person whose general opinion based on training or experience is relevant to some of the issues in dispute.

expiration *n* the act of breathing out air from the lungs — **expire** *vt, vi*.

expiratory reserve volume (ERV) *n* maximum amount of air that can be forcefully expelled from the lungs after normal expiration. ⇒ respiratory function tests.

expressed emotion see Box – Expressed emotion.

expression *n* **1.** expulsion by force, as of the placenta from the uterus, milk from the breast etc. **2.** facial disclosure of feelings, mood etc. **3.** in genetics, the appearance of a particular trait or characteristic.

expressive aphasia a type of aphasia characterized by difficulty in language production. Word finding difficulties and problems in producing sentence structures may occur. May occur with receptive aphasia. ⇒ receptive aphasia.

exsanguination *n* the process of rendering bloodless. ⇒ haemorrhage. ⇒ shock — **exsanguinate** *vt*.

Expressed emotion

Expressed emotion (EE) is a research concept that was developed by George Brown and Michael Rutter, over 30 years ago. Using a semi-structured interview known as the Camberwell family interview, they sought to ascertain the effects of certain environments upon the course of schizophrenia. Relatives of clients with schizophrenia were interviewed, and investigations found that when clients returned to live in hostile, critical or over protective high EE environments they relapsed more frequently than those who took regular medication and returned to live in low EE accepting, supportive environments. These studies have been replicated throughout the world and the measurement of EE is now recognized to be a robust predictor of relapse. Indeed, the characteristics of EE (see table below) are not exclusively found in rela-

tives as professional carers share similar attributes (Oliver and Kuipers, 1996) and neither are they specific to schizophrenia. The measurement of high EE can also predict relapse in other psychiatric and medical disorders such as, depression, anorexia (Butzlaff and Hooley, 1998) and obesity (Fischmann-Havstad and Marston, 1984).

References

Butzlaff R L, Hooley J M 1998 Expressed emotion and psychiatric relapse. Archives of General Psychiatry 55: 547–552
Fischmann-Havstad L, Marston A R 1984 Weight loss maintenance an aspect of family emotion process. British Journal of Clinical Psychology 23: 265–271
Leff J, Vaughn C 1985 Expressed Emotion in Families. Guildford Press, New York
Oliver N, Kuipers E 1996 Stress and its relationship to expressed emotion in community care workers. International Journal of Social Psychiatry 42(2) 150–159

Characteristics of Low and High EE

	Low EE	High EE
Cognitive	Carers recognize the condition/illness to be genuine and have lower expectations	Carers doubt the legitimacy of the condition/illness, they are generally critical and expect the individual to function as they did before diagnosis was made
Emotional	Carers have another focus to their lives and are empathetic, calmer and more objective	Carers have limited access to other interests or another focus in their lives, they are more likely to exhibit hostility, anger and/or distress
Behavioural	Carers are adaptive, use a problem solving approach, are generally nonintrusive and nonconfrontational	Carers are less flexible and are more likely to be overprotective, intrusive, dismissive and/or confrontational

(adapted from Leff & Vaughn, 1985)

extended family a term currently used to mean the wider group of family relations including aunts, uncles, cousins, grandparents, etc. It is used mainly in a comparative sense when considering the concept 'nuclear family'. ⇒ family.

extended scope physiotherapy practitioners (ESPs) *n* specialist physiotherapists whose role has been extended to include assessment, ordering certain investigations, making referrals, etc. See Box – Extended scope physiotherapy practitioners (ESPs).

extension *n* **1.** traction upon a fractured or dislocated limb. **2.** the increasing of the angle at a joint. ⇒ flexion.

extensor *n* a muscle which, on contraction, extends or straightens a part, e.g. extensor digitorum. ⇒ flexor *ant.*

external cephalic version (ECV) ⇒ version.

extirpation *n* complete removal or destruction of a part.

extra-anatomic bypass (EAB) a prosthetic vascular graft is threaded subcutaneously to carry a limb-preserving blood supply from an efficient proximal part of an artery to a distal one, thus bypassing the ineffective part of the artery.

extra-articular *adj* outside a joint.

extracapsular *adj* outside a capsule. ⇒ intracapsular *ant.*

extracardiac *adj* outside the heart.

extracellular *adj* outside the cell membrane. *extracellular fluid (ECF)* body fluid outside the cell, such as interstitial fluid, plasma, lymph, CSF and gastrointestinal fluid. ⇒ fluid compartment. ⇒ intracellular *ant.*

extracorporeal *adj* outside the body. *extracorporeal circulation* blood is taken from the body, directed through a machine ('heart-lung' or 'artificial - kidney') and returned to the general circulation. ⇒ cardiac bypass. ⇒ cardiopulmonary bypass. ⇒ extracorporeal membrane oxygenation (ECMO). ⇒ haemodialysis.

extracorporeal membrane oxygenation (ECMO) see Box – Extracorporeal membrane oxygenation.

extracorporeal shock-wave lithotripsy ⇒ Dornier lithotriptor.

extract *n* a preparation obtained by evaporating a solution of a drug.

extraction *n* removal. *dental extraction* removal of a tooth. *extraction of lens* surgical removal of the lens of the eye. *extracapsular extraction* the capsule is ruptured prior to delivery of the lens of the eye and preserved in part. *intracapsular extraction* the lens of the eye is removed within its capsule.

extradural *adj* external to the dura mater. *extradural haematoma* a collection of blood outside the dura.

Extended scope physiotherapy practitioners (ESPs)

Increasingly, nurses and physiotherapists are working together in multidisciplinary teams in orthopaedic clinics. Variously described as clinical assistants, orthopaedic assistants and clinical or orthopaedic physiotherapy specialists or practitioners, ESPs are the first contact for new referrals who are not considered to need the immediate attention of an orthopaedic surgeon. They provide timely and relevant assessment, identify patients for whom physiotherapy is appropriate, and allow consultants and registrars to devote their time to patients requiring a surgical opinion. Currently, ESPs work in about 50 centres in the UK, primarily in outpatient orthopaedic clinics but also with rheumatology consultants and neurosurgeons. ESPs in orthopaedic teams are specialists in soft tissue and joint mobilization (mobilisation), have considerable experience in the management of musculoskeletal disorders, have completed specialist continuing professional education and, like orthopaedic registrars, have usually received special training from the consultants with whom they work. They may order blood tests, X-rays and other tests, recommend bone scan or MRI scans, request physiotherapy, order appliances, send an opinion to the referring general practitioner or refer the patient to the orthopaedic surgeon. Best practice requires each patient to be reviewed by the surgeon and physiotherapist after the initial assessment. Tests used by ESPs are described in Magee (1997).

Reference
Magee D J 1997 Orthopaedic Physical Assessment, 3rd edn. W. B. Saunders, London

extragenital *adj* on areas of the body apart from genital organs. *extragenital chancre* is the primary ulcer of syphilis when it occurs on the finger, the lip, the breast, etc.

extrahepatic *adj* outside the liver.

extramural *adj* outside the wall of a vessel or organ — **extramurally** *adv.*

extraocular *adj* outside the eyeball. *extraocular (extrinsic) muscles* the six muscles that move each eyeball. The four rectus muscles: medial, lateral, superior and inferior, and two oblique muscles: superior and inferior. ⇒ strabismus.

extraperitoneal *adj* outside the peritoneum.

extrapleural *adj* outside the pleura, i.e. between the parietal pleura and the chest wall — **extrapleurally** *adv.*

extrapulmonary outside the lungs, such as tuberculosis affecting other organs, e.g. kidney, skin, etc.

extrapyramidal *adj* outside the pyramidal tracts. *extrapyramidal effects/disturbances* include the tremor and rigidity seen in parkinsonism and the side-effects of some drugs, e.g. phenothiazine neuroleptics that may cause a parkinsonian-like syndrome. ⇒ tardive dyskinesia. *extrapyramidal tracts* motor pathways that pass outside the internal capsule. They modify the motor functions of the pyramidal tracts that connect the cerebral cortex to other parts of the brain, muscles and sensory receptors. They influence coarse voluntary movement and affect balance, posture and coordination.

extrarenal *n* outside the kidney — **extrarenally** *adv.*

extrasensory outside the normally accepted senses. *extrasensory perception (ESP)* response to external stimuli in the absence of normal contact or communication.

extrasystole *n* premature beats (ectopic beats) in the pulse rhythm; the cardiac impulse is initiated in some focus apart from the sinoatrial node. *atrial extrasystole*, also called premature atrial contraction, produced by irritable cells in the atria and conducted via abnormal pathways. *ventricular extrasystole*, usually called ventricular ectopic, a common arrhythmia that occurs in normal individuals, but may be associated with heart disease. Premature ventricular contraction occurs without atrial contraction. It is initiated by an abnormal focus in the ventricle that is conducted via an abnormal pathway.

extrathoracic *adj* outside the thoracic cavity.

extrauterine *n* outside the uterus. *extrauterine pregnancy* ⇒ ectopic pregnancy.

extravasation *n* an escape of fluid from its normal enclosure into the surrounding tissues.

extravenous *adj* outside a vein.

extrinsic *adj* developing or having its origin from without; not internal. *extrinsic coagulation pathway* ⇒ coagulation.

Extracorporeal membrane oxygenation
The extracorporeal membrane oxygenation (ECMO) circuit is a cardiopulmonary bypass device which uses a membrane oxygenator or artificial lung. Blood circulates through the device by a roller pump at a rate of approximately 100 mL/kg/min. A fresh flow of oxygen into the device passes through a semipermeable membrane that enables the diffusion of oxygen whilst simultaneously removing carbon dioxide and water. Entry ports in the circuit allow the administration of drugs and the withdrawal of blood specimens. Normal blood temperature can be maintained by a heat exchanger.

A cannula is placed in either the jugular or femoral vein to allow blood to be diverted to the device. Once the blood has been oxygenated it is returned through a vein or an artery. A venoarterial circuit can be used.

Intensive care is required for ECMO, and nursing considerations include the prevention of complications such as infection, haemorrhage and air emboli. The child will be ventilated using low pressures but because paralyzing agents are often avoided so that neurological function can be monitored, regular assessment and treatment of pain and discomfort is essential.

Further reading
Kanto W P 1994 A decade of experience with neonatal extracorporeal membrane oxygenation. J. Pediatrics. 24 (3): 335–345.

extrinsic factor vitamin B_{12}, essential for the maturation of erythrocytes and nerve function, cannot be synthesized in the body but must be supplied in the diet, hence it is called the extrinsic factor. It is absorbed in the presence of the intrinsic factor secreted by the stomach.

extrinsic allergic alveolitis an allergic alveolitis resulting from occupational exposure to moulds, fungal spores or animal proteins, when working in agriculture, forestry, handling birds or animals. It includes: bird fancier's lung, farmer's lung, etc.

extrinsic sugar *npl* sugars, such as fructose in honey, lactose in milk and sucrose as table sugar, not contained in cell walls. ⇒ intrinsic sugar.

extroversion *n* turning inside out. In psychology, the direction of thoughts to the external world.

extrovert *adj* Jungian description of an individual whose characteristic interests and modes of behaviour are directed outwards to other people and the physical environment. ⇒ introvert *ant* — **extroversion** *n*.

extubation *n* removal of a tube from a hollow organ, e.g. removal of endotracheal tube following assisted ventilation. ⇒ intubation *ant*.

exudate *n* the product of exudation. Discharge from a wound containing protein and blood cells.

exudation *n* the oozing out of fluid (exudate) through the capillary walls, such as in the inflammatory response; the sweat through the pores of the skin — **exude** *vt, vi*.

eye *n* organ of vision situated within the bony orbit. It has three layers: sclera (outer fibrous layer), a middle layer, the uvea, that forms the pigmented choroid, ciliary body and iris, and the light-sensitive retina containing photoreceptors (cones and rods) and pigment cells. Light entering the eye is focused on the retina by the lens. Nerve endings in the retina convert the images and transmit them to the brain, in fibres of the optic nerve, for interpretation. (See Figure 22).

eye contact looking at the face of the person to whom one is talking. In many instances, it is a reciprocal activity and is such an important part of most cultures' nonverbal language that blind people are advised to turn their faces in the direction of the voice being heard. In some cultures, however, it is considered inappropriate to make or maintain eye contact during conversation, or when acknowledging a person on the street. *same-level eye contact* a term increasingly being used in nursing to remind nurses that sitting, when talking to a patient in bed or a chair, is good nursing practice.

eye-teeth the canine teeth in the upper jaw.

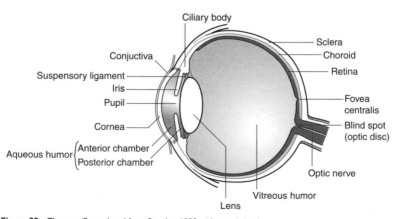

Figure 22 The eye. (Reproduced from Brooker 1998 with permission.)

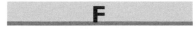

F

F v. West Berkshire Health Authority (1989) a professional who acts in the best interests of an incompetent person, who is incapable of giving consent, does not act unlawfully if he/she follows the accepted standard of care according to the Bolam test.

facet *n* a small, smooth, flat articulating-surface of a bone or a calculus.

facial *adj* pertaining to the face. *facial expression* part of non-verbal body language by which current mood can be conveyed. ⇒ Bell's palsy. ⇒ hemiparesis. ⇒ ptosis. *facial gesture* part of nonverbal body language usually used to reinforce spoken language. Some people, such as those with cerebral palsy, do not have control of the voluntary muscles involved, consequently nurses assessing a person with spasticities may have difficulty in interpreting facial gestures because of unfamiliarity with them. *facial nerve* the VIIth pair of cranial nerves, they supply the facial muscles, part of the tongue and glands including: salivary, lacrimal and nasal. *facial paralysis* paralysis of muscles supplied by the facial nerve.

facies *n* the surface of any structure; the face or its appearance or expression. *adenoid facies* open mouthed, vacant expression due to deafness from enlarged adenoids. *Parkinson facies* a mask-like appearance; saliva may trickle from the corners of the mouth.

facilitated diffusion *n* a process by which larger molecules (e.g. glucose), that are not fat-soluble, diffuse through the plasma membrane by using a protein carrier molecule. The process does not use energy, but requires a concentration gradient.

factor I *n* fibrinogen. ⇒ coagulation.

factor II *n* prothrombin. ⇒ coagulation.

factor III *n* thromboplastin. ⇒ coagulation.

factor IV *n* calcium ions. ⇒ coagulation.

factor V *n* labile factor (proaccelerin). ⇒ coagulation.

factor VII *n* stable factor (proconvertin). ⇒ coagulation.

factor VIII *n* antihaemophilic factor A (AHF) or antihaemophilic globulin. ⇒ coagulation.

factor IX *n* Christmas factor or anti-haemophilic factor B. ⇒ coagulation.

factor X *n* Stuart-Prower factor. ⇒ coagulation.

factor XI *n* plasma thromboplastin antecedent (PTA). ⇒ coagulation.

factor XII *n* Hageman factor. ⇒ coagulation.

factor XIII *n* fibrin stabilizing factor (FSF). ⇒ coagulation.

faecal fat collection collection of faeces over a given period, e.g. 3 days, so that the laboratory can estimate the amount of fat per weight of faeces.

faecal impaction the presence of a large amount of dried hardened faeces in the rectum and colon. After taking medication to soften the faeces, an evacuant enema is introduced into the rectum via the anus. ⇒ constipation ⇒ impacted. → manual evacuation of the bowel. → spurious diarrhoea.

faecalith *n* a concretion formed in the bowel from faecal matter; it can cause obstruction and/or inflammation.

faecal-oral route a term that describes the ingestion of micro-organisms from faeces which can be transmitted directly or indirectly by hands.

faeces *n* the waste matter excreted from the bowel, consisting mainly of indigestible cellulose, unabsorbed food, intestinal secretions and epithelial cells, mucus, water, electrolytes, stercobilin, bacteria and various chemicals producing odour. It is recommended that sufficient dietary fibre should be taken to produce 150–250 g of faeces daily — **faecal** *adj* pertaining to faeces. *faecal occult blood* ⇒ occult blood.

Fahrenheit *n* a thermometric scale, the freezing point of water is 32° and its boiling point 212°.

failure to thrive failure to grow and develop at the expected rate, ascertained by consistent measurement of weight and height plotted on a growth chart. The syndrome may be the result of an organic disorder or have nonorganic causes, such as inadequate feeding, maternal deprivation or psychosocial problems. Systematic investigation is required to establish the cause.

faint *n* syncope — **faint** *vi*.

falciform *adj* sickle-shaped. *falciform ligament* a fold of peritoneum separating the right and left lobes of the liver.

fallopian tubes *n* ⇒ uterine tubes.

Fallot's tetralogy a form of cyanotic congenital heart disease which comprises four abnormalities: a large ventricular septal defect; stenosis of the pulmonary valve; overriding of the aorta; right ventricular hypertrophy. Increasingly, total surgical correction is being used. Also known as tetralogy of Fallot.

false substrate substances, such as drugs, that disrupt a metabolic pathway by forming abnormal products.

falx *n* a sickle-shaped structure. *falx cerebri* that portion of the dura mater separating the two cerebral hemispheres.

familial *adj* pertaining to the family, as of a disease affecting several members of the same family.

family see Box – The family.

family-centred care a philosophy of nursing, usually applied to children, which takes into account the needs and circumstances of the whole family, not just the child.

Family Health Services (FHS) the community-based services provided by family doctors, dentists, opticians and pharmacists as independent contractors. They are not employed by the NHS, but have contractual arrangements to work in the NHS.

family planning the methods used to space or limit the number of children, or for enhancing conception. *natural family planning* methods of family planning that do not use drugs or appliances. They may use one or a combination of the following: temperature, cervical mucus and menstrual cycle calendar. ⇒ assisted fertility/conception. ⇒ contraceptive. ⇒ condom.

family therapy in psychotherapy, a technique which uses group or individual psychotherapy in an attempt to resolve the problems of a single family member.

Fanconi syndrome proximal renal tubular acidosis. An inherited or acquired dysfunction of the proximal kidney tubules. Large amounts of amino acids, glucose, uric acid and phosphates are excreted in the urine, yet the blood levels of these substances are normal. Symptoms may include thirst, polyuria, bone abnormalities and muscular weakness. ⇒ aminoaciduria. ⇒ cystinosis.

fantasy, phantasy *n* a 'day dream' in which the thinker's conscious or unconscious desires and impulses are fulfilled. May be accompanied by a feeling of unreality. Occurs pathologically in schizophrenia.

The Family

The family is assuming a higher profile in modern westernized societies as political leaders, policy-makers and social scientists argue for the institution of marriage to be maintained.

The family as a social organization has undergone many changes. Nowadays it is more common to use the term 'families' since there are many family types. For example, in addition to the conventional family types such as the nuclear family, the extended family, the step family, and the compound family (as in some African societies), one must also include lone parent families; cohabitation; gay and lesbian families. Perspectives on the family abound. Functionalists stress the role of the family in stress management and in its reproductive and economic activities for societies' benefit. Feminists, however, argue that women in families are being oppressed, in a patriarchal society. Marxist theorists on the other hand explain that the family participates in reproducing a workforce for the benefit of a capitalist society.

Families have an essential role to play in health care (Béphage 2000). The World Health Report (WHO 1998) stipulates that the family forms the basis of the healthcare system, together with personal responsibility and the community. Furthermore the role of the family in the maintenance of mental well-being, and in helping those with mental health problems is emphasized (DoH 1999).

References
Béphage G 2000 Social and Behavioural Sciences for Nurses: An integrated approach. Churchill Livingstone, Edinburgh
Department of Health 1999 Saving Lives: Our Healthier Nation. The Stationery Office, London
World Health Organization 1998 The World Health Report. Life in the 21st Century a vision for all. World Health Organization, Geneva

farinaceous *adj* pertaining to cereal substances, i.e. made of flour or grain. Starchy.

farmer's lung a form of extrinsic alveolitis due to allergy to certain spores (e.g. *Aspergillus fumigatus, Micropolyspora faeni*) that occur in the dust of mouldy hay or other mouldy vegetable produce. Management includes: avoiding the allergen, corticosteroids and oxygen in patients with hypoxia. Recognized as an industrial disease. → extrinsic allergic alveolitis.

FAS *abbr* fetal alcohol syndrome.

fascia *n* a fibrous connective tissue which attaches the skin to the underlying tissues. It also surrounds and separates many of the muscles, and, in some cases, holds them together — **fascial** *adj*.

fasciculation *n* visible flickering of muscle; can occur in the upper and lower eyelids.

fasciculus *n* a little bundle, as of muscle or nerve — **fasciculi** *pl*.

fasciotomy *n* incision of a fascia.

fastigium *n* the summit or height, e.g the highest point of a fever; the period of full development of a disease.

fat *n* 1. complex organic molecule of glycerol with fatty acids; known as triacylglycerol or triglyceride. May be of animal or vegetable origin. Fats and oils. *fat embolus* ⇒ embolism. *fat-soluble vitamins* vitamins A, D, E and K are fat-soluble. ⇒ adipose. ⇒ brown fat. ⇒ fatty acid. ⇒ glycerol. → kilojoule. → triacylglycerol. 2. adipose tissue, which acts as a reserve supply of energy, protects organs and smooths out body contours — **fatty** *adj*.

Fatal Accident Enquiry ⇒ coroner.

fatigue *n* weariness. Term used in physiological experiments on muscle to denote diminishing reaction to stimulus applied — **fatigability** *n*.

fatty acids *npl* hydrocarbon constituent of lipids. Classified as saturated or unsaturated (monounsaturated or polyunsaturated) according to the number of double chemical bonds in their structure. ⇒ essential fatty acids.

fatty degeneration degeneration of tissues which results in appearance of fatty droplets in the cytoplasm; found especially in diseases of liver, kidney and heart.

fauces *n* the opening from the mouth into the pharynx, bounded above by the soft palate, below by the tongue. Pillars of the fauces, anterior and posterior, lie laterally and enclose the palatine tonsil — **faucial** *adj*.

favism *n* describes the acute haemolytic anaemia resulting from eating or being in contact with the fava (broad) bean in people with the inherited X-linked disorder, where the enzyme glucose-6-phosphate dehydrogenase (G6PD) is deficient in the red blood cells. ⇒ glucose-6-phosphate dehydrogenase (G6PD).

favus *n* a type of ringworm not common in Britain; caused by *Trichophyton schoenleini*. Yellow cup-shaped crusts develop, especially on the scalp.

fear *n* an intense emotional state involving a feeling of unpleasant tension, and a strong impulse to escape, which is natural in response to a threat of danger but is unnatural as a continuous state. → anxiety. ⇒ fight or flight mechanism. ⇒ general adaptation syndrome.

Fear Questionnaire (FR) a 16 item questionnaire used in the assessment of anxiety. It uses a Likert scale. 0 (would not avoid it) to 8 (always avoid it) to assess how much a person avoids certain situations. It can be self administered or used by mental health nurses and other practitioners.

febrile *adj* feverish; accompanied by fever. *febrile convulsions* occur in children who have an increased body temperature. Most common between the ages of 6 months and 5 years. ⇒ convulsions.

fecundation *n* impregnation; fertilization.

fecundity *n* the power of reproduction; fertility.

feedback *n* homeostatic control mechanism whereby the rate at which a physiological process proceeds is controlled by the product of the process. *negative feedback* most commonly, a process is slowed or 'turned off' by an increasing amount of product, for example in the regulation of blood glucose. *positive feedback* much more rarely, the process is accelerated by high levels of the product. Examples include: normal blood clotting and the events of labour and childbirth.

feedback treatment → biofeedback.

Felty's syndrome adult rheumatoid arthritis with splenomegaly and neutropenia. Common clinical feature include: lymphadenopathy, vasculitis, leg ulcers, weight loss, skin pigmentation, recurrent infections and anaemia.

feminism a sociological doctrine that puts forward the idea that women have been disadvantaged in every area of society. It supports the idea of equal oportunities for women and men. Feminist sociologists have disputed the body of 'malestream' sociological research undertaken by men who failed to consider the sociological significance of women, for instance in the workforce. Feminism takes several forms including: liberal, black, radical and Marxist/socialist.

femoral hernia ⇒ hernia.

femur *n* the thigh bone; the longest and strongest bone in the body — **femoral** *adj* pertaining to the femur or thigh. Applied to the artery, vein, nerve and canal.

fenamates *npl* a group of nonsteroidal anti-inflammatory drugs, e.g. mefenamic acid.

fenestra *n* a window-like opening. *fenestra ovalis* an oval opening between the middle and internal ear. Below it lies the *fenestra rotunda* a round opening.

fenestration *n* 1. a perforation, pore or opening. The capillaries in the glomerulus of the kidney, which form part of the filtration membrane, are adapted for permeability and filtration by the presence of fenestrations. 2. the surgical creation of an opening (or fenestra) in the inner ear for the relief of deafness in otosclerosis.

fermentation *n* the process whereby enzymes in yeasts and bacteria break down sugars (glycolysis) and other substrates. Excellent examples are the making of bread, alcohol, vinegar and cheese.

ferric *adj* pertaining to trivalent iron and its salts. Ferric iron is converted to the absorbable ferrous state by gastric acid.

ferritin *n* a storage form of iron. Combined with proteins, the iron, which would be toxic alone, is stored safely in the liver and spleen. ⇒ haemosiderin.

ferrous *adj* pertaining to divalent iron, as of its salts and compounds. *ferrous carbonate, ferrous fumarate, ferrous glu-conate, ferrous succinate* and *ferrous sulphate* are oral preparations for iron-deficiency anaemias. ⇒ anaemia.

fertility the ability to produce young. *fertility control* ⇒ contraceptive. ⇒ familiy planning. *fertility rate* the number of live births occurring per 1000 women aged 15–44, e.g. 60 per 1000 women. It can also be described in terms of the total fertile period, i.e. the average number of live births that would occur per woman if the woman experienced the current age-specific fertility rate throughout her reproductive years, e.g. 1.9 per woman.

fertilization *n* the impregnation of an oocyte by a spermatozoon and the fusion of their two nuclei to form the diploid zygote.

FESS functional endoscopic sinus surgery.

fester *vi* to become inflamed; to suppurate.

festination *n* increasingly rapid gait, as in parkinsonism.

fetal alcohol syndrome (FAS) stillbirth and fetal abnormality due to prenatal growth retardation caused by maternal consumption of alcohol during pregnancy. It includes both physical and mental abnormalities and is characterized by poor growth, facial, cardiac and limb abnormalities, and learning disabilities.

fetishism *n* a condition in which a particular material object is regarded with irrational awe or has a strong emotional attachment. Can have a psychosexual dimension in which such an object is repeatedly or exclusively used in achieving sexual excitement and gratification.

fetoplacental unit *n* term used to describe the interdependence of fetal and placental tissues in hormone production, particularly oestrogen, during pregnancy.

fetor *n* offensive odour, stench. *fetor hepaticus* 'mousy' breath odour associated with hepatic encephalopathy. *fetor oris* bad breath.

fetoscopy *n* direct visual examination of the fetus by using a suitable fibreoptic endoscope.

fetus *n* the internationally preferred spelling. The developmental stage from the eighth week of gestation until birth. An unborn child. *fetus papyraceous* a dead fetus, one of twins which has become flattened and mummified — **fetal**

adj pertaining to the fetus. *fetal assessment* various methods used to assess fetal well-being, they include: physical examination, ultrasound scan, amniocentesis, chorionic villus sampling, blood tests, kick charts (fetal movement) and checks on placental function. *fetal circulation* circulation adapted for intrauterine life. Extra vessels and shunts (ductus arteriosus, ductus venosus, foramen ovale and umbilical vein) allows blood to largely bypass the lungs, liver and gastrointestinal tract, as their functions are dealt with by maternal systems and the placenta.

FEV *abbr* forced expiratory volume. ⇒ respiratory function tests.

fever *n* (*syn* pyrexia) an elevation of body temperature above normal. Designates some infectious conditions, e.g. *enteric fevers*, *scarlet fever*, *spotted fever*, etc. ⇒ pyrexia.

FHS *abbr* Family Health Services.

fibre *n* 1. a thread-like structure 2. ⇒ nonstarch polysaccharide — **fibrous** *adj*.

fibreoptics *n* the transmission of light via very fine glass or plastic fibres enclosed within a flexible tube. The technolgy utilized in endoscopic equipment

fibril *n* a component filament of a fibre; a small fibre.

fibrillation *n* uncoordinated quivering contraction of muscle, usually of the myocardium. → atrial fibrillation. → cardiac arrest. → ventricular fibrillation.

fibrin *n* the matrix on which a blood clot is formed. The substance is formed from soluble fibrinogen of the blood by the action of thrombin. ⇒ coagulation — **fibrinous** *adj*.

fibrin stabilizing factor (FSF) *n* factor XIII in coagulation.

fibrinogen *n* a soluble plasma protein produced by the liver. Factor I in blood coagulation. It is converted to fibrin by the action of thrombin. → coagulation.

fibrinogenopenia *n* (*syn* fibrinopenia) lack of fibrinogen in the blood. Causes include reduced synthesis in liver disease and abnormal coagulation, such as DIC. ⇒ afibrinogenaemia.

fibrinolysin *n* ⇒ plasmin. ⇒ plasminogen.

fibrinolysis *n* one of the four overlapping processes of haemostasis. The dissolution of the fibrin clot by plasmin (proteolytic

enzyme) when healing is complete. The debris is removed by phagocytosis. There is normally a balance between blood coagulation and fibrinolysis in the body. ⇒ coagulation. ⇒ platelet plug — **fibrinolytic** *adj* pertaining to the dissolution of fibrin clots. *fibrinolytic therapy* the use of plasminogen activators, e.g. alteplase and streptokinase, used to treat various thromboembolic conditions, such as myocardial infarction, severe venous thrombosis and pulmonary embolism. Also called thrombolytic therapy.

fibrinopenia *n* ⇒ fibrinogenopenia.

fibroadenoma *n* a benign tumour containing fibrous and glandular epithelial tissue. Commonly found in the breasts of young women under the age of 30 years. They present as small mobile lumps.

fibroblast *n* immature blast cell that forms some connective tissues. Active during development and tissue repair → chondroblast. → haemocytoblast. → osteoblast — **fibroblastic** *adj*.

fibrocartilage *n* cartilage containing fibrous tissue. ⇒ cartilage — **fibrocartilaginous** *adj*.

fibrocaseous *adj* a soft, cheesy mass infiltrated by fibrous tissue, formed by fibroblasts.

fibrochondritis *n* inflammation of fibrocartilage.

fibrocyst *n* a fibroma which has undergone cystic degeneration, i.e. cystic fibroma.

fibrocystic *adj* pertaining to a fibrocyst. *fibrocystic disease of bone* cysts may be solitary or characterized by an overgrowth of fibrous tissue and development of cystic spaces. It is symptomatic of hyperparathyroidism. ⇒ von Recklinghausen's disease. *fibrocystic disease of pancreas* cystic fibrosis.

fibrocyte *n* ⇒ fibroblast — **fibrocytic** *adj*.

fibroid *n* fibromyoma. A fibromuscular benign tumour usually found in the uterus. Frequently asymptomatic but may cause menorrhagia, pain and symptoms that depend on the location, such as pressure on the bladder. Classified according to location: *interstitial (intramural) uterine fibroid* is embedded in the wall of the uterus. *subperitoneal (subserous) fibroid* extends to the outer wall. *submucous fibroid* extends to the inner or endometrial surface. ⇒ endometrial destruction. ⇒ hysterectomy. → myomectomy.

fibroma *n* a benign tumour composed of fibrous tissue — **fibromatous** *adj*.

fibromuscular *adj* pertaining to fibrous and muscle tissue.

fibromyalgia *n* a syndrome of chronic musculoskeletal pain. It is characterized by pain, specific tender points, stiffness, fatigue, and may be accompanied by irritable bowel syndrome and tension headaches. ⇒ fibrositis.

fibromyoma *n* a benign tumour consisting of fibrous and muscle tissue. ⇒ fibroid — **fibromyomatous** *adj*.

fibroplasia *n* the production of fibrous tissue which is a normal part of healing. *retrolental fibroplasia* older term for retinopathy of prematurity. Describes the final stages of more severe cases. The presence of fibrous tissue in the vitreous humor and retina, extending in an area from the ciliary body to the optic disc, causing blindness. Associated with the administration of high concentration oxygen therapy to preterm or low birth weight babies.

fibrosarcoma *n* a malignant tumour of fibrous tissue — **fibrosarcomatous** *adj*.

fibrosis *n* the formation of excessive fibrous tissue in areas of cell damage, often as a result of inflammation. *pulmonary fibrosis* may be caused by serious lung disease, such as pneumoconiosis, radiation, or the use of certain drugs, some cytotoxic drugs — **fibrotic** *adj*.

fibrositis *n* inflammation of fibrous tissue. It is generally associated with stiffness and local tenderness and pain. ⇒ fibromyalgia.

fibrovascular *adj* pertaining to fibrous tissue which is well supplied with blood vessels.

fibula *n* one of the longest and thinnest bones of the body, situated on the outer side of the leg and articulating at the upper end with the lateral condyle of the tibia and at the lower end with the lateral surface of the talus and tibia — **fibular** *adj*.

field of vision the area in which objects can be seen by the fixed eye.

fight or flight mechanism the extreme physiological response to an immediate stressor such as perceived danger. Adrenaline (epinephrine) and noradrenaline (norepinephrine) the catecholamines are released. These stimulate an increase in heart rate, rise in blood pressure, vasoconstriction, increased respiration, increased blood glucose, and diversion of blood to the vital organs and skeletal muscles to deal with the stressor or remove the body from it.

FIGO staging a system devised by the International Federation of Gynaecology and Obstetrics to classify tumours of the ovary, cervix and uterus according to the extent of spread.

Filaria *n* a genus of parasitic, thread-like nematode worms, e.g. *Wuchereria bancrofti*, *Brugia malayi*, *Onchocerca volvulus* and *Loa Loa*. They are found mainly in the tropics and subtropics. ⇒ filariasis — **filarial** *adj*.

filariasis *n* infestation with Filaria. The adult worms may live in the lymphatics, connective tissues or mesentery, where they may cause obstruction, but the microfilariae migrate to the bloodstream and some invade the skin, eye or pulmonary capillaries. In some types, the completion of the lifecycle is dependent upon passage through a mosquito. ⇒ elephantiasis. ⇒ loiasis. ⇒ onchocerciasis.

filaricide *n* an agent which destroys *Filaria*, e.g. diethylcarbamazine.

file *n* in computing a discrete set of characters stored on a disk. Files may hold information in a variety of forms which include: a database, program, document or as a graphic image. Individual files and their contents are identified by a unique filename. ⇒ folder.

filiform *adj* thread-like. *filiform papillae* small projections ending in several minute processes; found on the tongue.

filipuncture *n* insertion of wire thread etc into an aneurysm to produce coagulation of contained blood.

filoviruses *npl* a family of RNA viruses that include the Ebola and Marburg viruses. ⇒ Ebola. ⇒ Marburg disease.

filter *n* a device designed to remove electromagnetic rays of specific wavelength or particles over a certain size while allowing others to pass through. Examples include fluid filters and optical filters.

filtrate *n* that part of a substance which passes through the filter.

filtration *n* the process of straining through a filter under gravity, pressure or vacuum. The act of passing fluid through a porous medium. *filtration under pressure* occurs in the kidneys, due to the high pressure of blood in the afferent arteriole of the glomerulus.

filum *n* any filamentous or thread-like structure. *filum terminale* modified pia mater forming a strong, fine cord that secures the spinal cord to the coccyx.

fimbria *n* a fringe or frond; resembling the fronds of a fern; e.g. the fimbriae of the uterine tubes **fimbrial, fimbriated** *adj.*

fine tremor *n* slight trembling as seen in the outstretched hands or tongue of a patient with hyperthyroidism.

finger *n* a digit. *clubbed finger* swelling of terminal phalanx which occurs in many lung and heart diseases.

finger spelling a means of communicating by spelling words using the fingers of either one hand (in one handed finger spelling) or two hands (in two-handed finger spelling) to make the letters of the alphabet.

first pass metabolism where drugs given orally are absorbed in the gastrointestinal tract and arrive in the liver via the hepatic portal vein to be rapidly metabolized, which results in a situation where the active drug does not reach the systemic circulation in sufficient amounts to produce a therapeutic effect. It can be avoided by use of other methods of administration, such as sublingual or transdermally. Many drugs are subject to partial first pass metabolism (first pass effect), e.g. oral contraceptive.

first/primary intention ⇒ wound healing.

fish oils such as cod liver oil, contain vitamins A and D and are good sources of *n*-3(omega-3) polyunsaturated fatty acids. May be beneficial in the prevention of heart disease.

fish skin disease ⇒ ichthyoses.

fission *n* a method of reproduction common among the bacteria and protozoa. ⇒ binary fission.

fissure *n* a split or cleft. *anal fissure* split in the anal mucosa causing severe pain on defaecation. *palpebral fissure* the opening between the eyelids. *fissure of Rolando* central sulcus, separating the parietal and frontal cerebral lobes. *fissure of Sylvius* lateral sulcus separating the frontal and temporal cerebral lobes. ⇒ sulcus.

fistula *n* an abnormal communication between two body surfaces or cavities, e.g. gastrocolic fistula between the stomach and colon, or a faecal fistula where faeces discharge on to the surface of the body via a wound or drain site. ⇒ biliary fistula. ⇒ rectovaginal fistula. ⇒ tracheo-oesophageal fistula. ⇒ vesicovaginal fistula — **fistular, fistulous** *adj.*

fistula-in-ano an abnormal track communicating with the skin around the anus. It is associated with bowel disease and ischiorectal abscess.

fistulogram *n* X-ray of a fistula after injection into it of a contrast medium.

Fitness for Practice a report prepared by the Commission for Education established by the UKCC to look at preregistration nursing and midwifery education and propose education that 'enabled fitness for practice based on healthcare need' (UKCC 1999). ⇒ Project 2000.

fixation *n* 1. as a psychoanalytical term, an incomplete separation from an earlier stage of psychosexual development. An emotional attachment, generally sexual, to a parent, which may cause difficulty in forming new attachments later in life. 2. in optics, the direct focusing of one or both eyes on an object so that the image falls on the retinal disc.

fixed costs the costs incurred regardless of the level of activity, e.g. related to the buildings and land, equipment maintenance.

flaccid *adj* soft, flabby, not firm. *flaccid paralysis* results mainly from lower motor neuron lesions. There are diminished or absent tendon reflexes — **flaccidity** *n.*

flagellation *n* the act of whipping oneself or others to gain sexual pleasure, or as a form of masochism or sadism.

flagellum *n* a microscopic, hair-like appendage of certain cells: spermatozoa, certain bacteria and protozoa. Used for movement — **flagella** *pl.*

flail chest unstable thoracic cage due to multiple rib fractures. ⇒ respiration.

flap *n* tissue used to repair defects in an adjacent or distant part of the body. *cross leg flap* a flap with vascular attachment raised from one leg to cover defect on other leg. *free flap* an island flap detached from the body and reattached at the distant recipient site by microvascular surgery. *myocutaneous flap* a compound flap of skin and muscle with vascular attachment to permit sufficient tissue to be transferred to recipient site, such as for breast reconstruction following mastectomy. *pedicle flap* a full thickness flap attached by a pedicle. *rotation flap* pedicle flap whose width is increased by transforming the edge of the flap distal to the defect into a curved line; the flap is then rotated. *skin flap* a full thickness mass of tissue containing epidermis, dermis and subcutaneous tissue.

flat-foot *n* (*syn* pes planus) a congenital or acquired deformity marked by flattening or complete loss of the longitudinal arches of the foot.

flat pelvis contracted pelvis. A pelvis in which the anteroposterior diameter of the brim is reduced. May cause problems during labour. ⇒ conjugate.

flatulence *n* gastric and intestinal distension with gas. Causes belching and discomfort — **flatulent** *adj*.

flatus *n* gas in the gastrointesinal tract, usually applied to that passed rectally.

flatus tube rarely used to relieve flatulent abdominal distension. It is a long openended tube which is passed along the bowel while the free end is immersed under water through which flatus (air) bubbles.

flea *n* a blood-sucking wingless insect of the order Siphonaptera; it acts as a host and can transmit disease. Its bite leaves a portal of entry for infection. *human flea Pulex irritans. rat flea Xenopsylla cheopis*, transmitter of plague.

flex *vi, vt* bend.

flexibilitas cerea literally, waxy flexibility. A condition of generalized hypertonia of muscles found in catatonic schizophrenia. When fully developed, the patient's limbs retain positions in which they are placed, remaining immobile for hours at a time.

flexion *n* the reduction of the angle at a joint. ⇒ extension.

Flexner's bacillus ⇒ *Shigella flexneri*.

flexor *n* a muscle which on contraction flexes or bends a part, e.g. biceps brachii ⇒ extensor *ant*.

flexure *n* a bend, as in a tube-like structure, e.g. the flexures in the colon, or a fold, as on the skin – it can be obliterated by extension or increased by flexion in the locomotor system. *left colic (splenic) flexure* is situated at the junction of the transverse and descending parts of the colon. It lies at a higher level than the *right colic* or *hepatic flexure* the bend between the ascending and transverse colon, beneath the liver. *sigmoid flexure* the S-shaped bend at the lower end of the descending colon. It is continuous with the rectum below. ⇒ colon — **flexural** *adj*.

flight of ideas succession of thoughts with no rational connection. A feature of manic disorders.

floaters *npl* floating bodies in the vitreous humor (of the eye) which are visible to the person.

floating kidney abnormally mobile kidney.

flocculation *n* the coalescence of colloidal particles in suspension resulting in their aggregation into larger discrete masses which are often visible to the naked eye as cloudiness (turbidity). *flocculation test* where abnormal protein concentrations in cerebrospinal fluid or serum cause flocculation of substances, such as colloidal gold, zinc sulphate, thymol and cephalincholesterol.

flooding *n* a popular term to describe excessive bleeding from the uterus.

floppy baby syndrome may be due to true muscle or nervous system disorder as opposed to benign hypotonia.

florid *adj* flushed, high coloured.

flowmeter *n* an instrument for measuring the flow rate of gases or liquids.

fluctuation *n* a wave-like motion felt on digital examination of a fluid-containing tumour, e.g. abscess — **fluctuant** *adj*.

fluid *n* a substance that flows, either liquid or gaseous. ⇒ fluid compartments.

fluid compartments *n* fluids in the body are either intracellular fluid (ICF) within the cells, or extracellular fluid (ECF) outside the cells. Extracellular fluids include: plasma, interstitial fluid, lymph, cerebrospinal fluid and gastrointestinal fluids. In the adult about two-thirds of body water is inside the cells (intracellular). The remaining third is outside the cells (extracellular). (See Figure 23.)

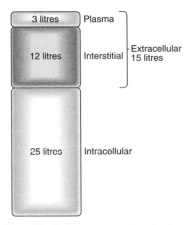

3 litres	Plasma
12 litres	Interstitial
25 litres	Intracellular

Extracellular 15 litres

3 litres Plasma
12 litres Interstitial
25 litres Intracellular

Figure 23 Fluid compartments (Reproduced from Brooker 1996 with permission.)

fluke *n* a trematode worm of the order Digenea. The *European* or *sheep fluke (Fasciola hepatica)* is usually ingested from watercress. There is fever, malaise, a large tender liver and eosinophilia. The *Chinese fluke (Clonorchis sinensis)* is usually ingested with raw fish. The adult fluke lives in the bile ducts and, while it may produce cholangitis, hepatitis and jaundice, it may be asymptomatic or be blamed for vague digestive symptoms. *lung fluke (Paragonimus)* usually ingested with raw crab in China and Far East. The symptoms are those of chronic bronchitis, including blood in the sputum. ⇒ Schistosoma.

fluorescein *n* red substance which forms a green fluorescent solution. Used as eye drops to detect corneal lesions, which stain green.

fluorescent treponemal antibody absorbed test (FTA-abs) a specific serological test for syphilis.

fluoridation *n* ⇒ fluoride.

fluoride *n* a salt of fluorine sometimes present in drinking water. It can be incorporated into the structure of bone and teeth, where it provides protection against dental caries, but in gross excess it causes mottling of the teeth. As a preventive measure it is often added to toothpaste and can be added to a water supply (fluoridation).

fluorine (F) *n* halogen element.

fluoroquinolones *npl* a group of synthetic antibiotics that include broad spectrum ciprofloxacin, which is effective against both Gram-positive and Gram-negative bacteria, and nalidixic acid, which is used for urinary tract infection.

fluoroscopy *n* X-ray examination of movement in the body, observed by means of fluorescent screen and TV system.

foam dressings *npl* wound dressing available as sheets, shaped for special areas, e.g. heels, or as cavity dressings (preformed or as a kit that is made up to fit a specific cavity). They are used for a large range of wounds to provide a moist wound environment with varying degree of absorption.

focus 1. point of maximum intensity. 2. point where light rays or sound waves converge.

focus groups *npl* research method where data are obtained by interviewing people in small interacting groups.

foetus *n* ⇒ fetus.

folate *n* collective name for the B vitamin compounds derived from folic acid. Folates occur naturally in foods such as liver, yeasts and leafy green vegetables and are absorbed from the small intestine. They are coenzymes involved in many biochemical reactions in the body, e.g. purine and pyrimidine synthesis, and adequate amounts, along with vitamin B_{12}, are required for normal red cells and cell division generally. A deficiency results in a megaloblastic anaemia. It is recommended that supplements are taken before and in the first weeks after conception, as this reduces the risk of neural tube defects in the fetus. All women of child-bearing age should ensure that their diet contains sufficient folate.

folder *n* in computing an area on the disk in which files are placed. Also known as directory. ⇒ file.

Foley catheter a self-retaining urinary catheter.

folic acid (*syn* pteroyl glutamic acid) the molecule that gives rise to a large group of molecules known as folates that form part of the vitamin B complex.

follicle *n* 1. a small secreting sac. 2. an epidermal invagination enclosing a hair. 3. a simple tubular gland. *follicle stimulating hormone (FSH)* a gonadotrophin secreted by the anterior pituitary gland; it acts on the ovaries in the female, where it stimulates the development of ovarian follicles containing oocytes during the ovarian cycle. ⇒ Graafian follicle. ⇒ ovulation. In the male, FSH stimulates the seminiferous tubules of the testes to produce spermatozoa — **follicular** *adj* pertaining to a follicle. *follicular phase* days 1–14 of the ovarian cycle which includes ovulation.

folliculitis *n* inflammation of follicles, such as the hair follicles. ⇒ alopecia.

fomentation *n* a hot, wet application to produce hyperaemia.

fomite *n* any article, such as bedding, which has been in contact with infection and is capable of transmitting same.

font describes the design, point size and style of a particular typeface.

fontanelles *npl* 'soft spots'. The membranous spaces between the cranial bones of an infant prior to complete bony ossification. The diamond-shaped anterior fontanelle (bregma) is at the junction of the frontal and two parietal bones. It usually closes in the second year of life. The triangular posterior fontanelle is at the junction of the occipital and two parietal bones. It closes within a few weeks of birth. The state of the fontanelles can be diagnostic, such as sunken fontanelles caused by dehydration or bulging caused by raised intracranial pressure. The timing of fontanelle closure is a guide to developmental progress. ⇒ suture.

food allergy *n* allergic reactions to substances present in foods, such as nuts (peanuts), strawberries, eggs and shellfish. The reaction happens immediately on contact with the food and can be very severe, leading to life-threatening anaphylaxis. Once identified, the food substance is removed from the diet and the person's immediate environment. Individuals who are at risk of suffering an extreme reaction usually carry prefilled devices of adrenaline (epinephrine) for injection. ⇒ allergy.

food intolerance *n* intolerance to particular foods. It has been estimated that as many as a third of people experience some form of intolerance. Diagnosis may take time whilst different foods are eliminated from the diet to trace the cause. ⇒ lactose intolerance.

food poisoning a group of diseases characterized by vomiting, with or without diarrhoea, resulting from eating food contaminated with chemical toxins, preformed bacterial toxin or live microorganisms (bacteria and viruses) or poisonous natural vegetation, e.g. berries, toadstools (fungi). Food poisoning is notifiable and may be caused by bacterial multiplication in the food, e.g. *Campylobacter jejuni*, *Bacillus cereus*, *Salmonella typhimurium* and viruses, or from toxins produced by bacteria, such as *Escherichia coli 0157*, *Staphylococcus aureus* and *Clostridium perfringens*.

food sensitivity *n* See Box – Food sensitivity.

Food Standards Agency *n* a UK body set up by the government to oversee food standards and safety.

foot *n* that portion of the lower limb below the ankle. *foot drop* inability to dorsiflex foot, as in severe sciatica and nervous disease affecting lower lumbar regions of the cord. Can arise as a complication of bedrest. *foot or footling presentation* an

---

Food sensitivity

Food sensitivity can be defined as an unpleasant reaction to a specific food or ingredient that is reproducible for a specific individual, but not necessarily the entire population. These signs and symptoms include gastrointestinal disturbance, asthma, urticaria, headache and behavioural changes.

There are five categories of food sensitivity:

- Toxic – food acts as a toxic substance, e.g. bacterial food poisoning;
- Metabolic – a specific component of the food cannot be metabolized normally, e.g.

lactose in milk in adults with lactase deficiency;

- Pharmacological – individuals are particularly sensitive to a substance in food, e.g. the caffeine and theobromine in tea and coffee;
- Idiosyncratic – no mechanism of action can be identified, but the sufferer responds with reproducible symptoms to a blind challenge of a particular food;
- Allergic – an abnormal immunological response is triggered by a particular food. Can result in potentially fatal food induced anaphylaxis, e.g. peanuts.

abnormal situation during labour when one or both legs are the presenting part.

foramen *n* a hole or opening. Generally used with reference to bones. *foramen magnum* the opening in the base of the skull (occipital bone) through which the spinal cord passes. *foramen ovale* an adaption of the fetal circulation. A communication between the cardiac atria that allows blood to bypass the pulmonary circulation. Normally it is occluded by a flap after the infant's first breath but takes some months to close completely. Surgical intervention may be required where the foramen fails to close — **foramina** *pl*.

forced expiratory volume (FEV) volume of air exhaled during a given time (usually the first second. FEV_1) whilst performing a forced vital capacity. ⇒ respiratory function tests.

forced vital capacity (FVC) the maximum gas volume that can be expelled from the lungs in a forced expiration following a maximal inspiratory effort. ⇒ respiratory function tests.

forceps *n* surgical instruments with two opposing blades which are used to grasp or compress tissues, swabs, needles and many other surgical appliances. The two blades are controlled by direct pressure on them (tong-like), or by handles (scissor-like). *forceps delivery* the use of various types of obstetric forceps applied to the infant and used to deliver the infant during the second stage of labour.

forensic medicine (*syn* medical jurisprudence) also called 'legal medicine'. The application of medical knowledge to questions of law.

forensic mental health services *npl* describes those mental health services that are concerned with the relevant laws, e.g. current Mental Health Act, and are concerned with legal matters/problems. They include: hospitals/clinics providing secure environments; the mental health nurses designated to work closely with the criminal justice system, such as court diversion schemes for offenders with mental health problems and nurses working within Youth Offending Teams.

foreskin *n* the prepuce or skin covering the glans penis.

formaldehyde *n* toxic, pungent smelling gas, used as a disinfectant. Dissolved in water (formalin), it is used to preserve histological specimens and for disinfection.

format in computing the structure which determines the way in which data are stored in a file. A program able to recognize the structure is required to read or write files. — **formatting** preparing a new disk to store data in the manner required by the operating system of the computer. ⇒ operating system.

formication *n* a sensation as of ants running over the skin. Occurs in nerve lesions, particularly in the regenerative phase.

formula *n* a prescription. A series of symbols denoting the chemical composition of a substance, e.g. $NaHCO_3$ is the formula for sodium hydrogen carbonate (sodium bicarbonate) — **formulae, formulas** *pl*.

formulary *n* a collection of formulas. The *British National Formulary (BNF)* is a description of licensed pharmaceutical preparations, produced by the Joint Formulary Committee of the British Medical Association and the Royal Pharmaceutical Society. *nurse prescribers' formulary (NPF)* a limited formulary available to suitably qualified nurses who have completed an approved course and demonstrated prescribing competence. ⇒ nurse prescribing.

fornix *n* an arch, particularly referred to the vagina, i.e. the space between the vaginal wall and the cervix of the uterus — **fornices** *pl*.

fossa *n* a depression or furrow. *olecranon fossa* in the humerus it receives the ulnar process during elbow extension. *pituitary fossa* in the sphenoid bone it accommodates the pituitary gland, the sella turcica — **fossae** *pl*.

fostering *n* placing a child in the care of a compatible family as a short or long term measure. The aims are: (a) to provide a child in need of care with the security of a home environment; (b) to reunite child and natural family as soon as practical. Long-term fosterings can be 'with a view to adoption'.

Fothergill's operation ⇒ Manchester repair.

fourchette *n* a membranous fold connecting the posterior ends of the labia minora.

'fourth-day blues' ⇒ postpartum blues.

fovea *n* a small depression or fossa; particularly the fovea centralis retinae, the site containing many cones, it is important for distinct colour vision.

FQ *abbr* Fear Questionnaire.

fractionation *n* **1.** in radiotherapy, the division of the total dose of radiation prescribed into smaller portions to be given over a period of time to minimize tissue damage. **2.** in chemistry, the division of a substance into its constituent parts.

fracture *n* breach in continuity of a bone, usually as a result of injury. The type of break in the bone may be: oblique, due to indirect violence, when a force applied at some distance causes the bone to break at its weakest point; spiral, when a limb is violently rotated; or transverse, due to direct violence at the point of fracture. Fractures may be characterized by pain, swelling, deformity, loss of function, shortening and crepitus, and can be classified as: *closed (simple) fracture* with no wound communicating with the outside. *comminuted fracture* where the bone is broken into two or more fragments. *complicated fracture* where the fracture is associated with injury to another structure, such as nerve, artery or organ, e.g. bladder damage from fractured pelvis. *compression fracture* usually of lumbar or dorsal region due to hyperflexion of spine; the anterior vertebral bodies are crushed together. *depressed fracture* when the bone is driven inwards, causing pressure on underlying structures, e.g. skull fracture pressing on the brain. *greenstick (incomplete) fracture* where the bone is fractured half through on the convex side of the bend (as in a green twig); seen only in children. *impacted fracture* where one fragment is driven into the other. *open (compound) fracture* where the fracture communicates with the surface via a wound. *pathological*

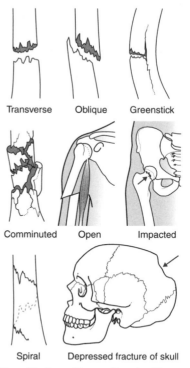

Transverse   Oblique   Greenstick

Comminuted   Open   Impacted

Spiral   Depressed fracture of skull

Figure 24   Types of fracture. (Reproduced from Brooker 1996 with permission.)

fracture associated with existing bone disease, e.g. metastatic malignancy. *spontaneous fracture* one occurring without appreciable violence; may be synonymous with pathological fracture. ⇒ Bennett's fracture. ⇒ Colles fracture. ⇒ supracondylar fracture. (See Figure 24).

fraenotomy *n* ⇒ frenotomy.

fragile-X syndrome *n* a genetic condition caused by a defective X chromosome. See Box – Fragile-X syndrome.

Fragile-X syndrome

This form of learning disability is mainly, but not exclusively, found in men. It was first identified in 1943 through studies of families in which a common, inherited set of clinical features including learning disabilities were found. The cause is a defect in the X chromosome, which is one of the sex chromosomes. In many cases the condition is passed from a carrier mother to an affected son. There is as yet no reliable antenatal test for this syndrome which research has shown to be present in 1 in every 2–4000 males. Physical features showing in around 80% of adult men who have the condition are enlarged testes and ears, a long and narrow face, and in a smaller percentage very smooth skin, flat feet and mitral valve prolapse. The physical features tend to come to prominence after puberty and learning disability is usually the most notable feature in childhood. It can range from borderline to severe. Because it is an inheritable disorder, genetic counselling for affected families is important.

fragilitas *n* brittleness. *fragilitas ossium* congenital abnormality with brittle bones, otosclerosis and blue sclerae. ⇒ osteogenesis imperfecta.

framboesia *n* ⇒ yaws.

FRC *abbr* functional residual capacity.

free-floating anxiety ⇒ anxiety.

free radical *n* activated oxygen species, such as the superoxide ion (O_2^-) and hydroxyl radical. They are extremely reactive chemicals (with unpaired electrons) produced as part of normal cell metabolism. They are normally dealt with by complex antioxidant enzyme defence mechanisms, but will cause oxidative damage to cells where defences are overwhelmed. → antioxidant.

Frei test an intradermal test for the diagnosis of lymphogranuloma venereum, using antigen from those infected and a control. A positive skin reaction to the killed antigen confirms diagnosis.

Freiberg's infarction an aseptic necrosis of bone tissue which most commonly occurs in the head of the second metatarsal bone.

Frenkel's exercises special repetitive exercises to improve muscle and joint sense.

frenotomy *n* surgical severance of a frenum, particularly for tongue-tie.

frenulum *n* a fold of membrane which checks or limits the movement of an organ. Also called frenum. *frenulum linguae* from the undersurface of the tongue to the floor of the mouth.

frenum → frenulum.

frequency *n* **1.** the need to pass urine more often than is acceptable to the patient, usually more often than was experienced in the past. The person passes small amounts of urine. It may be a sign of urinary tract infection. **2.** rate of vibration or cycles per second, such as sound waves, measured in hertz (Hz).

frequency distribution the number of times (frequency) each value in a variable is observed.

Freud, Sigmund Austrian psychiatrist/psychoanalyst (1856–1939) — **Freudian** *adj* pertaining to the work of Freud. Psychoanalysis and psychoanalytical theory of the causation of neuroses. ⇒ psychosexual development.

friable *adj* easily crumbled.

friction *n* rubbing. Can cause abrasion of skin, leading to a superficial pressure ulcer; the adhesive property of friction, increased in the presence of moisture, can contribute to a shearing force which can cause a more severe pressure ulcer. ⇒ frictions. *friction murmur* heard through the stethoscope when two rough or dry surfaces rub together, as in pleurisy and pericarditis.

frictions small, accurately localized, penetrating massage manipulations with the pads of the fingers and thumb in a circular direction on muscle and connective tissue, or transversely across tendons, to mobilize tissues, e.g. to maintain and restore mobility of tissues liable to develop adhesions after injury or strain.

Friedreich's ataxia a hereditary, degenerative disease of the spinocerebellar and pyramidal tracts and the posterior columns of the spinal cord, with onset in early childhood. Ataxia and muscular weakness occurs; the heart may also be affected. The disease progresses slowly, with patients becoming increasingly disabled and often using a wheelchair by early adult life.

frigidity *n* lack of normal sexual desire.

frog plaster conservative treatment of a developmental dysplasia of the hip (DDH) (congenital dislocation of the hip), whereby the dislocation is reduced by gentle manipulation and both hips are immobilised in plaster of Paris, the hips being abducted to 80 degrees and externally rotated.

Fröhlich's syndrome *n* adiposogenital dystrophy. A disorder with obesity, sexual infantilism, somnolence, disturbance of temperature regulation and diabetes insipidus due to damage of the pituitary and hypothalamus.

frontal *adj* **1.** pertaining to the front of a structure. **2.** the forehead bone. *frontal sinus* a cavity at the inner aspect of each orbital ridge on the frontal bone.

frostbite *n* injury to the skin or a body part from extreme cold. There is redness, swelling and pain. Necrosis and gangrene may occur. ⇒ trench foot.

frozen shoulder initial pain followed by stiffness in the shoulder, lasting several months. As pain subsides, exercises are intensified until full recovery is gained. Cause unknown.

fructose *n* (*syn* laevulose) fruit sugar, a monosaccharide found in some fruit and vegetables and in honey. It is intensely sweet and combines with glucose to form the disaccharide sucrose (cane or beet sugar). Fructose can be converted to glycogen in the body, without the presence of insulin.

FSF *abbr* fibrin stabilizing factor.

FSH *abbr* follicle stimulating hormone.

FTA-abs test *abbr* fluorescent treponemal antibody absorbed test.

fuel molecules glucose, fatty acids, gylcerol and amino acids oxidized in the body to release energy for cellular activities.

fugue *n* a state of altered awareness in which the person makes a journey and does certain actions of which they have no subsequent memory. The behaviour of the person involved may appear normal or unspectacular to the casual observer. May occur in some forms of epilepsy, hysteria or schizophrenia.

fulguration *n* destruction of tissue by diathermy.

full-term *adj* when pregnancy has lasted 40 weeks.

fulminant *adj* sudden, severe, rapid in course, such as fulminant glaucoma or fulminant hepatic failure.

fumigation *n* disinfection by exposure to the fumes of a vaporized disinfectant.

function *n* the special work performed by an organ or structure in its normal state.

functional *adj* **1.** in a general sense, pertaining to function. **2.** of a disorder, of the function but not the structure of an organ. **3.** as a psychiatric term, of neurotic origin, i.e. psychogenic, without primary organic disease.

functional assessment *n* usually includes ADL assessment, but may refer to specific aspects, such as range of movement, grip strength, balance and mobility.

functional endoscopic sinus surgery (FESS) *n* minimally invasive surgery performed on the sinuses via a fine nasal endoscope. It is possible to view the sinuses, improve drainage and remove abnormal tissue.

functional residual capacity (FRC) *n* volume of air in the lungs after normal expiration. ⇒ respiratory function tests.

functionalism a sociological perspective based on an idea that social sytems are analagous with organic systems where actions are interdependent. Social activity has consequences for other activities, social institutions and the smooth functioning of society.

fundoplication *n* surgical folding of the fundus of the stomach to prevent reflux of gastric contents into the oesophagus.

fundus *n* the enlarged portion of a hollow organ furthest away from the opening. *fundus of the eye* the back of the eye viewed through the pupil using an ophthalmoscope. *fundus of the stomach* at the top of the greater curvature. *fundus of the uterus* the top of the uterus — **fundal** *adj* *fundal height* palpation of the top of the uterus or measuring the distance from the symphysis pubis to the fundus to assess the period of gestation.

fungate very rapid growth of a fungus-like tumour, seen in the later stages of some cancers where it has involved the skin, e.g. breast.

fungating wound may occur when a cancer has involved the epithelium and has ulcerated through the skin. They are most commonly seen with breast cancer, melanoma, head and neck cancers and those affecting the cervix, vagina or vulva. They are characterized by pain, exudate, infection causing malodour, bleeding and considerable psychological distress. Management includes: local radiotherapy, specialist wound care and selection of appropriate dressings and topical antibiotics. ⇒ deodorant.

fungi *npl* simple plants. Mycophyta which include mushrooms, yeasts, moulds and rusts. Used in wine making, brewing, baking, pharmaceutical industry and as a food source. The fungi include many micro-organisms that cause superficial and systemic disease in humans, such as actinomycosis, aspergillosis, candidiasis and tinea — **fungal** *adj*.

fungicide *n* an agent which is lethal to fungi — **fungicidal** *adj*.

fungiform *adj* resembling a mushroom, like the fungiform papillae found chiefly in the dorsocentral area of the tongue.

fungistatic *adj* describes an agent which inhibits the growth of fungi.

funiculitis *n* inflammation of the spermatic cord.

funiculus *n* a cord-like structure.

funnel chest (*syn* pectus excavatum) a congenital deformity in which the sternum is depressed towards the spine.

furor *n* a sudden outburst of uncontrolled fury or rage, during which an irrational act of violence may be committed.

furuncle *n* ⇒ boil.

furunculus orientalis oriental sore.

furunuculosis *n* an affliction due to boils.

fusiform *adj* resembling a spindle.

FVC *abbr* forced vital capacity. ⇒ respiratory function tests.

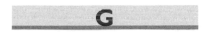

GABA *abbr* ⇒ gamma aminobutyric acid.

gag *n* 1. an instrument placed between the teeth to keep the mouth open. 2. reflex contraction of the pharyngeal muscles and elevation of the palate when the soft palate or posterior pharynx is touched.

gait *n* a manner or style of walking. *ataxic gait* an incoordinate or abnormal gait. *cerebellar gait* reeling, staggering, lurching. *scissors gait* one in which the legs cross each other in progressing. *spastic gait* stiff, shuffling, the legs being held together. *tabetic gait* the foot is raised high, then brought down suddenly, the whole foot striking the ground.

galactagogue *n* an agent inducing or increasing the flow of milk.

galactocele *n* a cyst containing milk, or fluid resembling milk.

galactorrhoea *n* excessive flow of milk. Usually reserved for abnormal or inappropriate secretion of milk.

galactosaemia *n* excess of galactose in the blood and other tissues. Normally the enzyme lactase in the small intestine converts lactose into glucose and galactose. In the liver another enzyme system converts galactose into glucose. Galactosaemia is inherited as an autosomal recessive disorder that results in enzyme deficiency in this system (two types). It is characterized by diarrhoea, failure to thrive, jaundice and cirrhosis, cataracts and learning disability. Early diagnosis is vital and management consists of excluding milk and foods containing lactose and galactose from the diet — **galactosaemic** *adj*.

galactose *n* a monosaccharide that combines with glucose to form the disaccharide lactose. Galactose can be converted to glycogen by the body.

gall *n* ⇒ bile.

gallbladder *n* a pear-shaped muscular bag on the undersurface of the liver. See Box – Gallbladder and bile ducts. → biliary. ⇒ cholecystokinin.

gallipot *n* a small vessel for lotions.

gallows traction ⇒ Bryant's traction.

gallstones *n* concretions (calculi) formed within the gallbladder or bile ducts; they are often multiple and faceted. Frequently associated with inflammation and infection; cholecystitis. The stones may consist of cholesterol, bile pigments or a mixture of these. The stone may move within the biliary ducts giving rise to severe pain or biliary colic, or become impacted in the common bile duct, causing obstruction to the flow of bile and jaundice.

Gallbladder and bile ducts

The gallbladder stores bile, which is manufactured in the liver, until it is due to be released into the small intestine. Bile, which is required for the emulsification of fats in food, is collected from the liver via the right and left hepatic ducts which unite as the common hepatic duct connecting in turn with the cystic duct which conducts bile into the gallbladder. When the gallbladder contracts, bile is expelled via the cystic duct and into the common bile duct which conveys the bile to the duodenum via the ampulla of Vater (hepatopancreatic ampulla). The smooth muscle of the gallbladder is innervated by the vagus nerve (Xth cranial nerve) which stimulates the contraction of the gallbladder. The gallbladder also constricts when it is stimulated by the hormones cholecystokinin and secretin which are released by the duodenum in the presence of food. Some individuals suffer from gallstones (biliary calculi) which may consist of crystals of cholesterol, bile pigments or a mixture of these, and this can be very painful if the gallstones prevent bile from leaving the gallbladder. When the gallbladder constricts and the pressure in the gallbladder increases the gallstones prevent the expulsion of bile by blocking the cystic duct.

galvanocauterization *n* ⇒ cauterize.

galvanometer *n* an instrument for measuring an electrical current.

Gamblers Anonymous an organization which exists to help compulsive gamblers to resist the compulsion.

gamete *n* a female or male reproductive cell having the haploid (n) number of chromosomes, an oocyte or spermatozoon. ⇒ gametogenesis. ⇒ ovum. ⇒ oocyte. ⇒ spermatozoon.

Gamete Intrafallopian Transfer (GIFT) an assisted fertility/conception technique. One patent uterine tube has to be identified. Oocytes and spermatozoa are mixed together and transferred to the uterine tube; fertilization takes place in vivo in the normal way. A simpler technique than IVF, but it still needs one functional uterine tube. It may be used to overcome hostile (to sperm) cervical mucus.

gametogenesis the formation of the gametes (oocytes and spermatozoa) in the ovary or testes. ⇒ oogenesis. ⇒ spermatogenesis.

gamma third letter of the Greek alphabet. *gamma aminobutyric acid (GABA)* an inhibitory neurotransmitter in the central nervous system and other locations. *gamma camera* equipment used in radionuclide imaging. After radioactive isotopes are introduced into the body the gamma camera detects the amount of radioactivity in a specific area. ⇒ nuclear medicine. ⇒ radionuclide imaging/ scanning. *gamma globulins* ⇒ globulins. ⇒ immunoglobulins. *gamma radiation* used in diagnosis, therapy and for the sterilization of disposable items, such as plastic syringes. *gamma rays* electromagnetic radiation of short wavelength emitted during the disintegration of the atomic nuclei of radioactive isotopes. ⇒ X-rays.

gamma-encephalography a small dose of radioactive isotope is given. It is concentrated in many cerebral tumours. The pattern of radioactivity is then measured.

gammaglobulinopathy *n* an abnormality of gamma globulin.

gamma-glutamyl transferase (gamma-GT) *n* an enzyme present in many body tissues. Increased plasma levels can indicate liver disease, but can be influenced by some drugs and alcohol.

ganglion *n* **1.** a collection of nerve cell bodies in the peripheral nervous system, such as those containing the cell bodies of the autonomic nervous system and the dorsal root ganglia which contain the cell bodies of sensory nerves — **ganglia** *pl.* **2.** localized synovial cyst-like swelling near a tendon, sheath or joint. Contains a clear, transparent, gelatinous or colloid substance; sometimes occurs on the back of the wrist due to strain such as excessive use of the piano or word processor — **ganglionic** *adj.*

ganglionectomy *n* surgical excision of a ganglion.

gangliosidosis ⇒ Tay-Sachs' disease.

gangrene *n* massive tissue necrosis (death) resulting from ischaemia, infection and occasionally due to direct injury (traumatic gangrene). It usually affects the extremities, but can occur in the gallbladder, bowel and appendix. Causes include: vessel disease, arterial embolus, frostbite, infection, external pressure, such as from a tourniquet, and trauma. Lower limb gangrene is a complication of diabetes mellitus and is also seen in heavy smokers. *dry gangrene* the arterial blood supply is gradually occluded, such as with arterial disease. The affected part is dry, cold and shrivelled. Infection and oedema are usually absent. Arteries are obstructed but veins are not. *gas gangrene* seen in contused wounds infected with anaerobes such as *Clostridium perfringens*. It is characterized by local swelling, discoloration, foul discharge, gas formation which crackles when the tissue is touched and severe systemic effects including circulatory collapse. *moist/wet gangrene* seen in a limb or the bowel when the arterial supply is suddenly occluded, often with impaired venous return. Infection and oedema usually present — **gangrenous** *adj.*

gangrenous stomatitis ⇒ cancrum oris.

Ganser syndrome a condition characterized by inappropriate actions, absurd answers to questions, hallucinations, disturbances of consciousness, and amnesia. Also known as 'prison psychosis' or 'hallucinatory mania'.

gap junction *n* a type of junction between cells, formed from an adaptation of the plasma membrane. It contains minute gaps that allow the movement of small water-soluble molecules, such as cells, between cells. It also permits the movement of ions between excitable cells, such as heart muscle, to allow the smooth passage of electrical impulses during contraction. ⇒ desmosome. ⇒ tight junction.

Gardnerella vaginalis *n* bacterium responsible for bacterial vaginosis. There is a grey frothy vaginal discharge and a 'fishy' odour. Its presence has been linked to late miscarriage or preterm delivery. Treatment is with metronidazole or clindamycin.

gargoylism *n* (*syn* Hunter-Hurler syndrome) congenital disorder of mucopolysaccharide metabolism with recessive or sex-linked inheritance. The polysaccharides chondroitin sulphate 'B' and heparitin sulphate are excreted in the urine. Characterized by skeletal abnormalities, coarse features, enlarged liver and spleen, learning disability. ⇒ Hunter's syndrome. ⇒ Hurler's syndrome. ⇒ mucopolysaccharidoses.

Gartner's bacillus *Salmonella enteritidis.*

gas *n* one of the three states of matter, the others being solid and liquid. A gas retains neither shape nor volume when released. *gas embolus* ⇒ caisson disease. → embolism. *gas gangrene* a wound infection caused by anaerobic microorganisms of the genus clostridium, especially *Clostridium perfringens*, a soil microbe often harboured in the intestine of humans and animals; consequently there are many sources from which infection can arise. → gangrene. *gas laws* → Boyle's law. ⇒ Charles' law. → Dalton's law. ⇒ Henry's law — **gaseous** *adj.*

GAS *abbr* general adaptation syndrome.

gastralgia *n* pain in the stomach.

gastrectomy *n* removal of a part or the whole of the stomach. Used mainly to remove cancers, but may be used for gastric ulcers that are resistant to drug therapy and rarely to manage uncontrolled haemorrhage. There are various complications following gastrectomy including: recurrent ulcer, small stomach syndrome, vomiting, dumping syndrome, diarrhoea, hypoglycaemia and anaemia due to poor iron absorption and lack of intrinsic factor required for vitamin B_{12} absorption. *Billroth I gastrectomy* is a partial gastrectomy where the remaining part of the stomach is joined to the duodenum. *Billroth II*

or *Polya's gastrectomy* part of the stomach and duodenum are removed, the gastric remnant is joined to the jejunum. *total gastrectomy* is carried out for cancers at the upper end of the stomach. ⇒ Roux-en-Y operation. ⇒ vagotomy.

gastric *adj* pertaining to the stomach. *gastric aspiration or suction* the removal of stomach contents via a nasogastric tube; may be used to obtain samples for analysis, where the bowel is obstructed or following gastrointestinal surgery. It may be continuous or intermittent. *gastric influenza* a term used when gastrointestinal symptoms predominate. *gastric juice* fluid produced by the stomach; contains hydrochloric acid, enzymes, mucus and the instrinsic factor is acid in reaction and contains two proteolytic enzymes. *gastric ulcer* an ulcer in the gastric mucosa. The aetiology includes a genetic predisposition and the majority are associated with the presence of the bacterium *Helicobacter pylori* in the stomach. Other factors may include slow gastric emptying and the reflux of bile into the stomach. Characteristically there is pain shortly after eating food which may be so severe that the person fails to eat adequately and loses weight. The ulcer can bleed, leading to haematemesis and/or melaena, or it can perforate, constituting an abdominal emergency. Severe scarring following chronic ulceration may produce pyloric stenosis and gastric outlet obstruction. Management includes: (a) general measures; smoking cessation, avoiding foods that cause pain, avoiding aspirin and NSAIDs; (b) drugs to irradicate *H. pylori*; specific anti-ulcer drugs, including H_2 receptor antagonists, e.g. ranitidine and the proton pump inhibitor, omeprazole and antacids based on calcium, magnesium or aluminium salts; (c) surgical treatment may be required where medical treatment fails, in an emergency, such as haemorrhage or perforation, or to improve gastric drainage. ⇒ gastrectomy.

gastric inhibitory peptide (GIP) *n* a regulatory peptide hormone secreted by the duodenal mucosa. It inhibits gastric secretion and stimulates insulin secretion by the pancreas. ⇒ enterogastric reflex.

gastrin *n* a hormone secreted by the hormone-secreting cells of the gastric mucosa on entry of food, which causes a further gastric secretion.

gastritis *n* inflammation of the stomach, especially the mucous membrane lining.

gastrocnemius *n* the large two-headed muscle of the calf.

gastrocolic *adj* pertaining to the stomach and the colon. *gastrocolic reflex* sensory stimulus arising on entry of food into stomach, resulting in strong peristaltic waves in the colon.

gastroduodenal *adj* pertaining to the stomach and the duodenum.

gastroduodenostomy a surgical anastomosis between the stomach and the duodenum.

gastrodynia *n* pain in the stomach.

gastroenteritis *n* food poisoning. Inflammation of mucous membranes of the stomach and the small intestine; mostly caused by micro-organisms, but may be due to chemicals, poisonous fungi etc. The signs and symptoms of diarrhoea and vomiting may be due to either the multiplication of micro-organisms (invasive intestinal gastroenteritis) ingested in food or from bacterial toxins (intoxication). The causative organism may be bacterial, e.g. *Campylobacter jejuni*, *Salmonella enteritidis*, *Bacillus cereus*, *Escherichia coli*, *Staphylococcus aureus*, *Clostridium perfringens* and *Clostridium botulinum*, or viral, e.g. Norwalk virus, rotovirus. Gastroenteritis is generally spread by faecal-oral route, either directly or indirectly, but some viruses are spread via droplets.

gastroenterology *n* study of the digestive tract, including the liver, biliary tract and pancreas and the accompanying diseases — **gastroenterologically** *adv*.

gastroenteropathy *n* disease of the stomach and intestine — **gastroenteropathic** *adj*.

gastroenteroscope *n* an endoscope for visualization of stomach and intestine — **gastroenteroscopically** *adv*.

gastroenterostomy *n* a surgical anastomosis between the stomach and small intestine.

gastrointestinal *adj* pertaining to the stomach and intestine. *gastrointestinal tract* ⇒ alimentary canal/tract.

gastrojejunostomy *n* a surgical anastomosis between the stomach and the jejunum.

gastro-oesophageal *adj* pertaining to the stomach and oesophagus. *gastro-oesophageal reflux* reflux of gastric acid contents into the oesophagus. See Box – Gastro-oesophageal reflux. *gastro-oesophageal sphincter* physiological sphincter between the oesophagus and the stomach (also known as cardiac sphincter).

gastro-oesophagostomy *n* a surgical operation in which the oesophagus is joined to the stomach to bypass the natural junction.

gastropathy *n* any disease of the stomach.

gastropexy *n* surgical fixation of a displaced stomach.

gastrophrenic *adj* pertaining to the stomach and diaphragm.

Gastro-oesophageal reflux

Gastro-oesophageal reflux (GOR) consists of an incompetent/malfunctioning lower oesophageal sphincter which allows the stomach contents to move into the oesophagus on inspiration. This results in vomiting, oesophagitis, scarring and stricture. There is also the danger of aspiration pneumonia. The exact cause is unknown but predisposing factors include: gastric distension, increased abdominal pressure caused by coughing, central nervous system disease, delayed gastric emptying, hiatus hernia and gastrostomy placement. Approximately 1 in 500 children have significant problems and those who have undergone oesophageal repairs or with neurological disorders, scoliosis, asthma or cystic fibrosis are especially at risk.

Management may be conservative with small frequent thickened feeds and a head elevated position after feeding and at night. H_2-receptor antagonists such as cimetidine, or ranitidine help to prevent oesophagitis. In some countries cisapride is used to promote gastric emptying. Surgical management, which consists of a 360° wrap of the fundus of the stomach around the distal oesophagus (Nissen fundoplication), is usually performed on those children with complications or for whom medical treatment has failed.

Further reading
Wong D 1999 Whaley & Wong's Nursing care of infants and children. 6th Edn. St Louis: Mosby.

gastroplasty *n* any plastic operation on the stomach. Currently used for reconstruction of the cardiac orifice of the stomach, where fibrosis prevents replacement of the stomach below the diaphragm in cases of hiatus hernia.

gastroptosis *n* downward displacement of the stomach.

gastroschisis *n* a congenital incomplete closure of the abdominal wall to the right of a normal umbilical cord, with consequent protrusion of the viscera uncovered by peritoneum.

gastroscope *n* ⇒ endoscope — **gastroscopy** *n*.

gastrostomy *n* a surgically established fistula between the stomach and the exterior abdominal wall; usually for long-term enteral feeding. (See Figure 25). ⇒ percutaneous endoscopic gastrostomy.

gastrotomy *n* incision into the stomach during an abdominal operation, for such purposes as removing a foreign body, securing a bleeding blood vessel, approaching the oesophagus from below

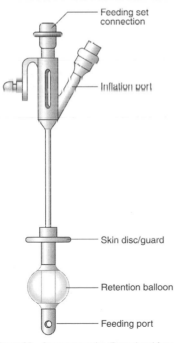

Figure 25   Gastrostomy tube. (Reproduced from Nicol et al 2000 with permission.)

to pull down a tube through a constricting growth.

gastrula *n* the next stage after blastocyst in early embryonic development. ⇒ gastrulation.

gastrulation *n* the process of massive change as the blastocyst becomes the gastrula. The three primary germ layers (ectoderm, endoderm and mesoderm) are formed and cells migrate to their correct positions in readiness for the start of structural development.

gate control theory a theory that seeks to explain how the transmission of pain impulses is modulated by 'gates' operating in the spinal cord.

Gaucher's disease very rare inherited disorder of fat metabolism, caused by the lack of an enzyme. Results in hepatosplenomegaly, enlarged lymph nodes and bone marrow malfunction. Diagnosis is confirmed by biopsy of the spleen, liver, or bone marrow.

gauze *n* a thin open-meshed absorbent material used in operations to dry the operative field and facilitate the procedure.

Gay-Lussac's law → Charles' law.

GCS *abbr* Glasgow coma scale.

Geiger counter a device for detecting and registering radioactivity.

gelatin(e) *n* the protein-containing, glue-like substance found in animal connective tissue, used in capsules, suppositories, culture medium and in food preparation. Vegans and some vegetarians may find medicines containing gelatin unacceptable — **gelatinous** *adj*.

gender different from biological sex. The term includes the concept of socially constructed views of feminine and masculine behaviour within individual cultural groups.

gene *n* hereditary factor located at a specific place (locus) of a specific chromosome; consisting of DNA. Genes are responsible for determining specific characteristics or traits and the precise replication of proteins. According to how they influence these characteristics, different forms of genes (alleles) may act as dominant (i.e. they manifest their presence in single doses of such alleles as are required). ⇒ dominant. ⇒ Mendel's law. ⇒ recessive.

general adaptation syndrome (GAS) *n* a triphasic response to a stressor: alarm, resistance/adaptation and exhaustion.

general anaesthetic ⇒ anaesthesia.

General Health Questionnaire (GHQ) an assessment that is used to measure neurotic symptoms. To ensure that it is not used inappropriately, it is not in the public domain.

General Medical Services the services provided by family doctors.

general practitioner a doctor who, as part of the primary healthcare team, provides personal, primary and continuing medical care, including prevention, which is accessible to individuals and families irrespective of age, sex and illness, and which is easily available at times of need. He or she will make initial decisions, give continuing medical care and refer patients for specialist advice and treatment.

general sales list in the UK. Drugs on sale to the public through a variety of retail outlets, e.g. mild analgesics. There are controls in place regarding the number of tablets that may be purchased, e.g. packs containing greater quantities may be sold by a pharmacy.

generative *adj* pertaining to reproduction.

genetic *adj* that which pertains to heredity, e.g. the inherited characteristics or disorders, the basis of which resides in abnormalities of the genetic material, genes and chromosomes. ⇒ congenital. *genetic counselling* specialized service available to people who have a history of genetic disease, where the risk of problems or of producing affected children can be assessed and discussed.

genetic code *n* the information carried on the DNA molecules of the chromosome. It is in this coded form that the information contained in the genes is transmitted to the cells to determine their activity through the precise replication of proteins.

genetic imprinting a form of inheritance caused by structural alterations to chromosomes during gametogenesis which may affect the way a particular allele is expressed. The effects depend on whether the chromosome is paternal or maternal. It results in two distinct conditions which arise from the same mutation, e.g. chromosome 15 change results in Prader-Willi syndrome if inherited via paternal chromosomes and Angleman syndrome when the chromosome is maternal.

genetically modified food *n* a particular food, such as soya beans, maize or tomatoes, containing genetic material from other organisms. The new material imparts a particular quality to the modified food, e.g. disease resistance or improved keeping properties.

genetics *n* the science of heredity and variation, namely the study of the genetic material, its transmission (from cell to cell and generation to generation) and its changes (mutations). *biochemical genetics* the science concerned with the chemical and physical nature of genes, and with the mechanism by which they control the development and maintenance of the organism. *clinical genetics* the study of the possible genetic factors influencing the occurrence of a pathological condition. ⇒ immunogenesis.

geniculate ganglion *n* ganglion of the facial nerve (VIIth cranial nerve).

genital *adj* pertaining to the generative or reproductive structure. *genital herpes* ⇒ herpes.

genital stage the final stage of psychosexual development, commencing during puberty and resulting in adult sexuality.

genital warts small raised lesions occurring on the skin or mucosa of the genitalia and perianal area. They are caused by the human papilloma virus.

genitalia *n* the generative structures. Divided into the external or internal genitalia.

genitocrural *adj* pertaining to the genital area and the leg.

genitourinary *adj* pertaining to the reproductive and urinary organs. *genitourinary medicine (GUM)* branch of medicine dealing with sexually transmitted infections in specialist GUM clinics within district general hospitals.

genome *n* the basic set of chromosomes, with the genes contained therein, equivalent to the sum total of gene types possessed by different organisms of a species.

genotype *n* the total genetic information encoded in the chromosomes of an individual. Also, the genetic constitution of an individual at a particular locus, namely the alleles present at that locus.

gentian violet ⇒ crystal violet.

genu *n* the knee.

genu valgum (knock knee) abnormal incurving of the legs so that there is a gap between the feet when the knees are in contact.

genu varum (bow legs) abnormal outward curving of the legs, resulting in separation of the knees.

genupectoral position the knee-chest position, i.e. the weight is taken by the knees, and by the upper chest, while the shoulder girdle and head are supported on a pillow in front.

genus *n* a classification ranking between the family (higher) and the species (lower).

geophagia *n* the habit of eating clay or earth.

geriatrician *n* one who specializes in old age and its diseases.

geriatrics *n* the branch of medical science dealing with old age and its diseases, together with the medical care. The nursing care of older people is the term now preferred in nursing. ⇒ ageism.

germ *n* lay term for a unicellular microorganism, especially used for a pathogen.

germ cell ⇒ gamete.

German measles ⇒ rubella.

germicide *n* an agent which kills germs — **germicidal** *adj*.

gerontology *n* the scientific study of ageing. See Box – Gerontology — **gerontological** *adj*

Gestalt theory Gestalt is a German word meaning 'organized whole'. A theory of behaviour developed in the first part of the twentieth century. It contends that perception and learning are active, creative processes that are part of an 'organized whole'.

gestation *n* pregnancy. *gestation sac* the contents of a pregnant uterus: embryo, membranes and decidua etc — **gestational** *adj*.

GFR *abbr* glomerular filtration rate. ⇒ glomerulus.

GH *abbr* growth hormone.

GHIH *abbr* growth hormone inhibiting hormone.

Ghon focus ⇒ primary complex.

GHQ *abbr* General Health Questionnaire.

GHRH *abbr* growth hormone releasing hormone.

giardiasis *n* (*syn* lambliasis) infection with the flagellate (protozoon) *Giardia intestinalis*. Often asymptomatic, especially in adults. Can cause diarrhoea and malabsorption with steatorrhoea. Treatment is tinidazole or metronidazole orally.

GIFT *acr* ⇒ Gamete Intrafallopian Transfer.

gigantism *n* an abnormal condition characterized by excessive growth and height due to excessive secretion of growth hormone (GH) prior to the ossification of the epiphyses. ⇒ acromegaly.

Gillick Competence see Box – Gillick Competence.

gingiva *n* the gum; the vascular tissue surrounding the necks of the erupted teeth — **gingival** *adj* pertaining to the gum. *gingival hypertrophy* overgrowth of the gum associated with certain antiseizure medication, e.g. phenytoin. *gingival sulcus* the invagination made by the gingiva as it joins with the tooth surface.

Gerontology

Gerontology is the study of ageing incorporating biology, psychology, sociology, economics, geography and other disciplines. At the turn of the last century the discipline of modern gerontology began with investigations into the process of biological ageing. There are a range of theories from the evolutionary and genetic, through cellular theories to physiological theories. Whatever the reason one of the major aspects of biological ageing is a decreased ability for homeostasis as we age and, thereby, a decreased ability to withstand physiological stresses such as those which accompany illness.

Psychologically, there are several theories which revolve around whether or not we gradually disengage from social activities as we age or whether we compensate for the loss of some activities, such as employment, with other activities. It is commonly misconceived that older people have poor memories and become less intelligent with age. Some aspects of intelligence and memory do alter with age but the net effect is negligible in the absence of disease. The remaining aspects of gerontology are more concerned with the consequences of ageing in terms of the place of older people in society and their effect on the economy than they are with the causes of ageing.

Gillick competence

In Gillick v West Norfolk and Wisbech Area Health Authority (1985) 3 All ER 402 the House of Lords ruled that children under 16 can give legally effective consent to medical treatment providing they can demonstrate that they have the "*sufficient maturity and intelligence to understand the proposed treatment*". Parental power is transferred to competent children not shared with them. The Children Act (1989) supports this by stating that adults "*should have regard in particu-lar to the ascertainable wishes and feelings of the child concerned*". The Gillick ruling has enabled children to have the right to be consulted about decisions which affect them: medical treatment, residence, contact with parents, their education, religion and welfare.... "*if the child is of sufficient understanding to make an informed decision*".

Further reading
Moules C, Ramsay J 1998 The textbook of children's nursing Module 8: Legal and ethical issues. London: Stanley Thornes.

---

gingivectomy *n* excision of a portion of the gum, usually for pyorrhoea.

gingivitis *n* inflammation of the gum or gingiva usually caused by irritation from dental plaque and calculus. May be associated with pregnancy, due to hormone changes.

girdle *n* usually a bony structure of oval shape such as the shoulder and pelvic girdles.

gland *n* an organ or structure composed of specialized cells capable of producing substances that are secreted or excreted via ducts or directly into the blood or lymph. ⇒ endocrine. ⇒ exocrine — **glandular** *adj.*

glanders *n* a contagious, febrile, ulcerative disease communicable from horses, mules and asses to man.

glandular fever ⇒ infectious mononucleosis.

glans *n* the bulbous termination of the clitoris and penis.

Glasgow coma scale (GCS) a standardized tool for evaluating responsiveness. It assesses eye opening according to four criteria, motor response using six criteria, and verbal response against five criteria. The lower the score the more 'serious' the patient's condition, i.e less responsive.

glaucoma *n* a condition where intraocular pressure is raised due to an obstruction to the outflow of aqueous humor or extra fluid. It may be primary or secondary to eye disease or trauma. Glaucoma may be acute (closed or narrow-angle) and the more common chronic (open or wide-angle) type. Regular screening of intraocular pressure is recommended for people over 40 years old (25 or over in Afro-Caribbean individuals) and where close relatives have glaucoma. ⇒ tonography. ⇒ tonometer. The presentation varies according to type and includes: eye pain which can be severe, red eye, blurred vision, loss of visual field, visual disturbances such as halos around lights, nausea and vomiting and eventual blindness if the optic nerve is damaged. Untreated acute glaucoma can lead to blindness in a matter of days. In some chronic cases the onset may be insidious with gradual loss of peripheral vision. The management again depends on type and severity and may be: (a) medical – with miotic eye drops, e.g. pilocarpine, which constricts the pupil and improves drainage, or eye drops that reduce aqueous humor production, e.g timolol a beta (β)-adrenoceptor anatagonist. Systemic mannitol or acetazolamide may be used in acute situations to reduce pressure; (b) surgery or laser treatment to improve drainage. ⇒ cyclodialysis. ⇒ cyclodiathermy. ⇒ goniotomy. ⇒ iridectomy. ⇒ trabeculotomy — **glaucomatous** *adj.*

glenohumeral *adj* pertaining to the glenoid cavity of scapula and the humerus.

glenoid *adj* a cavity on the scapula in which the head of the humerus articulates to form the shoulder joint.

glia *n* ⇒ neuroglia — **glial** *adj.*

glioblastoma multiforme a highly malignant brain tumour.

glioma *n* a malignant growth occurring in the brain which does not give rise to secondary deposits. It arises from neuroglia. One form, occurring in the retina, is sometimes inherited. ⇒ astrocytoma. ⇒ retinoblastoma — **gliomata** *pl.*

gliomyoma *n* a tumour of nerve and muscle tissue — **gliomyomata** *pl.*

globin *n* a protein which combines with haem to form haemoglobin.

globulins *npl* a group of proteins widely distributed in the body. Those in the plasma are classified as alpha, beta and gamma; their functions include transport of substances (alpha and beta) and protection against infection (gamma). The gammaglobulins are the immunoglobulins A, D, E, G and M. ⇒ antibodies. ⇒ immunoglobulins.

globus hystericus a subjective feeling of neurotic origin of a lump in the throat. Can also include difficulty in swallowing due to tension of muscles of deglutition. May accompany acute anxiety and emotional conflict. Sometimes follows slight trauma to throat, e.g. scratch by foreign body.

globus pallidus literally pale globe; a mass of motor nerve cell bodies (grey matter) situated deep within the cerebral hemispheres, forming part of the basal nuclei. Situated close to the internal capsule and the thalamus.

glomerulitis *n* inflammation of the glomeruli, usually of the kidney.

glomerulonephritis *n* describes a group of conditions characterized by inflammation of the renal glomeruli with the presence of antibodies and immune complexes; it may be acute or chronic. The diagnosis and classification has been greatly enhanced by techniques such as percutaneous kidney biopsy, electron microscopy and advances in immunohistological methods. May be idiopathic but many cases are associated with polyarteritis, Henoch-Schonlein purpura, certain drugs, e.g. gold salts, infections, cancers and systemic lupus erythematosus. Proteinuria and microscopic haematuria, hypertension and impaired renal function are features. Progression to chronic renal disease and eventual failure may occur. ⇒ Goodpastures syndrome. ⇒ nephrotic syndrome.

glomerulosclerosis *n* describes a condition where the glomeruli of the kidney are partially or completely replaced by hyaline material. The aetiology may be unknown, or it may occur with ischaemia or follow inflammation, such as acute glomerulonephritis. Patients may present with the nephrotic syndrome or later with hypertension, haematuria and declining renal function. Diabetic patients may have microalbuminuria during the early stages which can be reversed with good blood glucose control. ⇒ Kimmelsteil-Wilson syndrome — **glomerulosclerotic** *adj.*

glomerulus *n* a coil of capillaries formed from a wide-bore afferent arteriole which lies within the invaginated blind end of the renal tubule. The glomerulus forms part of the filtration membrane involved in filtration; the first process of urine production. The glomerulus and renal tubule form the nephron. ⇒ nephron — **glomeruli** *pl* — **glomerular** *adj* pertaining to the glomerulus. *glomerular filtration rate* the rate of filtration from blood in the capillaries of the glomerulus to the fluid in Bowman's capsule. A process driven by the hydrostatic pressure within the glomerulus. It is usually 120 mL per min and is an accurate index of renal function. ⇒ Bowman's capsule. ⇒ filtration. ⇒ hydrostatic.

glomus *n* vascular tumour in middle ear.

glossa *n* the tongue — **glossal** *adj.*

glossectomy *n* excision of the tongue.

glossitis *n* inflammation of the tongue.

glossodynia *n* a name used for a painful tongue when there is no visible change.

glossopharyngeal *adj* pertaining to the tongue and pharynx. The ninth pair of the 12 pairs of cranial nerves arising directly from the brain. They innervate the tongue and pharynx and are concerned with taste, salivation, swallowing and the gag reflex.

glossoplegia *n* paralysis of the tongue.

glottis *n* the space between the vocal folds of the larynx, when they are abducted. Allows air to enter the trachea and is concerned with sound production — **glottic** *adj.*

glucagon *n* hormone produced in alpha cells of pancreatic islets of Langerhans. It raises blood glucose levels by stimulating the release of glucose from the breakdown of liver glycogen. Given by injection to treat hypoglycaemia. ⇒ insulin.

glucocorticoid *n* any of a large group of steroid hormones that promote gluconeogenesis, glycogenesis and protein and fat breakdown. They are hyperglycaemic hormones. They are essential to life and provide longer term resistance to stressors. Occurring naturally in the adrenal cortex as cortisone and hydrocortisone, and produced synthetically as, e.g. prednisone and prednisolone.

glucogenesis *n* synthesis of glucose.

glucometer *n* an electronic meter used by people with diabetes to carry out home blood glucose monitoring (HBGM). There is a variety of makes available.

gluconeogenesis *n* the formation of glucose from noncarbohydrate sources, e.g. amino acids, lactate and glycerol. It takes place in the liver and to a limited extent in the kidney.

glucose *n* dextrose or grape sugar. A monosaccharide. It is present in some foods (fruit juices), but most is produced by the digestion of complex dietary carbohydrates. A constituent of the disaccharides: sucrose, maltose and lactose. It is the main metabolic fuel molecule for cell use. Amounts in excess of immediate requirements are stored as glycogen in the liver and skeletal muscle, or converted to fat. ⇒ blood sugar.

glucose-6-phosphate dehydrogenase (G6PD) *n* an enzyme of the metabolic pathway through which red cells obtain most of their energy. Deficiencies occurring in the red blood cell may be inherited. It affects Africans, and their descendants elsewhere, people living around the Mediterranean and in the Middle East. People lacking G6PD develop haemolytic anaemia when exposed to certain foods or drugs, such as antimalarial agents. ⇒ anaemia. ⇒ favism.

glucose tolerance test *n* after a period of fasting, a measured quantity of glucose is taken orally; thereafter blood and urine samples are tested for glucose at intervals. Higher than normal levels are indicative of diabetes mellitus. (See Figure 26).

glucuronic acid a carbohydrate derivative used in the liver for the conjugation of bile pigments. One of the main conjugating agents required for the metabolism of foreign compounds.

glue ear an accumulation of thick mucoid fluid behind the tympanic membrane in the middle ear. It impairs hearing. ⇒ grommet. ⇒ otitis media.

glue sniffing ⇒ solvent abuse.

glutamic oxaloacetic transaminase *n* ⇒ aminotransferases. ⇒ AST.

glutamic pyruvic transaminase ⇒ aminotransferases. ⇒ ALT.

glutaraldehyde a chemical used to decontaminate and disinfect delicate equipment such as endoscopes. It is effective against viruses, bacterial spores and acid fast bacilli, but exposure of three hours or more is needed for sterilization. It is highly toxic and must be used according to Control of Substances Hazardous to Health (COSHH) regulations, e.g. use of protective clothing and proper ventilation/extraction system. Where possible, substitute disinfectants should be used.

glutathione *n* a tripeptide required for red blood cell integrity and for conjugation in the liver. Liver stores are seriously depleted by paracetamol overdose.

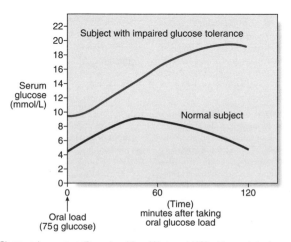

Figure 26 Glucose tolerance test. (Reproduced from Westwood 1999 with permission.)

gluteal *adj* pertaining to the buttocks.

gluten *n* a protein (formed from the proteins gliadin and glutenin) constituent of certain cereals: wheat, barley, rye and oats. It is a vital constituent of flours used to make well risen bread of good quality. ⇒ coeliac disease.

gluten-induced enteropathy ⇒ coeliac disease.

gluteus muscles three large muscles of the buttock – gluteus maximus, medius and minimus.

glycaemic index *n* a classification of foods according to their acute effect on blood sugar level. Foods such as simple sugars have a high glycaemic index as they cause an immediate rise in blood sugar. However, low glycaemic index foods such as complex carbohydrates (high in soluble fibre), e.g. wholegrain cereals, pasta and legumes, are absorbed more slowly and evenly, which avoids sudden swings in blood sugar.

glycerin *n* a clear, syrupy liquid used as an emollient and in suppositories and mouthwashes. It has a hygroscopic action. *glycerin suppository* a suppository incorporating glycerin, which, by its hygroscopic action, attracts fluid to soften hardened faeces in the rectum. The effectiveness of subsequent bowel evacuation is dependent on how long it has been retained.

glycerol *n* a sugar-alcohol that combines with fatty acids to form triacylglycerols (triglycerides) and phospholipids.

glycine *n* a nonessential (dispensable) amino acid.

glycogen *n* the main carbohydrate storage compound in animals. Glucose molecules are linked in branched chains to form a polysaccharide in a process called glyco genesis. The liver and skeletal muscle are the main sites of production. The conversion of liver glycogen back to glucose is known as glycogenolysis. *glycogen storage disease* a metabolic recessive inherited condition caused by various enzyme deficiencies, leading to the accumulation of glycogen in organs and tissues, such as the liver. Hypoglycaemia is a major problem. The body tends to metabolize fat rather than glucose, and ketosis and acidosis are prevalent.

glycogenesis *n* formation of glycogen from blood glucose (in excess of immediate requirements). It is stimulated by insulin. ⇒ glycogenolysis *ant*.

glycogenolysis *n* hydrolysis of glycogen stores to glucose within the liver. A process stimulated by glucagon and adrenaline (epinephrine). ⇒ glycogenesis *ant*.

glycogenosis *n* ⇒ glycogen storage disease.

glycolysis *n* a metabolic pathway consisting of a series of reversible reactions where glucose is broken down to form pyruvic acid and a small amount of energy (ATP) — **glycolytic** *adj*.

glycopeptide antibiotics *npl* a group of antibiotics that includes vancomycin that is mainly used for pseudomembranous colitis and in the treatment of MRSA, and teicoplanin which has similar actions but can only be given parenterally. ⇒ vancomycin resistant enterococci.

glycoprotein *n* a protein combined with a carbohydrate, such as collagen.

glycosides *npl* complex substance containing a sugar found in some plants. Many contain pharmacologically active substances, such as digitalis from foxgloves. *cardiac glycosides* digoxin is an example of a glycoside. It increases myocardial contractility and is described as being a positive inotrope. Digoxin slows heart rate by increasing vagal activity and by partially blocking impulse conduction; it inhibits the sodium-potassium pump, causing calcium to accumulate in the myocardial fibres, which increases contractility and improves cardiac output. It is used in heart failure with atrial fibrillation and other atrial arrhythmias. Although digoxin is a very useful therapeutic agent it does have serious side-effects, such as nausea and vomiting, heart block and other serious arrhythmias such as ventricular tachycardia, and, because it has a long half life, it can accumulate in the body. As it may cause bradycardia, the apex beat/radial pulse should be determined prior to administration. Should the apical rate fall below 60 beats/min the dose is withheld and medical advice is sought.

glycosuria *n* the presence of glucose in the urine. In some individuals, it follows a meal high in carbohydrate, but may indicate a low renal threshold for glucose or diabetes mellitus.

glycosylated haemoglobin (HbA$_1$) n haemoglobin plus glucose. The amount reflects blood sugar levels over a period of some months and can be used to assess the degree of control in diabetes mellitus.

GM *abbr* genetically modified.

GMS *abbr* General Medical Services.

gnathalgia n pain in the jaw.

gnathoplasty n plastic surgery of the jaw.

goal n a goal is set for each actual problem experienced by a patient/client which is amenable to nurse-initiated intervention. For each identified potential problem, the goal of the nurse-initiated intervention will be preventing it from becoming an actual problem. Goals may be short, medium or long-term.

goal setting an essential part of the process of nursing, which occurs after identification of the patient's actual and potential problems that are amenable to nurse-initiated intervention. Whenever possible, the patient/client and/or family participate in goal setting. ⇒ empowerment.

goals, patient the desired outcomes of care, planned by the nurse, with the patient and/or family where possible, as part of the nursing process. They form the basis for the later evaluating of care.

goblet cells special mucus secreting cells, shaped like a goblet, found in the mucous membranes of the respiratory and gastrointestinal tracts.

goitre n an enlargement of the thyroid gland. In *simple goitre* the patient does not show any signs of excessive thyroid activity. May occur during puberty and pregnancy. It is also associated with a deficiency of iodine in the diet, and in regions where it occurs frequently it is termed *endemic goitre.* ⇒ Derbyshire neck. In *toxic goitre* the enlarged gland secretes an excessive amount of thyroid hormone. The patient is nervous, loses weight and often has palpitations and exophthalmos. ⇒ colloid. ⇒ hyperthyroidism. Enlargement of the thyroid gland may also be caused by cysts, benign and malignant growths, infections and autoimmune disorders. ⇒ Hashimoto's disease.

goitrogens *npl* agents causing goitre. Some occur in plants, e.g. turnip, cabbage, brussels sprouts and peanuts.

gold (Au) n metallic element used in the treatment of rheumatoid arthritis. The radioactive isotope gold-198 (^{198}Au) is used in the treatment of some malignant conditions.

Goldthwait belt wide belt with steel support for back injuries.

Golgi apparatus n a subcellular organelle consisting mainly of membranous sacs. Involved in the synthesis of glycoproteins and lipoproteins. They are larger and more extensive in secretory cells.

gomphosis n a type of fibrous joint. There is very slight movement, such as the teeth in their sockets.

gonad n the primary reproductive structure; the female (ovary) or male (testis) sex gland. ⇒ ovary. ⇒ testis — **gonadal** *adj.*

gonadotrophic *adj* having an affinity for, or influence on, the gonads.

gonadotrophin n any gonad-stimulating hormone. ⇒ follicle stimulating hormone. ⇒ human chorionic gonadotrophin. ⇒ luteinizing hormone.

gonioscope n an instrument (ophthalmoscope) used to examine and measure the angle of the anterior chamber of the eye.

gonioscopy n measuring angle of anterior chamber of eye with a gonioscope.

goniotomy n operation for glaucoma. Incision through the anterior chamber angle to the canal of Schlemm, typically used in treating congenital glaucoma.

gonococcal complement fixation test a specific serological test for the diagnosis of gonorrhoea. ⇒ VDRL test.

Gonococcus n a Gram-negative diplococcus (*Neisseria gonorrhoea*), the causative organism of gonorrhoea. It is a strict parasite. Occurs characteristically inside polymorphonuclear leucocytes in the tissues — **gonococcal** *adj.*

gonorrhoea n a sexually transmitted infection caused by the gonococcus. It is notifiable and classified legally as venereal. An acute inflammation affecting the genital tract, urinary tract and the mucosa of the throat and anus. Usual sites are the cervix and urethra in females and the urethra in males; it presents with dysuria and discharge but it may be asymptomatic in females. Diagnostic tests include microscopy and culture of secretions. It may lead to sterility if the uterine tubes (i.e. pelvic inflammatory disease) or epididymis become involved. Rare systemic effects include arthritis and septicaemia. Nonsexual spread may occur, e.g. an infant's eyes infected during birth and vulvovaginitis in prepubertal girls. ⇒ ophthalmia neonatorum — **gonorrhoeal** *adj* resulting from gonorrhoea.

Goodpasture syndrome a haemorrhagic lung disorder associated with glomerulonephritis.

goose flesh contraction of the tiny muscles attached to the sheath of the hair follicles causes the hair to stand on end; it is a reaction to either cold or fear and occurs in the early stages of increasing core body temperature.

GOR *abbr* gastro-oesophageal reflux.

Gordh needle an obsolete intravenous needle with a rubber diaphragm through which repeated injections were given.

gouge *n* a chisel with a grooved blade for removing bone.

gout *n* group of metabolic disorders where serum uric acid levels are elevated (hyperuricaemia). It may be due to abnormal purine metabolism or increased intake, increased uric acid production and reduced renal excretion of uric acid. Urate crystals are deposited within joints, the ears and elsewhere. The big toe is characteristically involved and becomes acutely painful and swollen. Gout may occur in situations where there is increased purine turnover, such as in some types of leukaemia and severe psoriasis. Management involves NSAIDs and colchicine during an acute episode. Allopurinol and colchicine are used after the acute attack or to prevent gout occurring in situations where increased purine turnover is anticipated. Uricosuric agents, such as probenicid may be given to increase uric acid secretion. Patients are advised to rest the affected part and to limit their intake of purine-containing foods, such as offal, and restrict alcohol intake.

GPI *abbr* general paralysis of the insane. ⇒ neurosyphilis.

Graafian follicle a mature ovarian follicle, a minute vesicle in the stroma of an ovary. It contains fluid and a single oocyte which is released when it ruptures at ovulation. Usually one primordial follicle develops into a Graafian follicle each month under the influence of gonadotrophic hormones. Following ovulation, the Graafian follicle gives rise to the corpus luteum which, if fertilization occurs, maintains the pregnancy until the placenta is sufficiently developed. Where fertilization does not occur, the corpus luteum only persists for 12–14 days. Degenerates to become the corpus albicans.

grading a method of classifying a cancer based on its histopathological characteristics. The degree of malignancy of the tissue is calculated by comparing the amount of cellular abnormality and the rate of cell division with normal cells in the same tissue. High grade cancer is aggressive and spreads rapidly, whereas low grade cancer tends to have slow tumour growth and spread. For some cancers, the grade of the disease is more important than the stage as an indicator of prognosis and treatment. ⇒ differentiation. ⇒ staging.

graft *n* transplanted living tissue, e.g. skin, bone, bone marrow, cornea and organs such as kidney, heart, lungs, pancreas and liver; to implant or transplant such tissue. Grafts may be: autografts when tissue is moved from one site to another in the same individual; isografts between genetically identical individuals; allografts (homografts) where tissue is obtained from a suitable donor; and xenografts (heterograft) between different species. *graft versus host disease (GVHD)* may follow a successful transplant, especially bone marrow, where the graft 'attacks' the tissues of the immunologically compromised host, causing rashes, liver problems and diarrhoea. ⇒ transplant.

gram (g) *n* unit of mass. One thousand equals a kilogram.

Gram's stain a bacteriological stain for the identification and classification of microorganisms. Those staining violet are Gram-positive and those that stain pink are Gram-negative.

grand mal ⇒ convulsions. ⇒ epilepsy.

granulation *n* the outgrowth of new capillaries and connective tissue cells from the surface of an open wound. It occurs during the proliferative phase of wound healing. *granulation tissue* the new, soft tissue so formed. *hypergranulation/outgranulation* over-production of granulation tissue during healing — **granulate** *vi*.

granulocyte *n* white blood cell (leucocyte) which contains granules in its cytoplasm. These may be neutrophils, eosinophils or basophils.

granuloma *n* a tumour formed of granulation tissue. *granuloma venereum* granuloma inguinale.

granuloma inguinale a sexually transmitted infection caused by *Donovania granulomatis* (bipolar rods). It is characterized by a primary lesion on the genitalia and buboes in the regional lymph nodes.

graphics any printout or screen display that includes pictures made up of many small dots or pixels.

Graves' disease ⇒ hyperthyroidism.

gravid *adj* pregnant; carrying fertilized eggs or a fetus.

gravitational *adj* being attracted by force of gravity. *gravitational ulcer* ⇒ venous ulcer.

gravity *n* weight. The weight of a substance compared with that of an equal volume of water is termed *specific gravity*.

Grawitz tumour ⇒ hypernephroma.

gray (Gy) *n* the derived SI unit (International System of Units) for the absorbed dose of radiation. The unit has replaced the rad.

green monkey disease ⇒ Marburg disease.

green papers government consultation documents that address a range of issues, e.g. health, education, transport etc. They are distributed to interested parties to elicit opinion prior to implementation of action on a particular matter, e.g. Department of Health (1998) *Our Healthier Nation. A Contract for Health.* London: The Stationery Office. ⇒ white papers.

greenstick fracture ⇒ fracture.

gregarious *adj* showing a preference for living in a group, liking to mix. The gregarious or herd instinct is an inborn tendency on the part of various species, including humans.

grey matter nerve cell bodies and unmyelinated nerve fibres in the central nervous sysyem. ⇒ white matter.

grieving process the word 'process' has been added to what was traditionally known as grieving to signify increased knowledge about the stages (denial, anger, bargaining, depression, acceptance and possibly fear) which a person may experience in relation to bereavement and dying. Grieving is not only associated with these experiences, but also with any other loss including: loss of body function, such as paralysis or infertility; loss of body part, e.g. breast, limb, uterus. ⇒ bereavement.

Griffith's typing a subdivision of *Streptococcus pyogenes* (Lancefield group A) using differences in their antigenic structure.

gripe *n* abdominal colic.

grocer's itch ⇒ baker's itch.

groin *n* the junction of the thigh with the abdomen.

grommet *n* a type of ventilation tube inserted into the tympanic membrane. Frequently used in the treatment of glue ear in children. ⇒ myringotomy.

grounded theory research where a hypothesis is derived from the data obtained.

group activities (occupational therapy) *npl* working with people in groups, using a variety of recreational, social, creative and practical activities. See Box – Group activities (occupational therapy).

group C meningococcal disease *n* serious infection caused by *Neisseria meningitidis* of the serological group C. It

---

Group activities (occupational therapy)
In the context of occupational therapy (OT) an activity group will have a defined purpose and specified goals. For example, the group may be structured to promote skill development, to facilitate interactions between members, to stimulate cognition or to enable exploration of personal issues and meanings. There will be goals for the group as a whole and/or for individuals attending the group. A referral to the occupational therapist is normally required, and an OT assessment will be carried out before the client can be accepted for a group. The therapist selects activities to facilitate group processes and uses participation in the activity as a means of working towards the specified goals. Some groups take place for a number of sessions with the same group of people and new members are not accepted (closed group).

causes meningococcal meningitis and life-threatening septicaemia in children and young adults. Effective immunization is available. *group C meningococcal disease vaccines* injectable vaccine included in the routine immunization programme. Offered to high risk groups: infants, pre-school children, school children, and young people entering further and higher education. ⇒ meningitis. ⇒ septicaemia.

group psychotherapy ⇒ psychotherapy.

growth hormone (GH, somatotropin) a protein hormone secreted by the anterior pituitary gland under the influence of two hypothalamic hormones: growth hormone releasing hormone (GHRH) and growth hormone inhibiting hormone (GHIH) or somatostatin. Growth hormone has widespread effects on body tissues; it stimulates the growth of bone etc, and influences the metabolism of proteins, fats and carbohydrates. It is particularly important in protein synthesis which is essential for healing. More than half the daily amount is released during early sleep. ⇒ acromegaly. ⇒ dwarfism. ⇒ gigantism.

growth hormone inhibiting hormone (GHIH) somatostatin. Hypothalamic hormone that inhibits the secretion of growth hormone. It is also produced by pancreatic and intestinal cells.

growth hormone releasing hormone (GHRH) hypothalamic hormone that stimulates the release of growth hormone.

growth hormone test (GHT) there is a reciprocal relationship between growth hormone (secreted by the pituitary gland) and blood glucose. GH can also be measured during a standard 50 g oral glucose tolerance test. In acromegaly, not only is the resting level of GH higher, but it does not show normal suppression with glucose.

GSL *abbr* general sales list.

GTN *abbr* glyceryl trinitrate. ⇒ nitrates.

guanine *n* nitrogenous base derived from purine. A component of nucleic acids (DNA, RNA).

guar gum *n* fibre derived from natural sources. It is used commercially as a thickening and binding agent. Taken orally, it absorbs water from the gut and produces a feeling of fullness. It may help to stabilize blood sugar levels by slowing carbohydrate absorption and preventing sudden increases after meals.

guardian ad litem a person with a social work or childcare background who is appointed to ensure that the court is fully informed of the relevant facts which relate to a child, and that the wishes and feelings of the child are clearly established. The appointment is made from a panel set up by the local authority.

Guedel airway ⇒ airway.

Guillain-Barré syndrome *n* acute demyelinating peripheral polyneuropathy that may follow a viral or bacterial infection, or immunization. It results in pain, weakness, paralysis and possibly respiratory problems.

guillotine *n* a surgical instrument for excision of the tonsils.

Guinea worm ⇒ *Dracunculus medinensis.*

gullet *n* the oesophagus.

GUM *abbr* genitourinary medicine. ⇒ sexually transmitted infection.

gumboil *n* lay term for an abscess of gum tissue and periosteum (alveolar abscess) which is usually very painful.

gumma *n* a localized granuloma with fibrosis, necrosis and ulceration which develops in the later stages (tertiary) of syphilis. Gummata may affect any organ and those near a surface of the body tend to break down, forming chronic ulcers, that have a characteristic 'punched out' appearance — **gummata** *pl.*

gustation taste. A chemical sense that is closely linked to the individual's ability to smell.

gut *n* the intestine. *gut decontamination* the use of nonabsorbable antibiotics to suppress growth of micro-organisms to prevent endogenous infection for patients undergoing bowel surgery or those who are neutropenic or immunocompromised.

Guthrie test screening test. Assay of phenylalanine to test for phenylketonuria in the newborn. A drop of blood, usually taken from the heel, is dried on special filter paper. Carried out on the 6th day of life. It is necessary to confirm the diagnosis in those infants with a positive test.

GVHD *abbr* graft versus host disease. ⇒ graft.

gynaecologist *n* a surgeon who specializes in gynaecology.

gynaecology *n* the science dealing with the diseases of the female reproductive system — **gynaecological** *adj*.

gynaecomastia *n* enlargement of the male breasts (mammary glands). It may occur at puberty and in older men, in liver disease, when oestrogenic hormones accumulate in the blood, and with the use of anabolic steroids. Unilateral enlargement should always be investigated as breast cancer does affect the male breast.

gypsum *n* plaster of Paris (calcium sulphate).

gyrus *n* a convoluted portion of cerebral cortex — **gyri** *pl*.

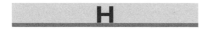

H

H₁-receptor antagonists antiemetic drugs that block histamine receptors, e.g. cyclizine, used for motion sickness, raised intracranial pressure etc.

H₂-receptor antagonists an agent which selectively blocks the H_2 histamine receptors that normally stimulate gastric secretion and thereby decrease the secretion of gastric juice, e.g. cimetidine, ranatidine. They are used in the management of peptic ulcer, hyperacidity and gastro-oesophageal reflux, and in the prophylaxis of gastrointestinal ulceration and bleeding in critically ill patients. ⇒ Curling's ulcer. ⇒ proton pump inhibitors.

habilitation *n* the means by which a child gradually progresses towards the maximum degree of physical, psychological and social independence, of which he or she is capable. A term often applied to the processes that assist people with learning disability, mental health problems or physical disability to achieve maximum levels of independence with the activities of daily living. ⇒ rehabilitation.

habit *n* any learned behaviour that has a relatively high probability of occurrence in response to a particular situation or stimulus. Acquisition of habits may depend on both reinforcement and associative learning. *habit training* used in the care of people with a learning disability or mental health problem which requires them to relearn personal hygiene by constant repetition with encouragement.

habit retraining the patient voids at set times, according to the baseline frequency/volume chart, but may use the lavatory at other times. ⇒ bladder retraining. ⇒ incontinence.

habitual abortion ⇒ abortion.

habituation *n* term to describe decreasing response to a stimulus when it becomes familiar through repeated presentation. It is often used in a negative sense in relation to drug use, where a psychological dependence develops through repeated use of a drug. ⇒ drug dependence.

haem *n* the iron-containing pigment part of the haemoglobin molecule. ⇒ haemoglobin.

haemangioma *n* a malformation of blood vessels which may occur in any part of the body. When in the skin, it is one form of birthmark, appearing as a red spot or a 'port wine stain' — **haemangiomata** *pl*.

haemarthrosis *n* the presence of blood in a joint cavity. ⇒ haemophilias. ⇒ haemophilic arthopathy — **haemarthroses** *pl*.

haematemesis *n* vomiting blood. It may be bright red when fresh, or dark brown with the appearance of 'coffee grounds' that results from partial digestion of the blood by gastric juice. The site of bleeding is usually gastrointestinal and causes include: peptic ulcer, varices, neoplasms, drug erosions and coagulation defects, but blood swallowed from elsewhere, e.g. after tonsil surgery, may be vomited.

haematin *n* a ferric iron-containing derivative of haemoglobin. It may crystallize in the kidney tubules when there is excessive haemolysis, such as in malaria.

haematinic *adj* any substance which is required for the production of the red blood cell and its constituents, e.g. iron.

haematocele *n* a swelling filled with blood.

haematocolpos *n* a collection of retained menstrual blood in the vagina. ⇒ cryptomenorrhoea.

haematocrit *n* ⇒ packed cell volume.

haematology *n* the science dealing with the formation, composition, functions and diseases of the blood — **haematological** *adj*.

haematoma *n* a swelling filled with blood — **haematomata** *pl*.

haematometra *n* an accumulation of blood (or menstrual fluid) in the uterus.

haematopoiesis *n* ⇒ haemopoiesis.

haematosalpinx *n* (*syn* haemosalpinx) blood in the uterine tube. Often associated with tubal pregnancy.

haematozoa *npl* parasites living in the blood — **haematozoon** *sing*.

haematuria *n* blood in the urine; it may be from the kidneys, one or both ureters, the bladder or the urethra, and may indicate trauma, infection or abnormal pathology, such as glomerulonephritis or renal calculi. Bleeding may also occur in coagulation defects or with anticoagulant drugs, such as warfarin. The bleeding may be gross: bright red in colour, dark red or smoky in appearance, or only detected by use of test sticks/strips or microscopy — **haematuric** *adj*.

haemochromatosis *n* bronzed diabetes. A condition caused by excess iron in the body. Iron is deposited in organs such as the liver, heart and pancreas, and in the skin, causing bronze pigmentation. The cause may be a *primary* hereditary defect of iron metabolism, or *secondary* to high intake, excessive haemolysis, alcohol related cirrhosis and frequent blood transfusion — **haemochromatotic** *adj*.

haemoconcentration *n* an increase in the volume of red blood cells relative to the volume of plasma.

haemocytoblast *n* primitive stem cell found in the bone marrow that gives rise to all blood cells. ⇒ chondroblast. ⇒ fibroblast. ⇒ osteoblast.

haemocytometer *n* a device used to count blood cells in a sample.

haemodiafiltration (CVVHD) *n* similar to haemofiltration, but with the addition of dialysate solution. This allows diffusion to occur enhancing the removal of molecules. See Box – Haemofiltration.

haemodialysis *n* removal of metabolic waste products, electrolytes, other toxic solutes and excess fluid from the blood by dialysis, which is achieved by putting a semipermeable membrane between the blood and a rinsing solution called dialysate within a dialyser (artificial kidney). It is undertaken in the management of the end stage of renal failure (irreversible), in acute renal failure (reversible) or after poisoning, such as a drugs overdose. ⇒ haemodiafiltration. ⇒ haemofiltration.

haemodilution *n* a decrease in the volume of red blood cells relative to the volume of plasma.

haemodynamics *npl* the forces involved in circulating blood round the body.

haemofiltration (CVVH) *n* a continuous form of renal replacement therapy that utilizes ultrafiltration to remove molecules. See Box – Haemofiltration (continuous venous-venous haemofiltration).

haemoglobin (Hb) *n* the red iron containing respiratory pigment in the red blood cells. A haemoglobin molecule has four haem groups containing ferrous iron and

---

Haemofiltration (continuous venous-venous haemofiltration)
Haemofiltration – continuous venous-venous haemofiltration (CVVH) was developed as a treatment for acute renal failure in the critically ill to overcome the complications associated with haemodialysis and peritoneal dialysis in this group of patients.

It is a continuous procedure where a large vein, commonly the femoral, subclavian or internal jugular, is cannulated using a double lumen catheter. Blood is pumped from one lumen of the catheter into an extracorporeal circuit and through an artificial kidney where semipermeable membranes filter the blood. Substances such as water, waste products (urea and creatinine) and electrolytes are removed from the blood and discarded, this is known as the filtrate. The blood is then returned to the patient via the other lumen of the catheter.

The technique utilizes ultrafiltration which is unselective; waste products can only be removed from the blood with an accompanying volume of water. To maintain fluid balance and haemodynamic stability, specially formulated fluid is concurrently infused into the patient.

The removal of waste products can be enhanced by passing a dialysate fluid through the artificial kidney which allows diffusion of waste products from the blood in addition to ultrafiltration. This technique is known as haemodiafiltration – continuous venous-venous haemodialfiltration (CVVHD).

four globin chains (see Figure 27). It has the reversible function of combining with and releasing oxygen to the tissues. Haemoglobin carries some carbon dioxide and buffers pH changes. There are several types of haemoglobin: fetal type (HbF) and two major forms of adult haemoglobin (HbA and HbA$_2$). Fetal haemoglobin, which has a high affinity for oxygen, is gradually replaced by adult haemoglobin during early childhood. ⇒ glycosylated haemoglobin. ⇒ haemoglobinopathies. ⇒ oxyhaemoglobin.

haemoglobinaemia *n* free haemoglobin in the blood plasma — **haemoglobinaemic** *adj*.

haemoglobinometer *n* an instrument for estimating the percentage of haemoglobin in the blood.

haemoglobinopathies *npl* inherited disorders of haemoglobin structure or production. ⇒ anaemia. ⇒ sickle cell disease. ⇒ thalassaemia — **haemoglobinopathic** *adj*.

haemoglobinuria *n* haemoglobin in the urine — **haemoglobinuric** *adj*.

haemolysin *n* an agent which causes disintegration of red blood cells. ⇒ immunoglobulins.

haemolysis *n* disintegration of red blood cells, with liberation of contained haemoglobin. Causes include: red cell defects, infections, drugs, chemicals, incompatible blood transfusion, antibodies and hypersplenism — **haemolytic** *adj* pertaining

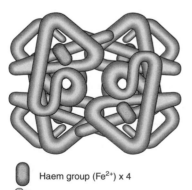

Haem group (Fe^{2+}) x 4

Globin chains x 4 (2α + 2β)

Figure 27 Structure of haemoglobin. (Reproduced from Brooker 1998 with permission.)

to haemolysis or the power to disrupt red blood cells. ⇒ anaemia. ⇒ jaundice.

haemolytic disease of the newborn (*syn* erythroblastosis fetalis) a pathological condition affecting the fetus and the newborn child, caused by Rhesus blood group incompatibility between the child's blood and that of the mother. Red blood cell destruction occurs with anaemia, jaundice and an excess of erythroblasts or primitive red blood cells in the circulating blood. Immunization of women at risk, using anti-D immunoglobulin, can prevent haemolytic disease of the newborn. Management of affected infants includes phototherapy, blood transfusion and exchange transfusion in severe cases. ABO incompatibility does occur, but is usually mild. Problems with other blood group systems occur very rarely. ⇒ blood groups. ⇒ hydrops fetalis. ⇒ icterus gravis. ⇒ kernicterus.

haemolytic uraemic syndrome (HUS) the potentially fatal intravascular haemolysis and acute renal failure that occurs secondary to some other condition, such as food poisoning with enterohaemorrhagic *Escherichia coli* type 0157. Affected individuals (mainly children) may require renal replacement therapy. Most make a full recovery, but some will have residual renal problems.

haemopericardium *n* blood in the pericardial sac.

haemoperitoneum *n* blood in the peritoneal cavity.

haemophilias *npl* a group of inherited blood coagulation defects. In clinical practice the most commonly encountered are: *haemophilia A*, blood clotting factor VIII deficiency; *haemophilia B* or Christmas disease, blood clotting factor IX deficiency. Both these conditions are X-linked recessive disorders primarily affecting males and resulting in abnormalities of the coagulation mechanism. The bleeding usually occurs into deeply lying structures, muscles and joints. Management involves replacement of the missing factor as required and specific treatment, such as splinting joints. ⇒ coagulation. ⇒ haemarthrosis. ⇒ haemophilic arthropathy. ⇒ von Willebrand's disease.

haemophilic arthropathy joint damage seen in people suffering from haemophilia. The extent of the damage is staged as follows: (a) synovial thickening; (b) epiphyseal overgrowth; (c) minor joint changes and cyst formation; (d) definite joint changes with loss of joint space; (e) end-stage joint destruction and secondary changes leading to deformity.

Haemophilus *n* a genus of bacteria. Small Gram-negative bacilli that show much variation in shape (pleomorphism). Characteristically intracellular in polymorphonuclear leucocytes in exudate. *Haemophilus aegyptius* causes a form of acute infectious conjunctivitis. *Haemophilus ducreyi* causes chancroid. *Haemophilus influenzae*, a major cause of epiglossitis and meningitis in young children, causes respiratory infections in people with chronic respiratory disease and may follow viral influenza infections. Effective immunization is available. ⇒ Hib. *Haemophilus pertussis* ⇒ *Bordetella pertussis*. ⇒ pertussis.

haemopneumothorax *n* the presence of blood and air in the pleural cavity.

haemopoiesis *n* (*syn* haematopoiesis) the formation of blood. ⇒ erythropoiesis. ⇒ leucopoiesis — **haemopoietic** *adj*.

haemoptysis *n* the coughing up of blood or blood stained mucus from the respiratory tract. Causes include: infections, cancers, trauma, pulmonary infarction, left heart failure, coagulation defects and anticoagulant drugs. The blood may be: bright red, frothy and pink, dark red or have a 'rusty' appearance — **haemoptyses** *pl*.

haemorrhage *n* the escape of blood from a vessel; usually refers to a rapid and considerable loss. Severe haemorrhage leads to hypovolaemic shock with hypotension, tachycardia, pallor, sweating, restlessness, air hunger, oliguria and eventually altered consciousness. Haemorrhage can be classified in a variety of ways. (a) by the type of vessel: arterial, capillary or venous; (b) by the time since surgery or injury: *primary haemorrhage* that which occurs at the time of injury or operation. *reactionary haemorrhage* occurring within 24 hours of the original event. *secondary haemorrhage* occurring more than 24 hours after the event, usually associated with sepsis. It may be some days after an injury or operation; (c) whether it is external (revealed) or internal (concealed). ⇒ antepartum haemorrhage. ⇒ intrapartum haemorrhage. ⇒ placental abruption. →

postpartum haemorrhage — **haemorrhagic** *adj*.

haemorrhagic disease of the newborn characterized by gastrointestinal, pulmonary or intracranial haemorrhage occurring during the first week of life. Lack of vitamin K causes a deficiency of the clotting factor prothrombin. Normal bacterial colonization of the gut results in synthesis of vitamin K, thus permitting formation of prothrombin by the liver. Responds to or prevented by administration of vitamin K.

haemorrhagic fever ⇒ mosquito-transmitted haemorrhagic fevers. ⇒ viral haemorrhagic fevers.

haemorrhoidal *adj* **1.** pertaining to haemorrhoids. **2.** applied to blood vessels and nerves in the anal region.

haemorrhoidectomy *n* surgical removal of haemorrhoids.

haemorrhoids *npl* (*syn* piles) varicosity of the veins around the anus. *external haemorrhoids* those outside the anal sphincter, covered with skin. *internal haemorrhoids* those inside the anal sphincter, covered with mucous membrane.

haemosalpinx *n* ⇒ haematosalpinx.

haemosiderin *n* a storage form of iron. Combined with proteins, the iron which would be toxic alone, is stored safely in the liver and spleen. ⇒ ferritin.

haemosiderosis *n* iron deposits in the tissues.

haemospermia *n* the discharge of blood-stained semen.

haemostasis *n* **1.** the physiological process whereby bleeding from small vessels is controlled. Damage to the endothelial lining of blood vessels initiates a complex series of reactions between substances in the blood and others released from damaged tissue and platelets. It involves the four overlapping stages: vasoconstriction, platelet plug formation, coagulation and fibrinolysis. Also describes the measures taken to arrest bleeding after injury or during surgery. **2.** stagnation of blood within its vessel.

haemostatic *adj* any agent which arrests bleeding, e.g. aprotinin. *haemostatic forceps* artery forceps.

haemothorax *n* blood in the pleural cavity.

Hageman factor *n* factor XII in coagulation.

HAI *abbr* hospital acquired infection. ⇒ infection. ⇒ nosocomial.

hair *n* a filamentous appendage of skin, present on all parts except palms, soles, lips, glans penis and terminal phalanges. It consists of keratinized cells and grows within a hair follicle. There are three types of hair: ⇒ lanugo. ⇒ terminal hair. ⇒ vellus hair. Hair has a minimal role in temperature regulation and has protective functions: protects the skin; eyebrows and lashes protect the eyes; and nasal hair traps large debris. The broken-off stump found at the periphery of spreading bald patches in alopecia areata is called an exclamation mark hair, from the characteristic shape caused by atrophic thinning of the hair shaft. *hair analysis* hair samples can be tested to measure the individual's exposure to various substances, such as toxic chemicals or pollutants, nutrients and illegal drugs. *hair follicle* the sheath derived from epidermal cells that grows down into the dermis. The hair grows within the follicle. *hair root* the internal end of a hair; it is attached to the papilla (dimpled end) of the hair follicle through which it receives its blood supply.

halal describes meat obtained from animals killed according to Islamic law.

half life (t$\frac{1}{2}$) the time taken for the radioactivity of a radioactive substance to decay by half of its initial value. The half life is a constant for each radioactive isotope, e.g. iodine-131 is eight days. Or the time taken for the concentration of a drug in the plasma to fall by half of its initial level. *biological half life* the time taken by the body to eliminate 50% of a dose of any substance by normal biological processes. *effective half life* the time taken for a combination of radioactive decay and biological processes to reduce radioactivity by 50%.

halibut liver oil a very rich source of vitamins A and D. The smaller dose required makes it more acceptable than cod liver oil.

halitosis *n* foul-smelling breath.

hallucination *n* a false perception occurring without any true sensory stimulus. A common symptom in severe psychoses, including schizophrenia, paraphrenia and confusional states. Also common in delirium, during toxic states and following head injuries. ⇒ Hallucinations Rating Scale.

Hallucinations Rating Scale (HRS) unpublished scale. An eleven item checklist for auditory hallucinations. It assesses distress control and beliefs regarding the origin of voices, in addition to how the client experiences voices.

hallucinogens *npl* any substance that produces hallucinations, e.g. MDMA. ⇒ Ecstasy.

hallucinosis *n* a psychosis in which the patient is grossly hallucinated. Usually a subacute delirious state; the predominant symptoms are auditory illusions and hallucinations.

hallux *n* the big toe. *hallux valgus* ⇒ bunion. *hallux varus* the big toe is displaced towards the other foot. *hallux rigidus* ankylosis of the metatarsophalangeal articulation caused by osteoarthritis.

halo *n* 1. a ring splint which encircles the head. ⇒ halopelvic traction. 2. circle of light such as that seen by people with glaucoma.

halogen *n* any one of the nonmetallic elements: bromine, chlorine, fluorine, iodine.

halopelvic traction a form of external fixation whereby traction can be applied to the spine between two fixed points. The device consists of three main parts: (a) a halo; (b) a pelvic loop and (c) four extension bars.

hamate *n* one of the carpals or wrist bones.

Hamilton-Russell traction *n* a form of skin traction on the femoral shaft with the knee flexed. ⇒ traction.

hammer toe a permanent hyperextension of the first phalanx and flexion of second and third phalanges.

hamstring group flexor muscles at the back of the thigh.

hand *n* that part of the upper limb below the wrist.

hand-arm vibration syndrome (HAVS) an occupational hazard of certain machine or tool operators. The effects include vascular blanching of terminal digits, known as Raynaud's phenomenon, and neurological numbness and tingling of terminal digits. It is a progressive disease and may lead to gangrene.

hand, foot and mouth disease an infectious disease affecting children. It is caused by a coxsackie virus and characterized by vesicles on hands, feet and mouth.

handicap *n* term formerly used to denote disadvantage arising from impairment or disability. It is no longer favoured by disability groups because this term carries negative connotations.

handicapped *adj* term, no longer considered acceptable, applied to a person with a condition that interferes with normal activity and achievement.

Hand-Schüller-Christian disease ⇒ histiocytosis X.

handwashing *n* the most important activity in preventing infection, both in hospital and community settings. It should include the wrists, the bulbar eminence of each thumb as well as between the fingers. The hands should be washed after patient contact, and both before and after certain interventions, such as aseptic procedures, tracheal suction and emptying urine from a closed drainage system. The Infection Control Committee usually advises about the circumstances to be followed by handwashing, in addition to those which have to be preceded, as well as followed, by handwashing. Local policies dictate when gloves are worn and when antiseptic hand rubs are used. (See Figure 28).

hangnail *n* a narrow strip of skin partly detached from the nailfold.

Hansen's bacillus ⇒ leprosy.

haploid *adj* describes a cell with a set of unpaired chromosomes seen in the gametes (oocytes and spermatozoa) following meiosis (reduction division). In humans the haploid number is 23 (n). There are 22 autosomes and 1 sex chromosome. Its normal multiple is diploid, but abnormally three or more chromosome sets can be found (triploid, tetraploid, etc). ⇒ diploid.

hapten *n* incomplete antigens. Small molecules, such as peptides, which combine with a body protein to become antigenic. Alone they cause no immunological response.

haptoglobin *n* an α globulin that combines with free haemoglobin in the plasma.

hard drugs a term used in relation to drug misuse. There is not a standard classification but many people include amfetamine (amphetamine) or Ecstasy, barbiturates, cocaine, heroin, lysergic acid diethylamide (LSD) and morphine in the category. Current concern is about those who inject the drug and share dirty needles and syringes, not only exposing themselves, but also others, to the dangers of blood borne viruses, e.g. hepatitis B and HIV. ⇒ drug.

hardware the computer (box) and associated peripherals including monitor, printer and modem.

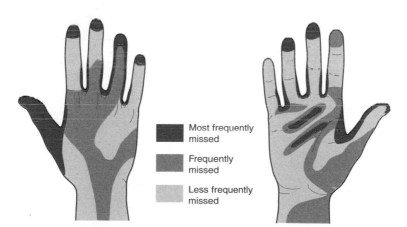

Most frequently missed

Frequently missed

Less frequently missed

Figure 28 Hand washing – areas missed. (Reproduced from Nicol et al 2000 with permission.)

Hardy-Weinberg equilibrium equation *n* the relationship between the frequency of a gene and genotype occurring in a given population.

Harrington rod used in operations for scoliosis: it provides internal fixation whereby the curve is held by the rod and is usually accompanied by a spinal fusion.

Hartmann's solution an electrolyte replacement solution for intravenous infusion. Contains sodium lactate and chloride, potassium chloride and calcium chloride.

Hartnup disease an inborn error of the metabolism of neutral amino acids, such as tryptophan from which nicotinamide is synthesized. It is associated with skin lesions, stomatitis, glossitis, dysphagia, diarrhoea, psychiatric symptoms or mild learning disability. It can be treated with nicotinamide. ⇒ pellagra.

Hashimoto's disease Hashimoto's thyroiditis. An autoimmune condition affecting the thyroid gland. Antithyroid antibodies are produced in response to antigens, and the gland is infiltrated by immune cells such as lymphocytes. It causes goitre with or without hypothyroidism.

hashish *n* ⇒ cannabis indica.

haustration *n* pouches or sacculations in the colon produced by puckering. It occurs because longitudinal muscle bands, the taenia coli, are shorter than the colon. ⇒ sacculation. ⇒ taenia coli — **haustra** *pl.*

HAV *abbr* hepatitis A virus.

haversian system *n* the basic unit of bone tissue (also known as an osteon). *haversian canal* central canal, which runs along the long axis of the bone within a haversian system; carries blood vessels, lymph vessels and nerve fibres.

HAVS *abbr* hand-arm vibration syndrome.

Hawthorne effect a positive result from introduction of change, of which people are less conscious with the passage of time. Nurses carrying out participant or nonparticipant observation in a research project allow for this reaction to their presence by not using the data collected in the first few days in the final analysis of the data. The term is derived from indus-trial management research at the Hawthorne factory in Illinois managed by the Western Electric Company.

hay fever ⇒ allergic rhinitis.

Haygarth's nodes swelling of joints, sometimes seen in the finger joints of patients suffering from arthritis.

HAZ *abbr* Health Action Zone.

HBcAg *abbr* hepatitis B core antigen. ⇒ hepatitis.

HBeAg *abbr* hepatitis B e antigen. It is associated with the core of the hepatitis B virus.

HBIG *abbr* hepatitis B immunoglobulin. Can be used in situations where accidental contamination, e.g. 'needlestick' injury, has occurred.

HBsAg *abbr* hepatitis B surface antigen. It is found in the serum of individuals with acute and chronic hepatitis B, or who are carriers of the disease. The chronic carriage state is associated with the development of cirrhosis and liver cancer. ⇒ hepatitis.

HBV *abbr* hepatitis B virus.

HCA *abbr* ⇒ healthcare assistant.

hCG *abbr* human chorionic gonadotrophin.

HCV *abbr* hepatitis C virus.

HDL *abbr* high-density lipoprotein.

HDU *abbr* high dependency unit.

HDV *abbr* hepatitis D virus.

head injury usually the result of a blow to the head; there may or may not be fracture of the skull. The injury may result in concussion, contusion of brain tissue and swelling (cerebral oedema), and bleeding from a damaged blood vessel may lead to an extradural or subdural haematoma. Swelling of the brain, or haematoma formation, may cause raised intracranial pressure (RIP) and further ischaemia and pressure on vital centres. Assessment and observation following head injury is vital to detect changes in condition that may indicate RIP. ⇒ Glasgow coma scale. ⇒ neurological assessment.

head lice (Pediculus capitis) lay their eggs (nits) at the junction of the hair and skin. They hatch in 1 week and are fully grown in 3 and live for 5 weeks. They pierce the scalp to suck blood and cause intense itching; subsequent scratching can introduce infection. They spread quickly in schools, and nurses can provide information for parents and children about head lice, how to be constantly vigilant for their presence, and how to treat an infestation.

headache *n* pain most commonly experienced in the frontal or occipital region; it can accompany many illnesses which do not involve head structures. Causes of severe headache include: stress and muscle tension, conditions of the brain and meninges, such as inflammation, new growths which can be benign or malignant, increased intracranial pressure from trauma, and cardiovascular conditions, e.g. hypertension and stroke. Nursing intervention is based on nursing assessment and may be pharmacological, or use complementary therapies or health education. → migraine.

Heaf test multiple skin puncture test with tuberculin purified protein derivative (PPD) using a special Heaf device (gun). It is generally used for routine screening, e.g. before BCG immunization. The inflammatory reaction grade (0–IV) is read after 3–7 days.

healing *n* 1. the natural process of cure or repair of the tissues. ⇒ wound healing. 2. a term used in complementary or integrated medicine that refers to a return to health; also the use of a therapy that may act as a catalyst in the healing process; a specific therapeutic form, such as healing, spiritual or remote healing and therapeutic touch, based on the concept of the direct transmission of some form of psychic energy for therapeutic purposes — **heal** *vt, vi* a return to health or a percep-

tion of enhanced physical, psychological or spiritual well-being.

health *n* see Box – Health.

Health Action Zone (HAZ) a geographical area targeted for focused multiprofessional collaboration between the NHS, local government authorities and other agencies for health improvement.

health and safety law *n* the law, common law and statute covering health and safety duties. The Health and Safety at Work Act 1974 sets out the responsibilities of the employer in relation to the workforce, work environment, equipment and substances, and those of individual employees to themselves and others.

health authority *n* the body that administers the NHS at local level. Recent changes have resulted in fewer health authorities, many of which have common boundaries with local government authorities, e.g. Norfolk Health Authority covers the whole county of Norfolk. This is likely to result in a more co-ordinated service for patients and clients as administration should be more straightforward.

Health Board in Scotland, the equivalent of a Health Authority.

health centre a building designated by a government to distribute its healthcare policies at local level. The personnel working in and from the centre are members of several health professions according to local needs and provisions.

Health Development Agency a statutory body set up to improve standards in public health. It is concerned with identifying the need for evidence and for commissioning research. Other roles include:

Health

Health is generally understood to identify a state of being to which we all aspire. The most common usage is health being the absence of disease or illness, the opposite of being sick. Health is thus a negative term, defined more by what it is not than what it is. There is also a positive definition interpreted by the World Health Organization in its constitution in 1948 as 'a state of complete physical, mental and social well-being'. During the Enlightenment period in the seventeenth century the body came to be viewed as a machine which could be reduced

down to component parts. This led to an era of laboratory medicine which focused not on the patient as a whole but rather on their organs, tissues or even cells. Modern society views the body more holistically and within its social, environmental and economic context. Health is thus seen broadly as encompassing a person's social and psychological resources as well as their physical capacities. An understanding of what constitutes good health may vary from one individual to another, from place to place as well as at different times. Health is therefore a very subjective concept.

standard setting, undertaking health promotion campaigns and distributing examples of good practice.

health education see Box – Health education. ⇒ behaviour change. ⇒ health promotion.

health gain a term used to describe health improvement. It might be used by health professionals and health managers in the context of their need to use limited resources to produce a tangible improvement or gain in health. ⇒ quality-adjusted life years.

Health Improvement Programme (HImP) a focused action plan aimed at improving health and health care at a local level. The lead organization is the Health Authority, in collaboration with Primary Care Groups/Acute Trusts, health professionals, local government authorities and other groups with an interest, e.g. Patient groups, voluntary sector etc.

Health of the Nation Outcome Scale (HoNOS) a twelve item health and social functioning scale. It measures risk behaviours, physical problems, deterioration and/or improvement in symptoms and social functioning. Can be completed by the mental healthcare team and/or the individual practitioner.

health promotion see Box – Health promotion.

health visitor a nurse with a specialist qualification in health visiting who is concerned with preventative care, mainly with the under fives, school-aged children, mothers and older people. ⇒ specialist community practitioner.

healthcare assistant (HCA) a health service employee who provides nursing support services under the direction of a qualified nurse, who remains accountable for the care given. Formerly known as nursing auxiliaries, HCAs can now receive a nationally co-ordinated training, based on national vocational qualifications (NVQ/SNVQs).

healthcare system the means by which a government organizes the finance and administration of its healthcare policies.

Healthy Living Centres *npl* in the UK. National Lottery funded centres that aim to meet the health and social needs of deprived and disadvantaged communities.

Health education
Health education aims to help people to make and sustain healthy actions and equip them with the skills to exercise choice. It may include a wide range of activities at different levels. For the individual, it may involve advice on how to follow a treatment schedule. For the wider population, it may involve a campaign to raise awareness about the importance of physical activity. A main focus of health education is the modification of those aspects of behaviour that are known to impact on health. The process includes imparting knowledge, clarifying attitudes and developing skills. Simply conveying information about risks is not effective. People's health behaviour may be a response to, and maintained by, the environment in which they live. Understanding their health beliefs and their perceptions about their own susceptibility and the seriousness of the disease is an important task of health education.

Health promotion
Health promotion is an umbrella term used to describe any measure aimed at health improvement in individuals, communities or the population as a whole. The health improvement may increase the length of life or the number of years people spend free of illness and it may narrow the health gap between the worst and better-off in society. Health promotion embraces many approaches including education and information to enable people to make informed decisions about healthy ways of living; personal counselling to support people to make changes in their health behaviour; legislative and fiscal measures and developing the capacity of communities to become involved in health decisions affecting them. The World Health Organization (WHO 1986) identified the broad components of a health promotion strategy as building public policy, creating supportive environments for health, strengthening community action, developing personal skills and reorienting health services from treatment to prevention.

Reference
World Health Organization 1986 Ottawa Charter for Health Promotion. World Health Organization, Geneva

hearing impairment ⇒ deafness. See Box – Hearing impairment.

heart *n* the hollow muscular organ which pumps the blood around the general and pulmonary ciculations. It is situated in the mediastinum behind the sternum. It is roughly cone-shaped, with its base uppermost and the apex inclined to the left. It is about the size of the owner's fist and weighs around 300 g. It is divided into a right and left side by the septum and has four chambers: two upper receiving chambers – the atria, and two large lower pumping chambers – the ventricles. The heart has three layers: the outer serous pericardium, a middle of cardiac muscle (myocardium) and an endothelial lining (endothelium). Valves control the flow of blood between the atria and ventricles; bicuspid on the left and tricuspid on the right, and semilunar valves prevent backflow from the pulmonary artery and aorta (see Figure 29). *heart block* partial or complete block to the passage of impulses through the conducting system. *heart failure* ⇒ cardiac failure. ⇒ congestive cardiac failure. *heart transplant* surgical transplantation of a heart from a suitable donor. May be combined with a lung transplant.

heartburn *n* lay term describing the burning sensation at the lower end of the oesophagus, due to reflux of acidic gastric contents. → pyrosis.

heart-lung machine ⇒ cardiopulmonary bypass. → extracorporeal.

heat exhaustion (*syn* heat syncope) collapse, with or without loss of consciousness, suffered in conditions of heat and high humidity; largely resulting from loss of fluid and electrolytes by sweating. If the surrounding air becomes saturated, heatstroke will ensue.

heatstroke *n* (*syn* sunstroke) final stage in heat exhaustion. When the body is unable to lose heat, hyperpyrexia occurs and death may ensue.

heat treatment the application of heat to a part of the body; either dry, in the form of an electric pad or poultice, or moist, in the form of a compress wrung out of hot water or an immersion bath.

hebephrenia *n* a common type of schizophrenia characterized by a general disintegration of the personality. The onset is sudden and usually occurs in the teenage years. There is thought disorder, and symptoms include meaningless behaviour, inappropriate emotional responses such as laughter, peculiar mannerisms, incoherent talk, and delusions — **hebephrenic** *adj*.

Heberden's node small osseous swellings at terminal phalangeal joints occurring in many types of arthritis.

hedonism *n* excessive devotion to pleasure, so that a person's conduct is determined by an unconscious drive to seek pleasure and avoid unpleasant things.

Hegar's sign marked softening of the cervix in early pregnancy.

Hearing Impairment

Hearing impairment results from hearing loss. Individuals can experience hearing loss at any time during their life. The most common causes of hearing loss are 'glue ear' which occurs most often in childhood resulting in a temporary and fluctuating conductive hearing loss, and presbycusis which is a permanent sensorineural hearing loss associated with ageing.

Facilitating communication with all hearing impaired individuals

- Make sure you are in front of, fairly close to, and on the same level as the hearing impaired person;
- Position yourself with your face to the light and avoid placing yourself in front of a bright window;
- Reduce background noise;
- Do not shout;
- Speak clearly and maintain normal rhythm of speech;
- Sentences are easier to understand than individual words;
- Stop talking if you turn away;
- Keep hands, pens and so forth away from your face while speaking;
- If the hearing impaired individual is accompanied by a hearing person, avoid conversing with the hearing person and ignoring the hearing impaired person;
- Make sure the hearing impaired person is looking at you before you begin to speak.

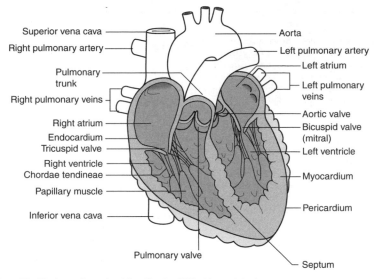

Superior vena cava
Right pulmonary artery
Pulmonary trunk
Right pulmonary veins
Right atrium
Endocardium
Tricuspid valve
Right ventricle
Chordae tendineae
Papillary muscle
Inferior vena cava
Pulmonary valve

Aorta
Left pulmonary artery
Left atrium
Left pulmonary veins
Aortic valve
Bicuspid valve (mitral)
Left ventricle
Myocardium
Pericardium
Septum

Figure 29 The heart. (Reproduced from Brooker 1996 with permission.)

Heimlich manoeuvre abdominal thrusts. An emergency technique to remove a foreign body from upper part of lower respiratory tract. It is achieved by a forceful compression of the upper abdomen.

Heinz body irregularly-shaped body present in red blood cells in some haemolytic anaemias and haemoglobinopathies.

Helicobacter pylori *n* a Gram-negative bacterium that causes gastric inflammation. The presence of the bacteria is associated with gastritis, peptic ulceration and possibly gastric cancer. It is transmitted by the oral-faecal and oral-oral routes and many people are asymptomatic carriers. Eradication involves a combination of drugs: bismuth, metronidazole, tetracycline or amoxicillin (amoxycillin) and a H_2-receptor antagonist, such as ranitidine. The administration of a proton pump inhibitor, e.g. omeprazole, aids the healing process.

helium *n* an inert gas. Medical uses include: the dilution of other gases and pulmonary function tests.

helix 1. spiral. Describes the structure of molecules, such as DNA. **2.** the outer ridge of the pinna of the outer ear.

Heller's operation *n* division of the muscle coat at the junction between the oesophagus and the stomach; used to relieve the difficulty in swallowing in cases of achalasia.

helminthiasis *n* the condition resulting from infestation with parasitic worms.

helminthology *n* the study of parasitic worms.

hemeralopia *n* day blindness; poor vision in bright light that improves in dim light.

hemianopia *n* blindness in one half of the visual field of one or both eyes.

hemiatrophy *n* atrophy of one half or one side. *hemiatrophy facialis* a congenital condition, or a manifestation of scleroderma in which the structures on one side of the face are shrunken.

hemichorea *n* choreiform movements limited to one side of the body. ⇒ chorea.

hemicolectomy *n* removal of approximately half the colon.

hemicrania *n* unilateral headache, as in migraine.

hemidiaphoresis *n* unilateral sweating of the body.

hemiglossectomy *n* removal of approximately half the tongue.

hemiparesis *n* a paralysis or weakness of one half of face or body.

hemiplegia *n* paralysis of one side of the body, usually resulting from a cerebrovascular accident on the opposite side — **hemiplegic** *adj.*

Henderson definition of nursing a much used definition of nursing, put forward by Virginia Henderson in 1969. The unique function of the nurse is to assist the individual, sick or well, in the performance of those activities contributing to health or recovery (or to a peaceful death) that the person would perform unaided if he or she had the necessary strength, will or knowledge, and to do this in such a way as to help him or her gain independence as rapidly as possible.

Henderson-Hasselbalch equation *n* the equation that explains how the ratio between a weak acid and weak alkali influences the pH of a solution, e.g. blood.

$pH = 6.1 + \log[HCO_3^-]$ hydrogen carbonate / $[CO_2]$ carbon dioxide in solution.

Henle's loop part of the renal tubule, important in the production of variable concentration urine. ⇒ nephron.

Henoch-Schönlein purpura (anaphylactoid purpura) *n* a small vessel vasculitis, mainly affecting children. It is due to hypersensitivity which may follow a streptococcal respiratory infection, or a drug allergy, but it may be idiopathic. Immune complexes are formed which damage capillaries in the skin, gut and elsewhere. It is characterized by purpuric bleeding into the skin, particularly shins and buttocks, and from the wall of the gut, resulting in abdominal colic and rectal bleeding; and bruising around joints with arthritis. The vasculitis may involve the kidneys, leading to haematuria, proteinuria, acute glomerulonephritis, nephrotic syndrome or acute renal failure.

Henry's law states that the amount of gas dissolving in a fluid is proportional to its partial pressure and solubility at a constant temperature.

hepadnaviruses *npl* a family of DNA viruses that include the hepatitis B virus (HBV).

hepar *n* the liver — **hepatic** *adj.*

heparin *n* a group of naturally occurring anticoagulant substances produced by mast cells and present in liver and lung tissue. In the body it is concerned with preventing inappropriate blood coagulation. Used therapeutically, it inhibits blood coagulation in several ways; primarily by the prevention of fibrin formation by inhibiting thrombin activity and the activity of other coagulation factors, and altering platelet aggregation. Heparin is used in the management of thromboembolic conditions, such as deep vein thrombosis and in prophylaxis, e.g. perioperatively. Heparin is given by intravenous or subcutaneous injection. A side-effect of therapy is haemorrhage. The effects of heparin can be reversed with the antidote protamine sulphate. *low molecular weight heparin* given subcutaneously it has a more sustained action and fewer side-effects. ⇒ coagulation.

hepatectomy *n* excision of the liver, or more usually part of the liver.

hepatic *adj* pertaining to the liver. *hepatic ducts* two main bile ducts draining bile from the liver.

hepatic encephalopathy there is impaired function of the central nervous system due to liver disease (cirrhosis and fulminant hepatic failure) which prevents detoxication of many chemicals, particularly nitrogenous substances. It is characterized by changes to emotions, behaviour, intellect and consciousness, and convulsions, flapping tremor and a 'mousy' odour of the breath (fetor hepaticus) is usually present. Nursing aims to keep the person as reality oriented as possible and prevent the potential problems of accident, infection, injury, malnutrition and pressure ulcers from becoming actual ones. Management involves the restriction of dietary protein, oral neomycin to reduce the bowel flora responsible for producing nitrogenous chemicals, and oral lactulose helps to decrease intestinal ammonia production.

hepatic portal circulation *n* that of venous blood from the gastrointestinal tract, pancreas and spleen to the liver before return to the heart.

hepatic portal hypertension increased pressure in the hepatic portal vein. Usually caused by cirrhosis of the liver; results in splenomegaly, with hypersplenism and alimentary bleeding. ⇒ oesophageal varices.

hepatic portal vein *n* conveying blood into the liver, it is about 75 mm long and is formed by the union of the superior mesenteric and splenic veins.

hepaticocholedochostomy *n* end-to-end union of the severed hepatic and common bile ducts.

hepaticoenteric *adj* pertaining to the liver and intestine.

hepaticojejunostomy *n* anastomosis of the common hepatic duct to a loop of proximal jejunum.

hepaticolenticular *adj* pertaining to the liver and the lentiform nucleus (one of the basal nuclei). ⇒ Wilson's disease.

hepatitis *n* inflammation of the liver, commonly associated with viral infection but can be due to toxic agents, such as alcohol, drugs and chemicals, or metabolic disorders, e.g. Wilson's disease. The onset is usually accompanied by vague symptoms, such as loss of appetite, nausea, vomiting and general fatigue. As the disease progresses, the patient becomes jaundiced and develops abdominal tenderness and pain in the right upper quadrant. Hepatitis is currently a serious public health problem. It is associated with a number of hepatitis viral types, most commonly hepatitis-A virus (HAV), hepatitis-B virus (HBV), hepatitis-C virus (HCV) and hepatitis-D virus (delta virus). Other types of hepatitis identified include: hepatitis-E virus, hepatitis-F virus and hepatitis-G virus. *hepatitis-A* caused by an RNA enterovirus of the family *Picornaviruses*. Relatively common and may be epidemic, especially in institutions, e.g. schools. The incubation period is short (10–50 days) and the virus is transmitted by the faeco-oral route, due to poor hygiene or contaminated food. Signs and symptoms range from mild to severe and occasionally can be fatal. *hepatitis-B* caused by a DNA virus of the family *Hepadnaviruses*. Long incubation period (40–160 days), usually transmitted sexually (vaginal or anal intercourse), injection of infected blood or blood products, or via contaminated equipment, e.g. needles. The virus is shed in saliva, semen and vaginal secretions. Those at high risk include: intravenous drug users, homosexual or bisexual men, prostitutes and healthcare professionals. Hepatitis-B virus may persist, causing chronic hepatitis, or a carrier state can develop. Virus particles carry the hepatitis-B surface antigen (HBsAg) and, at times when there is active viral replication, hepatitis B e antigen (HBeAg) can be detected free in the plasma, indicating a high degree of infectivity. An effective vaccine exists. *hepatitis-C* (previously called nonA, nonB hepatitis). It has an incubation period between 30–90 days. It is an RNA virus and is most common in intravenous drug users and in people who have had a transfusion of blood or blood products. Virus particles may remain in the blood for years and in 30–50% of infected people lead to chronic hepatitis, cirrhosis, liver failure and possibly cancer of the liver. The carrier state also exists. *hepatitis-D (delta virus)* can only replicate in the presence of hepatitis-B and is therefore found infecting simultaneously with hepatitis-B, or as a superinfection in a person chronically carrying hepatitis-B. Delta virus may increase the severity of a hepatitis-B infection, increasing the risk of chronic liver disease. *hepatitis-E* is transmitted via the faeco-oral route. It has been reported in travellers returning from Asia, Africa, USA and Mexico.

hepatocellular *adj* pertaining to or affecting liver cells.

hepatocirrhosis *n* ⇒ cirrhosis.

hepatocyte *n* the parenchymal or functional cell type of the liver, it carries out the functions performed by the liver, e.g. synthesis, bile production, detoxification.

hepatoma *n* primary carcinoma of the liver — **hepatomata** *pl*.

hepatomegaly *n* enlargement of the liver, palpable below the costal margin.

hepatorenal syndrome *n* renal failure resulting from cirrhosis and hepatic failure.

hepatosplenic *adj* pertaining to the liver and spleen.

hepatosplenomegaly *n* enlargement of the liver and the spleen, so that each is palpable below the costal margin.

hepatotoxic *adj* having an injurious effect on liver cells, such as alcohol — **hepatotoxicity** *n*.

herbalism *n* the therapeutic use of herbs or mineral remedies. The use of plant material by trained practitioners to promote health and recovery from illness.

hereditary *adj* inherited; capable of being inherited.

heredity *n* transmission from parents to offspring of genetic characteristics and traits by means of the genetic material; the process by which this occurs, and its study.

Hering-Breuer reflex *n* a stretch reflex that prevents lung overinflation. It operates through the vagus nerve and causes a short period of apnoea if the lungs are overinflated. Probably only significant as a protective mechanism in adults, but for newborns it may be an important control of ventilation.

hermaphrodite *n* individual possessing both ovarian and testicular tissue. May be associated with an ambiguity of the external genitalia.

hermaphroditism ⇒ intersexuality.

hermetic *adj* sealed by fusion to make airtight. Such a seal ensures that a wound is not exposed to air.

hernia *n* the abnormal protrusion of an organ, or part of an organ, through an aperture in the surrounding structures; commonly the protrusion of an abdominal organ through a 'weak spot' in the abdominal wall. *diaphragmatic hernia* (*syn* hiatus hernia) protrusion through the diaphragm, the commonest one, involving the stomach at the oesophageal opening. *femoral hernia* protrusion through the femoral canal, alongside the femoral blood vessels as they pass into the thigh. *incisional hernia* protrusion through an abdominal wound. *inguinal hernia* protrusion through the inguinal canal. *irreducible hernia* when the contents of the sac cannot be returned to the appropriate cavity without surgical intervention. *strangulated hernia* hernia in which the blood supply to the organ involved is impaired, usually due to constriction by surrounding structures. *umbilical hernia* (*syn* omphalocele) protrusion of a portion of intestine through the area of the umbilical scar.

herniation *n* the formation of a hernia; rupture.

hernioplasty *n* an operation for hernia in which an attempt is made to prevent recurrence by refashioning the structures to give greater strength — **hernioplastic** *adj*.

herniorrhaphy *n* an operation for hernia in which the weak area is reinforced by some of the patient's own tissues or by some other material.

herniotomy *n* an operation to cure hernia by the return of its contents to their normal position and removal of the hernial sac.

heroin *n* diamorphine. It is addictive and subject to considerable criminal misuse. ⇒ controlled drug. ⇒ drug.

herpangina *n* minute vesicles and ulcers at the back of the palate. Short, febrile form of pharyngitis in children, caused by a coxsackie virus.

herpes *n* a vesicular eruption due to infection with herpes simplex virus (HSV) types 1 and 2. HSV-1 usually causes skin ulceration around the mouth, but can cause genital herpes. HSV-2, a related virus, usually infects the genitalia. It produces genital herpes with lesions, dysuria and systemic illness. Spread is usually through sexual contact, but infants born to infected women may be affected. In the female, ulcers and vesicles can occur on the cervix, vagina and labia. The presence of HSV-2 infection correlates with cervical malignancy, but any link remains unproven. In the male, the lesions occur on the glans, prepuce and penile shaft and less commonly on the scrotum. In both sexes, lesions may be seen on the pharynx, thighs, buttocks and perianal regions. *herpes gestationis* a rare skin disease peculiar to pregnancy. It clears in about 30 days after delivery. ⇒ cytomegalovirus. → Epstein-Barr virus.

herpes simplex virus (HSV) consists of two biologically and immunologically distinct types designated Type 1, which generally causes oral disease and lesions above the waist, and Type 2, most commonly associated with genital disease and lesions below the waist. Recurrent episodes are common as the virus remains latent in nerve ganglia after the initial infection. → herpes.

herpesviruses *npl* group of DNA viruses that include: herpes simplex virus (HSV) type 1 and 2, varicella/zoster virus (VZV), Epstein-Barr virus (EBV), human herpesvirus 6 (HHV6) and cytomegalovirus (CMV).

herpes zoster *n* caused by varicella/zoster virus (VZV), which also causes chickenpox. Affects the sensory nerves causing pain and skin eruption along the course of the nerve. Also known as shingles.

herpetiform *adj* resembling herpes.

hertz (Hz) *n* the derived SI unit (International System of Units) for wave frequency. It equals one cycle per second.

hesitancy *n* a delay in starting to pass urine, even when responding to a strong desire to void. A symptom of outflow obstruction, such as in prostatic enlargement.

Hess test a sphygmomanometer cuff is applied to the arm and is inflated. Petechial eruption in the surrounding area after 5 min denotes weakness of the capillary walls, characteristic of purpura.

heterogenous *adj* of unlike origin; not originating within the body; derived from a different species. ⇒ homogenous *ant*.

heterograft *n* ⇒ xenograft.

heterologous *adj* of different origin; from a different species. ⇒ homologous *ant*.

heterophile *n* a product of one species which acts against that of another, e.g. human antigen against sheep's red blood cells.

heterosexual *adj, n* literally, of different sexes; used to describe a person who is sexually attracted towards the opposite sex. ⇒ homosexual *ant*.

heterozygous *adj* having different genes or alleles at the same locus on both chromosomes of a pair (one of maternal and the other of paternal origin). ⇒ homozygous *ant*.

HEV *abbr* hepatitis E virus.

hexose *n* a class of simple sugars. A six carbon monosaccharide, such as glucose, mannose, galactose.

HGH *abbr* human growth hormone. ⇒ growth hormone.

hiatus *n* a space or opening. *hiatus hernia* ⇒ hernia — **hiatal** *adj*.

Hib vaccine *abbr* Haemophilus influenzae type B vaccine. An injectable vaccine offered to infants at 2, 3 and 4 months as protection against the serious respiratory infection, epiglottitis, otitis media and meningitis caused by *Haemophilus influenzae*.

hiccough *n* (*syn* hiccup). Repeated spasmodic inspiration associated with diaphragmatic contraction, a sudden closure of the glottis with the production of a characteristic sound. Mainly mild and transient, but can be painful after surgery. When they occur over long periods, the person is unable to eat and drink or sleep and may become exhausted.

hiccup ⇒ hiccough.

Hickman line a type of central venous catheter designed for long term use, commonly used to deliver chemotherapy or total parenteral nutrition.

hidrosis *n* sweat secretion.

Higginson's syringe a rubber bulb with tubes leading to and from it. One tube rested in a container of fluid, e.g. saline. Compression of the bulb forced fluid through the nozzle of the other tube for irrigation of a body cavity. Rarely used and now mostly replaced by single-use items of equipment.

high-density lipoprotein (HDL) *n* ⇒ lipoprotein.

high dependency unit (HDU) *n* a unit that provides specialist monitoring and care to patients requiring more care than is available on general wards, but who do not require intensive care. ⇒ intensive care unit.

higher level practice (advanced) see Box – Higher level practice. ⇒ specialist nursing practice.

hilum *n* a depression on the surface of an organ where vessels, ducts and nerves etc enter and leave, such as the hilum of the lung — **hilar** *adj* hilar adenitis ⇒ adenitis.

HImP *abbr* Health Improvement Programme.

hindgut an embryonic structure destined to become part of the small and large bowel and other structures.

hip bone innominate bone formed by the fusion of three separate bones: the ilium, ischium and pubis.

hip joint articulation of the head of femur within the acetabulum to form a synovial, freely movable joint. *hip replacement* ⇒ arthroplasty.

hip replacement ⇒ arthroplasty.

hip spica enclosure of the lower trunk and one (single spica) or both (double spica) lower limb(s) in a plaster cast. ⇒ spica.

Hippocrates *n* Greek physician and philosopher (460–367 BC) who established a school of medicine. He is often termed the 'Father of Medicine'.

Higher level practice
The UKCC has stated that "the nature, organization and delivery of health care is changing and the professional practice of nurses, midwives and health visitors across the United Kingdom will continue to evolve in response to the needs of those in their care." (UKCC 1999). George Castledine, Chair of the UKCC Higher level practice steering group, suggests that "the UKCC recognizes that the issues associated with role developments ..... are complex and have been a concern to the public, employers and the professions."

Practitioners working at a higher level of practice not only use their original knowledge and skills as a basis on which to develop practice, but demonstrate that this development includes their understanding of much wider issues including the implications of the social, economic and political context of health care. More importantly, practitioners working at this level then have the capacity and ability to bring about change and development within their own and others' practice and within the services and environments in which they work.

After extensive consultation, the UKCC identified seven key themes, all of which practitioners claiming 'higher level practice' must demonstrate evidence to support their claim. The key elements are:

- Providing effective health care;
- Improving quality and health outcomes;
- Evaluation and research;
- Leading and developing practice;
- Innovation and changing practice;
- Developing self and others;
- Working across professional and organizational boundaries.

The standards and assessment processes have been piloted amongst volunteers from across the nursing and midwifery professions encompassing the whole of the UK, and across all disciplines. The results of the pilot were reported to the council in June 2001.

Reference
UKCC 1999 A Higher Level of Practice. Report of the consultation on the UKCC's proposals for a revised regulatory framework for post-registration clinical practice. UKCC, London

Hirschsprung's disease congenital intestinal aganglionosis, leading to intractable constipation or even intestinal obstruction. There is marked hypertrophy and dilation of the colon (megacolon) above the aganglionic segment. There is an association with Down's syndrome. Treatment involves surgical removal of the aganglionic segment. ⇒ aganglionosis.

hirsute *adj* hairy or shaggy.

hirsuties, hirsutism *n* excessive growth of hair in sites in which body hair is normally found. ⇒ hypertrichosis.

hirudin *n* a substance secreted by the medicinal leech, which prevents the clotting of blood by acting as an antithrombin.

hirudo *n* ⇒ leech.

histamine *n* an amine released in a variety of tissues where it causes smooth muscle constriction, gastric secretion and vasodilation. Its release from mast cells as part of the inflammatory response leads to capillary dilatation and increased vessel permeability. ⇒ allergy. ⇒ inflammatory. *histamine receptors* there are three types in the body, H_1 in the bronchial muscle, H_2 in the secreting cells in the stomach and H_3 present in neural tissue. In humans the main effects of histamine on the different receptors include: H_1 – smooth muscle contraction, apart from that in blood vessels, vasodilatation and increased permeability, and H_2 – gastric secretion and an increase in heart rate and output. *histamine test* test previously used to determine the maximal gastric secretion of hydrochloric acid.

histidine *n* an amino acid. Essential (indispensable) during childhood.

histiocytes *npl* phagocytic tissue cells. More commonly known as macrophages.

histiocytosis X *n* a rare disorder of the monocyte-macrophage system (reticuloendothelial system) in which there is an abnormal proliferation of histiocytes associated with local inflammatory reaction. Clinical features depend upon the organs or tissues involved. Three classical syndromes have been described: eosinophilic granuloma of bone, Hand-Schüller-Christian disease, and Letterer-Siwe disease. Treatment varies according to the type of disease. Local lesions may be excised or treated with radiotherapy; cytotoxic therapy may be required for more severe forms of the disease.

histogram a bar chart. Graphical representation of variables plotted against frequency or time.

histology *n* microscopic study of tissues — **histologically** *adv.*

histolysis *n* disintegration of organic tissue — **histolytic** *adj.*

histones *npl* a special set of proteins closely associated with the chromosomal DNA of higher organisms, which coils and supercoils around histone molecules. These are therefore part of the way the DNA is organized to form the chromosomes.

histopathology the study of disease involving tissues.

histoplasmosis *n* an infection caused by inhaling spores of the fungus *Histoplasma capsulatum.* The primary lung lesion may go unnoticed or be accompanied by fever, malaise, cough and adenopathy. Progressive histoplasmosis can be fatal.

histrionic personality disorder tends to be characterized by a person who needs to be physically attractive and have the interest of others, and they will act in ways that ensure that they are the centre of attention. They can be manipulative, easily influenced and self indulgent. Their moods are labile and emotions tend to be dramatized.

HIV *abbr* human immunodeficiency virus. ⇒ acquired immune deficiency syndrome.

hives *n* nettlerash; urticaria.

HLA *abbr* human leucocyte antigens. ⇒ major histocompatibility complex (MHC).

HMG-CoA reductase inhibitors *npl* 3-hydroxy-3-methylglutaryl-coenzyme A. Group of drugs used to reduce blood cholesterol level by inhibiting its synthesis in the. liver, e.g. pravastatin, simvastatin. Known colloquially as 'statins', they are used in the management of the hyperlipidaemias.

hoarseness *n* roughness of voice which can have many causes from laryngitis (acute or chronic) to cancer. Where no improvement occurs, patients are advised to consult a doctor because a cancer may be present. Nurses can offer steam inhalations and provide alternative means of communication to rest the larynx.   ·

hobnail liver firm nodular liver which may be found in cirrhosis.

Hodgkin's disease ⇒ lymphoma.

holistic *adj* relating to the theory of holism. It considers that individuals function as a whole rather than as separate parts or systems. Holistic nursing care takes account of physical, psychological, emotional, social and spiritual aspects. ⇒ total patient care.

Homans' sign passive dorsiflexion of foot causes pain in calf muscles. Indicative of incipient or established venous thrombosis of leg.

home assessment made by an occupational therapist to evaluate the home environment and determine the need for adaptations or services.

home carers previously called home helps. Important members of social services community care teams who provide care for older and/or disabled people living in their own homes, in bathing, dressing, shopping and cooking meals. Less likely than formerly to do domestic work. A charge for home care services is usually made.

home page the first page or starting point of an internet web site. ⇒ internet. ⇒ web site.

home visit made by an occupational therapist to a client's home to assess or provide services. *predischarge home visit* the occupational therapist takes a hospital patient home in order to assess the person's level of independence and ability to cope in the home environment. The individual returns to hospital whilst appropriate arrangements can be made to facilitate discharge.

homeostasis *n* body equilibrium. The autoregulatory processes that maintain a stable internal body environment. Controls functions such as blood pressure, body temperature and electrolytes which are maintained within set parameters — **homeostatic** *adj* pertaining to homeostasis. *homeostatic control* operates through receptors, control area and effectors. Communication between the components is neural or hormonal. (See Figure 30).

homicide *n* killing of another person: manslaughter (culpable homicide in Scotland) if accidental, murder if intentional. See Box – Homicide and euthanasia.

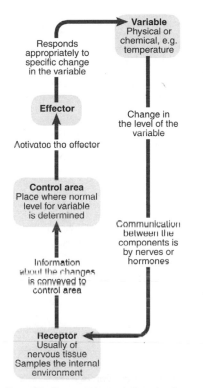

Figure 30 Homeostatic control. (Reproduced from Brooker 1998 with permission.)

The diagram labels:

- **Variable** Physical or chemical, e.g. temperature
- Responds appropriately to specific change in the variable
- **Effector**
- Activates the effector
- Change in the level of the variable
- **Control area** Place where normal level for variable is determined
- Communication between the components is by nerves or hormones
- Information about the changes is conveyed to control area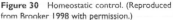
- **Receptor** Usually of nervous tissue Samples the internal environment

homocysteine *n* an intermediate which reacts with serine to form cysteine. It is also a precursor for methionine regeneration in reactions requiring folates and cobalamins. A deficiency in folates is associated with increased homocysteine level in the blood and an increased risk of CHD.

homocystinuria *n* recessively inherited inborn error of metabolism. There is excretion of homocystine (a sulphur-containing amino acid, homologue of cystine) in the urine. Gives rise to slow development of varying degree; associated with lens dislocation, overgrowth of long bones, osteoporosis, pathological features, widespread vascular thrombosis, and other symptoms. May be diagnosed by a biochemical screening test — **homocystinuric** *adj*.

homoeopathy *n* a method of treating illness and disease by prescribing minute amounts of medicines or remedies to stimulate the body's own healing mechanisms. See Box = Homoeopathy. → allopathic — **homoeopathic** *adj*.

homogeneous *adj* of the same kind; of the same quality or consistency throughout.

homogenize *vt* to make into the same consistency throughout.

Homicide and euthanasia

Homicide is the act of killing a human being and includes murder, manslaughter and infanticide. Murder is a death of a person (which does not include a fetus) resulting from an act where the perpetrator intended to kill or do serious harm. There is no longer a time limit that death should occur within a year and a day from the act. (Law Reform (Year and a Day Rule) Act 1996) If a health professional carries out an act intended to shorten the life of a person, then that would constitute murder. A conviction for murder is followed by a sentence of life imprisonment. The fact that recognized and medically supported treatment may incidentally shorten the life of a patient will not amount to the crime of murder if the treatment is given in the patient's interests to relieve pain and suffering. (R. v. Bodkin Adams [1957] Crim LR 365)

Homicide that does not amount to murder may be manslaughter. Manslaughter can be voluntary, i.e. there was the mental intention to kill or cause serious harm but there are certain mitigating circumstances which prevent a charge of murder arising, e.g. diminished responsibility, death in a suicide pact or provocation. Involuntary manslaughter exists where there was no intention on the part of the accused to cause death or serious harm, but the accused has acted with such gross recklessness or negligence as to the safety of the victim that it amounts to the criminal offence of manslaughter. (R. v Adomako [1994] 5 Med LR 27)

Whilst it is unlawful to carry out any act to shorten the life of a person, care can be withheld where there is no longer a duty in law to continue intrusive life support of a patient. (Airedale NHS Trust v. Bland [1993] 1 All ER 821) The law therefore distinguishes between killing and letting die. Euthanasia is not recognized as lawful in this country.

To attempt to commit suicide ceased to be unlawful following Section 1 of the Suicide Act 1961 but a person who aids, abets, counsels or procures the suicide of another or an attempt by another to commit suicide would be guilty of an offence under Section 2.

Homoeopathy

Homoeopathy is based upon a *Law of Similars* – let like be cured with like. Whilst this principle can be found in the writings of Hippocrates in the 5th century BC, the founding father of homoeopathy is generally accepted to be Samuel Hahnemann who worked in the 18th century.

Hahnemann experimented upon himself to discover that doses of quinine used to treat malaria could produce malaria-like effects. He concluded that it was this reaction that made it effective against the disease. His subsequent work pursued this theory observing that the more a remedy was diluted, the more specific the effect. Homeopathic remedies were termed *Nosodes* produced to counteract miasma, alleged weaknesses that impede an individual's response to treatment (Woodham & Peters 1997). Isopathic treatment used remedies that cause like illnesses – a concept not dissimilar to immunization. For example, minute doses of pollen may be given to treat hay fever.

Homoeopathic medicines or remedies are produced from a range of natural sources, for example plants, venoms, minerals or bacteria. Effectiveness results from the process by which remedies are made. The original substances are diluted many times in a water and alcohol base. At each dilution the mixture is shaken vigorously. This process is known as succussion, which homoeopaths believe enhances the healing potential of side-effects (or aggravations) although some patients may still experience these (Woodham & Peters 1997).

Homoeopathy seeks to work by attempting to reharmonize health by stimulating the vital force in order to maintain health. In the 17th century, the concept of *Vitalism* predominated – the notion that a vital force regulated the body and maintained it in a state of health. Illness is the result of an imbalance of the vital force. Homoeopaths perceive symptoms as the body's attempt to restore health, for example pyrexia is a result of the body's attempt to fight infection. Treatment is to redress the balance of health by stimulating the body's innate predisposition towards health rather than to treat symptoms.

For many years critics have attributed the success of homoeopathy treatment to the placebo effect. However, increasing research particularly in the field of veterinary medicine seems to suggest otherwise (Atherton 1995). Currently there is no definitive rationale explaining how homoeopathy works. One theory is that of 'water memory' whereby an electromagnetic imprint or memory of the original substance is retained through each dilution. This may be similar to the way in which a drop of water retains an ability to recreate a unique symmetrical pattern when frozen (as a snow flake) despite having been diluted in lakes, waterfalls or turned into water vapor. However, more research is needed to substantiate such claims.

References
Atherton K 1995 Homoeopathy. In: Rankin-Box D (ed) The Nurses' Handbook of Complementary Therapies. Churchill Livingstone, Edinburgh
Woodham A, Peters D (eds) 1997 Encyclopedia of Complementary Medicine. Dorling Kindersley, London

homogenous *adj* having a like nature, e.g. a tissue graft from another human being. ⇒ heterogenous *ant.*

homograft *n* ⇒ allograft.

homolateral *adj* on the same side.

homologous *adj* corresponding in origin and structure. ⇒ heterologous *ant.* *homologous chromosomes* those that pair during reduction division (meiosis) whereby mature gametes are formed.

homonymous *adj* consisting of corresponding halves.

homosexual *adj, n* literally, of the same sex; used to describe a person who is sexually attracted to a member of the same sex. Homosexuals themselves prefer to be called 'gay' or 'lesbian'. Male homosexuals who have unprotected sex are at particular risk of contracting infection with hepatitis B virus (HBV), cytomegalovirus (CMV), Epstein-Barr virus (EBV), human immunodeficiency virus (HIV). ⇒ heterosexual *ant.*

homosexuality *n* attraction for, and desire to establish an emotional and sexual relationship with, a member of the same sex.

homozygous *adj* having identical genes or alleles in the same locus on both chromosomes of a pair (one of maternal and the other of paternal origin). ⇒ heterozygous *ant.*

HoNOS *abbr* Health of the Nation Outcome Scale.

hookworm *n* ⇒ Ancylostoma.

hoop traction fixed skin traction used in the management of fractures of the femur in children. It is also used to achieve gradual abduction of the hip in children with developmental dysplasia of the hip.

hordeolum *n* ⇒ stye.

hormone *n* specific chemical messengers secreted by an endocrine gland and conveyed in the blood or lymph to regulate the functions of tissues and organs elsewhere in the body. They are usually steroids, or amino acid based, but other substances can act as hormones. ⇒ paracrines.

hormone replacement therapy (HRT) generally applied to the oestrogen treatment given to women for the relief of menopausal symptoms and the prevention of osteoporosis. Women with an intact uterus should also be prescribed progesterone to prevent endometrial hyperplasia. Hormone replacement is administered orally, transdermally by patch or gel, or by implant.

Horner's syndrome clinical picture following paralysis of cervical sympathetic nerves on one side. There is miosis (myosis), slight ptosis with enophthalmos, facial vasodilation with anhidrosis. Caused by apical bronchial cancers and brainstem lesions.

Horton's syndrome severe headache due to the release of histamine in the body. To be differentiated from migraine.

hospice care *n* system of care available to the chronically or terminally ill person and their family. It is designed specially for the purpose of family-centred care and may involve care at home, in a day unit and in the actual hospice premises. The multidisciplinary team have experience and special expertise in caring for people, their family and friends at the end of life. Patient and family participation is encouraged and individualized symptom (especially pain) control programmes are implemented. The aim is to minimize the physical, emotional and spiritual problems and reduce distress.

hospital acquired infection (HAI) ⇒ infection.

Hospital Sterilization and Disinfection Units (HSDU) central sterile supply units (CSSUs) which have extended their work to include disinfection of equipment.

host *n* the organic structure upon which parasites or bacteria thrive. *intermediate host* one in which the parasite passes its larval or cystic stage.

hot-fat heartburn syndrome due to reflux from stomach to oesophagus producing hypersensitivity in the oesophageal mucosa; tends to be worse after fatty or fried food or drinking coffee. May be associated with hiatus hernia.

hour-glass contraction a circular constriction in the middle of a hollow organ (usually the stomach or uterus), dividing it into two portions following scar formation.

housemaid's knee ⇒ bursitis.

HPV *abbr* ⇒ human papilloma viruses.

HRS *abbr* Hallucinations Rating Scale.

HRT *abbr* hormone replacement therapy.

HSDU *abbr* hospital sterilization and disinfection unit.

HSV *abbr* herpes simplex virus.

5-HT₃-receptor antagonists *npl* antiemetic drugs that block 5-hydroxytryptamine receptors, e.g. ondansetron, used for the vomiting associated with cytotoxic drugs.

HTLV *abbr* human T-cell lymphotropic viruses.

HTML *abbr* for hyper text markup language. Language used to write pages on most web sites. ⇒ web site.

human chorionic gonadotrophin (hCG) a hormone produced by the trophoblast cells and later the chorion. ⇒ chorionic gonadotrophin. Used therapeutically for cryptorchism, and sometimes for female infertility. Also a tumour marker for testicular and chorion cancer.

human immunodeficiency viruses (HIV) retroviruses. Currently designates the AIDS virus. There are two types: HIV-1 (many strains), responsible for HIV disease in North America, Western Europe and Central Africa, and HIV-2, causing similar disease in West Africa.

human leucocyte antigens (HLA) *npl* human major histocompatibility complexes, so called because they were first described on leucocytes.

human needs the concept has been widely used in nursing; it is based on Maslow's analysis of human needs. The basic physiological needs for food, breathing and eliminating are at the bottom of the hierarchy and have to be at least minimally fulfilled before motivation is established to deal with safety and security needs; then love and belonging, and self-esteem needs are attended to; and at the top level, achievement of self-actualization brings satisfaction with living and a sense of fulfilment.

human papilloma viruses (HPV) belong to a group of wart viruses affecting human beings. HPV_{16} and HPV_{18} are implicated in genital warts and cervical cancer.

human T-cell lymphotropic viruses (HTLV) retroviruses. There are two types: HTLV-1 and HTLV-2, both of which are associated with some forms of leukaemia.

human tetanus antitoxin immunoglobulin that confers artificial passive immunity in situations where there is a risk of tetanus. It should be in addition to proper wound toilet, tetanus toxoid vaccine and antimicrobial drugs, such as penicillin.

humanism *n* humanism is a philosophical movement which focuses on the nature and essence of the human individual. It explores and promotes the central importance of the human individual and has underpinned the reasonings behind human rights movements, patients' rights campaigns and patient-centred approaches to health care. It is one of the main philosophical movements underlying current theories of nursing practice.

humerus *n* the bone of the upper arm, between the elbow and shoulder joint — **humeral** *adj*.

humidity *n* the amount of moisture in the atmosphere, as measured by a hygrometer. *relative humidity* the ratio of the amount of moisture present in the air to the amount which would saturate it (at the same temperature).

humor *n* any fluid of the body. ⇒ aqueous. ⇒ vitreous.

humoral immunity that part of the immune response initiated by B-lymphocytes and the production of antibodies (immunoglobulins). ⇒ immunity.

Hunter-Hurler syndrome ⇒ gargoylism.

Hunter's syndrome one of the mucopolysaccharidoses, designated Type II. A sex-linked recessive condition. ⇒ gargoylism.

Huntington's disease an inherited condition. The transmission is autosomal dominant affecting both sexes. The condition

usually appears in adult life (30s and 40s) and is caused by a destruction of the basal nuclei and a deficiency of the neurotransmitter GABA. It is characterized by choreiform movements, progressive dementia, sometimes seizures and eventual death. The management is based on symptom control and support for the person and their family and carers. Genetic testing and counselling is available for affected families. ⇒ chorea.

Hurler's syndrome one of the mucopolysaccharidoses; designated Type II. Inherited as an autosomal recessive trait. ⇒ gargoylism.

HUS *abbr* haemolytic uraemic syndrome.

Hutchinson's teeth defect of the upper central incisors (second dentition) which is part of the facies of congenital syphilis. The teeth are broader at the gum than at the cutting edge, with the latter showing an elliptical notch.

hyaline *adj* like glass; transparent, such as hyaline cartilage. ⇒ cartilage. *hyaline degeneration* degeneration of connective tissue especially that of blood vessels in which tissue takes on a homogenous or formless appearance. *hyaline membrane disease* ⇒ neonatal respiratory distress syndrome.

hyaloid *adj* resembling hyaline tissue. ⇒ hyaline. *hyaloid membrane* ⇒ membrane.

hyaluronic acid *n* mucopolysaccharide found in the extracellular matrix which holds cells together. Also a constituent of synovial fluid where it contributes to viscosity.

hyaluronidase *n* enzyme that breaks down hyaluronic acid. It is among the enzymes present in the acrosome from where its release by many spermatozoa allows one to penetrate and fertilize the oocyte. Hyaluronidase may be used therapeutically to improve the absorption and dispersion of some drugs or fluids administered parenterally.

hydatid cyst *n* the cyst formed by larvae of a tapeworm, *Echinococcus granulosa*, found in dogs and other canines. The encysted stage normally occurs in sheep but can occur in humans after eating with soiled hands from contact with dogs or infected sheep. The cysts are commonest in the liver, but also occur in the lungs, brain and bone; they grow slowly and only do damage by the space they occupy. If they leak, or become infected, urticaria and fever supervene and 'daughter' cysts can result. The treatment is surgical excision of cysts and anthelmintic drugs, e.g. albendazole, praziquantel.

hydatidiform *adj* pertaining to or resembling a hydatid cyst. *hydatidiform mole* a condition in which the chorionic villi of the placenta undergo cystic degeneration to form grape-like vesicles and the fetus is absorbed. The villi penetrate and destroy only the decidual layer of the uterus, but a hydatidiform mole may progress to become an invasive mole in which the villi penetrate the myometrium and can destroy the uterine wall and metastasize to the vagina or even the lungs and brain. It is associated with the secretion of high levels of human chorionic gonadotrophin (hCG) that is excreted in the urine. An invasive mole may convert to a choriocarcinoma.

hydraemia *n* a relative excess of plasma volume compared with cell volume of the blood; it is normally present in late pregnancy — **hydraemic** *adj.*

hydramnios *n* an excess of amniotic fluid. May be associated with multiple pregnancy, certain fetal abnormalites, such as oesophageal atresia, or maternal conditions.

hydrarthrosis *n* a collection of watery fluid in a joint cavity.

hydrate *vi* combine with water — **hydration** *n.*

hydroa *n* 1. a vesicular or bullous disease occurring in children. It affects exposed parts and probably results from photosensitivity. 2. sun-induced skin blistering and scarring in some forms of porphyria.

hydrocarbon *n* a compound formed from hydrogen and carbon.

hydrocele *n* a swelling containing clear fluid. Most often applied to the accumulation of serous fluid in the tunica vaginalis of the testis.

hydrocephalus *n* (*syn* 'water on the brain') an excess of cerebrospinal fluid inside the skull due to an obstruction to normal CSF circulation. It may be congenital, when it is often associated with spina bifida, or acquired, following infection, trauma or tumours. Treatment is usually based on diverting the excess fluid back to the circulation via various types of shunt. ⇒ Spitz-Holter valve. ⇒ ventriculoatrial shunt. ⇒ ventriculocisternostomy. ⇒ ventriculoperitoneal shunt — **hydrocephalic** *adj.*

hydrochloric acid *n* an acid formed from hydrogen and chlorine. It is secreted by the gastric oxyntic cells.

hydrocolloid dressings *npl* absorbent dressings available in sheets and shaped for heels and sacral area. They form a soft gel consistency on contact with exudate. They reduce pain, rehydrate wounds, encourage autolytic debridement and can be used at all phases of healing on wounds with low or moderate amounts of exudate.

hydrocortisone ⇒ cortisol.

hydrogel dressings *npl* sheet or amorphous gels (for cavities) used as wound dressings. They rehydrate dry necrotic tissue, reduce pain and can be used at all phases of healing on dehydrated wounds or those with moderate exudate.

hydrogen (H) *n* a colourless, odourless, combustible gas. A constituent of all organic compounds. *hydrogen bond* a weak chemical bond between water molecules, and in certain complex biological molecules, such as nucleic acids (DNA, RNA) and proteins. They are vital in maintaining the three-dimensional structure necessary for the functioning of proteins such as enzymes. ⇒ covalent bond. ⇒ ionic bond. *hydrogen ion concentration (pH)* a measure of the acidity (concentration of hydrogen ions) or alkalinity (concentration of hydroxyl ions) of a solution. The pH is measured on a logarithmic scale ranging from 0 to 14 and representing the indices of the concentration rather than the actual number of hydrogen ions. A pH below 7 is acid having an excess of hydrogen ions, 7 being approximately neutral, and a pH above 7 is alkaline having an excess of hydroxyl ions. *hydrogen peroxide* H_2O_2, a powerful oxidizing and deodorizing agent, used in suitable dilution as a mouthwash.

hydrogenation the addition of hydrogen to a substance. ⇒ reduction.

hydrolysis *n* the splitting into more simple substances by the addition of water — **hydrolyse** *vt.*

hydrometer *n* an instrument for determining the specific gravity of fluids — **hydrometry** *n*.

hydronephrosis *n* distension of the renal pelvis and calyces with urine, from obstructed outflow. Causes include: calculi, tumour and prostatic enlargement. If unrelieved, pressure eventually causes damage to kidney tissue. Surgical operations include nephroplasty and pyeloplasty on the kidney.

hydropericarditis *n* pericarditis with effusion.

hydropericardium *n* fluid in the pericardial sac in the absence of inflammation. Can occur in heart and kidney failure.

hydroperitoneum *n* ⇒ ascites.

hydrophilic *adj* having an affinity for water.

hydrophobia *n* fear of water. ⇒ rabies.

hydrophobic *adj* having an aversion to water. ⇒rabies.

hydropneumopericardium *n* the presence of air and fluid in the membranous pericardial sac surrounding the heart. It may accompany pericardiocentesis.

hydropneumoperitoneum *n* the presence of fluid and gas in the peritoneal cavity: it may accompany aspiration of that cavity; it may be due to perforation of the gut; or it may be due to gas-forming micro-organisms in the peritoneal fluid.

hydropneumothorax *n* fluid and air in the pleural cavity. ⇒ pneumothorax.

hydrops *n* oedema. *hydrops fetalis* generalized oedema associated with severe haemolytic anaemia in the fetus or newborn due to rhesus incompatibility. A severe form of haemolytic disease of the newborn — **hydropic** *adj*.

hydrosalpinx *n* distension of a uterine tube with watery fluid.

hydrostatic pressure the pressure exerted by a fluid on the walls of its container, such as a blood vessel.

hydrotherapy *n* the science of therapeutic bathing and/or exercise for diagnosed conditions.

hydrothorax *n* the presence of fluid in the pleural cavity.

hydroureter *n* abnormal distension of the ureter with urine.

hydroxocobalamin *n* a commercially produced substance with vitamin B_{12} activity. ⇒ cobalamin. ⇒ cyanocobalamin.

hydroxyapatite *n* a constituent of bone conferring extreme hardness. It comprises inorganic calcium salts: carbonate, phosphate and hydroxide.

hydroxybutyrate dehydrogenase (HBD) the heart isoenzyme of lactate dehydrogenase.

5-hydroxyindoleacetic acid (5-HIAA) *n* a metabolite of 5-hydroxytryptamine. High levels found in the urine are associated with carcinoid tumour.

hydroxyl (OH) *n* a chemical group consisting of a hydrogen atom linked to an oxygen atom. Acts as a free radical so can cause tissue damage. ⇒ hydrogen ion concentration.

5-hydroxytryptamine (5-HT) *n* a monoamine neurotransmitter. Also present in high concentration in platelets and the gastrointestinal tract. ⇒ serotonin.

hygiene *n* the science dealing with the maintenance and preservation of health by the promotion of cleanliness including handwashing — **hygienic** *adj*.

hygroma *n* a swelling containing watery fluid. It may be caused by a malformation of the lymphatic vessels, causing a cystic swelling. *cystic hygroma* usually situated at the neck and present at birth, sometimes interfering with birth. Surgical excision is necessary before complications associated with infection develop — **hygromatous** *adj*.

hygrometer *n* an instrument for measuring the amount of moisture in the air. ⇒ humidity.

hygroscopic *adj* readily absorbing water, e.g. glycerine.

hymen *n* a membranous perforated structure stretching across the vaginal entrance. *imperforate hymen* a congenital condition leading to haematocolpos. ⇒ cryptomenorrhoea.

hymenectomy *n* surgical excision of the hymen.

hymenotomy *n* surgical incision of an imperforate hymen. ⇒ haematocolpos.

hyoid *n* a U-shaped bone at the root of the tongue.

hyperacidity *n* excessive acidity. ⇒ hyperchlorhydria.

hyperactivity *n* excessive activity and distractibility; modes of treatment incorporate techniques such as behaviour modification, dietary restrictions and drugs. ⇒ attention deficit hyperactivity disorder.

hyperaemia *n* excess of blood in an area. *active hyperaemia* caused by an increased flow of blood to a part. *passive hyperaemia* occurs when there is restricted flow of venous blood from a part — **hyperaemic** *adj*.

hyperaesthesia *n* excessive sensitiveness of a part — **hyperaesthetic** *adj*.

hyperaldosteronism *n* an excess secretion of the mineralocorticoid aldosterone, resulting in hypokalaemia, hypertension and sometimes tetany resulting from metabolic acidosis. It may be: *primary hyperaldosteronism* due to adrenal disease when it is called Conn's syndrome, or *secondary hyperaldosteronism* when it is caused by another condition, e.g. cardiac failure.

hyperalgesia *n* excessive sensitivity to pain — **hyperalgesic** *adj*.

hyperalimentation *n* total parenteral nutrition.

hyperbaric term applied to gas at greater pressure than normal. *hyperbaric oxygen therapy* a form of treatment in which a patient is entirely enclosed in a pressure chamber breathing 100% oxygen at greater than one atmospheric pressure. Used for patients with carbon monoxide poisoning, decompression sickness (caisson disease) and clostridial infections such as gas gangrene etc.

hyperbilirubinaemia *n* excessive bilirubin in the blood — **hyperbilirubinaemic** *adj*.

hypercalcaemia *n* excessive calcium in the blood, usually resulting from bone resorption as occurs in prolonged immobility, hyperparathyroidism, metastatic tumours of bone, Paget's disease and osteoporosis. It results in anorexia, abdominal pain, nausea, vomiting, lethargy, muscle pain and weakness and cardiac arrhythmias leading to cardiac arrest. It is accompanied by hypercalciuria and can lead to nephrolithiasis and renal failure — **hypercalcaemic** *adj*.

hypercalciuria *n* greatly increased excretion of calcium in the urine. Occurs in diseases which result in bone resorption. *idiopathic hypercalciuria* is the term used when there is no known metabolic cause. Hypercalciuria is of importance in the pathogenesis of nephrolithiasis.

hypercapnia *n* raised CO_2 tension in arterial blood ($PaCO_2$) — **hypercapnic** *adj*.

hypercatabolism *n* excessive breakdown of body protein. Amino acids are used as an energy source where intake is insufficient for physiological needs. It occurs in situations where nutritional requirements are increased, e.g. major trauma, surgery, burns and sepsis. ⇒ catabolism. ⇒ nitrogen balance — **hypercatabolic** *adj*.

hyperchloraemia *n* excessive chloride in the blood. It is associated with hyperkalaemia and where chloride intake is high. Leads to metabolic acidosis as the acid-base balance is disrupted — **hyperchloraemic** *adj*.

hyperchlorhydria *n* excessive hydrochloric acid in the gastric juice — **hyperchlorhydric** *adj*.

hypercholesterolaemia *n* excessive cholesterol in the blood. Predisposes to atheroma and gallstones. Also associated with hypothyroidism — **hypercholesterolaemic** *adj*.

hyperemesis *n* excessive vomiting. *hyperemesis gravidarum* excessive vomiting in pregnancy, necessitating medical intervention.

hyperextension *n* overextension.

hyperflexion *n* excessive flexion.

hyperglycaemia *n* excessive glucose in the blood, usually indicative of diabetes mellitus. The discovery of isolated high blood glucose readings in an otherwise symptomless diabetic is of little value, but during illness raised blood glucose readings may be a valuable guide to the need for extra insulin — **hyperglycaemic** *adj*.

hyperglycaemic coma ⇒ coma. ⇒ diabetes mellitus. ⇒ hyperosmolar diabetic coma.

hyperhidrosis *n* excessive sweating — **hyperhidrotic** *adj*.

hyperinsulinism *n* intermittent or continuous loss of consciousness, with or without convulsions (a) due to excessive insulin from the pancreatic islets lowering the blood sugar. ⇒ insulinoma; (b) due to administration of excessive insulin.

hyperkalaemia (*syn* hyperpotassaemia) excessive potassium in the blood as occurs in renal failure, excess intake of potassium, acidosis, tissue damage, catabolic states and where aldosterone is deficient; early signs are nausea, diarrhoea and muscular weakness. Very high levels cause arrhythmias and cardiac arrest — **hyperkalaemic** *adj*.

hyperkeratosis *n* hypertrophy of the stratum corneum, the horny layer of the skin. Also called keratosis — **hyperkeratotic** *adj*.

hyperkinesis *n* excessive movement — **hyperkinetic** *adj*.

hyperkinetic syndrome also known as hyperactivity syndrome. Usually appears between the ages of 2 and 4 years. The child is slow to develop intellectually and displays a marked degree of distractability and a tireless unrelenting perambulation of the environment, together with aggressiveness (especially towards siblings) even if unprovoked. The parents complain of his or her cold unaffectionate character, disrupted sleep patterns, poor eating and destructive behaviour. The child's history may suggest the possibility of minimal brain dysfunction. Careful management is required, with an individual programme arranged for each family. Drugs may be prescribed for some children; the exclusion of certain foods from the diet may relieve the hyperactivity. ⇒ attention deficit hyperactivity disorder.

hyperlipaemia *n* ⇒ hyperlipidaemia.

hyperlipidaemia *n* excessive total fat in the blood. May be due to an inherited disorder or secondary to dietary intake and conditions, such as diabetes mellitus — **hyperlipidaemic** *adj*.

hypermagnesaemia *n* excessive magnesium in the blood, found in kidney failure and in people who take excessive magnesium-containing antacids. It is characterized by lethargy — **hypermagnesaemic** *adj*.

hypermetabolism *n* production of excessive body heat. Characteristic of hyperthyroidism — **hypermetabolic** *adj*.

hypermetropia *n* long/far sightedness caused by faulty accommodation of the eye, with the result that the light rays are focused beyond, instead of on, the retina. It is corrected by use of a convergent biconvex lens. (See Figure 31). — **hypermetropic** *adj*.

hypermnesia an exaggerated memory involving minute detail.

hypermobility *n* excessive mobility.

hypermotility *n* increased movement, as peristalsis.

hypernatraemia *n* high levels of sodium in the blood, caused by excessive loss of water and electrolytes through polyuria, diarrhoea, excessive sweating or inadequate fluid intake and by high sodium intake. It causes cellular dehydration with thirst, muscle weakness and neurological effects that include: dizziness, confusion and behaviour changes — **hypernatraemic** *adj*.

hypernephroma *n* (*syn* Grawitz tumour) a malignant neoplasm of the kidney — **hypernephromatous** *adj*.

hyperonychia *n* excessive growth or thickening of the nails.

hyperosmolar diabetic coma coma characterized by a very high blood sugar (hyperglycaemia) and dehydration without accompanying ketoacidosis.

hyperosmolarity *n* (*syn* hypertonicity) a solution exerting a higher osmotic pressure than another is said to have a hyperosmolarity, with reference to it. In medicine, the comparison is usually made with normal plasma.

hyperostosis *n* overgrowth of bone tissue. ⇒ exostosis.

hyperoxaluria *n* excessive calcium oxalate in the urine. May be associated with a

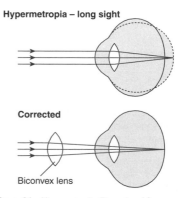

Hypermetropia – long sight

Corrected

Biconvex lens

Figure 31 Hypermetropia. (Reproduced from Brooker 1998 with permission.)

high intake of fruit and vegetables containing oxalates and increased intestinal absorption of oxalates. May lead to the formation of calcium oxalate kidney stones — **hyperoxaluric** *adj.*

hyperparathyroidism *n* excessive secretion of the parathyroid glands due to adenoma or hyperplasia. The resultant increase in serum calcium levels may result in osteitis fibrosa cystica with decalcification, leading to backache, joint and bone pain and possible spontaneous fracture of bones. The increase in urinary excretion of calcium leads to renal damage. ⇒ hypercalcaemia. ⇒ hypercalciuria. ⇒ von Recklinghausen's disease.

hyperperistalsis *n* excessive peristalsis — **hyperperistaltic** *adj.*

hyperphenylalaninaemia *n* excess of phenylalanine in the blood, which results in phenylketonuria.

hyperphosphataemia *n* excessive phosphates in the blood. It is associated with renal failure and extensive necrosis or tissue damage. Patients complain of pruritus, and calcium homeostasis is usually disturbed — **hyperphosphataemic** *adj.*

hyperpigmentation *n* increased or excessive pigmentation, such as in Addison's disease or with drugs, e.g. oral contraceptives. → chloasma.

hyperpituitarism *n* overactivity of the anterior lobe of the pituitary gland. ⇒ acromegaly. ⇒ Cushing's disease. ⇒ gigantism. ⇒ hyperprolactinaemia.

hyperplasia *n* an increase in the number of cells, such as bone marrow hyperplasia that increases red blood cell production in some types of anaemia, or prostatic hyperplasia. ⇒ hypertrophy — **hyperplastic** *adj.*

hyperpnoea *n* increased depth and rate of respiration — **hyperpnoeic** *adj.*

hyperpotassaemia *n* ⇒ hyperkalaemia — **hyperpotassaemic** *adj.*

hyperprolactinaemia *n* excessive prolactin in the blood. May be due to a pituitary tumour, but can occur as an endocrine side-effect from certain antipsychotic drugs. In women, there may be breast enlargement, galactorrhoea and secondary amenorrhoea. In men, there may be gynaecomastia, loss of libido and impotence.

hyperpyrexia *n* very high body temperature above 40–4°C (105°F). *malignant hyperpyrexia* an inherited condition which presents in response to certain drugs used during general anaesthesia and neuroleptic drugs; there is progressive rise in body temperature and, if untreated, may be fatal — **hyperpyrexial** *adj.*

hyperreflexia abnormally increased reflexes.

hypersecretion *n* excessive secretion.

hypersensitivity *n* a state of being unduly sensitive to a stimulus or an allergen. *hypersentivity reactions* may be classified by the timing and whether it involves antibodies or is cell mediated: (a) antibody-mediated type I reaction (anaphylaxis) occurs when IgE binds to an allergen such as pollen; (b) antibody-mediated type II reaction (cytotoxic) involves IgG or IgM. An example would be the agglutination of donated red cells occurring after a mismatched blood transfusion; (c) antibody-mediated type III reaction (immune complex) involves antibodies and complement activation, such as in extrinsic allergic alveolitis or the Arthus reaction; (d) cell-mediated type IV reaction which occurs 24–48 hours after exposure to the antigen. Examples include chronic skin inflammation caused by exposure to nickel, cosmetics and plants, such as poison ivy. It is also seen in the local reaction to skin testing with tuberculin; (e) mixed antibody/cell-mediated type V reaction involving antibodies, T lymphocytes and phagocytes, which may be seen in some autoimmune diseases — **hypersensitive** *adj.*

hypersplenism *n* overactivity of an enlarged spleen, especially haemolytic activity. It leads to depression of erythrocyte, granulocyte and platelet counts in presence of active bone marrow. The causes include: hepatic portal hypertension, haemolytic anaemia and malaria. ⇒ anaemia.

hypertelorism *n* genetically determined cranial anomaly (low forehead and pronounced vertex) associated with learning disability.

hypertension *n* abnormally high tension, by custom abnormally high systemic blood pressure involving systolic and/or diastolic levels. There is no universal agreement of their upper limits of normal, especially in increasing age. Many cardiologists consider a resting systolic pressure of 140 mmHg and/or a resting diastolic pressure of 90 mmHg to be abnormal at age 20 years, whereas 160 mmHg and/or a resting diastolic pressure of 95 mmHg to be pathological at 50 years of age. In the vast majority of cases, no cause is found and it is termed 'essential hypertension'. Secondary hypertension may result from coarctation of the aorta, renal artery stenosis, renal disease, phaeochromocytoma, Cushing's disease/syndrome, Conn's syndrome, various drugs, such as oral contraceptives, NSAIDs, and the pre-eclampsia associated with pregnancy. The management involves: (a) lifestyle changes, such as weight reduction, smoking cessation, increasing exercise and limiting sodium intake; (b) drugs that include: thiazide diuretics, beta (β)-adrenoceptor antagonists, angiotensin converting enzyme inhibitors (ACE), calcium antagonists, vasodilators and low dose aspirin to reduce the risk of complications, e.g. stroke; (c) treating the cause, if known. ⇒ hepatic portal hypertension. ⇒ pulmonary hypertension — **hypertensive** *adj.*

hyperthermia *n* ⇒ hyperpyrexia — **hyperthermic** *adj.*

hyperthyroidism *n* a condition caused when body tissues are exposed to an excessive amount of thyroxine (T$_4$), one of the thyroid gland hormones. A common endocrine disorder that affects women much more often than men. The causes include: Graves' disease where abnormal antibodies stimulate thyroxine production; nodular goitre; adenoma; thyroiditis; thyroid cancer. Classically, patients present with goitre, anxiety, emotional lability, tachycardia, palpitations, atrial fibrillation, dyspnoea, sweating, heat intolerance, increased appetite with weight loss, diarrhoea, amenorrhoea, reduced libido, fatigue, fine tremor of the outstretched hands, and lid lag and exophthalmos in Graves' disease. Treatment depends on the cause and may include: antithyroid drugs such as carbimazole, subtotal thyroidectomy, beta (β)-adrenoceptor antagonists or radioactive iodine.

hypertonia *n* increased tone in a muscular structure, such as a muscle or artery — **hypertonicity** *n.*

hypertonic *adj* **1.** pertaining to hypertonia. **2.** having a higher osmotic pressure relative to the fluid with which it is being compared. *hypertonic saline* has a greater osmotic pressure than normal physiological (body) fluid. ⇒ hypotonic. ⇒ isotonic.

hypertonicity *n* ⇒ hyperosmolarity.

hypertrichosis *n* excessive growth of normally sited hair, or hair growth in sites not usually bearing prominent hair, e.g. the forehead. May occur in conditions that include: hormone disturbance, porphyria and some medication.

hypertrophy *n* increase in the size of tissues or structures such as organs, due to individual cells enlarging. It may occur as a normal process, or in response to increased use, e.g. leg muscles enlarge in a cyclist, or as part of compensation mechanisms by which the body tries to minimize the effects of declining function, such as myocardial enlargement in heart failure. ⇒ hyperplasia — **hypertrophic** *adj.*

hyperuricaemia *n* excessive uric acid in the blood. Characteristic of gout. ⇒ Lesch-Nyhan disease — **hyperuricaemic** *adj.*

hyperventilation *n* overbreathing. Increased respiration rate above the body's metabolic requirements; may occur during anxiety attacks, in salicylate poisoning or head injury, or passively as part of a technique of general anaesthesia in intensive care.

hypervitaminosis *n* any condition arising from an excess of vitamins, especially the fat soluble vitamins A and D. Excess vitamin A is toxic to the liver and causes hyperostosis. Too much vitamin D leads to hypercalcaemia and renal damage.

hypervolaemia *n* an increase in the volume of circulating blood.

hyphae *npl* tubular filaments of some fungi. ⇒ mycelium.

hyphaema *n* blood in the anterior chamber of the eye.

hypnogogic stage the stage between being awake and asleep. Hallucinations may occur.

hypnosis *n* the deliberate use of a trance state; an altered state of consciousness. This may be initiated by a therapist or by the patient (self hypnosis) utilizing the mental mechanism of suggestion to bring about a state of relaxation or an improvement in health and well-being. It may also be used to facilitate smoking cessation, symptom reduction in irritable bowel disease and forms of anaesthesia, as in dental extractions, skin suturing and pain relief — **hypnotic** *adj*.

hypnotherapy *n* treatment by a sleeplike state, hypnosis.

hypnotic *adj* 1. pertaining to hypnotism. An experience inducing a state of trance. 2. a drug which produces a sleep resembling natural sleep, e.g. temazepam. ⇒ narcotic. ⇒ sedative.

hypoaesthesia *n* diminished sensitiveness of a part — **hypoaesthetic** *adj*.

hypoalbulimaemia *n* low level of albumin in the blood.

hypocalcaemia *n* decreased calcium in the blood. It may be due to lack of vitamin D and impaired renal metabolism, excess calcium excretion by the kidneys, alkalosis, where the amount of available ionised calcium is decreased, and hypoparathyroidism. It is characterized by tingling in the hands and feet, carpopedal spasm, with stridor and convulsions in children. ⇒ tetany. ⇒ hyperventilation — **hypocalcaemic** *adj*.

hypocapnia *n* reduced CO_2 tension in arterial blood ($PaCO_2$); can be produced by hyperventilation — **hypocapnic** *adj*.

hypochloraemia *n* reduced chlorides in the circulating blood. It occurs after vomiting of hydrochloric acid from the stomach, with prolonged use of alkali indigestion medicines and in association with hypokalaemia. Leads to metabolic alkalosis as the acid-base balance is disrupted — **hypochloraemic** *adj*.

hypochlorhydria *n* decreased hydrochloric acid in the gastric juice — **hypochlorhydric** *adj*.

hypochlorite *n* salts of hypochlorous acid. Widely used as disinfectants. ⇒ chlorine.

hypochondria *n* excessive anxiety about one's health. Common in depressive and anxiety states — **hypochondriasis** *n*.

hypochondrium *n* the upper lateral regions (left and right) of the abdomen, either side of the epigastrium and below the lower ribs (see Figure 1) — **hypochondriac** *adj*.

hypochromic *adj* deficient in colouring or pigmentation. Of a red blood cell, having decreased haemoglobin. It is associated with the microcytic anaemia caused by iron deficiency. ⇒ anaemia.

hypodermic *adj* below the skin; subcutaneous — **hypodermically** *adv*.

hypofibrinogenaemia *n* low fibrin levels in blood. ⇒ afibrinogenaemia — **hypofibrinogenaemic** *adj*.

hypofunction *n* diminished performance.

hypogammaglobulinaemia *n* decreased gammaglobulin in the blood, occurring either congenitally or, more commonly, as a sporadic disease in adults. Lessens resistance to infection. ⇒ agammaglobulinaemia. ⇒ globulins — **hypogammaglobulinaemic** *adj*.

hypogastrium *n* the abdominal region which lies immediately below the umbilical region. It is flanked on either side by the iliac regions/fossae (see Figure 1) — **hypogastric** *adj*.

hypoglossal *adj* under the tongue. *hypoglossal nerve* the 12th pair of cranial nerves which arise directly from the brain. They innervate tongue movements required for speaking, moving food and swallowing.

hypoglycaemia *n* decreased blood glucose levels, attended by anxiety, excitement, confusion, nausea, headache, perspiration, hunger and altered consciousness. Hypoglycaemia commonly occurs in diabetes mellitus, when it is due to insulin overdosage, strenuous exercise or to inadequate intake of carbohydrate, but can occur in non-diabetics — **hypoglycaemic** *adj* pertaining to hypoglycaemia *hypoglycaemic coma* loss of consciousness caused by low blood glucose. May happen to people with diabetes who have no early warning signs of hypoglycaemia, and can occur at night. People are educated about prevention and always carrying a source of carbohydrate with them. If it occurs the treatment depends on whether the person is able to swallow oral carbohydrate; otherwise they are given parenteral glucagon or glucose. ⇒ coma. ⇒ diabetes mellitus.

hypoglycaemic drugs *npl* oral drugs that lower blood glucose in some types of diabetes mellitus. The sulphonylureas, e.g. glipizide, glibenclamide, act by stimulating insulin secretion. Biguanides, e.g. metformin, increase glucose uptake by muscle cells, but they may cause lactic acidosis. A further group, the α-glucosidase inhibitors, e.g acarbose, delays the absorption of carbohydrate from the intestine. Where blood sugar control is difficult in people with type 2 diabetes, they may be prescribed the drug rosiglitazone in conjunction with another hypoglycaemic as an alternative to insulin therapy.

hypokalaemia *n* abnormally low potassium level of the blood. The causes include: vomiting, gastrointestinal drainage, diarrhoea, starvation, excess renal loss in Cushing's syndrome or aldosteronism and with prolonged use of diuretics. Leads to muscle weakness, arrhythmias and cardiac arrest — **hypokalaemic** *adj.*

hypokinesis *n* diminished movement.

hypomania *n* a less intense form of mania in which there is a milder elevation of mood with restlessness, distractibility, increased energy and pressure of speech. The flight of ideas and grandiose delusions of frank mania are usually absent — **hypomanic** *adj.*

hypometabolism *n* decreased production of body heat. Characteristic of hypothyroidism.

hypomotility *n* decreased movement, as of the gastrointestinal tract.

hyponatraemia *n* decreased sodium in the blood. Causes include: sodium loss in vomiting, diarrhoea, sweating and burns; diuretics, aldosterone deficiency, excess ADH, renal disease and diabetes mellitus or a failure to excrete water or excess intake. Leads to cerebral oedema with convulsions and altered consciousness. When there is associated water loss, it can lead to hypovolaemic shock — **hyponatraemic** *adj.*

hypo-osmolarity *n* (*syn* hypotonicity) a solution exerting a lower osmotic pressure than another is said to have a hypo-osmolarity, with reference to it. In medicine, the comparison is usually made with normal plasma.

hypoparathyroidism *n* undersecretion of the parathyroid glands with decrease in serum calcium levels, producing tetany. Causes include damage to the parathyroid glands during thyroid surgery, idiopathic

forms and autoimmune disease. Management includes: treatment of tetany with intravenous calcium gluconate and maintenance with calcitriol (1,25-dihydroxycholecalciferol). ⇒ hypocalcaemia.

hypopharynx *n* that portion of the pharynx lying below and behind the larynx, more correctly called the laryngopharynx.

hypophoria *n* a state in which the visual axis in one eye is lower than the other.

hypophosphataemia *n* decreased phosphates in the blood. Results from alkalosis, dialysis, inadequate intake during parenteral nutrition, and hyperparathyroidism. Leads to muscle weakness and pain, breathing problems, confusion, convulsions and cardiac arrhythmias — **hypophosphataemic** *adj.*

hypophysectomy *n* surgical removal of the pituitary gland.

hypophysis cerebri *n* ⇒ pituitary gland — **hypophyseal** *adj.*

hypopigmentation *n* decreased or poor pigmentation, such as seen in phenylketonuria, vitiligo and albinism.

hypopituitarism *n* undersecretion of pituitary gland hormones, especially of the anterior lobe. Absence of gonadotrophins leads to failure of ovulation, uterine atrophy and amenorrhoea in women, gynaecomastia, impotence and reduced facial hair in men, and loss of libido, pubic and axillary hair in both sexes. Lack of growth hormone in children results in short stature. Lack of adrenocorticotrophic hormone (ACTH) results in decreased cortisol secretion and signs of adrenal insufficiency. A reduction in thyroid stimululating hormone (TSH) results in secondary hypothyroidism. Usually due to tumour of or involving pituitary gland or hypothalamus, but other causes include: postpartum necrosis of the pituitary gland, head injury, haemorrhage following surgery and radiotherapy. Management involves replacement therapy for the missing hormones. ⇒ Sheehan's syndrome.

hypoplasia *n* incomplete development of any tissue, a less severe form of aplasia — **hypoplastic** *adj.*

hypopnoea shallow respirations.

hypopotassaemia *n* ⇒ hypokalaemia.

hypoproteinaemia *n* reduced amounts of serum proteins, from dietary deficiency or excessive loss, such as in albuminuria — **hypoproteinaemic** *adj.*

hypopyon *n* a collection of pus in the anterior chamber of the eye.

hyporeflexia *n* diminished reflexes.

hyposecretion *n* deficient secretion.

hyposensitivity *n* lacking sensitivity to a stimulus.

hyposmia *n* decrease in the normal sensitivity to smell. Has been observed in patients following laryngectomy.

hypospadias *n* a congenital malformation of the male urethra. Subdivided into two types: (a) penile, when the terminal urethral orifice opens at any point along the ventral surface of the penis; (b) perineal, when the orifice opens on the perineum. → epispadias.

hypostasis *n* 1. a sediment 2. congestion of blood in a part, due to impaired circulation — **hypostatic** *adj.*

hypotension *n* abnormally low blood pressure that is not sufficient for adequate tissue perfusion and oxygenation; may be primary or secondary (e.g. caused by hypovolaemic shock, decreased cardiac output, Addison's disease) or postural — **hypotensive** *adj.*

hypothalamus *n* literally, below the thalamus. An area of grey matter situated in the brain, just above the pituitary gland and combines functions of the nervous and endocrine systems. It is the main centre of the autonomic nervous system and controls various physiological functions such as emotion, hunger, thirst and circadian rhythms. Also has an important endocrine function as it produces releasing and some inhibiting hormones that act on the anterior pituitary and regulate the release of its hormones. Also produces the hormones oxytocin and antidiuretic hormone (vasopressin) that are stored and released by the posterior pituitary — **hypothalamic** *adj.*

hypothermia *n* a core body temperature below 35°C. Accidental hypothermia with very low temperatures is seen in older people, associated with hypothyroidism, and in infants and individuals inappropriately prepared for severe climatic conditions. Hypothermia may be artificially induced to reduce metabolic rate and hence oxygen demands, such as during cardiac surgery.

hypothesis a statement that can be tested by a statistical (inferential) test. It is a prediction based on the relationship between the dependent and independent variables.

hypothetico-deductive method theories are considered and hypotheses for testing are derived in a deductive manner. The research study tests the hypotheses by data analysis that either supports or rejects the original theory.

hypothyroidism *n* conditions caused by low circulating levels of one or both thyroid hormones. It is much more common in women than men and may be: (a) due to spontaneous atrophy; (b) associated with a goitre, such as autoimmune Hashimoto's thyroiditis, iodine deficiency or drug-induced, e.g. with lithium; (c) following surgery for hyperthyroidism. Some people have a transient form and in others the condition is subclinical. It results in decreased metabolic rate and may be characterized by some of the following: tiredness, somnolence, bradycardia, angina, hypertension, aches and pains, carpal tunnel syndrome, low temperature and cold intolerance, weight gain, goitre, constipation, thin hair, dry coarse skin, facial swelling, anaemia, hoarseness, slow speech, menorrhagia and depression. Treatment is with replacement thyroxine. Congenital hypothyroidism can be detected (by routine blood testing) soon after birth and treated successfully with thyroxine. Untreated, it leads to impaired mental and physical development with a failure to achieve normal milestones. It is characterized by coarse facies and protruding tongue. Previously known as cretinism.

hypotonia decreased tone in a body structure, such as a muscle or artery — **hypotonicity** *n.*

hypotonic *adj* 1. relating to hypotonia. 2. having a lower osmotic pressure relative to the fluid with which it is being compared. ⇒ hypertonic. ⇒ isotonic.

hypotonicity *n* ⇒ hypo-osmolarity.

hypoventilation *n* diminished breathing or underventilation.

hypovitaminosis *n* a lack of vitamins in the body due to deficient intake or poor absorption.

hypovolaemia a reduction in the volume of circulating blood — **hypovolaemic** *adj* relating to hypovolaemia.

hypovolaemic shock *adj* the shock syndrome caused by a reduced blood volume. It may be due to loss of blood or other body fluids, or due to increased vessel permeability such as in sepsis or anaphylaxis.

hypoxaemia *n* diminished amount of oxygen in the arterial blood, shown by decreased arterial oxygen tension (PaO_2) and reduced saturation. ⇒ oxygenation — **hypoxaemic** *adj*.

hypoxia *n* diminished amount of oxygen in the tissues. *anaemic hypoxia* resulting from a deficiency of haemoglobin or a reduced number of erythrocytes. *histotoxic hypoxia* interference with the cells in their utilization of O_2, e.g. in cyanide poisioning. *hypoxic hypoxia* interference with pulmonary oxygenation. *stagnant hypoxia* tissue blood volume is normal but blood flow is reduced due to impairment of venous outflow or, in some cases, reduced arterial flow — **hypoxic** *adj*.

hysterectomy *n* surgical removal of the uterus. *abdominal hysterectomy* effected via a lower abdominal incision. *subtotal hysterectomy* removal of the uterine body, leaving the cervix in the vaginal vault. *total hysterectomy* complete removal of the uterine body and cervix. *vaginal hysterectomy* carried out through the vagina. *Wertheim's hysterectomy* a radical operation for advanced cancer. It involves total removal of the uterus, the adjacent lymphatic vessels and nodes, with a cuff of the vagina and both uterine tubes and ovaries.

hysteria *n* **1.** the term previously used for conversion disorder. **2.** a state of tension or excitement in a person or group which results in a temporary loss of control over emotions — **hysterical** *adj*.

hysterosalpingectomy *n* surgical removal of the uterus and of one or both uterine tubes.

hysterosalpingography *n* ⇒ uterosalpingography.

hysterosalpingostomy *n* anastomosis between a uterine tube and the uterus.

hysteroscopy *n* an endoscopic examination of the cavity of the uterus. It provides a direct view and the opportunity to biopsy abnormal areas.

hysterotomy *n* incision into the uterus. It usually excludes caesarean section. It may be performed for a late termination of pregnancy.

hysterotrachelorrhaphy *n* repair of a lacerated cervix uteri.

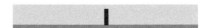

IAA *abbr* indispensable amino acid.

IADL *abbr* Instrumental Activities of Daily Living. ⇒ Activities of Daily Living.

iatrogenic *adj* describes a secondary condition arising from medical or surgical treatment of a primary condition, e.g. drug side-effects.

IBD *abbr* inflammatory bowel disease.

IBS *abbr* irritable bowel syndrome.

IC *abbr* inspiratory capacity.

ICD *abbr* International Classification of Disease.

ICE *acr* ice, compress and elevation. Used in the first aid treatment of bruises and swellings on the limbs. An ice compress is placed on the injured part which is then elevated to aid venous return. ⇒ RICE.

ICF *abbr* intracellular fluid.

ichthyoses *npl* a group of inherited conditions in which the skin is dry, hyperkeratotic with fissures and scaly appearance. Also called fish skin disease or xeroderma. Similar, but acquired, skin changes may be produced by defective nutrition.

ICN *abbr* **1.** International Council of Nurses. **2.** Infection Control Nurse.

ICP *abbr* intracranial pressure.

ICSH *abbr* interstitial-cell stimulating hormone. ⇒ luteinizing hormone.

ICSI *abbr* intracytoplasmic sperm injection.

icterus *n* ⇒ jaundice. *icterus gravis* acute diffuse necrosis of the liver. *icterus gravis neonatorum* one of the clinical forms of haemolytic disease of the newborn. *icterus neonatorum* excess of the normal, or physiological, jaundice occurring in the first week of life as a result of excessive destruction of haemoglobin. ⇒ phototherapy. *icterus index* measurement of concentration of bilirubin in the plasma. Used in diagnosis of jaundice.

id *n* that part of the unconscious mind which consists of a system of primitive urges (instincts) and, according to Freud, persists unrecognized into adult life.

IDDM *abbr* insulin dependent diabetes mellitus.

ideation *n* the process concerned with the highest function of awareness, the formation of ideas. It includes thought, intellect and memory.

identical twins uniovular. Twins of the same gender derived from a single fertilized ovum (zygote). They are genetically identical. ⇒ monozygotic.

identification *n* recognition. In psychology, the way in which we form our personality by modelling it on a chosen person, e.g. identification with the parent of same sex helping to form one's sex role; identification with a person of own sex in the hero worship of adolescence. A mental defence mechanism where individuals take on the characteristics of the admired role model figure.

ideomotor *n* mental energy, in the form of ideas, producing automatic movement of muscles, e.g. mental agitation producing agitated movements of limbs.

idiopathic *adj* without apparent cause.

idiopathic thrombocytopenic purpura (ITP) a syndrome characterized by the presence of auto-antibodies that cause low blood platelet count that results in intermittent mucosal bleeding and purpura. In children it can occur after viral illness. Adults tend to have an insidious onset. Treatment may include: platelet transfusion, corticosteroids, immunoglobulin and, in severe cases, a splenectomy. ⇒ transfusion.

idiosyncrasy *n* an individual character or property. It may relate to an unusual response to a particular drug or food.

idioventricular *adj* pertaining to the cardiac ventricles and not affecting the atria.

IHD *abbr* ⇒ ischaemic heart disease.

ileal bladder ⇒ ileoureterostomy.

ileal conduit ⇒ ileoureterostomy.

ileitis *n* inflammation of the ileum.

ileocaecal *adj* pertaining to the ileum and the caecum. *ileocaecal valve* a valve between the ileum (small bowel) and the caecum (large bowel).

ileocolic *adj* pertaining to the ileum and the colon.

ileocolitis *n* inflammation of the ileum and the colon.

ileocolostomy *n* a surgically made fistula between the ileum and the colon, usually the transverse colon. Most often used to bypass an obstruction or inflammation in the caecum or ascending colon. ⇒ colon.

ileoproctostomy *n* an anastomosis between the ileum and rectum; used when disease extends to the sigmoid colon.

ileorectal *adj* pertaining to the ileum and the rectum.

ileosigmoidostomy *n* an anastomosis between the ileum and sigmoid colon; used where most of the colon has to be removed.

ileostomy *n* a surgically made fistula between the ileum and the anterior abdominal wall; usually a permanent form of artificial anus when the whole of the large bowel has to be removed, e.g. in severe inflammatory bowel disease. ⇒ panproctocolectomy. *ileostomy bags* disposable bags used to collect the liquid discharge from an ileostomy.

ileoureterostomy *n* (*syn* ureteroileostomy) transplantation of the lower ends of the ureters from the bladder to an isolated loop of small bowel (ileal bladder) which, in turn, is made to open on the abdominal wall (ileal conduit).

ileum *n* the lower three-fifths of the small intestine, lying between the jejunum and the caecum. It is important in the absorption of vitamin B_{12} and other nutrients, such as amino acids. ⇒ intrinsic factor — **ileal** *adj*.

ileus *n* obstruction of the intestine. Usually applied to paralytic ileus rather than a mechanical obstruction. Causes include: peritonitis, following bowel surgery, spinal injuries and hypokalaemia. Peristalsis ceases, there is stasis of intestinal contents, toxin absorption, vomiting, distension, varying degrees of pain and constipation. ⇒ meconium.

iliacus muscles of the loin.

iliococcygeal *adj* pertaining to the ilium and coccyx.

iliofemoral *adj* pertaining to the ilium and the femur.

iliopectineal *adj* pertaining to the ilium and the pubis.

iliopsoas *adj* pertaining to the ilium and the loin. *iliopsoas muscle* the psoas and iliacus muscles.

ilium *n* the upper part of the innominate (hip) bone; it is a separate bone in the fetus — **iliac** *adj* pertaining to the ilium. *iliac arteries* supply blood to the pelvis and legs. *iliac crest* the highest point of the ilium. *iliac region/fossa* the abdominal region situated either side of the hypogastrium (see Figure 1). *iliac veins* drain blood from the legs and pelvis.

illusion *n* a deceptive appearance. A misidentification of a sensation, e.g. of sight, a white sheet being mistaken for a ghost, the sheet being misrepresented in consciousness as a figure.

IM&T *abbr* information management and technology. See Box – Information management.

image *n* a revived experience of a percept recalled from memory (smell and taste). Also applied to the optical reproduction of an object formed on the retina as light is focused through the eye.

imagery *n* imagination. The recall of vivid mental images of various types depending upon the special sense organs involved when the images were formed, e.g. *auditory imagery* sound. *motor imagery* movement. *olfactory imagery* smell. *tactile imagery* touch. *visual imagery* sight. The technique of *guided imagery*, in which the patient is asked to imagine a particular situation or state, can be used with other interventions as a coping strategy in the control of pain and other symptoms.

imaging techniques the diagnostic techniques used to investigate the state and functioning of body structures, e.g. radiographic examination, radionuclide scans, ultrasonography, computed tomography, magnetic resonance and positron emission tomography.

imbalance *n* lack of balance. Term refers commonly to the upset of acid-base relationship, water and the electrolytes in body fluids. ⇒ Menière's disease. ⇒ vertigo.

immersion foot ⇒ trench foot.

immune *adj* possessing the capacity to resist infection. *immune complexes* antigen-antibody complexes. *immune respo-* nse the antigen-specific adaptive defences provided by humoral immunity (B-lymphocytes) and cell mediated immunity (T-lymphocytes). Together they protect against foreign particles, such as micro-organisms, transplanted cells and abnormal cells arising in the body, e.g. cancer. *immune surveillance* the function of certain lymphocytes that are able to detect and react to the presence of abnormal cells, such as those showing early malignant changes. *immune system* a functional system which is able to recognize antigens (foreign substances) and use various methods of preventing them from causing damage in the body, e.g. antigen destruction.

immunity *n* an intrinsic or acquired state of resistance to an infectious agent. *active immunity* is acquired, naturally during an infection or artificially by immunization. It involves the production of antibodies in response to exposure to an antigenic stimulus. The primary response to exposure is followed by a 2–3 week lag phase before enough antibodies are produced, but the secondary reponse following a subsequent exposure is more intense and has a much reduced lag phase because the memory cells are able to produce antibodies very quickly. This type of immunity tends to be of long duration. (See Figure 32). *cell mediated immunity* T-lymphocyte-dependent responses which cause graft rejection, immunity to some infectious agents and tumour rejection. *humoral immunity* from immunoglobulins produced by plasma cells derived from B-lymphocytes. Immunity can be innate (from inherited qualities), or it can be acquired, actively or passively, naturally or artificially. *passive immunity* is acquired, naturally when maternal antibody passes to the child via the placenta or in colostrum and breast milk, or artificially by administering immunoglobulins (usually human in origin). This type of immunity tends to be short-lived because the immune response is not stimulated to produce antibodies.

immunization *n* artificial means by which immunity is initiated or augmented. Achieved by using vaccines containing attenuated micro-organisms or inactive micro-organisms or bacterial products such as toxins. This results in antibody production (active immunity) and is gen-

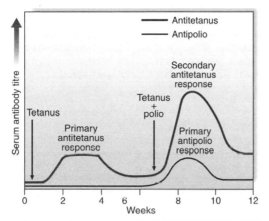

Figure 32 Primary and secondary immune response. (Reproduced from Westwood 1999 with permission.)

erally long-lasting. In certain situations, such as during an epidemic, the injection of immunoglobulins obtained from immune humans, or rarely sera from animals, can give temporary protection. *immunization programme* a routine programme of immunization offered during childhood and to special groups such as healthcare workers and those travelling abroad.

immunocompetence the ability to initiate a specific immune response following exposure to an antigen.

immunocompromised patient an individual with defective immune responses or where their immune system is prevented from responding normally, often produced by treatment with drugs or irradiation or by AIDS. Also occurs in patients undergoing invasive procedures and some patients with cancer and other diseases affecting the immune system. Patients are liable to develop infections with opportunistic organisms such as *Candida albicans*, *Pneumocystis carinii* and *Cryptococcus neoformans*. ⇒ immunosuppression.

immunodeficiency *n* an impairment of the humoral or cell mediated immune responses, leading to increased susceptibility to infectious diseases, opportunistic infections and malignant conditions, such as Kaposi's sarcoma.

immunodeficiency diseases inherited or acquired disorders of the immune system, e.g. deficiency of immunoglobulin synthesis, AIDS.

immunofluorescence techniques *npl* immunological diagnostic techniques that use fluorescent dyes to identify specific antibodies etc.

immunogenesis *n* the process of production of immunity — **immunogenetic** *adj*.

immunogenetics *n* **1.** the study of the interrelationship between immunity to disease and genetic makeup. **2.** the branch of immunology that deals with the molecular and genetic bases of the immune response.

immunogenicity *n* the ability to produce immunity — **immunogenic** *adj*.

immunoglobulins (Igs) *n* (*syn* antibodies) high molecular weight Y-shaped proteins produced by plasma cells (derived from B lymphocytes) in response to specific antigens. They are found in the blood and other body fluids where they form part of body defences. Immunoglobulins function in a variety of ways, but all involve combining with the antigen to form an immune complex. There are five classes of immunoglobulins – IgG, IgA, IgD, IgM and IgE – each with different characteristics, locations and functions.

immunological response ⇒ immunity.

immunology *n* the study of the immune system and immunity — **immunologically** *adv*.

immunopathology *n* the study of tissue injury involving the immune system.

immunosuppressant drugs *npl* drugs used to suppress the immune responses, such as to prevent transplant rejection or suppress some cancers and rheumatoid arthritis. They include azathioprine, ciclosporin (cyclosporin) etc.

immunosuppression *n* deliberate inhibition of the immune response with drugs, radiation or antilymphocyte immunoglobulin to prevent rejection of transplanted tissue.

immunosuppressive *n* that which reduces immunological responsiveness.

immunotherapy a term used to describe immunization, and specific treatments aimed at the immune system including: (a) desensitization treatments for allergies, and (b) the use of biological response modifier (BRM) therapies, e.g. interferons, interleukins and anti-tumour necrosis factor (TNF)monoclonal antibody, used in the management of some cancers, multiple sclerosis, rheumatoid arthritis, Crohn's disease, etc.

impacted *adj* firmly wedged; abnormal immobility, as of faeces in the rectum, fracture, a fetus in the pelvis, a tooth in its socket or a calculus in a duct. ⇒ faecal impaction. ⇒ fracture.

impairment *n* loss or lack of part (e.g. a limb) or physiological function (e.g. hearing, walking).

impalpable *adj* not palpable; incapable of being felt by touch (palpation).

imperforate *adj* lacking a normal opening. *imperforate anus* a congenital absence of an opening into the rectum. *imperforate hymen* a fold of mucous membrane at the vaginal entrance which has no natural outlet for the menstrual fluid. ⇒ haematocolpos.

impetigo *n* a streptococcal or staphylococcal inflammatory, pustular skin disease, usually affecting the face with local spread. *impetigo contagiosa* a highly contagious form of impetigo, commonest on the face and scalp, characterized by vesicles which become pustules and then honey-coloured crusts. ⇒ ecthyma.

implantation *n* the insertion of living cells or solid materials into the tissues, e.g. accidental implantation of tumour cells in a wound; implantation of radium or solid drugs; implantation of the fertilized ovum into the endometrium.

implants *npl* substances or drugs inserted surgically into the human body, e.g.

implantation of pellets containing various hormones, e.g. oestrogens and progesterones for HRT, or synthetic implants used in plastic surgery, e.g in breast reconstruction.

implementing *v* the third phase of the nursing process, when planned interventions to achieve the set goals are implemented and recorded on the patient's nursing notes, which provide cumulative information on the date set for evaluating.

impotence *n* inability to participate in sexual intercourse, by custom referring to the male. It can be due to lack of erection, failure to maintain an erection, or premature ejaculation.

impregnate *vt* fill; saturate; render pregnant.

imprinting describes very early learning where a newborn becomes attached to a model, usually a parent, but may be a carer.

impulse *n* 1. a sudden inclination, sometimes irresistible urge to act without deliberation. 2. the transmission of electrochemical energy occurring along nerve fibres as electrical and concentration gradients result from ion movement across membranes.

impulsive action ⇒ action.

IMV *abbr* intermittent mandatory ventilation.

in extremis at the point of death.

in situ in the correct position, undisturbed. Also describes a cancer which has not invaded adjoining tissue.

in vitro literally in glass, as in a test tube. *in vitro fertilization (IVF)* an assisted fertility/conception technique used for both male and female infertility, e.g. low sperm count, blocked uterine tubes etc. Oocytes collected from the ovaries via a laporoscope are fertilized, using the partner's semen under specialized laboratory conditions, outside the body. Up to three of the resulting embryos are later introduced into the hormonally prepared uterus for a potentially normal gestation, with varying degrees of success. Oocytes or spermatozoa may be donated for IVF.

in vivo in living tissue.

inaccessibility *n* in psychiatry, absence of patient response.

inattention a negative symptom associated with mental illness. It is characterized by:

becoming easily distracted during conversations; difficulty focusing attention on a task, such as reading a magazine or getting dressed; and stopping midway through a task or conversation.

incarcerated *adj* describes the abnormal imprisonment of a part, as in a hernia which is irreducible or a pregnant uterus held beneath the sacral promontory.

incest *n* sexual intercourse between close blood relatives. The most common type of sexual abuse occurs between father and daughter; other types between mother and son and between siblings are known to occur. ⇒ abuse.

incidence *n* number of new cases of a disease that occur in a population over a defined time period.

incipient *adj* initial, beginning, in its early stages.

incision *n* the result of cutting into body tissue, using a sharp instrument — **incise** *vt*.

incisors *npl* the teeth first and second from the midline, four in each jaw, used for cutting food.

inclusion bodies round, oval or irregularly shaped bodies found in the cytoplasm and nuclei of cells affected by viral infections such as rabies.

incompatibility *n* not capable of association, lacking compatibility. Usually applied to the bloods of donor and recipient in transfusion, when antigenic differences in the red cells result in adverse reactions such as agglutination, or drugs or tissue for transplantation.

incompetence *n* inadequacy to perform a natural function, e.g. mitral incompetence — **incompetent** *adj*.

incomplete abortion ⇒ abortion.

incomplete fracture ⇒ fracture.

incontinence *n* loss of continence. Inability to control the evacuation of urine or, less commonly, faeces. ⇒ encopresis. ⇒ enuresis. *faecal incontinence* loss of anal sphincter control may be due to faecal impaction, neurological problems, rectal prolapse, drugs causing diarrhoea and certain bowel diseases. ⇒ spurious diarrhoea. *urinary incontinence* nursing aims include prevention through promoting pelvic floor awareness, and, where loss of continence is present, the assess-

ment of voiding pattern and urodynamic investigations so that appropriate nursing or medical interventions can be planned. These depend on the type of incontinence and may include: pelvic floor exercises, treatment of urinary tract infections, bladder/habit training for continence, condom drainage for male patients, teaching and supervising self-catheterization, preventing nosocomial infection, managing untreatable incontinence by using protective clothing and bedding, or using a self-retaining catheter and a closed urinary drainage system. The various types of urinary incontinence include: *functional incontinence* where there is involuntary and erratic urine loss without any physical problems in the bladder or nervous system. It may occur in cognitive problems and immobility. *neurological or neurogenic incontinence* occurs in conditions that include spinal injuries, multiple sclerosis, diabetes mellitus and where the nerves supplying the bladder have been damaged. Presentation depends on the cause but may include an atonic or hypotonic bladder with overflow, reflex emptying of the full bladder or urge incontinence. *overflow incontinence* dribbling of urine from an overfull bladder. Occurs where there is outflow obstruction such as with an enlarged prostate gland. *stress incontinence* characterized by a leakage of urine when intra-abdominal pressure rises, e.g. coughing or laughing. It generally affects women and is caused by bladder neck displacement due to a weakening of the pelvic floor which follows childbirth, uterine prolapse and the climacteric. *urge incontinence* detrusor instability with erratic bladder contraction leads to urgency and involuntary leakage of urine on the way to the lavatory. ⇒ atonic bladder. ⇒ unstable bladder.

incoordination *n* inability to produce smooth, harmonious muscular movements.

incubation *n* 1. the period from contact with an infectious condition to the appearance of the first signs and symptoms. 2. the process of development, of an egg or of a bacterial culture, by means of artificial heat.

incubator *n* 1. low temperature oven used to provide optimum conditions for the culture (growth) of micro-organisms in the laboratory. 2. apparatus in which preterm or sick infants can be provided with an environment with controlled temperature and oxygen concentration.

incus *n* an anvil-shaped bone. One of the three middle ear ossicles. ⇒ malleus. ⇒ stapes.

independent component of nursing assessing, planning, setting goals and evaluating, in relation to problems which the patient is experiencing in everyday living activities which are amenable to nursing intervention; they may or may not be the product of the medical diagnosis.

indicanuria *n* excess indican in the urine, associated with increased bacterial breakdown of tryptophan in the bowel, as in blind loop syndrome. ⇒ indole.

indicator *n* a substance which, when added in small quantities, is used to make visible the completion of a chemical reaction or the attainment of a certain pH.

indigenous *adj* of a disease etc, native to a certain locality or country, e.g. simple endemic goitre seen in people living in isolated mountainous regions where iodine is deficient.

indigestion *n* (*syn* dyspepsia) a feeling of gastric discomfort, including fullness and gaseous distension, which is not necessarily a manifestation of disease.

indirect cost a cost that cannot be attributed to a specifc department and its budget. It is shared between various budgets, e.g. the cost of heating a building.

individualized nursing nursing care that is planned and implemented according to an assessment of the patient's individual needs and agreed goals. Wherever possible, the patient is involved in care planning.

indole *n* a product of the decomposition of tryptophan in the intestine; it is oxidized to indoxyl in the liver and excreted in urine as indican. ⇒ indicanuria.

indolent *adj* a term applied to a sluggish ulcer which is generally painless and slow to heal.

induction *n* the act of bringing on or causing to occur, as applied to anaesthesia and labour.

induration *n* the hardening of tissue, as in hyperaemia, infiltration by neoplasm, etc — **indurated** *adj*.

industrial dermatitis ⇒ contact dermatitis.

industrial disease (*syn* occupational disease) a disease contracted by reason of occupational exposure to an industrial agent known to be hazardous, e.g. dust, fumes, chemicals, irradiation, etc, the notification of safety precautions against which and compensation for which are controlled by law.

industrial therapy current organization of simulated outside industrial working conditions within a unit in a psychiatric hospital. The main purpose is preparation of patients for their return to the working community.

inequalities in health see Box – Inequalities in health.

inertia *n* inactivity. *uterine inertia* lack of contraction of parturient uterus during

---

Inequalities in health

An extensive body of evidence shows that health and disease are socially patterned and not merely the result of luck or chance. There is a clear relationship between deprivation (whether measured by income level, education level or position in the labour market) and poor health. The less well-off in society experience higher levels of premature death, acute and chronic illness and long term disability. This pattern affects many other industrialized countries and there has been a range of different explanations. These include the direct effect of low income on people's ability to acquire basic resources for health such as warmth, food and adequate housing. Insecure employment or unemployment and social isolation have been shown to contribute to stress which, in the long term, predisposes to poor health and mortality. Health damaging behaviours such as cigarette smoking, excessive alcohol consumption and the consumption of fats and sugars are more common in lower social groups but individual behaviour should not be seen in isolation from a social and material context. Programmes to reduce health inequalities have been widely debated and recommendations include raising income levels of the least well-off, maintaining the mobility, independence and social contacts of older people and expanding childcare and preschool education to support children and families living in poverty.

the second and third stages of labour. It may be due to exhaustion caused by frequent and forcible contractions.

inevitable abortion ⇒ abortion.

infant *n* a baby or a child of less than 1 year old.

infantile paralysis ⇒ poliomyelitis.

infantile spasms *npl* occurring in infants aged three to twelve months. They are characterized by sudden and repeated flexion of the limbs, causing the infant to fall backwards.

infantilism *n* general retardation of development with persistence of child-like characteristics into adolescence and adult life.

infarct *n* area of tissue affected when the end artery supplying it is occluded by atheroma, thrombosis or embolism, e.g. in kidney or heart muscle.

infarction *n* necrosis (death) of a section of tissue because the blood supply has been cut off. ⇒ myocardial infarction. ⇒ pulmonary infarction.

infection *n* the successful invasion, establishment and multiplication of micro-organisms in the tissues of the host. It may be of an acute or chronic nature. *cross infection* occurs when pathogens are transferred from one person to another, or from animal to person. *endogenous infection* one caused by organisms originating from the patient's own body, resulting in disease at another site. *hospital-acquired (nosocomial) infection (HAI)* one which occurs in a patient who has been in hospital for more than 48 h and who did not have signs and symptoms of such infection on admission; approximately 10% of hospital patients develop a hospital-acquired infection. Urinary tract, respiratory, wound and skin infections are the most common types. *opportunistic infection* an infection with a micro-organism which normally has little or no pathogenic activity but which becomes pathogenic when the host's resistance is lowered, e.g. through disease, invasive treatments or drugs — **infectious** *adj*.

Infection Control Committee (ICC) a multidisciplinary committee which should consist of a medical microbiologist, an infection control nurse, a representative from each of the areas in which patients are nursed; a representative from the chief executive, pharmacy, occupational health department, public health department, domestic and portering staff, catering department and sterile supply department. The committee formulates procedures to be carried out throughout the district to prevent hospital or community acquired infection and may meet to co-ordinate the control of outbreaks of infection.

Infection Control Nurse (ICN) a nurse who uses specialized knowledge and skills to support and encourage nurses in the clinical areas to carry out efficiently the policy of the Infection Control Committee. The pattern of incidents of nosocomial infection is studied, and if it clusters in a particular ward, or in a particular group of patients, e.g. those whose operation was performed in a particular theatre, further investigation is carried out to identify the source of infection.

infection, prevention of an essential role of nurses and all healthcare workers. It involves all activities which achieve social cleanliness of articles which come into contact with patients; personal hygiene of patients and staff; measures to protect staff; as well as aseptic techniques. ⇒ closed urinary drainage. ⇒ disinfection. ⇒ handwashing. ⇒infection. ⇒ infection control committee. ⇒ infection control nurse. ⇒ sterilization. ⇒ universal precautions.

infectious disease a disease caused by a specific, pathogenic organism and capable of being transmitted to another individual by direct or indirect contact.

infectious mononucleosis (*syn* glandular fever) a contagious self-limiting disease caused by the Epstein-Barr virus. It mainly affects teenagers and young adults and is characterized by tiredness, headache, fever, sore throat, lymphadenopathy, splenomegaly and appearance of atypical lymphocytes resembling monocytes. Specific antibodies to Epstein-Barr virus are present in the blood, as well as an abnormal antibody that forms the basis of the Paul-Bunnell test which confirms a diagnosis of infectious mononucleosis.

infective *adj* infectious. Disease transmissible from one host to another. *infective hepatitis* ⇒ hepatitis.

infective rhinitis *n* rhinitis following an infection, usually viral, such as a cold, but it may be bacterial.

inferential statistics also called inductive statistics. That which uses the observations of a sample to make a prediction about other samples. It generalizes from the sample. ⇒ descriptive statistics.

inferior *adj* lower; beneath.

inferiority complex feelings of inferiority compensated for by aggressive extrovert behaviour.

infertility *n* lack of ability to reproduce. Psychological and physical causes play their part. The problem can be in either or both parties and may be primary or secondary. Specialist services are required for investigation, diagnosis, treatment and counselling. ⇒ assisted fertility/conception.

infestation *n* the presence of animal parasites in or on the human body — **infest** *vt*.

infibulation *n* an extreme form of female circumcision where the clitoris, labia minora and part of the labia majora are removed. The sides are sutured together, leaving a small opening for urine and menstrual blood. ⇒ circumcision.

infiltration *n* the entry into cells, tissues and organs of abnormal substances or cells, e.g. fat, cancer cells. Penetration of the surrounding tissues; the oozing or leaking of fluid into the tissues. *infiltration anaesthesia* analgesia produced by infiltrating the tissues with a local anaesthetic.

inflammation *n* a nonspecific local defence mechanism initiated by tissue injury. The injury may be caused by trauma, microorganisms, extremes of temperature, U-V light, extremes of pH or ionizing radiation. It is characterized by heat, redness, swelling, pain and loss of function. ⇒ calor. ⇒ dolor. ⇒ rubor. ⇒ tumor — **inflammatory** *adj* pertaining to inflammation. *inflammatory chemical mediators* chemicals released from blood cells that trigger many of the events of the inflammatory response. They include prostaglandins, histamine and kinins. *inflammatory response* the tissue changes of inflammation, caused by chemical mediators, blood cells, vascular changes and the production of exudate.

inflammatory bowel disease (IBD) *n* non-specific inflammatory conditions affecting the alimentary canal/tract. *Crohn's disease* a nonspecific chronic recurrent granulomatous disease commonly affecting the terminal ileum, but lesions occur elsewhere in the small bowel and in the colon, rectum and anus. Affecting mainly young adults and characterized by a necrotizing, ulcerating inflammatory process, there usually being an abrupt demarcation between it and healthy bowel. There can be healthy bowel ('skip' area) intervening between two diseased segments. It causes pain, diarrhoea, steatorrhoea, malabsorption, anaemia, weight loss and fever. Complications include: abscess formation, obstruction, fistula formation and bowel perforation. Management includes: high protein/energy diet, enteral or parenteral feeding, correction of anaemia and vitamin deficiency, antidiarrheal drugs, e.g. loperamide, corticosteroids, an aminosalicylate, e.g. the sulphonamide and salicylic acid compound sulfasalazine (sulphasalazine) or mesalazine, the immunosuppressant azathioprine and metronidazole an antimicrobial drug. Recently treatment with an anti-tumour necrosis factor (TNF) monoclonal antibody has been introduced for severe forms of Crohn's disease. Surgery is indicated where medical treatment fails or to treat complications, such as obstruction. *ulcerative colitis* an inflammatory and ulcerative condition of the rectum and colon. The aetiology is complex and it appears to include genetic, immunological and possibly infective agent factors. Characteristically it affects young and early middle-aged adults and causes diarrhoea with blood and mucus, pain, tenesmus, anaemia, weight loss and serious complications which include: toxic dilatation, perforation, dehydration, electrolyte disturbances, malignant changes and liver damage. Management may include: general supportive measures, such as parenteral nutrition, drugs; corticosteroids (rectal and systemic), sulfasalazine (sulphasalazine) and an immunosuppressant ciclosporin (cyclosporin) or azathioprine. Surgery is indicated where medical treatment fails or as emergency treatment for toxic dilatation, haemorrhage or bowel perforation. ⇒ ileostomy. ⇒ proctocolectomy.

influenza *n* an acute illness caused by a group of myxoviruses of which there are several strains. Sporadic cases may occur but epidemics or occasional pandemics are more usual. Characterized by aches and pains, anorexia, pyrexia, headache, extreme fatigue and cough. It may be associated with considerable mortality caused by complications, such as pneumonia, especially in the very young, older adults and people with chronic diseases that include asthma, heart disease and diabetes. Immunization is offered to older adults and those with chronic conditions — **influenzal** adj.

informal patient n a patient who has entered hospital without any statutory requirements. ⇒ detained patient.

informatics information management and technology (IM&T). See Box – Information management.

information technology use of technology, usually meaning computers, to collect, store, process and manage information. ⇒ informatics.

informed choice the means by which patients/clients can make decisions about their own care and management. Nurses and other healthcare professionals provide accurate, appropriate information about the person's condition, and about the treatment options available, and on this the client decides how to proceed. Professionals may not always agree with the client's decisions, but the latter takes precedence where the adult patient is mentally competent.

informed consent in the UK, the Medical Defence Union recommends consent forms which include a signed declaration by the doctor that he/she has explained the nature and purpose of the operation or treatment to the patient in nontechnical terms. Informed consent is not recognized in English law. Should a patient, after signing the form, ask the nurse about the operation or treatment, the question should be referred to the doctor or other health professional who is to carry out the treatment.

infrared rays long wavelength, invisible rays of the electromagnetic spectrum.

infundibulum n any funnel-shaped passage, such as the end of the uterine tubes — **infundibular** adj.

infusion n 1. fluid flowing by gravity into the body, either intravenously or subcutaneously. 2. an aqueous solution containing the active principle of a drug, made by pouring boiling water on the crude drug.

ingestion n 1. the act of taking food or medicine into the stomach. 2. the means by which a phagocytic cell takes in surrounding solid material such as microorganisms. ⇒ phagocytosis.

ingrowing toenail spreading of the nail into the lateral tissue, causing inflammation.

inguinal adj pertaining to the groin. inguinal canal a tubular opening through the lower part of the anterior abdominal wall, parallel to and a little above the inguinal (Poupart's) ligament. In the male it contains spermatic cord; in the female the uterine round ligaments. inguinal hernia ⇒ hernia.

inhalation n a medicinal substance which is inhaled, such as the aerosols used in the management of asthma.

inhalation anaesthetic n inhaled drug, used in conjunction with intravenous

---

Information management

Information management is a process by which any sort of information is managed. Information is a resource which is needed to ensure the effective running of any organization. Data (singular: datum) are pieces of material which, when compiled appropriately, form information. This information may be managed in a number of different ways. Increasingly information is managed via technological approaches (Information technology, IT), but there are other means which may be more appropriate for the target group/recipient. For example, telephone calls, meetings, notice boards are all ways in which information might be managed. Using an inappropriate management technique will result in the information not being received by those for whom it is intended. Information sent via technology is of no use to those groups who have not the means, nor skills, to access technology.

Information management is achieving a higher profile as the public is more information-aware in every way. There is commitment to 'transparent systems' and patients and clients expect to be kept well informed. The White Paper *Information for health – an information strategy for the modern NHS 1998-2005* (Department of Health 1998) considers all aspects of information management, and demonstrates the importance of information in ensuring a quality service.

drugs, to induce and maintain general anaesthesia. They include desflurane, enflurane, halothane, isoflurane, nitrous oxide and sevoflurane.

inherent *adj* innate; inborn.

inhibition *n* the process of restraining one's impulses or behaviour as a result of conscious or unconscious influences.

injection *n* **1.** the introduction of fluid material into the body under pressure, usually by syringe. It may be: intra-arterial, intra-articular, intradermal, intramuscular, intrathecal, intravenous, subcutaneous or into a hollow structure or cavity. (See Figure 33). **2.** the substance injected.

injunction *n* an order of the court restraining a person.

innate *adj* inborn, dependent on genetic constitution.

innervation *n* the nerve supply to a part.

innocent *adj* benign; not malignant.

innocuous *adj* harmless.

innominate *adj* unnamed ⇒ hip bone. *innominate artery* ⇒ brachiocephalic artery.

inoculation *n* **1.** the injection of antigenic materials, especially vaccine, into the body. **2.** introduction of micro-organisms into culture medium for propagation. *accidental inoculation* a term pertaining to healthcare staff and others who have contact with contaminated material, it includes contamination of an abrasion or burn, heavy soiling of skin or mucosa

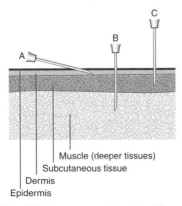

Figure 33 Injection routes. A Intradermal. B Intramuscular. C Subcutaneous. (Reproduced from Brooker 1996 with permission.)

(eyes and mouth) with blood or body fluid, as well as needlestick injury.

inorganic *adj* neither animal nor vegetable in origin. In chemistry, a compound that generally contains no carbon or hydrogen.

inotropes *npl* describes substances, such as drugs, that have an effect on myocardial contractility. Those that increase contractility are positive inotropes, e.g. digoxin, dobutamine, dopamine etc. ⇒ beta (β)-adrenoceptor agonists (stimulants). ⇒ glycosides. Drugs, such as atenolol, nifedipine, verapamil etc, reduce contractility and are negative inotropes. ⇒ beta (β)-adrenoceptor antagonists. ⇒ calcium antagonists (channel blockers).

inquest *n* in England and Wales, a legal enquiry, held by a coroner into the cause of sudden or unexpected death.

insecticide *n* an agent which kills insects — **insecticidal** *adj*.

insemination *n* introduction of semen into the vagina, normally by sexual intercourse. *artificial insemination* instrumental injection of semen into the vagina. ⇒ AID. ⇒ AIH. ⇒ DI.

insensible *adj* without sensation or consciousness. Too small or gradual to be perceived, as insensible perspiration.

insertion *n* **1.** the act of setting or placing in. **2.** the attachment of a muscle to the bone it moves.

insidious *adj* having an imperceptible commencement, as of a disease with a late manifestation of definite symptoms.

insight *n* ability to accept one's limitations but at the same time to develop one's potentialities. Also: (a) knowing that one is ill; (b) a developing knowledge of one's present attitudes and past experiences and the connection between them.

Insight Scale (IS) a self-reporting assessment scale for delusions. It consists of eight statements (four negative and four positive). Clients can agree, disagree or be unsure. The statements include the need for: medication; to see a doctor; illness recognition; and relabelling of psychotic experiences.

insomnia *n* sleeplessness. It may be short or long-term.

inspiration *n* breathing in; inhalation — **inspire** *vt*.

inspiratory capacity (IC) *n* maximum amount of air inspired after a normal expiratory effort.

inspissated *adj* thickened, as by evaporation or withdrawal of water, applied to sputum and culture media used in the laboratory.

instep *n* the arch of the foot on the dorsal surface.

instillation *n* insertion of drops into a body cavity, e.g. conjunctival sac, external auditory meatus.

instinct *n* an inborn tendency to act in a certain way in a given situation, e.g. *paternal, maternal instinct* to protect children — **instinctively** *adv*.

institutionalization *n* a condition of apathy resulting from lack of motivation, characterizing people living (or working) in institutions, who have been subjected to a rigid routine with deprivation of decision making.

insufflation *n* the blowing of air along a tube (pharyngotympanic, uterine) to establish patency. The blowing of powder into a body cavity.

insulin *n* a polypeptide hormone produced by the beta cells in the islets of Langerhans of the pancreas. Its secretion is regulated by the level of glucose in the bloodstream, i.e. a negative feedback mechanism. Its action is opposite to that of glucagon produced in the alpha cells and it has an effect on the metabolism of carbohydrate, protein and fat by stimulating the transport of glucose into cells. An absolute or relative lack of insulin results in hyperglycaemia, a high blood glucose with decreased utilization of carbohydrate and increased breakdown of fat and protein. This condition is known as diabetes mellitus. Three types of insulin are produced: from the pancreas of cows (bovine), from pigs (porcine), and human insulin, produced using genetic engineering techniques. Clear insulins have a shorter span of action (8–10 hours) than the cloudy insulins, which have an intermediate or longer activity span (12–24 hours). Mixtures of clear and cloudy insulins in varying proportions are also available. Insulin is produced in U100 strength, i.e. 100 units per mL, a standardization replacing the previous 20, 40 and 80 unit strengths. The most common method of administration is by subcutaneous injection using disposable plastic syringes. Preloaded pen devices are also popular, containing cartridges of insulin and allowing the dose to be dialled in 1 or 2 unit increments. Click count and preset syringes are also available for those having difficulty in drawing up the correct dosage, e.g. due to poor eyesight. Common injection sites are abdomen, buttocks, thigh, arm and sometimes calves. Rotation of sites is advised to prevent lipoatrophy or lipohypertrophy, i.e. hollows or swelling of fatty tissue. Subcutaneous injection of insulin using a syringe drive or infusion pump may have a limited use in some patients. Insulin may also be administered intravenously, e.g. prior to surgery or during an acute ketoacidotic episode. Diluted soluble insulin is given via an infusion pump, the amount being dictated by blood glucose levels. An excess of insulin administration may lead to hypoglycaemia, i.e. a low blood glucose. ⇒ diabetes mellitus.

insulin dependent diabetes mellitus *n* ⇒ diabetes mellitus.

insulinoma *n* an islet cell tumour. Adenoma of the βcells in the islets of Langerhans of the pancreas, which secrete insulin, resulting in hypoglycaemia.

intake and output a crude measure of a person's fluid balance. The amount of fluid taken orally, intravenously, by nasogastric tube or gastrostomy, is recorded on a special chart. All urine plus all output, in the form of vomit, diarrhoea and gastrointestinal drainage, is measured and recorded; some charts advise how much has to be added for estimated loss by perspiration, respiration and defaecation. The amount of intake and output is usually totalled over 24 h.

integrated medicine *n* a term ascribed to complementary medicine to reflect a harmonious integration of particular complementary therapies within orthodox healthcare practice. An emphasis is placed upon team work and efficacious therapies (both allopathic and complementary) towards promoting the health and well-being of individuals.

integration processes by which a person with a learning disability is able to function as an equal member of the community, e.g. attend mainstream school or college, or live and work within the community.

integument *n* a covering, especially the skin.

intellect *n* reasoning power, thinking faculty.

intellectualization an unconscious mental defence mechanism where individuals seek to detach themselves from emotionally difficult or threatening situations by managing the issues in an abstract, intellectual manner.

intelligence *n* inborn mental ability. *intelligence tests* designed to determine the level of intelligence. *intelligence quotient (IQ)* the ratio of mental age to chronological (actual) age.

intensive therapy unit (ITU) a unit in which highly specialized monitoring, resuscitation and therapeutic techniques are used to support critically ill patients. ⇒ high dependency unit.

intention tremor ⇒ tremor.

interaction *n* when two or more things or people have a reciprocal influence on each other. ⇒ care. ⇒ drug interaction.

interarticular *adj* between joints.

interatrial *adj* between the two atria of the heart.

intercellular *adj* between cells.

intercostal *adj* between the ribs. *intercostal muscles* muscles of respiration.

intercourse *n* communication. *sexual intercourse* coitus.

intercurrent *adj* describes a second disease arising in a person already suffering from one disease.

interference in psychology, describes the competition between items of information that may prevent learning and retrieval from long term memory. It occurs when different items of information are associated with the same retrieval clue. *proactive interference* when previously learned material makes it more difficult to learn and recall new information. *retroactive interference* when recent experiences prevent the recall of previously learned material from memory.

interferons (IFNs) *npl* protein mediators that enhance cellular resistance to viruses. When a virus infects a cell, it triggers interferon production. This then interacts with surrounding cells and renders them resist-

ant to virus attack. Interferons also act as cytokines to modulate the immune response. Interferon has caused regression of some tumours and is used in the management of some types of multiple sclerosis.

interleukins *npl* one of the large group of signalling molecules or cytokines. They are nonspecific immune chemicals produced by macrophages and activated T-lymphocytes. Interleukins also act with other cytokines in the regulation of haemopoiesis.

interlobar *adj* between the lobes, e.g. interlobar pleurisy.

interlobular *adj* between the lobules.

intermenstrual *adj* between the menstrual periods, such as bleeding.

intermittent *adj* occurring at intervals. *intermittent claudication* ⇒ claudication. *intermittent peritoneal dialysis* ⇒ dialysis. *intermittent pneumatic compression* a stocking worn to prevent deep vein thrombosis of upper and lower limb. ⇒ phlebothrombosis. *intermittent positive pressure* ⇒ mechanical ventilation. ⇒ positive pressure ventilation. *intermittent self-catheterization* ⇒ self-catheterization.

intermittent mandatory ventilation (IMV) *n* a type of assisted ventilation where a mandatory number of respirations are mechanically imposed on spontaneous breathing. It can be used to wean patients off mechanical ventilation.

intermittent positive pressure ventilation (IPPV) ⇒ mechanical ventilation.

internal *adj* inside. *internal capsule* area in the brain between the basal nuclei and the thalamus; it is formed by the efferent and afferent fibres that connect the cerebral cortex with other parts of the brain, muscles and sensory receptors. *internal ear* ⇒ ear. *internal respiration* ⇒ respiration. *internal secretions* those produced by the ductless or endocrine glands and passed directly into the bloodstream; hormones. *internal version* ⇒ version.

International and British Standards in Quality Systems *n* an audit programme used to monitor quality in organizations including those providing health care.

International Classification of Disease (ICD) list of disease categories compiled by the World Health Organization.

International Council of Nurses (ICN) at international level, the ICN, founded in 1899, represents worldwide national nurses' associations. The headquarters are in Geneva and, among its many duties, it organizes a quadrennial congress (each in a different country) which is open to nurses throughout the world.

internet a worldwide connection of many computer networks providing access to information sources and transmission of electronic mail. ⇒ E-mail.

interneuron(e) *n* a connecting or linking neuron.

interosseous *adj* between bones. *interosseous membrane* a membrane between two bones, such as the tibia and fibula.

interphalangeal *adj* between the phalanges.

interphase *n* phase between mitotic divisions during which the cell performs its normal metabolic processes and prepares for mitosis.

interpretive approach a research approach used by social scientists that includes the meaning and significance people attach to situations and behaviour.

interserosal *adj* between serous membrane, as in the pleural, peritoneal and pericardial cavities — **interserosally** *adv*.

intersexuality *n* hermaphroditism or pseudohermaphroditism. The condition where an individual has both male and female anatomical characteristics to varying degrees, or the external genitalia are ambiguous or are not those of their genetic sex.

interspinous *adj* between spinous processes, especially those of the vertebrae.

interstices *npl* spaces.

interstitial *adj* situated in the interstices of a part; distributed through the connective structures. *interstitial-cell stimulating hormone (ICSH)* (*syn* luteinizing hormone) a hormone released from the anterior lobe of the pituitary gland; which in the male causes the testes to produce testosterone. *interstitial fluid* the extracellular fluid in the tissue spaces surrounding the cells. *interstitial keratitis* ⇒ keratitis.

intertrigo *n* superficial inflammation occurring in moist skin folds, such as in the groin or under the breasts. It may result from poor hygiene or inadequate drying — **intertrigenous** *adj*.

intertrochanteric *adj* between trochanters, usually referring to those on the proximal femur.

interval cancer *n* a cancer that is diagnosed in the interval between screening appointments, such as breast cancer detected between mammography examinations.

interval data measurement data with a numerical score, e.g. temperature, that has an arbitary zero. The intervals between successive values are the same, e.g. a one degree increase from 36 to 37 is the same as from 37 to 38. ⇒ ratio data.

interventricular *adj* between ventricles, as those of the brain or heart.

intervertebral *adj* between the vertebrae. *intervertebral discs* pad of fibrocartilage between the vertebrae. Prolapse of a disc causes severe pain due to pressure on the nerve root. ⇒ nucleus pulposus. ⇒ prolapse.

interviewing *v* one of the methods used to collect data at the initial assessment. Prompting and reflecting techniques may be required to help the patient give the necessary information.

intestine *n* a part of the alimentary canal/tract extending from the stomach to the anus. It comprises the small intestine and the large intestine. ⇒ bowel. **intestinal** *adj*.

intima *n* the internal coat of an artery or vein. It consists of very smooth endothelium — **intimal** *adj*.

intolerance *n* the manifestation of various unusual reactions to particular substances such as nutrients or medications.

intra-abdominal *adj* within the abdominal cavity.

intra-amniotic *adj* within, or into, the amniotic fluid.

intra-aortic *adj* within the aorta. *intra-aortic balloon pump (IABP)* a device used to enhance the cardiac output in cardiogenic shock and ventricular failure.

intra-arterial *adj* within an artery.

intra-articular *adj* within a joint.

intrabronchial *adj* within a bronchus.

intracanalicular *adj* within a canaliculus.

intracapillary *adj* within a capillary.

intracapsular *adj* within a capsule, e.g. that of the lens or a joint. ⇒ extracapsular *ant*.

intracardiac *adj* within the heart.

intracaval *adj* within the vena cava — **intracavally** *adv*.

intracellular *adj* within cells. *intracellular fluid (ICF)* fluid inside the cells of the body. ⇒ extracellular *ant*. ⇒ fluid compartment.

intracerebral *adj* within the cerebrum. *intracerebral haemorrhage* bleeding into the cerebrum.

intracranial *adj* within the skull. ⇒ intracranial pressure.

intracranial pressure (ICP) maintained at a normal level by brain tissue, intracellular and extracellular fluid, cerebrospinal fluid and blood. A change in any of these compartments can increase the pressure. Raised intracranial pressure (RIP) may occur in conditions that include: brain tumours, haemorrhage and head injury.

intracutaneous *adj* within the skin tissues — **intracutaneously** *adv*.

intracytoplasmic sperm injection (ICSI) an assisted fertility/conception technique useful for low sperm counts. It involves the direct insertion in vitro of a single chosen spermatozoon into the female gamete (oocyte). Fertilized ova are then placed in the uterus.

intradermal *adj* within the skin — **intradermally** *adv*.

intradural *adj* inside the dura mater.

intragastric *adj* within the stomach.

intragluteal *adj* within the gluteal muscles comprising the buttock — **intragluteally** *adv*.

intrahepatic *adj* within the liver.

intralobular *adj* within the lobule, as the vein draining a hepatic lobule.

intraluminal *adj* within the hollow of a tube-like structure — **intraluminally** *adv*.

intralymphatic *adj* within a lymphatic gland or vessel.

intramedullary *adj* within the medullary cavity of a bone. *intramedullary nail* used for the fixation of certain fractures.

intramural *adj* within the layers of the wall of a hollow tube or organ — **intramurally** *adv*.

intramuscular *adj* within a muscle. Frequently used route for the injection of drugs — **intramuscularly** *adv*.

intranasal *adj* within the nasal cavity, such as packing used to stop nose bleeds.

intranatal *adj* ⇒ intrapartum — **intranatally** *adv*.

intranet connection of computer networks within an organisation, such as the NHS. ⇒ LAN. ⇒ WAN.

intraocular *adj* within the globe of the eye. *intraocular lens (IOL)* artificial lens implanted in the eye to provide correction of vision following cataract surgery.

intraoral *adj* within the mouth, as an intra-oral appliance.

intraorbital *adj* within the orbit.

intraosseous *adj* inside a bone. See Box – Intraosseous.

Intraosseous

The intraosseous route has developed as a means of giving fluids when rapid establishment of systemic access is vital and venous access is impossible. It provides an alternative route for the administration of drugs and fluids until venous access can be established. Any intravenous drug or fluid required during a paediatric resuscitation can be safely administered by this route. Onset of action and drug levels are similar to those achieved when using the intravenous route.

Paediatric advanced life support (PALS) courses recommend that the intraosseous access should be established if reliable venous access cannot be achieved within 3 attempts or 90 seconds, whichever comes first.

An intraosseous needle is a wide bore needle which is inserted into the medullary cavity of a long bone. The preferred site for children under 6 years is the flat anteromedial surface of the tibia, 1–3 cm below the tibial tuberosity. In children of this age the marrow cavity is very large, minimizing potential injury to adjacent tissues. The main contraindication to this route is a fracture of the pelvis, or the extremity proximal to or of the chosen site.

Further reading
Chamedides L, Hazinski M (Eds) 1988 Textbook of pediatric life support. Dallas: American Heart Association.

intrapartum *adj* (*syn* intranatal) at the time of birth; during labour, as asphyxia or infection. *intrapartum haemorrhage* bleeding occurring during labour, usually describes that from the uterus.

intraperitoneal *adj* within the peritoneal cavity.

intrapersonal skills those skills which operate within the mind and emotions of the individual.

intrapharyngeal *adj* within the pharynx.

intrapleural *adj* within the pleural cavity.

intrapulmonary *adj* within the lungs, as intrapulmonary pressure.

intrapunitive *adj* a tendency to blame oneself.

intraretinal *adj* within the retina.

intraspinal *adj* within the spinal canal.

intrasplenic *adj* within the spleen.

intrasynovial *adj* within a synovial membrane or cavity.

intrathecal *adj* within the meninges; into the subarachnoid space. Drugs may be administered via this route, e.g. antimicrobial drugs for meningitis.

intrathoracic *adj* within the cavity of the thorax, as in intrathoracic pressures.

intratracheal *adj* within the trachea.

intrauterine *adj* within the uterus. *intrauterine contraceptive device (IUCD, IUD)* a device which is implanted in the cavity of the uterus to prevent conception. Its exact mode of action is not known. *intrauterine growth retardation (IUGR)* associated with a poor delivery of maternal blood to the placental bed, diminished placental exchange or a poor fetal transfer from the placental area. Serial ultrasonography has been shown to be beneficial in high-risk pregnancies to measure fetal growth and well-being. *intrauterine insemination (IUI)* prepared, fresh semen sample is inserted into the uterus via the cervix, ovulation having usually already been induced using hormone injections and under ultrasound supervision. Fertilization should take place naturally in the uterine tubes.

intravaginal *adj* within the vagina — **intravaginally** *adv.*

intravascular *adj* within the blood vessels — **intravascularly** *adv.*

intravenous *adj* within or into a vein. *intravenous feeding* ⇒ parenteral. *intravenous infusion* commonly referred to as a 'drip'; the closed administration of fluids from a containing vessel into a vein for such purposes as hydrating the body, correcting electrolyte imbalance, administering drugs or introducing nutrients. *intravenous injection* the introduction of drugs, including anaesthetics, into a vein. It is not a continuous procedure. ⇒ eutetic mixture of local anaesthetics (EMLA). *intravenous pyelogram* ⇒ urography. ⇒ venepuncture.

intravenous anaesthetic *n* drugs administered for the induction of anaesthesia, including thiopental (thiopentone), etomidate, propofol, midazolam and ketamine. Drugs such as diazepam and ketamine can be used to produce basal anaesthesia and sedation prior to anaesthesia.

intraventricular *adj* within a ventricle, especially a cerebral ventricle.

intrinsic *adj* inherent or inside; from within; real; natural. *Intrinsic coagulation pathway* → coagulation. *intrinsic factor* a glycoprotein released by gastric oxyntic (parietal) cells, essential for the satisfactory absorption of the extrinsic factor vitamin B_{12} in the small intestine.

intrinsic sugars *npl* sugars found in the cell walls of various foods of plant origin. ⇒ extrinsic.

introitus *n* any opening in the body, an entrance to a cavity, particularly the vagina.

introjection *n* a mental process whereby a person incorporates another person's or group's standards and values into his own personality.

introspection *n* looking inwards. A state of mental self-examination where an individual attempts to analyse their conscious mental processes. May be seen in exaggerated form in some serious mental health disorders, such as schizophrenia.

introversion *n* 1. the direction of thoughts and interest inwards to the world of ideas, instead of outwards to the external world. 2. a hollow structure that invaginates or turns in on itself.

introvert *n* an individual whose characteristic interests and modes of behaviour are directed inwards towards the self. ⇒ extrovert *ant.*

intubation *n* insertion of a tube into a hollow organ. Tracheal intubation is used during anaesthesia to maintain an airway and to permit suction of the respiratory tract. *duodenal intubation* a double tube is passed as far as the pyloric region of the stomach under fluoroscopy. The inner tube is then passed along to the duodeno-jejunal flexure. Barium sulphate suspension can then be passed to outline the small bowel. ⇒ extubation *ant*.

intussusception *n* a condition in which one part of the bowel telescopes (invaginates) into the adjoining distal bowel, causing severe colic, intestinal obstruction, vomiting and the passage of blood and mucus rectally ('redcurrant jelly' stools). It occurs most commonly in infants around the time of weaning, presenting as an acute emergency. The intussusception may be reduced by performing a nonsurgical hydrostatic reduction, usually by barium enema, but may sometimes require surgical treatment. (See Figure 34).

intussusceptum *n* the invaginated portion of an intussusception.

inunction *n* the act of rubbing an oily or fatty substance into the skin.

invagination *n* the act or condition of being ensheathed; a pushing inward, forming a pouch — **invaginate** *vt*.

invasion *n* the entry of micro-organisms into the body or the spread of cancer cells.

inversion turning inside out, as inversion of the uterus. ⇒ procidentia.

investigations *npl* procedures which are done either to establish diagnosis or to monitor the course of a disease or its treatment. They are classified as invasive, e.g. a barium enema, or noninvasive, for instance taking the blood pressure using a sphygmomanometer. They all have poten-

tial for increasing patient anxiety and research has shown that well-informed patients are less anxious.

involucrum *n* a sheath of new bone, which forms around a necrosed bone (sequestrum), in such conditions as osteomyelitis. ⇒ cloaca.

involuntary *adj* independent of the will, as muscle of the thoracic and abdominal organs.

involution *n* **1.** the normal shrinkage of an organ after fulfilling its functional purpose, e.g. uterus after pregnancy and labour. **2.** the period of progressive decline occurring after midlife when tissues and organs reduce in size and functional ability declines. ⇒ subinvolution — **involutional** *adj*.

iodine (I) *n* an element essential for the production of thyroid hormones. It is a powerful bactericide and is used as povidone iodine for skin preparation prior to invasive procedures, and it is incorporated within various commercial wound dressings. An oral preparation is used preoperatively for patients with hyperthyroidism to decrease release of the thyroid hormones and reduce vascularity of the gland before surgery. *radioactive iodine* radioactive isotopes of iodine, e.g. [131]I, are used for the diagnosis and treatment of thyroid conditions, such as thyroid cancer.

iodism *n* poisoning by iodine or iodides; the symptoms are those of a common cold and the appearance of a rash.

ion *n* an electrically charged atom or radical. In electrolysis, ions in solution pass to one or the other pole, or electrode. *ion channel* water-filled channels in cell membranes that allow the passage of certain ions, e.g. in the transmission of a nerve impulse. They may be the site of drug action where the drug, e.g. local anaesthetic, blocks the channel, or the drug modulates channel function in some way. ⇒ anion. ⇒ cation — **ionic** *adj* pertaining to ions. *ionic bond* a chemical bond where electrons move between the reacting atoms, i.e. electrons are donated and accepted. Atoms donating electrons become positively charged and those accepting become negatively charged. The attraction between the charged ions holds the two together, such as with sodium

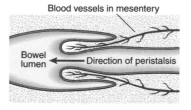

Blood vessels in mesentery

Bowel lumen ← Direction of peristalsis

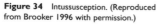

Figure 34 Intussusception. (Reproduced from Brooker 1996 with permission.)

chloride. ⇒ covalent bond. ⇒ hydrogen bond.

ion-exchange resins *npl* polystyrene resins used orally to reduce the level of specific ions (calcium and potassium) in the body. ⇒ ion.

ionization *n* the dissociation of a substance in solution into electrically charged ions.

ionizing radiation a form of radiation which destabilizes an atom, forming an ion. X-rays, gamma rays and particle radiation are all examples of ionizing radiation. Has the ability to cause tissue damage. ⇒ radiation.

iontophoresis *n* treatment whereby ions of various soluble salts are introduced into the tissues by means of a constant electrical current. The drug pilocarpine can be introduced into the skin by this method during a sweat test for cystic fibrosis.

IPD *abbr* intermittent peritoneal dialysis.

ipecacuanha *n* dried root from South America. Used as an emetic and contained in some expectorants.

IPP *abbr* intermittent positive pressure.

IPPV *abbr* intermittent positive pressure ventilation.

ipsilateral *adj* on the same side — **ipsilaterally** *adv.*

IQ *abbr* intelligence quotient.

iridectomy *n* excision of a part of the iris, thus forming an artificial pupil to improve drainage of aqueous humor.

iridencleisis *n* an older type of filtering operation. Scleral incision made at angle of anterior chamber; meridian cut in iris; either one or both pillars are left in scleral wound to contract as scar tissue. Decreases intraocular tension in glaucoma.

iridium-192 (¹⁹²Ir) *n* a radioactive element used in brachytherapy to treat cancers in anus, tongue, breast as implanted wires or hair pins.

iridocele *n* (*syn* iridoptosis) protrusion of part of the iris through a corneal wound (prolapsed iris).

iridocyclitis *n* inflammation of the iris and ciliary body.

iridodialysis *n* a separation of the iris from its ciliary attachment. Often as a result of trauma.

iridoplegia *n* paralysis of the iris.

iridoptosis ⇒ iridocele.

iridotomy *n* an incision into the iris.

iris *n* the circular coloured structure forming the anterior one-sixth of the middle coat of the eyeball. It is perforated in the centre by an opening, the pupil. Contraction of its muscle fibres controls the size of the pupil to regulate the amount of light entering the eye. Situated behind the cornea and in front of the lens it forms a division between the anterior and posterior chambers. *iris bombe* bulging forward of the iris due to pressure of the aqueous humor behind, when posterior synechiae are present around the pupil.

iritis *n* inflammation of the iris.

iron (Fe) *n* a metallic element required in the body for the formation of haemoglobin and several enzymes. *iron deficiency anaemia* ⇒ anaemia. ⇒ haemochromatosis.

irradiation *n* exposure to any form of radiant energy, e.g. heat, light or X ray.

irreducible *adj* unable to be brought to desired condition. *irreducible hernia* ⇒ hernia.

irritable *adj* capable of being excited to activity; responding easily to stimuli. *irritable bowel syndrome* common bowel dysfunction for which no organic cause can be found. It is characterized by unusual motility of both small and large bowel which produces discomfort and intermittent pain, alternating constipation and diarrhoea and the passage of mucus rectally — **irritability** *n.*

irritant *adj, n* describes any agent which causes irritation.

IS *acr* Insight Scale.

ISC *abbr* intermittent self-catheterization.

ischaemia *n* deficient blood supply to any part of the body. ⇒ angina. ⇒ Volkmann's ischaemic contracture — **ischaemic** *adj.*

ischaemic heart disease (IHD) insufficient supply of oxygenated blood to the myocardium, causing central chest pain of varying intensity which may radiate to arms, neck and jaw. The lumen of the blood vessels is usually narrowed by atheromatous plaques. ⇒ angina pectoris. ⇒ angioplasty. ⇒ coronary artery bypass graft. ⇒ myocardial infarction.

ischiofemoral *adj* pertaining to the ischium and the femur. *ischiofemoral ligaments* strong ligament which runs from the ischium to the greater trochanter of the femur.

ischiorectal *adj* pertaining to the ischium and the rectum, as in ischiorectal abscess which occurs between these two structures.

ischium *n* the lower and hind part of the innominate bone of the pelvis; the bone on which the body rests when sitting — **ischial** *adj*.

Ishihara colour test *n* test for colour blindness, using a series of charts with dots in a variety of colours that display specific numbers or shapes to an individual with normal colour vision.

islet cell tumour *n* a tumour affecting the islets of Langerhans of the pancreas. Usually secrete insulin. ⇒ insulinoma. More rarely, a tumour that secretes gastrin. ⇒ Zollinger-Ellison syndrome.

islets of Langerhans *n* collections of special cells scattered throughout the pancreas, mainly concerned with endocrine function. The pancreatic islets contain four types of hormone-secreting cells: alpha cells which secrete glucagon; beta cells which secrete insulin and amylin; the delta cells which secrete several substances, including somatostatin or growth hormone inhibiting hormone (GHIH); and other cells which secrete regulatory pancreatic polypeptide.

ISO 9000/BS 5750 *abbr* International and British Standards in Quality Systems.

isoantibody *n* an antibody produced by one individual that reacts with the isoantigen of another individual of the same species.

isoantigen *n* an antigen existing in an alternative form in a species, thus inducing an immune response when one form is transferred to a member of the species that lacks it; typical antigens are the blood group antigens; also called *alloantigens*.

isoenzyme *n* an enzyme that catalyses the same reaction, but exists in several forms and in different sites, such as lactate dehydrogenase and alkaline phosphatase.

isograft graft with material obtained from a donor of identical genotype, e.g. an identical twin.

isoimmunization *n* the formation of antibodies following exposure to an antigen from an individual of the same species, such as anti-D formation when a rhesus (Rh) negative person is exposed to Rh-positive blood. ⇒ blood groups. This occurs if a Rh-negative person is given Rh-positive blood, or a Rh-negative woman is carrying a Rh-positive fetus.

isolation *n* separation of a patient from others for a variety of reasons. ⇒ containment isolation. ⇒ protective isolation. ⇒ source isolation.

isoleucine *n* one of the essential (indispensable) amino acids.

isomers *npl* compounds which are formed from the same elements, but different atomic structure confers differing properties.

isometric *adj* of equal measure. *isometric contraction* a muscle contracts while its attachments remain stationary and, therefore, it stays the same length and joints do not move. *isometric exercises* carried out without movement; static contractions; increasing tension to maintain muscle tone.

isotonic *adj* equal tension; applied to any solution which has the same osmotic pressure as the fluid with which it is being compared. *isotonic muscle contraction* muscle contraction that results in a change in muscle length and movement of its attachments. *isotonic exercises* carried out with movement; to increase muscle strength and endurance. *isotonic saline* (*syn* normal saline, physiological saline), 0.9% solution of sodium chloride in water.

isotope scanning injection of a radioactive isotope before a scan. ⇒ isotopes.

isotopes *npl* two or more forms of the same element having identical chemical properties and the same atomic number but different mass numbers, such as hydrogen which has three forms. ⇒ radioactive isotopes.

ispaghula *n* ⇒ laxatives.

isthmus *n* a narrowed part of an organ or tissue such as that connecting the two lobes of the thyroid gland.

IT *acr* information technology.

itch *n* a sensation on the skin which makes one want to scratch. *itch mite Sarcoptes scabiei* ⇒ scabies.

ITU *abbr* intensive therapy unit.

IUCD *abbr* intrauterine contraceptive device.

IUD *abbr* intrauterine (contraceptive) device.

IUGR *abbr* ⇒ intrauterine growth retardation.

IUI *abbr* intrauterine insemination.

IVC *abbr* inferior vena cava. ⇒ vena cava.

IVF *abbr* in vitro fertilization.

IVU *abbr* intravenous urogram. ⇒ urography.

Jacksonian epilepsy ⇒ epilepsy.

Jacquemier's sign blueness of the vaginal mucosa seen in early pregnancy.

jargon *n* specialized or technical language which is only understood by a particular group. The word is often used to describe the use of obscure and pretentious language, together with a roundabout way of expression.

Jarisch-Herxheimer reaction *n* a situation where the symptoms of a disease are initially worsened by drug treatment, such as seen in the treatment of syphilis with penicillin. It occurs with other diseases, e.g. relapsing fever.

Jarman index an index that uses a set of factors that indicate health needs in a population, e.g. percentage of people belonging to minority ethnic groups, percentage of lone parent families etc. It was first devised to assess the workload of general practitioners.

jaundice *n* (*syn* icterus) a condition characterized by a raised bilirubin level in the blood (hyperbilirubinaemia). Minor degrees are only detectable chemically. Major degrees are visible in the yellow discoloration of skin, sclerae and mucosae. Pruritus occurs as bile salts also accumulate in the blood. Jaundice without the excretion of bilirubin in the urine is termed acholuric. Jaundice may be classified as: (a) *haemolytic or prehepatic jaundice* where excessive breakdown of red blood cells releases bilirubin into the blood, such as with physiological jaundice of the newborn and haemolytic anaemia. ⇒ haemolysis. ⇒ haemolytic disease of the newborn; (b) *hepatocellular jaundice* arises when liver cell function is impaired, such as with hepatitis or cirrhosis; (c) *obstructive or cholestatic jaundice* where the flow of bile is obstructed either within the liver (intrahepatic) or in the larger ducts of the biliary tract (extrahepatic). Causes include: cirrhosis, tumours, parasites and gallstones. (See Figure 35).

Java *n* a computer language. ⇒ computer language.

jaw-bone *n* either the maxilla (upper jaw) or mandible (lower jaw).

JCA *abbr* juvenile chronic arthritis.

jejunal biopsy a test used in the diagnosis of coeliac disease. A tube is passed through the mouth and into the jejunum. A small piece of jejunal mucosa is removed and sent for histological and enzyme examinations.

jejunostomy *n* a surgically made fistula between the jejunum and the anterior abdominal wall; used temporarily for feeding where passage of food through the stomach is impossible or undesirable.

jejunum *n* that middle part of the small intestine between the duodenum and the ileum. ⇒ bowel — **jejunal** *adj*.

jet lag disruption of biological processes which normally follow diurnal rhythms, occurs after travel through different time zones. There are problems with sleep, appetite, concentration and memory and tiredness for some days until body rhythms return to normal. Similar physical effects are reported by people whose work involves different shift patterns.

jigger *n* a sand flea, *Tunga penetrans*, prevalent in the tropics. It burrows under the skin to lay its eggs, causing intense irritation. Secondary infection is usual.

joint *n* the articulation of two or more bones (arthrosis). There are three main classes: (a) fibrous (synarthroses), immovable joints, e.g. the sutures of the skull; (b) cartilaginous (amphiarthroses), slightly movable joints of two types; synchondroses formed from the epiphyseal plates of long bones during growth and

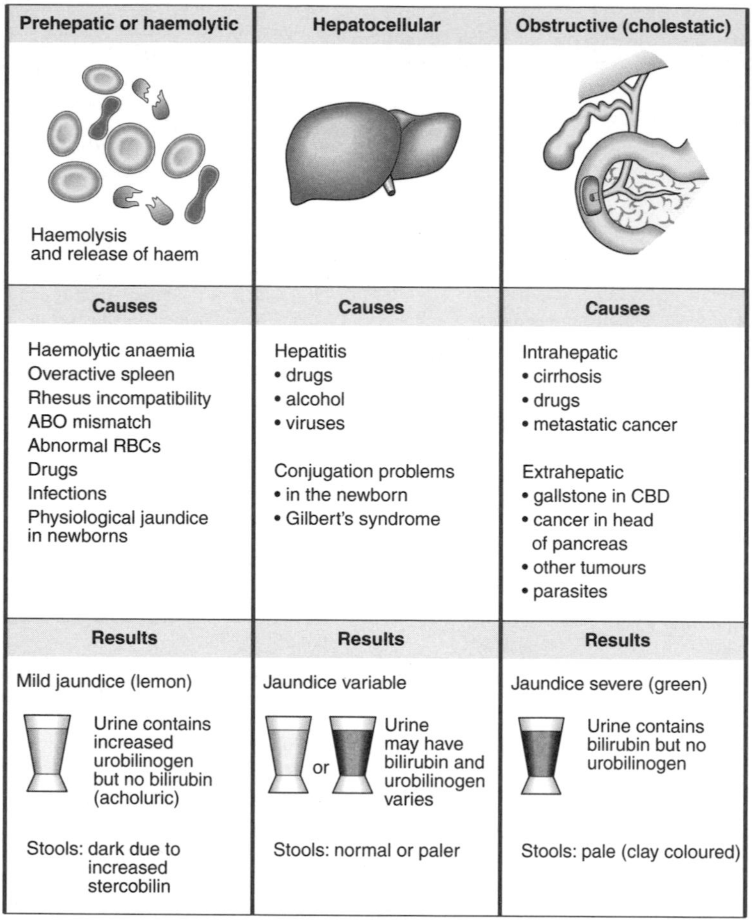

Prehepatic or haemolytic	Hepatocellular	Obstructive (cholestatic)
Haemolysis and release of haem		
Causes	**Causes**	**Causes**
Haemolytic anaemia Overactive spleen Rhesus incompatibility ABO mismatch Abnormal RBCs Drugs Infections Physiological jaundice in newborns	Hepatitis • drugs • alcohol • viruses Conjugation problems • in the newborn • Gilbert's syndrome	Intrahepatic • cirrhosis • drugs • metastatic cancer Extrahepatic • gallstone in CBD • cancer in head of pancreas • other tumours • parasites
Results	**Results**	**Results**
Mild jaundice (lemon) Urine contains increased urobilinogen but no bilirubin (acholuric) Stools: dark due to increased stercobilin	Jaundice variable Urine may have bilirubin and urobilinogen varies or Stools: normal or paler	Jaundice severe (green) Urine contains bilirubin but no urobilinogen Stools: pale (clay coloured)

Figure 35 Types and causes of jaundice. (Reproduced from Brooker 1996 with permission.)

symphyses, e.g. between the manubrium and the body of the sternum and (c) synovial (diarthoses), freely movable joints, e.g. elbow or hip. ⇒ Charcot's joint.

joule (J) *n* a derived SI unit (International System of Units) for energy, work and quantity of heat. The unit is the energy expended when 1 kg (kilogram) is moved 1 m (metre) by a force of gravity. The kilojoule (kJ = 10^3J) and the megajoule (MJ = 10^6J) are used by physiologists and nutritionists for measuring large amounts of energy.

jugular *adj* pertaining to the throat. *jugular veins* two large veins passing down either side of the neck which carry most blood from the head. *jugular venous pressure (JVP)* the pressure in the jugular veins – a guide to the pressure in the right side of the heart.

Jung, Carl Swiss psychiatrist/psychoanalyst (1875–1961) — **Jungian** *adj* pertaining to the work of Jung, especially his theories of psychoanalysis and 'collective unconscious'.

justice ethical principle involving concepts of fairness and justness. It may be described as acting within a set of moral laws, respecting the views and rights of others, or equity in the distribution of resources.

juvenile chronic arthritis (JCA) a form of inflammatory arthritis occurring in children. There are varying degrees of inflammation in joints with loss of articular cartilage and premature ossification of the epiphyseal growing plates. Management includes: relief of pain and inflammation with warmth and drugs that include NSAIDs; attention to nutrition and general well-being; adequate rest, both general and for specific joints with splints; good positioning and posture with expert physiotherapy.

juxtaglomerular near the glomerulus. *juxtaglomerular apparatus (JGA)* specialized cells in the distal convoluted tubule and the afferent arteriole of the nephron. Concerned with monitoring pressure changes and sodium levels in the blood and initiating the release of renin that converts an inactive precursor to angiotensin when blood pressure falls, or when sodium levels fall or blood flow is slow. ⇒ macula densa.

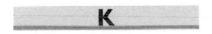

Kahn test *n* an obsolete serological test for syphilis.

kala-azar *n* a generalized form of leishmaniasis (visceral) occurring in the tropics. There is anaemia, fever, splenomegaly and wasting. It is caused by the parasitic protozoon *Leishmania donovani* and is spread by sandflies.

Kanner's syndrome a form of autism. ⇒ autistic disorders.

kaolin *n* natural aluminium silicate. When given orally, it absorbs toxic substances, hence useful in diarrhoea, colitis and food poisoning. Also used in dusting powders and poultices.

Kaposi's disease ⇒ xeroderma pigmentosum.

Kaposi's sarcoma a malignancy characterized by the growth of new blood vessels which appear as red, purple or brown patches on the skin. It metastasizes to the lymph nodes, liver and spleen. Originally common in Africa, it is usually only seen in individuals who are immunocompromised, such as those with acquired immune deficiency syndrome. According to the WHO/CDC classication, it is an AIDS-defining condition.

Kaposi's varicelliform eruption ⇒ eczema herpeticum.

Kardex *n* a proprietary piece of stationery which permits the storing of a given number of patients' nursing or medication records.

Kartagener's syndrome primary ciliary dyskinesia. A rare inherited autosomal recessive condition that causes abnormal movement of the respiratory cilia. It causes repeated sinusitis and respiratory tract infection leading to bronchiectasis.

karyotype *n* creation of an orderly array of chromosomes, usually derived from the study of cultured cells. This is usually done for diagnostic purposes, or persons at risk of producing children with chromosomal abnormalities, or for the prenatal detection of fetal abnormality in women at risk of producing chromosomally abnormal fetuses, for example because of advancing age.

KASI *abbr* Knowledge About Schizophrenia Interview.

katal *n* the amount of an enzyme required to catalyse a mole (mol) of substrate per second under defined physical conditions.

Kawasaki disease an inflammatory disease affecting small blood vessels (vasculitis). The aetiology is not well understood, but it is a cause of secondary cardiac disease in children. Occurs mainly in Japan and the US. ⇒ mucocutaneous lymph node syndrome (MLNS).

Kayer-Fleischer ring *n* brownish-green rings seen around the cornea in patients with Wilson's disease.

Kell factor a blood group factor found in about 10% of Caucasians; inherited according to Mendelian laws of inheritance. Anti-Kell antibodies can cross the placenta. ⇒ blood groups.

Keller's operation for hallux valgus or rigidus. Excision of the proximal half of the proximal phalanx, plus any osteophytes and exostoses on the metatarsal head. The toe is fixed in the corrected position; after healing a pseudarthrosis results.

Kelly-Paterson syndrome ⇒ Plummer-Vinson syndrome.

keloid *n* an overgrowth of scar tissue, which may produce a contraction deformity or large bulbous scar. Keloid scarring occurs in some pigmented skins; it tends to get progressively worse. ⇒ disfigurement. ⇒ pressure garment.

keratectasia protrusion of the cornea.

keratectomy *n* surgical excision of a portion of the cornea. ⇒ photorefractive keratectomy. ⇒ radial keratectomy.

keratin *n* a fibrous protein found in tissues such as the outer layer of the skin, nails, horn and hooves.

keratinization *n* the process by which tissue is converted to keratin (horny tissue). Occurs as a pathological process in vitamin A deficiency.

keratinocytes cells of the epidermis that produce keratin and other proteins.

keratitic precipitates (KP) large cells adherent to the posterior surface of the cornea; present in inflammation of iris, ciliary body and choroid.

keratitis *n* inflammation of the cornea. *interstitial keratitis* inflammation of the deeper layers of the cornea. May be a feature of syphilis or tuberculosis.

keratocele *n* protrusion of Descemet's membrane of the cornea.

keratoconjunctivitis *n* inflammation of the cornea and conjunctiva. *epidemic keratoconjunctivitis* due to an adenovirus. *keratoconjunctivitis sicca* ⇒ Sjögren syndrome.

keratoconus *n* a cone-like protrusion of the cornea, usually due to a noninflammatory thinning.

keratoiritis *n* inflammation of the cornea and iris.

keratolytic *adj* having the property of breaking down keratinized epidermis.

keratoma *n* ⇒ callosity — **keratomata** *pl.*

keratomalacia *n* softening of the cornea; ulceration may occur; frequently caused by lack of vitamin A.

keratome *n* a special knife with a trowel-like blade for incising the cornea.

keratopathy *n* any disease of the cornea — **keratopathic** *adj.*

keratophakia *n* surgical introduction of a biological 'lens' into the cornea to correct hypermetropia.

keratoplasty *n* ⇒ corneal graft — **keratoplastic** *adj.*

keratosis *n* thickening of the horny layer of the skin. Also referred to as hyperkeratosis. Has the appearance of warty excrescences. *keratosis palmaris et plantaris* (*syn* tylosis) a congenital thickening of the horny layer of the palms and soles.

keratotomy *n* incision into the cornea.

kerion *n* a boggy suppurative mass of the scalp associated with ringworm of the hair.

kernicterus *n* staining of brain cells, especially the basal nuclei, with bilirubin. A complication of jaundice in preterm infants and in haemolytic disease of the newborn. It may result in learning disability. ⇒ icterus gravis neonatorum.

Kernig's sign inability to straighten the leg at the knee joint when the thigh is flexed at right angles to the trunk. Occurs in meningeal irritation, such as in meningitis.

ketoacidosis *n* (*syn* ketosis) acidosis due to accumulation of ketone bodies β-hydroxybutyric acid, acetoacetic acid and acetone, products of the metabolism of fat. Primarily a serious complication of insulin dependent diabetes, but also occurs in starvation. Symptoms include drowsiness, headache and deep sighing respiration. *diabetic ketoacidosis* ketone bodies are formed as fatty acids are incompletely oxidized when glucose is unavailable as an energy source. There is acidosis and dehydration occurring with hyperglycaemia. ⇒ Kussmaul's respiration — **ketoacidotic** *adj.*

ketogenic diet a high fat content producing ketosis (acidosis).

ketonaemia *n* ketone bodies in the blood — **ketonaemic** *adj.*

ketones *npl* organic compounds (e.g. ketosteroids) containing a keto group (–C=O). *ketone bodies* include acetone, acetoacetic acid (acetoacetate) and β-hydroxybutyric acid produced during normal fat oxidation. Small amounts can be used as fuel but excess production leads to ketoacidosis. This may occur when blood glucose level is high, but unavailable for metabolism, such as in uncontrolled diabetes mellitus.

ketonuria *n* ketone bodies in the urine — **ketonuric** *adj.*

ketosis *n* ketoacidosis — **ketotic** *adj.*

ketosteroids *npl* steroid hormones which contain a ketone group, formed by the addition of an oxygen molecule to the basic ring structure. The 17-ketosteroids (which have this oxygen at carbon-17) are excreted in normal urine and are present in excess in overactivity of the adrenal glands and the gonads.

KGV ⇒ Manchester Symptom Severity Scale.

khat *n* the leaves contain two psychostimulants structurally similar to amfetamine (amphetamine). Chewing the leaves is a widespread habit in East Africa and the Middle East. It is becoming increasingly available in the UK.

kidneys *npl* paired retroperitoneal organs situated on the upper posterior abdominal wall in the lumbar region. Concerned with homeostasis, they produce urine to excrete waste such as urea, control water and electrolyte balance and blood pH. They also secrete renin and renal erythropoietic factor (REF) and are involved in vitamin D metabolism. *artificial kidney* ⇒ dialyser. *horseshoe kidney* a congenital anatomical variation in which the inner lower border of each kidney is joined to give a horseshoe shape. Usually symptomless and only rarely interferes with drainage of urine into ureters. *kidney failure* → renal failure. *kidney function tests* ⇒ renal function tests. *kidney transplant* replacement of diseased kidneys with a single well-matched donor organ (living donor or cadaveric). Kidneys may also be transplanted from the renal bed to other sites in the same individual in cases of ureteric disease or trauma.

kilogram (kg) *n* a measurement of mass. One of the seven base units of the International System of Units (SI). One thousand grams.

kilojoule (kJ) *n* a unit equal to 1000 joules, used by physiologists and nutritionists for measuring large amounts of energy. It replaces the kilocaloric (kcal) which is still in use (1 kcal = 4.2 kJ). 1 g of fat yields 38 kJ, 1 g of protein 17 kJ, and 1 g of carbohydrate yields 16 kJ.

Kimmelstiel-Wilson syndrome diabetic nephropathy, a glomerulosclerosis caused by damage to the glomerular capillaries. It is characterized by hypertension, proteinuria and the nephrotic syndrome leading to renal failure.

kinaesthesis *n* muscle sense; perception of movement, body weight and position — **kinaesthetic** *adj.*

kinase *n* enzymes which catalyse the transfer of a high-energy group of a donor, usually adenosine triphosphate, to some acceptor, usually named after the acceptor (e.g. fructokinase).

kineplastic surgery operative measures, whereby certain muscle groups are isolated and utilized to work certain modified prostheses.

kinetic *adj* pertaining to or producing motion.

King's Fund Audit process an organizational audit programme developed by the King's Fund (London) for use in healthcare settings.

kinins *npl* biologically active polypeptides, e.g. bradykinin, which initiate vasodilation, vessel permeability and pain.

Kirschner wire a wire drilled into a bone to apply skeletal traction. A hand or electric drill is used, a stirrup is attached and the wire is rendered taut by means of a special wire-tightener.

Klebsiella spp *n* a genus of anaerobic Gram-negative bacteria of the family Enterobacteriaceae. They are part of the normal flora in the bowel. They are opportunists and commonly cause respiratory, urinary and wound infections. Some strains are resistant to several antibiotics. *Klebsiella pneumoniae* is the cause of severe pneumonia in patients requiring respiratory support in intensive care settings.

Klebs-Loeffler bacillus old term for *Corynebacterium diphtheriae.*

kleptomania *n* compulsive stealing due to mental disturbance, usually of the obsessional type — **kleptomaniac** *n, adj.*

Klinefelter syndrome a chromosomal abnormality affecting males, usually with 47 chromosomes including XXY sex chromosomes. Puberty is frequently delayed, the person has male external genitalia but the testes remain small and firm. There is often obesity, gynaecomastia, female body hair distribution, eunuchoid build and infertility.

Klumpke's paralysis paralysis and atrophy of muscles of the forearm and hand which may be caused by a birth injury to the lower brachial plexus. It is often accompanied by Horner's syndrome which gives rise to sensory and pupillary disturbances due to injury to the cervical sympathetic nerves.

knee *n* the hinge joint formed by the lower end of the femur and the head of the tibia. *kneecap* the patella. *knee jerk* a deep tendon reflex where the relaxed quadriceps muscle contracts when the patellar tendon is tapped; usually performed with the lower femur supported behind, the knee bent and the leg limp. Persistent variation from normal usually signifies organic nervous disorder, e.g. exaggerated in lesions of the upper motor neurons.

Knowledge About Schizophrenia Interview (KASI) used by mental health nurses and others to assess and evaluate relatives' knowledge, beliefs and attitudes about six broad aspects of schizophrenia: diagnosis; symptomatology; aetiology; medication; prognosis and management.

knuckles *npl* the dorsal aspect of any of the joints between the phalanges and the metacarpal bones, or between the phalanges.

Koch's bacillus old term for *Mycobacterium tuberculosis*, the organism that causes tuberculosis.

Koch-Weeks bacillus old term for *Haemophilus aegyptius*.

Köhler disease osteochondritis of the tarsal navicular bone. Confined to children of 3–5 years. Tenderness, redness, swelling and sometimes pain occur over the tarsal navicular bone on the medial side of the foot.

koilonychia *npl* spoon-shaped nails, characteristic of iron deficiency anaemia. ⇒ anaemia.

Koplik's spots small white spots inside the mouth, during the first few days of the invasion (prodromal) stage of measles, often before the rash appears.

Korotkoff sounds (Korotkov) *npl* the sounds heard whilst recording noninvasive arterial blood pressure with a sphygmomanometer and stethoscope. The phases are: (1) a sharp thud which represents systolic pressure (2) a swishing sound (3) a soft thud (4) a soft blowing, becoming muffled (5) silence. In practice, opinion is divided as to whether phase 4 or 5 should represent diastolic pressure. (See Figure 36).

Korsakoff's psychosis, syndrome a condition which follows delirium and toxic states. Often due to alcohol misuse. The consciousness is clear and alert, but the patient is disorientated for time and place, with grossly impaired memory, especially for recent events (patient often confabulates to fill in the gaps). Associated with the thiamine (vitamin B_1) deficiency that occurs in malnutrition or chronic alcohol misuse. ⇒ Wernicke's encephalopathy.

kosher describes food that conforms to and is prepared according to the laws of Judaism.

KP *abbr* keratitic precipitates.

Krabbe's disease a rare inherited disorder of lipid metabolism that causes degeneration of the central nervous system.

kraurosis *n* skin changes characterized by atrophy and shrinking. *kraurosis vulvae* itching and dryness affecting the vulva in postmenopausal women. It is associated with a lack of oestrogen and may predispose to leukoplakia and malignant changes.

Krebs' cycle *n* final common pathway for the oxidation of fuel molecules: glucose, fatty acids, gylcerol and amino acids. Most enter the cycle as acetyl CoA and are oxidized to liberate energy (ATP), carbon dioxide and water. Various intermediates of these reactions are used for biosynthesis of other metabolic molecules, such as amino acids. Also called citric acid cycle and tricarboxylic acid cycle.

Krukenberg's tumour metastatic tumour in the ovary, usually from a primary cancer in the stomach.

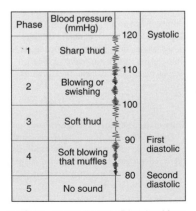

Phase	Blood pressure (mmHg)		
1	Sharp thud	120	Systolic
2	Blowing or swishing	110	
3	Soft thud	100	
4	Soft blowing that muffles	90	First diastolic
5	No sound	80	Second diastolic

Figure 36 Korotkoff sounds. (Reproduced from Brooker 1998 with permission.)

krypton (Kr) *n* an inert gas.

Küntscher nail used for intramedullary fixation of fractured long bones, especially the femur. The nail has a 'clover-leaf' cross-section.

Kupffer's cells *npl* large phagocytic cells of the liver. Part of the monocyte-macrophage system (reticuloendothelial) they are concerned with phagocytosis of bacterial and worn out erythrocytes.

Kussmaul's respiration *n* deep sighing respirations associated with diabetic ketoacidosis.

Kussmaul's sign venous pulsus paradoxus. A paradoxical rise in venous pressure during inspiration. It is characterized by distention of jugular veins and may indicate constrictive pericarditis.

Kveim test an intracutaneous test for sarcoidosis using tissue prepared from a person known to be suffering from the condition.

kwashiorkor *n* form of protein-energy malnutrition occurring when children are weaned onto a low protein diet with adequate amounts of energy from carbohydrate sources. It is characterized by a miserable child who fails to thrive. Weight loss may not be marked, but the child fails to grow. There is generalized oedema, anaemia, changes in hair and skin pigmentation, diarrhoea and hepatomegaly.

kymograph *n* an apparatus for recording movements, e.g. of muscles, columns of blood. Used in physiological experiments — **kymographically** *adv*.

kypholordosis *n* coexistence of kyphosis and lordosis.

kyphoscoliosis *n* coexistence of kyphosis and scoliosis. Combined anteroposterior and lateral deformity of the spine. May lead to difficulties with lung expansion and respiratory problems.

kyphosis *n* an excessive curvature of the thoracic spine, seen as round shoulder deformity, humpback. A common feature of osteoporosis — **kyphotic** *adj*.

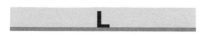

labelling 1. using a term to describe a person in terms of a characteristic or type of behaviour, such as individuals with a learning disability. **2.** provision of data regarding the composition of food, drugs and other items. ⇒ additive. ⇒ E-number.

labelling theory process by which socially defined labels or identities are assigned or accepted. These are often associated with deviant behaviour and may make it difficult for individuals to escape that identity. ⇒ stigma.

labia *npl* lips. *labia majora* two large lip-like folds of skin forming the vulva. They extend from the mons veneris to encircle the vagina. *labia minora* two smaller folds lying within the labia majora — **labial** *adj*.

labile *adj* unstable; readily changed, as many drugs when in solution; blood pressure and mood, especially in some mental health problems. *labile factor (proaccelerin)* factor V in blood coagulation.

labioglossolaryngeal *adj* relating to the lips, tongue and larynx. *labioglossolaryngeal paralysis* a nervous disease characterized by progressive paralysis of the lips, tongue and larynx.

labioglossopharyngeal *adj* relating to the lips, tongue and pharynx. ⇒ bulbar palsy.

labour *n* (*syn* parturition) the act of giving birth to a child. The first stage lasts from onset until there is full dilation of the cervical os; the second stage lasts until the baby is delivered; the third stage until the placenta and membranes are expelled with control of bleeding. *induced labour* one that has been initiated with drugs and/or artificial rupture of the fetal membranes. May be performed for a variety of reasons including: eclampsia. *precipitate labour* very rapid labour. *premature or preterm labour* occurring before term, usually taken to be before the 37th week of pregnancy.

labyrinth *n* part of the inner ear which includes the semicircular canals and the cochlea. *bony labyrinth* that part which is directly hollowed out of the temporal bone. *membranous labyrinth* the membrane which lines the bony labyrinth. ⇒ ear — **labyrinthine** *adj*.

labyrinthectomy *n* surgical removal of part or the whole of the membranous labyrinth of the internal ear. Sometimes carried out for Menière's disease.

labyrinthitis *n* inflammation of the internal ear.

lacerated wound one in which the edges are torn or irregular; not clean cut. It may be caused by a blunt instrument, biting or pressure, and is more likely to become infected and heal by second or third intention. ⇒ wound healing.

lacrimal, lachrymal, lacrymal *adj* pertaining to tears. *lacrimal apparatus* the glands, ducts, sacs and canaliculi that produce and convey tears. *lacrimal bone* a tiny bone at the inner side of the orbital cavity. *lacrimal duct* connects lacrimal gland to upper conjunctival sac. *lacrimal gland* situated above the upper, outer canthus of the eye. ⇒ dacryocyst.

lacrimation *n* an outflow of tears; weeping.

lacrimonasal *adj* pertaining to the lacrimal and nasal bones and ducts. ⇒ nasolacrimal.

lactagogue *n* any substance given to stimulate lactation. ⇒ galactagogue.

lactalbumin *n* the more easily digested of the two milk proteins. ⇒ caseinogen.

lactase *n* digestive enzyme present in the brush border of the small intestine mucosa. It catalyzes the hydrolysis of lactose to glucose and galactose. *lactase deficiency* an inherited condition common in Afro-Caribbean and Asian individuals. It causes an intolerance to lactose (milk sugar) resulting in bloating, colic, diarrhoea and increased flatus. Secondary lactase deficiency may be associated with conditions of the small intestine that include coeliac disease and Crohn's disease. It may arise on a temporary basis following a gastrointestinal tract infection. The management depends on severity and may involve the exclusion of lactose-containing foods or a lactose-restricted diet.

lactate dehydrogenase (LDH) an enzyme, of which there are five isoenzymes, that catalyses the interconversion of lactate and pyruvate in the heart muscle, skeletal muscle and the liver. The five isoenzymes consist of different amounts of heart type (H) or muscle type (M). When tissue of high metabolic activity dies, the ensuing tissue necrosis, such as after myocardial infarction, is quickly reflected by an increase in the serum of lactate dehydrogenase.

lactation *n* 1. secretion of milk. 2. the period during which the child is nourished from the breast.

lacteals *npl* blind ending lymphatic ducts in the intestinal villi; they absorb digested fat particles and convey them to the cisterna (receptaculum) chyli.

lactic pertaining to milk. *lactic acid* an organic acid formed from the fermentation of lactose (when milk sours). It is produced naturally in the body through the anaerobic metabolism of glucose in strenuously contracting skeletal muscle. A build up of the acid in the muscles can cause cramp and aching. *lactic acidosis* acidosis resulting from a build up of lactic acid in the blood and the lowering of the pH. Occurs in any condition causing tissue hypoxia, such as shock or respiratory failure, and diabetes mellitus, liver failure, some drugs (e.g. biguanides) and toxins, such as alcohol.

lactiferous *adj* conveying or secreting milk. *lactiferous ducts* channels draining milk from a breast lobule.

Lactobacillus *n* a genus of nonpathogenic Gram-positive bacteria of the family Lactobacillaceae. They form part of the normal flora of the body, such as in the vagina. ⇒ Döderlein's bacillus. They ferment sugars and are important in the production of yoghurt and other foods.

lactoferrin *n* an acute phase protein found in many body fluids. It is involved with nonspecific body defences.

lactogenic *adj* stimulating milk production. *lactogenic hormone* ⇒ prolactin.

lacto-ovovegetarian *n* an individual whose diet consists of milk, milk products, eggs, grain, fruit and vegetables, but no meat, poultry or fish.

lactose *n* milk sugar. A disaccharide present in milk, it consists of glucose and galactose. *lactose intolerance* ⇒ lactase deficiency.

lactovegetarian *n* an individual whose diet consists of milk, milk products, grain, fruit and vegetables, but no meat, poultry, fish or eggs.

lactulose *n* a disaccharide that is not metabolized so that it reaches the colon unchanged. ⇒ laxative.

lacuna *n* a space between cells; usually used in the description of bone — **lacunar** *adj*.

Laënnec's cirrhosis *n* a type of liver cirrhosis associated with alcohol misuse.

laevulose obsolete term for fructose.

lambdoid like the Greek letter λ, chiefly applied to the suture between the occipital and parietal bones. ⇒ fontanelles.

lambliasis *n* ⇒ giardiasis.

lamella *n* a thin plate-like scale or partition, such as bone in a haversian system — **lamellae** *pl.*

lamina *n* a thin plate or layer — **laminae** *pl.*

laminar flow method of controlling airflow as part of reducing infection risk in special units, e.g. those for immunosuppressed individuals.

laminectomy *n* removal of vertebral laminae to expose the spinal cord nerve roots and meninges. Most often performed in the lumbar region, for removal of degenerated invertebral disc.

LAN *abbr* for Local Area Network. A single site network where all the participating computers are directly linked to share files and resources. ⇒ WAN.

Lancefield's groups a serological classification of the genus *Streptococcus* into groups A–S on the basis of their antigenic characteristics. The members of each group have a characteristic capsular polysaccharide. *Streptococcus pyogenes*, belonging to group A, causes serious infections, such as sore throats, scarlet fever and skin and wound infections. ⇒ necrotizing fasciitis. Rheumatic fever or glomerulonephritis may result from a reaction to streptococcal toxin. Group B streptococci are part of the normal flora of the bowel and vagina, but may cause neonatal meningitis. ⇒ Griffith's typing.

Landry's paralysis ⇒ Guillain-Barré syndrome. ⇒ paralysis.

Langerhans' cells *npl* dendritic cells. An antigen presenting cell found in the epidermis. They are part of the biological barrier formed by the skin and are concerned with protecting the body against micro-organisms that breach the chemical and physical barriers.

Langer's cleavage lines *npl* natural linear striations in the skin arising from the arrangement of fibres in the dermis. They correspond to the natural skin creases. Postoperative scarring is reduced if surgical incisions are made parallel to the cleavage lines.

language *n* a communication system based on symbols (letters) and gestures. The usual interpretation involves verbal language (spoken and written), which uses a set of letters from which many thousands of words can be computed. Also using these letters, particular groups of people, such as health professionals, may construct a verbal language to explain their work and inadvertently confuse and exclude the service users. Body or nonverbal language conveys accurately the person's current mood. Dysphasic and deaf people can learn to use sign language. Profoundly deaf people benefit from the use of sign language, both personally and by their family, friends and colleagues.

lanolin *n* the fat obtained from sheep's wool. Used in ointment bases, as such bases can form water in oil emulsions with aqueous constituents, and are readily absorbed by the skin. Contact sensitivity to lanolin products may occur with long-term use.

lanugo *n* the soft, downy hair that covers the fetus from around the 5th month of gestation; it has mostly disappeared by term. It is sometimes present on newborn infants, especially when they are premature. Usually replaced before birth by vellus hair.

laparoscope *n* a type of endoscope inserted through the abdominal wall to facilitate examination of or surgery to the peritoneal cavity.

laparoscopy *n* endoscopic examination of, or surgery to, internal organs by the transperitoneal route. Specially designed instruments are introduced through the abdominal wall via small incisions into a preformed pneumoperitoneum, under video control. A variety of surgical procedures can now be performed in this way, including biopsy, aspiration of cysts, division of adhesions, tubal ligation, assisted fertility/conception techniques, appendicectomy and cholecystectomy. The procedure minimizes trauma of access, reduces morbidity and shortens the length of hospital stay. ⇒ minimally invasive surgery — **laparoscopically** *adv.*

laparotomy *n* incision of the abdominal wall. Usually reserved for exploratory operation.

large granular lymphocytes (LGLs) *npl* lymphocytes that lack the surface antigens characteristic of B and T-lymphocytes. They contain lysosomes within their cytoplasm and are important in the nonspecific defences against virus-infected cells and cancer cells. Also known as natural killer (NK) cells.

Larsen syndrome multiple joint dislocations and deformities.

larva *n* an embryo which is independent before it has assumed the characteristic features of its parents. *larva migrans* itching tracks in the skin with formation of blisters; caused by the burrowing of larvae of some species of fly, and the normally animal-infesting *Ancylostoma* — **larval** *adj*.

laryngeal *adj* pertaining to the larynx.

laryngectomy *n* surgical removal of the larynx. Usually performed for cancer of the larynx.

laryngismus stridulus momentary sudden attack of laryngeal spasm with closure of the glottis. It is characterized by a crowing sound on inspiration. It is associated with inflammation of the larynx, foreign bodies and the hypocalcaemia of childhood rickets.

laryngitis *n* inflammation of the larynx; can be acute or chronic. ⇒ hoarseness.

laryngologist *n* a specialist in diseases of the larynx.

laryngology *n* the study of diseases affecting the larynx.

laryngoparalysis *n* paralysis of the larynx.

laryngopharyngectomy *n* excision of the larynx and lower part of pharynx.

laryngopharynx *n* the lower portion of the pharynx — **laryngopharyngeal** *adj* ⇒ hypopharynx.

laryngoscope *n* instrument for exposure and visualization of the larynx, for diagnostic or therapeutic purposes or to facilitate tracheal intubation.

laryngoscopy *n* examination of the larynx, either indirectly using a mirror or with a laryngoscope.

laryngospasm *n* convulsive involuntary muscular contraction of the larynx, usually accompanied by spasmodic closure of the glottis. Causes an obstruction to air flow.

laryngostenosis *n* narrowing of the glottic aperture.

laryngotomy *n* the operation of opening the larynx.

laryngotracheal *adj* pertaining to the larynx and trachea.

laryngotracheitis *n* inflammation of the larynx and trachea.

laryngotracheobronchitis *n* an acute viral inflammation of the larynx, trachea and bronchi that may be complicated by a secondary bacterial infection. Particularly serious when it occurs in small children. ⇒ croup.

laryngotracheoplasty *n* an operation to widen a stenosed airway — **laryngotracheoplastic** *adj*.

larynx *n* the larynx is in front of the pharynx and opens into the trachea. It is formed from cartilages joined by membranes and ligaments. The larynx contains the vocal cords and produces sound. ⇒ arytenoid. ⇒ cricoid. ⇒ epiglottis. ⇒ thyroid cartilage — **laryngeal** *adj*.

LASER *acr* Light Amplification by Stimulated Emission of Radiation. Energy is transmitted as heat which can coagulate tissue. Has been used for detached retina, cancer and removal of skin lesions. Protective precautions must be taken by those using lasers as eye damage can be an occupational hazard.

Lassa fever one of the viral haemorrhagic fevers. Occurs as isolated cases and small outbreaks in West Africa. Mortality is as high as 50%. Infected people must be nursed in strict isolation.

latency stage the fourth stage of psychosexual development, occurring in middle childhood (6–12 years). The need for sexual gratification is minimal.

latent heat that heat which is used to bring about a change in state, not in temperature.

lateral *adj* at or belonging to the side; away from the midline. *lateral position* lying on one or other side. The left lateral position is used for rectal examination and giving enemas and suppositories. — **laterally** *adv*.

latex senstivity an allergy to latex, present in some medical gloves and other items such as urinary catheters. A particular problem for healthcare workers.

lavage *n* irrigation of or washing out a body cavity, such as gastric or peritoneal.

laxatives *npl* (*syn* aperients) drugs used to prevent or treat constipation. They may be given orally, or rectally as suppositories or an enema. They may be classified as: (a) bulking agents, e.g. methylcellulose, ispaghula, that retain water and form a soft bulky stool; (b) softeners, e.g. arachis oil enema, liquid paraffin, that lubricate or soften the faeces; (c) stimulants, e.g. docusate (softener as well), senna, sodium picosulfate (picosulphate), bisacodyl and glycerin suppositories, that cause peristalsis by stimulating local nerves; (d) osmotic laxatives, e.g. lactulose, phosphate enemas, that increase fluid in the bowel lumen through osmosis; (e) combined softeners and stimulants, e.g. co-danthramer is both softener and stimulant.

LDL *abbr* low-density lipoprotein.

LDQ *abbr* Leeds Dependence Questionnaire.

lead (Pb) *n* a soft heavy metal with toxic salts. *lead poisoning* (*syn* plumbism) acute poisoning is unusual, but chronic poisoning due to absorption of small amounts over a period is less uncommon. This can occur in young children by sucking articles made of lead alloys, or painted with lead paint. Where the water supply is soft, lead poisoning may occur because drinking water picks up lead from water pipes or cooking pots. Abnormally high levels of lead in the environment have been linked to the use of lead in petrol. Industrial poisoning is still the commonest cause in spite of legislation and safety precautions. The clinical presentation of poisoning includes: anaemia, colic, loss of appetite, and the formation of a blue line round the gums is characteristic. Nervous symptoms, including convulsions, are seen in severe cases.

learning difficulty sometimes used as an alternative for learning disability, although technically it will include a wider range of educational problems as well as impairments associated with incomplete or arrested development of the brain.

learning disability replaces the outdated term 'mental handicap'. It can be defined as a reduced ability to understand new or complicated material, experiencing problems with learning new skills, and in some instances being unable to function independently. The disability is present during childhood and affects development on a permanent basis.

lecithinase *n* an enzyme which catalyses the decomposition of lecithin (phosphatidylcholine) and occurs in the toxin of *Clostridium perfringens*.

lecithins *npl* a group of phospholipids found in animal tissues, mainly in cell membranes. They are present in surfactant.

lecturer practitioner a health professional, such as a nurse, midwife or health visitor, who has a dual educational and clinical role. They spend part of the working week in a college or university and part working in a clinical setting.

leech *n* *Hirudo medicinalis*. An aquatic worm which can be applied to the human body to suck blood. Its saliva contains hirudin, an anticoagulant.

Leeds Dependence Questionnaire (LDQ) a questionnaire designed to detect and rate the severity of illicit substance misuse. It contains ten items which are rated on a four point scale.

left occipitoanterior used to describe the position where the fetal occiput is against the left anterior part of the maternal pelvis.

left occipitoposterior used to describe the position where the fetal occiput is against the left posterior part of the maternal pelvis.

left ventricular assist device (LVAD) mechanical pump used to augment the output of blood from the left venticle of the heart. Used in various situations such as short-term support for critically ill patients, those waiting for a heart transplant, or to allow the heart to recover.

leg ulcer *n* ⇒ arterial ulcer. ⇒ venous ulcer.

Legionella pneumophila a tiny Gram-negative bacillus normally present in soil and water. It causes Legionnaires' disease.

Legionnaires' disease a severe and often fatal pneumonia caused by *Legionella pneumophila*; the outbreak first affected an American Legion convention. There is pneumonia, dry cough, and often nonpulmonary involvement such as gastrointestinal symptoms, renal impairment and confusion. A cause of both community and hospital-acquired pneumonia, it is often associated with an infected water supply in hotels, hospitals and other public buildings.

legumes *npl* pulse vegetables, e.g. peas, beans, lentils. Major source of protein.

Leishman-Donovan bodies the oval intracellular parasites *Leishmania donovani* found in the monocyte-macrophage system of patients suffering from leishmaniasis.

Leishmania *n* genus of flagellated protozoon *Leishmania donovani* responsible for several types of leishmaniasis. ⇒ kala-azar.

leishmaniasis *n* infestation by *Leishmania*, spread by sandflies. It may be generalized (visceral) as in kala-azar, or cutaneous. In the old world, cutaneous forms are known as an oriental sore. New world cutaneous forms may spread to involve the mucosa of the nose and mouth (lesion is termed an espundia).

lens *n* **1.** avascular, biconvex transparent structure immediately behind the iris of the eye. It separates the anterior and posterior cavities of the eye. The lens is supported by the suspensory ligaments and enclosed in a capsule. It alters shape to focus light on the retina. **2.** transparent material; glass or plastic used in optical equipment or to correct refractive errors in spectacles or contact lens.

lenticular *adj* pertaining to or resembling a lens.

lentigo *n* a freckle with an increased number of pigment cells. ⇒ ephelides — **lentigines** *pl*.

lentil *n* a nutritious legume containing a large amount of protein.

leontiasis *n* enlargement of the face and head giving a lion-like appearance; most often caused by fibrous dysplasia of bone. A feature of some types of leprosy.

leprologist *n* one who specializes in the study and treatment of leprosy.

leprology *n* the study of leprosy and its treatment.

lepromata *npl* the granulomatous cutaneous eruption of leprosy — **lepromatous** *adj*.

leprosy *n* a progressive and contagious disease, endemic in warmer climates but also seen in Europe. It is characterized by granulomatous formations affecting nerves (causing peripheral neuritis), the skin, mucous membranes and bones with tissue destruction. Caused by *Mycobacterium leprae* (Hansen's bacillus) and spread occurs through prolonged intimate contact. BCG vaccination conferred variable protection in different trials. The management of leprosy includes specific care, such as that required for impaired sensation and the long-term treatment with various antimicrobial drugs, including dapsone and rifampicin — **leprous** *adj*.

leptocytosis *n* ⇒ target cells.

leptomeningitis *n* inflammation of the inner meninges (arachnoid and pia mater) of brain or spinal cord.

Leptospira *n* a genus of spirochaete bacteria. Very thin, finely coiled bacteria which require dark ground microscopy for visualization. Common in water as saprophytes; pathogenic species are numerous in many animals and may infect humans. *Leptospira interrogans* serotype *icterohaemorrhagiae* causes Weil's disease in humans; *Leptospira interrogans* serotype *canicola* causes canicola fever in dogs and pigs; transmissible to humans. ⇒ leptospirosis — **leptospiral** *adj* pertaining to leptospira.

leptospiral agglutination tests serological tests used in the diagnosis of specific leptospiral infections, e.g. Weil's disease.

leptospirosis *n* infection of humans by bacteria of the leptospira group found in rats and other rodents, cattle, dogs, pigs and foxes. Those at risk include water sports enthusiasts, abattoir workers and farm workers. Presentation varies according to which leptospira is responsible, but may include: high fever, headache, myalgia, conjunctival congestion, rash, anorexia, jaundice, severe muscular pains, rigors and vomiting. Severe infections may cause hepatitis, myocarditis, renal tubular necrosis and meningitis with an associated mortality rate of 15–20%. ⇒ canicola fever. ⇒ Leptospira. ⇒ Weil's disease.

lesbianism *n* sexual attraction of one woman to another.

Lesch-Nyhan disease X-linked recessive genetic disorder of purine metabolism. It leads to an overproduction of uric acid, associated with poor physical development, impaired kidney function and brain damage, resulting in cerebral palsy and learning disability. There is self-mutilation with the urge to bite the mouth, lips and fingers.

lesion *n* pathological change in a bodily tissue.

lethargy *n* apathy, indifference and sluggishness in an environment to which the person usually responds positively.

Letterer-Siwe disease ⇒ histiocytosis X.

leucine *n* an essential (indispensable) amino acid.

leucocytes *npl* general name for white blood cells. Leucocytes have a nucleus, are mobile and are all concerned with body defences in some way, e.g. some are phagocytic and others produce antibodies. There are two main groups: (a) the polymorphonuclear cells or granulocytes: neutrophils, basophils and eosinophils; these have a many-lobed nucleus and granules in their cytoplasm; (b) the agranulocytes: monocytes and lymphocytes; these generally have no granules, but some lymphocytes are granular. → natural killer cells (see Figure 37) **leucocytic** *adj*.

leucocytolysis *n* destruction and disintegration of white blood cells — **leucocytolytic** *adj*.

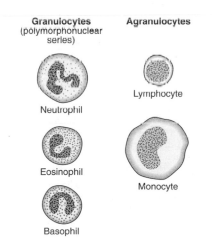

Granulocytes
(polymorphonuclear series)

Neutrophil

Eosinophil

Basophil

Agranulocytes

Lymphocyte

Monocyte

Figure 37 Types of leucocytes. (Reproduced from Brooker 1998 with permission.)

leucocytosis *n* increased number of leucocytes in the blood, usually neutrophils. Often a response to infection and haematological disorders — **leucocytotic** *adj*.

leucodepleted *n* describes donated blood from which the leucocytes have been removed.

leucoderma *n* defective skin pigmentation, especially when it occurs in patches or bands. ⇒ vitiligo.

leucoerythroblastosis *n* a condition characterized by the presence of primitive granulocytes and erythroblasts (immature erythrocytes) in the blood. The causes include cancer infiltration of the bone marrow and myelofibrosis.

leucoma (leukoma) *n* white opaque spot on the cornea — **leukomatous** *adj*.

leuconychia *n* white marks on the nails.

leucopenia *n* decreased number of white blood cells in the blood — **leucopenic** *adj*.

leucopoiesis *n* the formation of white blood cells from stem cells. Regulated by several cytokines and colony-stimulating factors — **leucopoietic** *adj*.

leucorrhoea *n* a white vaginal discharge. Normal unless it becomes copious, malodorous or abnormal in colour — **leucorrhoeal** *adj*.

leukaemia *n* a group of neoplastic diseases of haemopoeitic tissue characterized by an abnormal proliferation of immature white cells. This results in disruption of haemopoiesis with anaemia, thrombocytopenia causing bleeding and neutropenia causing infection. Factors associated with the development of leukaemia include: ionizing radiation, cytotoxic chemotherapy, retroviruses (human T-cell lymphotropic virus), chemicals, such as benzene, genetic predisposition, such as Down's syndrome. Leukaemias are classified by the cell type involved, its course and duration. *acute leukaemias* onset is rapid and early immature cells are produced (blast cells), commonly of the lymphoid and myeloid series. The acute leukaemias include acute lymphoblastic leukaemia (ALL) in children and acute myeloblastic leukaemia (AML) in adults. *chronic leukaemias* here the onset is insidious and the cells produced are more mature, commonly lymphocytes and granulocytes. Chronic forms can become acute with blast cell proliferation. Chronic leukaemias include chronic lymphocytic leukaemia and chronic granulocytic (myeloid) leukaemia, both of which affect adults. Less common leukaemias include: monocytic, eosinophilic, basophilic and hairy cell. The management depends upon: the cell type, whether acute or chronic and the aim of treatment: remission or palliation. Treatments include: bone marrow transplant, chemotherapy, interferon alpha, radiotherapy, corticosteroids and supportive measures such as antimicrobial drugs, blood components transfusion and protective isolation. ⇒ myeloproliferative disorders. ⇒ lymphoma — **leukaemic** *adj*.

leukoplakia *n* white, thickened patch occurring on mucous membranes. Occurs on lips, inside mouth or on genitalia. Sometimes denotes carcinoma-in-situ.

leukotrienes part of a group of regulatory lipids derived from arachidonic acid (fatty acid). They act as signalling molecules and mediators of the inflammatory response and are involved in some allergic responses. ⇒ prostaglandins. ⇒ thromboxanes.

levator *adj* **1.** a muscle which acts by raising a part, e.g. levator palpebrae superioris, which raises the upper eyelid. **2.** an instrument for lifting a depressed part (bone).

Levin tube a French plastic catheter used for gastric intubation; it has a closed weighted tip and an opening on the side.

Leydig cells *npl* interstitial cells in the testes which produce androgens such as testosterone. ⇒ interstitial cell stimulating hormone.

LGLs *abbr* large granular lymphocytes.

LGVCFT *abbr* lymphogranuloma venereum complement fixation test.

LHBI *abbr* lower hemibody irradiation.

LHG *abbr* Local Health Group.

liaison nurse may refer to a nurse who is appointed to organize the necessary resources in the community so that when a person is discharged from hospital these resources will be available.

libido *n* Freud's name for the urge to obtain sensual satisfaction, which he believed to be the mainspring of human behaviour. Sometimes more loosely used to mean sexual urge. Freud's meaning was satisfaction through all the senses.

lice *npl* ⇒ Pediculus.

lichen *n* a group of skin diseases characterized by aggregations of papular skin lesions. *lichen nitidus* characterized by minute, shiny, flat-topped, pink papules of pinhead size. *lichen planus* an eruption of unknown cause showing purple, angulated, shiny, flat-topped papules that are very itchy. *lichen simplex* a form of neurodermatitis characterized by pruritic papules forming a patch — **lichenoid** *adj*.

lichenification *n* thickening of the skin, usually secondary to scratching. Skin markings become more prominent and the area affected appears to be composed of small, shiny rhomboids. ⇒ neurodermatitis.

lienitis *n* inflammation of the spleen.

life crisis a term which describes an unexpected unpleasant happening, such as an accident, sudden illness or life event (such as divorce).

life event a sociological term which describes the major happenings in a lifetime, such as starting or changing school, getting married or divorced, changing house or work, or suffering a bereavement, etc.

life expectancy the average age at which death occurs. It is not only affected by health/illness, but also by social factors, such as education and industry, and environmental factors, such as housing, sanitation and a piped water supply.

lifelong learning continuing development of individuals and teams. ⇒ continuing professional development.

lifespan *n* the span of human life from birth to death, however long or short it might be. From collected data, different countries can predict the expected lifespan, which is increasing in the West and is lower in the developing countries. Some nursing specialities are predicated on patients' stage on the lifespan, e.g. neonatal nursing, paediatric nursing, midwifery and the nursing of older people.

lifestyle *n* the pattern which each individual has developed in relation to the everyday activities of living. These are investigated at the initial assessment of a person entering the healthcare service, so that the nursing contribution can be individualized.

lifestyle planning *n* occupational therapy techniques that help a person to achieve a balance between the occupational elements (self-care, work, rest and leisure) of their life in order to reduce stress, enhance quality of life, develop potential and achieve personal goals.

lifting *v* in nursing, an outdated term that was previously used in the context of moving patients. However, it is important to remember that nurses and other healthcare staff are still required to consider the health and safety implications of moving or lifting items of equipment etc. ⇒ manual handling. ⇒ safe-handling or no-lifting policies.

ligament *n* band of tough fibrous tissue which connects bones or other structures together. Provides strength and support at joints — **ligamentous** *adj*.

ligand *n* specific signalling chemicals, such as hormones, cytokines or neurotransmitters, that bind to cell membrane receptors to influence cell function in a variety of ways. Many drugs are designed to mimic the naturally occurring ligand.

ligate *vt* to tie off blood vessels etc at operation — **ligation** *n* tying off; usually reserved for *ligation of the uterine tubes* a method of sterilization.

ligature *n* the material used for tying vessels. Silk, catgut and man-made absorbable and nonabsorbable materials can be used.

light adaptation adjustments required by the eye to facilitate vision in bright light, e.g. chemical changes to photosensitive retinal pigments. The pupils constrict in bright light, the breakdown of rhodopsin reduces retinal sensitivity and the activity of the cones increases. ⇒ rhodopsin.

lightening *n* a word used to denote the relief of pressure on the diaphragm by the abdominal viscera, when the presenting part of the fetus descends into the pelvis in the last 3 weeks of a first pregnancy.

lightning pains symptomatic of tabes dorsalis. Occur as paroxysms of swift-cutting (lightning) stabs in the lower limbs.

Likert scale *n* a scale used in questionnaire surveys where the participants are asked to indicate their level of agreement of a particular statement: strongly agree, agree, unsure, disagree and strongly disagree.

limbic system *n* a diffuse collection of nuclei and fibres in the cerebral hemispheres. Part of the 'primitive' brain, they influence feelings and emotions.

lime *n* calcium oxide.

liminal *adj* of a stimulus, of the lowest intensity which can be perceived by the human senses. ⇒ subliminal.

linctus *n* a sweet, syrupy liquid, used to soothe coughing.

linea *n* a line. *linea alba* the white line visible after removal of the skin in the centre of the abdomen, stretching from the ensiform cartilage to the pubis, its position on the surface being indicated by a slight depression. *linea nigra* pigmented line from umbilicus to pubis which appears in pregnancy. *lineae albicantes* white lines which appear on the abdomen after reduction of tension as after childbirth, tapping of the abdomen, etc. → striae gravidarum.

linear accelerator a mega voltage machine which accelerates electrons and produces high energy X-rays which are used in the treatment of malignant disease.

lingua *n* the tongue — **lingual** *adj*.

liniment *n* a liquid to be applied to the skin by gentle friction.

linoleic acid *n* a polyunsaturated, essential fatty acid containing two double bonds. It is found in vegetable seed oils, such as sunflower, corn and soya bean. ⇒ essential fatty acids.

linolenic acid a polyunsaturated, essential fatty acid containing three double bonds. It is found in vegetable oils. ⇒ essential fatty acids.

lipaemia *n* increased lipoids (especially cholesterol) in the blood — **lipaemic** *adj*.

lipases *npl* any fat-splitting enzyme, such as that secreted by the pancreas. They split fats into fatty acids and glycerol.

lipids *npl* large and diverse group of fat-like organic molecules which include: neutral fats, such as triglycerides (triacylglycerols), phospholipids, lipoproteins, fat soluble vitamins, steroids, prostaglandins, leukotrienes, and thromboxanes. They consist of carbon, oxygen and hydrogen, and some contain phosphorus and nitrogen. They are insoluble in water, but they can be dissolved in organic solvents such as alcohol. Lipids are important in the body both structurally and functionally. Fat deposits provide an energy store, insulate and offer some protection. Other lipids are important constituents of cell membranes, are precursors for steroid hormones, act as regulatory molecules, e.g. prostaglandins, and transport fats around the body, and the fat soluble vitamins are concerned with blood clotting, vision and antioxidant functions etc. (See Figure 38).

lipoatrophy loss of subcutaneous fat. A complication that may arise at sites of insulin injections.

lipogenesis *n* a process stimulated by insulin, whereby amino acids and glucose are converted to triacylgylcerols (triglycerides) prior to storage in adipose tissue.

lipohypertrophy increase in the size of fat cells. A complication that may arise at sites of insulin injections.

lipoid *adj, n* (a substance) resembling fats or oil. Serum lipoids are raised in thyroid deficiency.

lipoidosis *n* disease due to disorder of fat metabolism — **lipoidoses** *pl.*

lipolysis *n* the chemical breakdown of fat. A process stimulated by glucocorticoid hormones such as cortisol, by which stored triacylglycerols (triglycerides) are released from adipose tissue to provide energy — **lipolytic** *adj.*

lipoma *n* a benign tumour of fat cells — **lipomatous** *adj.*

lipoprotein *n* lipids combined with an apoprotein in the liver prior to their release into the blood where they trans-

Types of lipids (with examples)	Outline of functions in the body
Neutral fats (triglycerides)	Energy store as fat deposits Insulation and protection
Steroids	
Cholesterol	Component of cell membranes and precursor of other steroid molecules
Sex hormones (testosterone, oestrogen and progesterone)	Control of reproductive function
Adrenal cortical hormones (corticosteroids such as cortisol and aldosterone)	Control metabolism of nutrients and electrolyte–water balance
Bile salts	Important for the digestion and absorption of fats
Vitamin D	Calcium homeostasis – bone growth and remodelling
Phospholipids	Component of the cell membrane – bilayer
Prostaglandins, thromboxanes and leukotrienes	Group of regulatory lipids concerned with blood clotting, inflammatory processes, reproduction and many other functions
Lipoproteins (high-density lipoproteins – HDLs and low density lipoproteins – LDLs)	Transport of fatty acids and cholesterol in the blood
Fat-soluble vitamins (Vitamin D, see above)	
Vitamin A	Visual functions, acts as antioxidant
Vitamin E	Acts as an antioxidant, in wound healing and possibly has a role in reproduction
Vitamin K	Blood clotting

Figure 38 Types of lipids and roles in the body. (Reproduced from Brooker 1998 with permission.)

port triacylglycerols (triglycerides) and cholesterol around the body. They are classified according to composition and density as chylomicrons: high-density lipoproteins (HDLs), low-density lipoproteins (LDLs) or very-low-density lipoproteins (VLDLs). In general, a high level of LDL in the blood is associated with arterial disease and HDLs are considered to be protective. A high HDL:LDL is associated with a reduced risk of atherosclerosis. ⇒ hyperlipidaemia. ⇒ lipids.

liposome drug delivery a method of packaging drugs in vesicles for administration. They are not released until the liposome is broken down by the monocyte-macrophage cells in the liver. This delivery system may allow drugs to be targeted at specific sites.

lipotrophic substances factors which cause the removal of fat from the liver by transmethylation.

liquor *n* a solution. *liquor amnii* the fluid surrounding the fetus. *liquor folliculi* the fluid surrounding a developing oocyte in a Graafian follicle.

listening *v* a cluster of complex skills used in communicating; health professionals give their whole attention to what is being said, as well as how it is being said, and whether or not it is congruent with non-verbal signals.

listeria *n* a genus of bacteria present in soil and animal faeces. *Listeria monocytogenes* causes meningitis, septicaemia and intrauterine or perinatal infections. → listeriosis.

listeriosis infection caused by bacteria of the genus listeria. It may be transmitted via contaminated soil, contact with infected animals and by the consumption of unpasteurized foods, such as soft cheeses which may be infected. It may cause a flu-like illness but groups at particular risk of serious consequences include: young infants, older people, debilitated people, pregnant women and immunosuppressed individuals. Infection during pregnancy may lead to flu-like illness in women, miscarriage, stillbirth, premature labour and septicaemia and meningitis in the neonate with a high mortality rate.

literature review a thorough and comprehensive examination of the papers relevant to a topic. Research methods and results are analysed and presented crit

ically. The literature review should state how the search was undertaken, e.g. bibliographical databases such as Medline.

lithiasis *n* any condition in which there are calculi, such as gallstones and kidney stones.

lithium (Li) *n* a metallic element. Lithium salts are used in the treatment of bipolar disorders.

lithopaedion *n* a fetus that has died and been retained becomes calcified. A rare occurrence.

lithotomy *n* surgical incision of the bladder for the removal of calculi. *lithotomy position* patient is lying supine, with hips and knees flexed. The thighs are abducted and the feet supported in stirrups. Used for a variety of procedures, especially urinary, obstetric or gynaecological. To avoid injury, it is essential that the legs are raised and lowered together. Maintaining privacy and patient dignity during procedures using this position is a vital nursing role.

lithotripsy *n* a method of removing a renal calculus by dissolving or crushing it in situ. Modern noninvasive techniques include the use of shock waves to disintegrate renal, and sometimes biliary, calculi. ⇒ lithotriptor.

lithotriptor (er) *n* a machine which sends shock waves through renal calculi, causing them to crumble and leave the body naturally via the urine. Can be used to disintegrate gallstones, in suitable patients, followed by a course of bile salt therapy to dissolve the stone fragments.

lithotrite *n* an instrument for crushing a stone in the urinary bladder.

lithotrity operation of crushing a stone in the urinary bladder.

litigation civil proceedings.

litmus *n* a vegetable pigment used as an indicator of acidity (red) or alkalinity (blue). Often stored as paper strips impregnated with blue or red litmus: blue litmus paper turns red when in contact with an acid; red litmus paper turns blue when in contact with an alkali.

litre (l/L) *n* unit of volume for fluids and gases. It is based on the volume of a cube (10 cm × 10 cm × 10 cm).

Little's area *n* anterior part of nasal septum with an abundant blood supply. A common site for epistaxis.

Little's disease diplegia of spastic type causing 'scissor leg' deformity. A congenital disease in which there is cerebral atrophy or agenesis.

liver *n* the largest gland in the body, varying in weight in the adult from 1.2–1.5 kg. It is relatively much larger in the fetus and neonate. It is situated in the right upper part of the abdominal cavity. It is vital to homeostasis and its functions include: metabolism of nutrients, protein synthesis, detoxification, storage of glycogen, vitamins and minerals and breakdown of red blood cells with the production of bile. With all these functions occurring the liver is the site of considerable heat generation. *liver function tests* blood tests used to assess liver function which include: serum bilirubin, alkaline phosphatase, alanine aminotransferase, aspartate aminotransferase, gamma- glutamyl transferase, coagulation tests and serum proteins. ⇒aminotransferases. *liver transplant* surgical transplantation of a liver from a suitable donor for the treatment of liver failure.

Liverpool University Neuroleptic Side Effect Rating Scale (LUNSERS) a simple self-rating scale for measuring neuroleptic side effects. It covers fifty one side effects; ten of these are 'red herrings', such as hair loss. Allows clients to rate their own side effects.

livid *adj* showing blue discoloration due to bruising, congestion or insufficient oxygenation.

living will *n* ⇒ advance directive.

LMP *abbr* last menstrual period.

LOA *abbr* left occipitoanterior.

Loa loa *n* a nematode parasite causing loiasis (filariasis).

lobar pneumonia a primary pneumonia affecting isolated lobes of the lung, usually caused by the bacterium *Streptococcus pneumoniae*. It frequently affects young or middle aged people. The onset is rapid and the person has a high temperature, tachycardia, headache, general aches, painful cough and localized chest pain. The breathing is rapid and shallow and later there is rust-coloured sputum. Management includes: antibiotics, pain relief, oxygen and physiotherapy. Patients may be very ill.

lobe *n* a rounded section of an organ, separated from neighbouring sections by a fissure or septum, such as in the lung — **lobar** *adj*.

lobectomy removal of a lobe, e.g. of the lung for tumour, lung abscess or localized bronchiectasis.

lobule *n* a small lobe or a subdivision of a lobe — **lobular, lobulated** *adj*.

local anaesthesia ⇒ anaesthesia.

local anaesthetics *n* drugs that cause local insensibility to painful stimuli when injected or applied topically, e.g. lidocaine (lignocaine). It is used in various strengths for infiltration anaesthesia and nerve blocks. Adrenaline (epinephrine) is usually added to delay absorption. Also effective for surface anaesthesia as ointment and for urethral anaesthesia as a gel. Now widely accepted as an antiarrhythmic agent, especially in the management of ventricular tachycardia and ventricular ectopic beats occurring as complications of acute myocardial infarction.

local authority in the UK, local government, e.g. regional councils, county councils, city councils, district and town councils and parish councils. They have the powers to raise taxes and some have statutory duties to provide services within a locality, such as environmental health, social services, housing, policing and crime prevention, education etc.

Local Commissioning Groups a collective term for various groups, e.g. Primary Care Groups (PCGs), Local Health Co-operatives and Local Health Groups (LHGs), that work together to commission local health services more efficiently. ⇒ commissioning.

local government ⇒ local authority.

Local Health Co-operative in Scotland, equivalent to a Primary Care Group.

Local Health Group (LHG) *n* in Wales, equivalent to a Primary Care Group.

localize *vt* 1. to limit the spread. 2. to determine the site of a lesion — **localization** *n*.

lochia *n* the vaginal discharge which occurs during the puerperium. At first pure blood, it later becomes paler, diminishes in quantity and finally ceases. It has three stages: *lochia rubra* which is red or brown, *lochia serosa* which is pink, and *lochia alba* which is a white discharge — **lochial** *adj*.

lockjaw *n* ⇒ tetanus.

locomotor *adj* can be applied to any tissue or system used in human movement. Usually refers to nerves and muscles. Sometimes includes the bones and joints. *locomotor ataxia* the disordered gait and loss of position sense (proprioception) in the lower limbs, which occurs in tabes dorsalis. ⇒ syphilis.

loculated *adj* divided into numerous cavities.

locus *n* specific site, such as a gene on a chromosome — **loci** *pl*.

locus of control the beliefs that people have about the degree of control and choice they have about issues that affect their lives, such as their health behaviours. An internal locus of control is associated with people who see themselves as making these decisions and taking responsibility for their health, whereas those with an external locus of control see themselves as being powerless and tend to be fatalistic about health.

log roll the patient lies on his back with legs extended and arms folded across chest and is rolled by the nurse on to one or other side. Used to facilitate washing, pressure area care and sheet changing, where patients are confined to bed.

Logan bow a thin metal device, shaped like a bow; it is used after cleft lip surgery to reduce tension on the suture line.

loiasis *n* a form of filariasis (caused by the worm *Loa loa*) which occurs in West Africa. The vector, a large fly *Chrysops*, bites in the daytime. Larvae take 2–3 years to develop and adult worms may live for up to 15 years. The infection causes eosinophilia. The worms move about the subcutaneous tissues and cause irritation and localized swellings (Calabar swelling). Sometimes a worm crosses the eye. Treatment is with the anthelmintic diethylcarbamazine which may precipitate a severe allergic reaction to substances released by the dead worms.

loin *n* that part of the back between the lower ribs and the iliac crest; the area immediately above the buttocks.

lone/single parent family a family formed from one parent with dependent children. It may result from death of a partner, divorce, separation or choice.

loneliness *n* a feeling which some people describe as devastating; it is sometimes accompanied by one of hopelessness. It can be experienced by people who are physically in the presence of others whom they find incompatible, as well as by those in the community who have few social contacts. Others can be alone for long periods, yet do not experience loneliness. When the assessment data reveal that a person lives alone and has few social contacts, nurses should explore with him the significance of these facts. Special arrangements may need to be made to overcome their negative effects after discharge from hospital or other healthcare settings. → liaison nurse. ⇒ suicide.

long term memory (LTM) the part of memory that deals with the retention of information for longer periods. It is potentially permanent and has a much greater capacity than STM.

longsighted *adj* hypermetropic. ⇒ hypermetropia.

longtitudinal study research study that collects data on more than one occasion, e.g. may study a cohort of people over many years. ⇒ cohort study.

loop diuretics *npl* diuretics that act by preventing reabsorption of sodium, chloride and potassium in the thick segment of the ascending limb of the loop of Henle (of the nephron) by chloride carrier inhibition. They include: furosemide (frusemide) and bumetanide, and are used for hypertension, oedema and oliguria caused by renal failure. Concurrent therapy with potassium is required.

LOP *abbr* left occipitoposterior.

lordoscoliosis *n* lordosis complicated by the presence of scoliosis.

lordosis *n* an exaggerated forward, convex curve of the lumbar spine **lordotic** *adj*.

loupe *n* a magnifying lens used in ophthalmology.

louse *n* ⇒ Pediculus — **lice** *pl*.

low birthweight term used to indicate a weight of 2.5 kg or less at birth, indicating the baby is preterm and/or 'small-for-dates'.

low-density lipoprotein (LDL) ⇒ lipoprotein.

low reading thermometer a thermometer used to record temperatures in a lower than normal range, such as in patients with hypothermia.

lower reference nutrient intake (LRNI) *n* a dietary reference value. See Box – Dietary reference values.

lower respiratory tract infection (LRTI) ⇒ pneumonia. ⇒ bronchitis.

LP *abbr* lumbar puncture.

LRNI *abbr* lower reference nutrient intake.

LRTI *abbr* lower respiratory tract infection.

LTM *abbr* long term memory.

lubb-dupp *n* words descriptive of the heart sounds as appreciated in auscultation.

lubricants *npl* faecal softeners. ⇒ laxatives.

lucid *adj* clear; describing mental clarity. *lucid interval* a period of mental clarity which can be of variable length, occurring in people with organic mental disorder, such as dementia.

Ludwig's angina ⇒ cellulitis.

lumbar *adj* pertaining to the loin or lower region of spine. *lumbar nerves* five pairs of spinal nerves (LI–L5). *lumbar puncture (LP)* the withdrawal of cerebrospinal fluid through a hollow needle inserted into the subarachnoid space in the lumbar region. The fluid can be examined for its chemical, cellular and bacterial content; its pressure can be measured by the attachment of a manometer. The procedure is hazardous if the intracranial pressure is high, but the pressure for an adult has a wide range – 50–200 mm water, so a better guide is examination of the optic fundi for papilloedema. *lumbar sympathectomy* surgical removal of the sympathetic chain in the lumbar region; used to improve the blood supply to the lower limbs by allowing the blood vessels to dilate. *lumbar vertebrae* five bones. They are the largest vertebrae, which reflects their weight-bearing role.

lumbocostal *adj* pertaining to the loin and ribs.

lumbosacral *adj* pertaining to the loin or lumbar vertebrae and the sacrum.

Lumbricus *n* a genus of earthworms. ⇒ ascarides. ⇒ ascariasis.

lumen *n* the space inside a tubular structure — **luminal** *adj*.

lumpectomy *n* the surgical excision of a tumour with removal of minimal surrounding tissue. Increasingly used, in conjunction with radiotherapy and sometimes chemotherapy, for breast cancer.

lunate *n* one of the carpals or wrist bones.

Lund and Browder's chart *n* a chart for calculating the percentage of body surface area affected by a burn in infants and children. ⇒ Wallace's rule of nines.

lungs *npl* the two main organs of respiration which occupy the greater part of the thoracic cavity; they are separated from each other by the heart and other contents of the mediastinum. They are concerned with gaseous exchange – the oxygenation of blood and excretion of carbon dioxide.

LUNSERS *abbr* Liverpool University Neuroleptic Side Effect Rating Scale.

lunula *n* the crescent-shaped pale area at the root of the nail.

lupus pernio *n* skin lesions on the fingers and nose associated with systemic sarcoidosis. They affect around a third of people with sarcoidosis.

lupus vulgaris *n* a form of extrapulmonary tuberculosis that affects the skin. It is characterized by ulceration that heals slowly with scarring.

luteal *adj* pertaining to the corpus luteum. *luteal phase* that part of the ovarian cycle occurring after ovulation. Its length is constant at around 14 days irrespective of overall cycle length.

luteinizing hormone (LH) *n* a gonadotrophin secreted by the anterior pituitary gland. In females high levels midway in the menstrual cycle cause ovulation and formation of the corpus luteum. In males the same hormone, known as interstitial-cell stimulating hormone (ICSH), stimulates Leydig cells of the testes to produce testosterone.

luxation *n* dislocation of bone at a joint site. ⇒ subluxation.

LVAD *abbr* left ventricular assist device.

Lyme disease ⇒ Borrelia. ⇒ relapsing fever.

lymph *n* the fluid contained in the lymphatic vessels. It is derived from tissue (interstitial) fluid and has a composition similar to blood plasma. *lymph circulation* that of lymph collected from the tissue spaces which returns to the blood via lymph capillaries, vessels, nodes and ducts. *lymph nodes* accumulations of lymphoid tissue at strategic intervals, e.g. axilla, along lymphatic vessels. They filter lymph and remove extraneous particles such as micro-organisms and tumour cells. They are a site of B and T-lymphocyte proliferation and antibody production.

lymphadenectomy *n* excision of one or more lymph nodes.

lymphadenitis *n* inflammation of a lymph node.

lymphadenopathy *n* any disease of the lymph nodes. ⇒ persistent generalized lymphadenopathy — **lymphadenopathic** *adj*.

lymphangiectasis *n* dilation of the lymph vessels — **lymphangiectatic** *adj*.

lymphangiography *n* ⇒ lymphography.

lymphangioma *n* a simple tumour of lymph vessels — **lymphangiomatous** *adj*.

lymphangioplasty *n* any plastic operation on lymph vessels, such as to improve drainage — **lymphangioplastic** *adj*.

lymphangitis *n* inflammation of a lymph vessel.

lymphatic *adj* pertaining to, conveying or containing lymph. *lymphatic system* the lymph vessels, nodes, tissues and organs, e.g. spleen.

lymphoblast *n* immature lymphocyte. Present in the blood and marrow in acute lymphoblastic leukaemia (ALL).

lymphocytes *npl* a group of white blood cells found in the blood and lymphoid tissues. *B lymphocytes (bursa dependent)* part of humoral immunity, they become plasma cells which produce antibodies (immunoglobulins) or memory cells. *T-lymphocytes (thymus dependent)* involved in cell-mediated immunity responses such as destroying transplanted cells, cancer cells and virus infected cells. T-lymphocytes may be classified according to the presence of a surface molecule; CD4 or CD8. T-helper and delayed hypersensitivity cells are CD4 (T4) cells and T-suppressor and T-cytotoxic/killer cells are CD8 (T8) cells — **lymphocytic** *adj*.

lymphocytopenia *n* decreased number of lymphocytes in the blood.

lymphocytosis *n* an increase in lymphocytes in the blood.

lymphoedema *n* excess of fluid in the tissues from obstruction of lymph vessels. May be primary due to a structural abnormality in lymph vessels or second-ary obstruction, e.g. following surgery for breast cancer. ⇒ elephantiasis. ⇒ filariasis.

lymphoepithelioma *n* rapidly growing malignant tumour of the epithelial tissue covering lymphoid tissue (tonsils) in the nasopharynx — **lymphoepitheliomata** *pl*.

lymphogranuloma venereum *n* a sexually transmitted infection caused by *Chlamydia trachomatis*. It is characterized by genital ulcers and lymph node enlargement. Occurs worldwide but mainly in tropical regions.

lymphography *n* X-ray examination of the lymphatic system after it has been rendered radiopaque. Largely replaced by CT scanning.

lymphoid *adj* pertaining to lymph. *lymphoid tissue* collections of tissue similar in structure to lymph nodes found in the spleen, liver, gut, bone marrow, tonsils and thymus.

lymphokines *npl* general term for cytokines produced by activated T-lymphocytes. They function during the immune response as intercellular mediators.

lymphology *n* study of the lymphatic system.

lymphoma *n* a group of malignant tumours arising from lymphoid tissue. They are classified as either Hodgkin's disease or nonHodgkin's lymphoma (NHL) which has many similarities with lymphoblastic and lymphocytic leukaemias. People with HIV infections may develop NHL which is classified as an AIDS-defining condition by WHO/CDC. The presenting features of lymphoma include: lymph node enlargement, splenomegaly, hepatomegaly and systemic effects, such as weight loss, night sweats and fever etc. Treatment depends on the type and stage of the disease but includes radiotherapy, chemotherapy, interferon alpha, bone marrow transplant and supportive measures, such as blood product transfusion and antibiotics. ⇒ Burkitt's lymphoma.

lymphorrhagia *n* an outpouring of lymph from a severed lymphatic vessel.

lyophilization *n* freeze drying. A method of preserving such biological substances as plasma, sera, bacteria and tissue.

lyophilized skin skin which has been subjected to lyophilization. It is reconstituted and used for temporary skin replacement.

lysin *n* a cell dissolving substance in blood. ⇒ bacteriolysin. ⇒ haemolysin.

lysine *n* an essential (indispensable) amino acid.

lysis *n* **1.** destruction or decomposition of a cell, or other substances, under the influence of a specific agent. ⇒ haemolysis. **2.** gradual abatement of the symptoms of an infectious disease. ⇒ crisis *ant*. **3.** surgery to loosen from restraining adhesions — **lytic** *adj*.

lysosome *n* membranous intracelluar sacs that contain lytic enzymes. Involved with breaking down substances and particles that enter the cell, and in clearing up after cell damage.

lysozyme *n* an enzyme which acts as an antibacterial agent and is present in various body fluids such as tears and saliva.

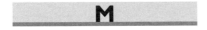

M

maceration *n* softening of the horny layer of the skin caused by prolonged exposure to moisture. Maceration reduces the protection afforded by an intact integument and so predisposes to penetration by micro-organisms.

Mackenrodt's ligaments (cardinal) ⇒ uterine supports.

Macmillan Cancer Relief a charity founded in 1911, to improve the quality of life for people with cancer and their families. It provides nurses, cancer care units, grants, medical support and education programmes, and finances for other charities. *Macmillan Nurses* clinical nurse specialists experienced and skilled in symptom control and general palliative care. They provide advice and support to patients and their families in a variety of settings. They also provide specialist information, advice and support for colleagues in the multidisciplinary team.

macrocephalic, megalocephalic *adj* ⇒ megacephalic.

macrocephaly *n* excessive size of the head — **macrocephalic** *adj*.

macrocheilia *n* enlargement of the lips.

macrocyte *n* abnormally large red blood cell. ⇒ anaemia. ⇒ megaloblast — **macrocytic** *adj* relating to macrocytes.

macrocytosis *n* an increased number of macrocytes.

macrodactyly *n* excessive development of the fingers or toes.

macroglobulinaemia *n* condition where there are large amounts of macroglobulins (high molecular weight globulins) in the blood. *Waldenström's macroglobulinaemia* overproduction of monoclonal IgM which results in increased blood viscosity. ⇒ immunoglobulins. ⇒ monoclonal.

macroglossia *n* an abnormally large tongue.

macrolides *npl* group of antibiotics that include erythromycin which is often prescribed for patients with penicillin hypersensitivity. Other examples include: azithromycin and clarithromycin.

macromastia *n* an abnormally large breast.

macronutrients *npl* nutrients, such as protein, carbohydrate and fats, required by the body in relatively large amounts. Each fulfils a vital role and the relative amounts of each taken in the diet are important. They consist of carbon, oxygen and hydrogen in different proportions, and proteins contain nitrogen, and some amino acids contain phosphorus and sulphur. ⇒ micronutrients.

macrophages *npl* cells of the monocyte-macrophage system (reticuloendothelial). They are derived from monocytes and have an important defensive role which includes phagocytosis of foreign bodies and cell debris and in the immune response. ⇒ histiocytes.

macroscopic *adj* visible to the naked eye; gross. ⇒ microscopic *ant*.

macula *n* a spot. *macula densa* specialized cells of the distal convoluted tubule of the nephron. Forms part of the juxtaglomerular apparatus. *macula lutea* the yellow spot on the retina that contains a small depression called the fovea centralis, which contains only cones. The area of clearest central vision — **macular** *adj*.

macular degeneration *n* loss of retinal pigment cells and damage to the macula. It occurs with aging and results in loss of colour vision and progressive visual impairment.

macule *n* a nonpalpable localized area of change in skin colour — **macular** *adj*.

maculopapular *adj* describes a rash having both macules and raised palpable spots (papules) on the skin.

MADEL *abbr* Medical and Dental Education Levy.

madura foot ⇒ mycetoma.

magnesium (Mg) *n* a metallic element required by the body as a cofactor for many enzyme reactions. It is found in bone and is an intracellular cation. Magnesium metabolism is closely linked to that of calcium.

magnesium salts widely used for their medicinal properties. *magnesium carbonate* used as an antacid. *magnesium chloride* used intravenously for magnesium deficiency. *magnesium hydroxide* used as an antacid and osmotic laxative. *magnesium sulphate* (*syn* Epsom salts) an effective rapid-acting osmotic laxative. It is used as a 25% solution as a wet dressing for inflamed conditions of the skin, and as a paste with glycerin for the treatment of boils and carbuncles. Used intravenously to correct magnesium deficiency. *magnesium trisilicate* used as an antacid.

magnetic resonance imaging (MRI) *n* (*syn* nuclear magnetic resonance (NMR)) is a noninvasive technique that does not use ionizing radiation. It uses radiofrequency radiation in the presence of a powerful magnetic field to produce high-quality images of the body in any plane. See Box – Magnetic Resonance Imaging.

MAI *abbr* Mycobacterium avium intracellulare.

major histocompatibilty complex (MHC) *n* a collection of genes that code for the MHC proteins (antigens) found as cell surface molecules. These molecules act as 'self' markers and normally the T-lymphocytes learn to recognize them as belonging to the body. They are involved in the complex processes involved when grafted tissue is rejected. ⇒ human leucocyte antigens.

Makaton *n* a form of sign language, more basic than British Sign Language and probably more commonly used. Especially useful for people with some forms of learning disability. ⇒ sign language.

mal *n* disease. *mal de mer* seasickness. *grand mal, petit mal* ⇒ epilepsy.

malabsorption *n* poor or disordered absorption of nutrients from the small bowel. *malabsorption syndrome* loss of

---

Magnetic resonance imaging

Magnetic resonance imaging (MRI) is an innovative diagnostic imaging system, which uses a powerful magnetic field combined with radiofrequency pulses to excite hydrogen nuclei in the body. When the nuclei relax the signal from the body is measured and reconstructed by computers into two dimensional or three dimensional images. MRI can demonstrate anatomy and pathology in any plane, providing superior soft-tissue contrast and functional information (some procedures require the injection of contrast media).

It is an established method of imaging the central nervous and musculoskeletal systems and more recently for investigations of the cardiovascular system, liver, and breast. Although MRI is often the imaging modality of choice, facilities may not be readily available.

There are no known harmful biological effects, and MRI scanning is noninvasive, painless and safe (no ionizing radiation is used). However, there are still major safety issues to consider. Contraindications to the use of MRI include:

heart pacemakers, intracerebral aneurysm clips, and other metallic implants. There have been reports in the literature (Kanal and Shellock 1996, Medical Devices Agency DoH 1993) of fatalities in patients with pacemakers, and injuries caused by metallic objects (keys, coins, oxygen cylinders).

MR scanners look similar to CT and the majority of patients tolerate MRI well, although some patients may experience anxiety.

Further reading
Lufkin R B (1990) *The MRI Manual*. USA: Year Book Medical Publishers.
Medical Devices Agency, Department of Health. (1998) *MRI Static magnetic field: Considerations – the projectile effect*. London: HMSO.

References
Kanal E, Shellock F 1996 MR Bioeffects, Safety and Patient Management, 2nd edn. Lippencott-Raven, New York
Medical Devices Agency, Department of Health (DoH) 1993 Guidelines for MR diagnostic equipment in clinical use with particular reference to safety. HMSO, London

weight and steatorrhoea of varying severity. Causes include: enzyme deficiency in cystic fibrosis, coeliac disease (gluten-induced enteropathy), Crohn's disease, lack of bile salts, infection and following surgical operations where small bowel is resected.

malacia *n* softening of a part. ⇒ keratomalacia. ⇒ osteomalacia.

maladaptation an abnormal or maladaptive response to a situation or change. It may relate to social interactions or to a response to stress that results in ill health, e.g. tension headaches, alterations in blood chemistry etc.

maladjustment *n* poor adaptation to environment, socially, mentally or physically.

malaise *n* a feeling of illness and discomfort.

malalignment *n* faulty alignment as of the teeth, or bones after a fracture.

malar *adj* relating to the cheek.

malaria *n* a serious disease caused by protozoa of the genus *Plasmodium* and carried by infected mosquitoes of the genus Anopheles. It occurs in tropical and subtropical regions and is encountered in people returning from malarial areas. The parasite causes haemolysis during a complex life cycle. *Plasmodium falciparum* causes the most severe disease with complications that include anaemia, shock and organ damage. *Plasmodium malariae* causes quartan malaria. *Plasmodium ovale* and *Plasmodium vivax* cause tertian malaria. The signs and symptoms depend on the type of malaria, but include: bouts of fever, rigors, headache, vomiting, cough, anaemia, jaundice, hepatosplenomegaly. Relapses are common in malaria. Various antimalarial drugs are available for both chemoprophylaxis and treatment. Drug resistance has occurred and many of the drugs have serious side effects. Efforts to eliminate the mosquito and its habitat are important in prevention — **malarial** *adj*.

malathion *n* organophosphorus compound, used as an insecticide in agriculture. Powerful and irreversible anticholinesterase action follows excessive inhalation; potentially dangerous to humans for this reason. Used in suitable dilution to treat head lice and scabies.

malformation *n* abnormal shape or structure; deformity.

malignant *adj* virulent and dangerous. The term is generally used to describe cancers, which, in the absence of effective treatment, usually spread locally and to distant sites (metastasize) and eventually kill the person. *malignant hyperpyrexia* ⇒ hyperpyrexia. *malignant hypertension* form of accelerated severe hypertension that causes papilloedema, headaches and kidney failure. *malignant pustule* ⇒ anthrax — **malignancy** *n*.

malingering *n* deliberate (volitional) production of symptoms to evade an unpleasant situation.

malleolus *n* a part or process of a bone shaped like a hammer. *external malleolus* at the lower end of the fibula. *internal malleolus* situated at the lower end of the tibia — **malleolar** *adj*.

malleus (hammer) *n* a hammer-shaped bone. One of the three middle ear ossicles. ⇒ incus. ⇒ stapes.

Mallory-Weiss syndrome *n* unusual cause of haematemesis where persistent vomiting causes small tears in the gastro-oesophageal mucosa.

malnutrition *n* the state of being poorly nourished. May be caused by a diet that is defective in either quantity or content, malabsorption or an inability to utilize the nutrients.

malocclusion *n* failure of the upper and lower teeth to meet properly when the jaws are closed.

malodour *n* an unpleasant odour, usually due to decomposing discharge from an infected wound, faeces or urine. ⇒ deodorants.

malposition *n* any abnormal position of a part.

malpractice *n* improper or injurious medical or nursing treatment. Professional practice which falls short of accepted standards and causes harm. It may involve unethical professional behaviour, negligence, abuse or criminal activities.

malpresentation *n* any presentation, other than the vertex, of the fetus at the onset of labour. Includes breech, face, shoulder, brow presentation etc.

Malta fever ⇒ brucellosis.

maltase *n* an enzyme found especially in intestinal juice that converts maltose to glucose.

maltose *n* malt sugar. A disaccharide consisting of two glucose molecules. Formed by the hydrolysis of starch by pancreatic amylase during digestion. Used as a nutrient and sweetener.

malunion *n* the union of a fracture in a bad position.

mamma *n* the breast **mammary** *adj.*

mammaplasty *n* plastic surgery reconstruction of the breast as may be done following mastectomy, or to augment or reduce breast size — **mammaplastic** *adj.*

mammilla *n* 1. the nipple. 2. a small papilla — **mammillae** *pl.*

mammogram *n* the product of mammography.

mammography *n* radiographic demonstration of the breast by use of specially low penetration (long wavelength) X-rays. Used in the diagnosis of or screening for breast cancer — **mammographically** *adv.*

mammotrophic *adj* having an effect upon the breast.

Manchester repair operation performed for uterine prolapse. It involves: anterior colporrhaphy, shortening of Mackenrodt's (cardinal) ligaments, amputation of part of the cervix and posterior colpoperineorrhaphy. Also known as Fothergill's operation.

Manchester Symptom Severity Scale a simplified version of the BPRS used to identify the type and severity of psychiatric symptoms. It has twelve items, of which five are rated on verbal responses and the remainder are rated on observation at interview. Also known as KGV.

mandatory minute volume in respiratory support that utilizes mechanical means to impose breaths to augment spontaneous respirations to produce a minimum preset minute volume or pulmonary ventilation.

mandible the lower jawbone — **mandibular** *adj.*

manganese (Mn) *n* a metallic element required by the body as a cofactor for many enzyme reactions.

mania *n* one phase of manic depressive psychosis in which the prevailing mood is one of undue elation and there is pronounced psychomotor overactivity and often pathological excitement. Flight of ideas and grandiose delusions are common — **manic** *adj.*

manic depressive psychosis/manic depression a type of mental disorder in which the patient's mood alternates between phases of excitement and phases of depression. Often between these phases there are periods of complete normality. Also known as bipolar depression or bipolar affective disorder. ⇒ depression.

manipulation *n* using the hands skilfully as in reducing a fracture or hernia, or changing the fetal position.

Mann Whitney test *n* a nonparametric alternative to Student's t test for independent groups.

mannitol *n* a natural sugar that is not metabolized in the body. ⇒ osmotic diuretic.

manometer *n* an instrument for measuring the pressure exerted by liquids or gases.

Mantoux reaction intradermal injection of old tuberculin or PPD (purified protein derivative, a purified type of tuberculin) into the anterior aspect of forearm. Inspection after 48–72 h. If positive, there will be an area of induration and inflammation greater than 5 mm in diameter. ⇒ Heaf test.

manual evacuation of bowel rarely undertaken nursing intervention because of risk of trauma to the rectum and the psychological distress caused. After oral medication to lubricate/soften hardened faeces, the nurse introduces a gloved finger into the rectum and tries to dislodge pieces of faeces. It is important that training is received before attempting this technique.

manual handling the moving, lifting or supporting of a load subject to legal regulations. See Box – Manual handling.

manubrium *n* a handle-shaped structure; the upper part of the breast bone or sternum.

MAOI *abbr* monoamine oxidase inhibitor.

maple syrup urine disease recessively inherited disorder of amino acid metabolism. An enzyme required for the

---

Manual handling

Back injuries are a major concern in the health and safety of health professionals, especially nursing and midwifery staff. Employers have a duty of care at common law (judge made law) and by statute (Health and Safety at Work Act 1974) to take reasonable care for the health and safety of their employees. Specific requirements have been laid down in respect of manual handling (MH).

Following a Directive of the European Community, regulations were made in 1992 and brought into force in January 1993 requiring employers to implement rules relating to MH operations. MH is defined as "any transporting or supporting of a load (including the lifting, putting down, pushing, pulling, carrying or moving thereof) by hand or by bodily force." (Regulation 2(1)).

The regulations require the employer:

• So far as is reasonably practicable, to avoid the need for his employees to undertake any MH operations at work which involve a risk of their being injured;

• Where it is not reasonably practicable to avoid the need for MH, to carry out a suitable and sufficient assessment of any MH operations;

• Where it is not reasonably practicable to avoid the need for MH, to take appropriate steps to reduce the risk of injury to those employees arising out of their undertaking any such MH to the lowest level reasonably practicable;

• To provide to the employee, where it is reasonably practicable, precise information on the weight of each load and the heaviest side of any load, whose centre of gravity is not positioned centrally;

• To review any assessment, where there is reason to suspect that it is no longer valid or there has been a significant change in the MH operations.

The MH regulations are enforced by the Health and Safety Executive which can prosecute for any infringements in the criminal courts. In addition if any employee or other person, can show that they have suffered harm as a result of failures by the employer or other employees in following the regulations, then action can be brought in the civil courts for compensation. For guidance on the Manual Handling regulations see the Manual Handling Guidance on Regulations by the Health and Safety Executive Stationery Office 1992.

---

breakdown of certain amino acids is deficient, and leucine, isoleucine and valine are excreted in the urine, giving rise to the characteristic odour of maple syrup. It is characterized by spasticity, poor feeding, convulsions, neurological damage and learning disability.

marasmus *n* severe form of protein-energy malnutrition, caused by insufficient protein and energy (calories) in the diet. It affects young children who become very thin with muscle wasting and have a distended abdomen and diarrhoea. Rarely seen in developed Western societies but still common in developing countries when famine occurs. ⇒ failure to thrive. ⇒ Kwashiorkor — **marasmic** *adj*.

marble bone disease ⇒ osteopetrosis.

Marburg disease a severe and highly infectious haemorrhagic fever caused by the Marburg/Ebola virus (first cases were amongst laboratory workers in Marburg, Germany, who had handled monkey tissue from Uganda). Incubation period is 5–9 days and there is a wide range of symptoms, including fever, severe headache and malaise, vomiting, diarrhoea, pharyngitis, generalized rash and bleeding from mucous membranes. No specific treatment is available and the mortality rate is 25–90%. ⇒ filoviruses.

Marfan's syndrome a hereditary genetic disorder of unknown cause which affects connective tissue. There is dislocation of the lens, congenital heart disease and arachnodactyly with hypotonic musculature and lax ligaments, occasionally excessive height and abnormalities of the iris.

marginal cost the cost of providing the extra resources required to carry out activity above a baseline figure.

marihuana *n* ⇒ cannabis indica.

marker *n* ⇒ tumour marker.

Marshall-Marchetti-Krantz operation an operation to relieve stress incontinence. A form of abdominal cystourethropexy usually undertaken where a colporrhaphy has failed to achieve continence for the woman.

marsupialization *n* operative procedure where a cyst is drained and its edges are sutured to form a patent opening.

masculinization the development of male secondary sexual charateristics in the female.

Maslow's hierarchy of human needs a list (pyramid) of human needs that range from basic physiological needs, such as food, to self-actualization. ⇒ human needs. (See Figure 39).

masochism *n* the deriving of pleasure from pain inflicted on self by others or occasionally by oneself. It may be a conscious or unconscious process and is frequently of a sexual nature. ⇒ sadism *ant*.

mass number the total mass of protons and neutrons in an atom.

massage *n* 1. the soft tissues are manipulated in different ways (kneaded, rubbed, stroked, tapped, etc) and at different depths and rates for various purposes. to improve circulation, metabolism and muscle tone, to break down adhesions, to expel gases, and to either relax or stimulate the patient. *cardiac massage* done for cardiac arrest. With the patient on his or her back on a firm surface, the lower portion of sternum is depressed to massage the heart. ⇒ cardiopulmonary resuscitation (CPR). 2. a complementary therapy. Conscious use of gentle muscle manipulation, employing stroking or light kneading in order to promote a sensation of relaxation.

MAST *acr* Michigan Alcoholism Screening Test.

mast cells *n* basophils that have migrated to the tissues. They are found around small blood vessels, where they bind to immunoglobulins (IgE) prior to releasing

chemical mediators, e.g. histamine, involved in the inflammatory response and anaphylaxis. ⇒ inflammatory.

mastalgia *n* pain in the breast. Also called mastodynia.

mastectomy *n* surgical removal of the breast. Usually performed for the treatment of breast cancer in conjunction with chemotherapy and radiotherapy. May also be used as prophylaxis for women at high risk of developing breast cancer. Women having mastectomy are offered some form of breast reconstruction, either immediate or later. ⇒ lumpectomy. ⇒ mammoplasty. *simple mastectomy* removal of the entire breast. *modified radical mastectomy* removal of the entire breast and division or excision of the pectoralis minor muscle with axillary lymph node clearance. *radical mastectomy* rarely performed operation that involves removal of the breast, pectoralis major muscle and clearance of the the axillary lymph nodes ⇒ pectoral.

mastication *n* the act of chewing.

mastitis *n* inflammation of the breast. May occur during lactation.

mastodynia *n* pain in the breast. Also called mastalgia.

mastoid *adj* nipple-shaped. *mastoid air cells* extend in a backward and downward direction from the antrum. *mastoid antrum* the air space within the mastoid process, lined by mucous membrane continuous with that of the tympanum and mastoid cells. *mastoid process* the prominence of the mastoid portion of the temporal bone just behind the ear.

mastoidectomy *n* drainage of the mastoid air cells and excision of diseased tissue. *cortical mastoidectomy* all the mastoid cells are removed, making one cavity which drains through an opening (aditus) into the middle ear. The external meatus and middle ear are untouched. *radical mastoidectomy* the mastoid antrum and middle ear are made into one continuous cavity for drainage of infection. Loss of hearing is inevitable. *modified radical mastoidectomy* tympanic membrane preserved.

mastoiditis *n* inflammation of the mastoid air cells. An infective process affecting the mastoid air cells.

masturbation *n* non-coital stimulation of the genitalia to produce sexual excitement and orgasm.

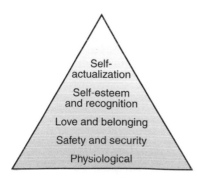

Figure 39 Maslow's hierarchy of needs.
(Reproduced from Brooker 1996 with permission.)

materia medica the science dealing with the origin, action and dosage of drugs.

maternal deprivation ⇒ abuse. ⇒ failure to thrive. ⇒ neglect.

matriarchy a community or social structure where a female (wife, mother or daughter) inherits, dominates and controls.

matrix *n* the foundation substance in which the tissue cells are embedded.

maturation *n* the process of attaining full development. The last stage in wound healing, during which the scar is reformed, the wound is strengthened and the scar gradually fades and shrinks.

Maurice Lee tube a double-bore tube which combines nasogastric aspiration and jejunal feeding.

maxilla *n* the upper jawbone — **maxillary** *adj maxillary antrum* a large paranasal sinus in the maxilla. ⇒ sinus. Also know as the antrum of Highmore.

maxillofacial *adj* pertaining to the maxilla and face.

maximal breathing capacity *n* the amount of gas exchanged in one minute when the person is breathing at the maximal depth and rate.

MBC *abbr* maximal breathing capacity. ⇒ respiratory function tests.

MCA *abbr* Medicines Control Agency.

McBurney's point a point one-third of the way between the right anterior superior iliac spine and the umbilicus, the site of maximum tenderness in cases of acute appendicitis.

MCH *n* mean cell haemoglobin.

MCHC *n* mean cell haemoglobin concentration.

McMurray's osteotomy division of femur between lesser and greater trochanter. Shaft displaced inwards beneath the head and abducted. This position maintained by a nail plate. Restores painless weight bearing.

MCV *n* mean cell volume.

MDA *abbr* Medical Devices Agency.

MDM *abbr* mental defence mechanism.

MDMA *abbr* methylenedioxymethamphetamine. ⇒ Ecstasy.

MDR-TB *abbr* multidrug resistant tuberculosis.

ME *abbr* myalgic encephalomyelitis. Also known as chronic fatigue syndrome and post-viral syndrome.

meals-on-wheels element of community care provided by social services for disabled and/or older clients in their own homes. Provides either a ready-cooked meal, or packs of frozen meals (to be cooked by the client), throughout the week. A charge is usually made.

mean the average. *arithmetric mean* figure calculated by dividing the sum of a set of values by the number of items in the group. ⇒ central tendency statistic.

mean cell haemoglobin (MCH) *n* a red cell parameter measured during a full blood count. It is the amount of haemoglobin in an individual red cell.

mean cell haemoglobin concentration (MCHC) *n* a red cell parameter measured during a full blood count. It is an estimation of the amount of haemoglobin, in grams, present in 100 mL of packed red cells.

mean cell volume (MCV) *n* a red cell parameter measured during a full blood count. It is the mean volume of red cells which provides information about cell size.

means-tested describes a nonuniversal benefit. Only those with income and/or savings below a predetermined level are entitled to certain benefits.

measles *n* (*syn* morbilli) an acute infectious disease caused by a paramyxovirus. Measles is endemic and worldwide in distribution and usually affects children. It is highly contagious and spreads via droplets. The incubation period is about 10 days. The disease has an initial catarrhal stage; with a cold-like illness, fever, sore and watery eyes, cough, Koplik's spots and photophobia. After 3 to 4 days a maculopapular rash appears. It may be complicated by a secondary bacterial infection such as otitis media or pneumonia. Other effects include eye damage from corneal ulcers and encephalitis. The mortality rate is very low in previously healthy and well nourished individuals, but in developing countries the mortality is high. Active immunity is offered as part of the routine immunization programme, in conjunction with protection against mumps and rubella (MMR), and passive immunity is available in special cases. *German measles* ⇒ rubella.

meatotomy *n* surgery to the urinary meatus for meatal ulcer and stricture in men.

meatus *n* an opening or channel, as in urinary meatus — **meatal** *adj*.

mechanical ventilation describes various mechanical methods used to support patients where spontaneous respirations have ceased or are inadequate to maintain sufficient gas exchange of oxygen and carbon dioxide, such as respiratory failure or during general anaesthetic. See Box – Mechanical ventilation.

mechanoreceptors *n* receptors that are sensitive to mechanical forces. They include: proprioceptors, receptors in the ear, baroreceptors, pressure and touch receptors in the skin and stretch receptors in structures such as the bladder.

Meckel's diverticulum a blind, pouch-like sac sometimes arising from the free border of the lower ileum. It is an embryonic remnant and occurs in 2% of population; usually symptomless. May cause obstruction, intussusception or be a site of peptic ulceration if it contains ectopic gastric mucosa.

meconium *n* black-green viscid material formed in the fetal bowel. It is discharged as the infant's first stool, normally soon after birth and during the next day or two, passed shortly after birth. *meconium aspiration* aspiration of meconium into the respiratory passages before or during birth. *meconium ileus* obstruction of the bowel by extremely thick meconium; may be associated with cystic fibrosis which can present in this way.

media 1. *n* the middle coat of a vessel. 2. *npl* nutritive jellies used for culturing bacteria. ⇒ medium.

medial *adj* pertaining to or near the middle — **medially** *adv*.

median *adj* 1. the middle. *median line* an imaginary line passing through the centre of the body from a point between the eyes to between the apposed feet. 2. a central tendency statistic; the middle or midway value in a series of scores when arranged in ascending order. ⇒ mean. ⇒ mode.

mediastinoscopy *n* endoscopic examination of the mediastinum and its contents. May be combined with biopsy of lymph nodes for histological examination.

mediastinum *n* the space between the lungs containing the oesophagus, heart and great vessels — **mediastinal** *adj*.

Medical and Dental Education Levy (MADEL) the budget used to fund prequalification dental and medical education.

Medical Devices Agency (MDA) in the UK, a government agency that works with government, users and manufacturers to ensure that medical devices meet the appropriate safety, quality and efficacy standards, and that they comply with European Union Directives. *Medical Devices Advisory Group (Committee of Safety of Devices Group)* a committee that provides external expert advice on medical devices.

medical diagnosis attribution of the disease exhibited by a patient into a specific category, using an international classification of same. Some people have multiple med-

---

Mechanical ventilation

Mechanical ventilation may be required to support breathing in respiratory failure. There are many causes of respiratory failure; those immediately associated with the lungs such as pneumonia, pulmonary oedema or severe acute asthma (status asthmaticus) and those that can affect the mechanics of breathing such as flail chest, Guillain-Barré syndrome or during anaesthesia. Mechanical ventilation can also be used to reduce the workload of the heart in certain conditions.

A ventilator takes a mixture of oxygen and air and passes it into the lungs, commonly via an endotracheal tube or tracheostomy tube, providing inspiration. Expiration, as in normal physiology, is reliant on the natural recoil of the lungs,

not the ventilator. Ventilators have controls that can alter parameters such as respiratory rate, the size of breath (tidal volume) and the percentage of inspired oxygen to suit the requirements of individual patients.

Most ventilators have the capacity to provide different modes or methods of ventilation. If the patient is completely unable to breathe, the ventilator will provide all of the breathing required. This mode is commonly called controlled mandatory ventilation (CMV). Alternatively, if the patient can provide some of the breathing, a ventilator mode can be chosen that supplements the patient's efforts. Such modes include: pressure support ventilation (PSV) or synchronized intermittent ventilation (SIMV).

ical diagnoses and occasionally a patient's characteristics cannot be allocated to a specific disease category, an example being pyrexia of unknown origin.

medical history the main objective of a history taken by a doctor is to enable the making of a medical diagnosis, according to an international classification.

medical jurisprudence ⇒ forensic medicine.

medical model in a nursing context, the term signifies that the focus of nursing is the medical diagnosis allocated by the doctor. ⇒ diagnosis.

medicament *n* a remedy or medicine. ⇒ drug.

medicated *adj* impregnated with a drug or medicine.

medication *n* therapeutic substance, taken orally or administered by injection subcutaneously, intramuscularly, intravenously; also by inhalation, suppository and topical application. ⇒ drug.

medicinal *adj* pertaining to a medicine.

medicine *n* **1.** science or art of healing, especially as distinguished from surgery. **2.** a therapeutic substance. ⇒ drug.

Medicines Control Agency (MCA) in the UK, a government agency that licenses new drugs. Decisions are based on safety, quality and efficacy.

medicochirurgical *adj* pertaining to both medicine and surgery.

medicosocial *adj* pertaining to medicine and sociology. For example, pertaining to the medical conditions caused by social factors, such as coronary heart disease due to a specific lifestyle.

mediolateral *adj* pertaining to the middle and one side.

meditation an altered state achieved by various exercises and rituals. The aim is mental and physical relaxation. It may be used as part of stress management.

medium *n* a substance used in bacteriology for the growth of organisms — **media** *pl.*

Medline *n* computerized database of medical science literature.

medulla *n* **1.** the marrow in the centre of a long bone. **2.** the central part of some structures, e.g. kidneys, adrenals, lymph nodes, etc. *medulla oblongata* the lowest part of the brainstem where it passes through the foramen magnum to become the spinal cord. It contains the nerve centres controlling various vital functions, e.g. respiratory and cardiac centres — **medullary** *adj.*

medullated *adj* containing or surrounded by a medulla or marrow. Particularly referring to nerve fibres insulated by a myelin sheath.

medulloblastoma *n* malignant, rapidly growing tumour of the cerebellum; arising from embryonic cells, it affects children. Treatment is by excision, and combination of radiotherapy and chemotherapy.

megacephalic *adj* (*syn* macrocephalic, megalocephalic) large headed.

megacolon *n* dilatation of the colon with constipation. *congenital megacolon or Hirschsprung's disease* due to congenital absence of the nerve plexus in the pelvic colon and rectum with loss of motor function, resulting in hypertrophic dilatation of the normal proximal colon. *acquired megacolon* associated with chronic constipation in the presence of normal innervation; it can be caused by hypothyroidism, misuse of laxatives, neurological problems and mental health problems where people ignore the urge to defaecate.

megakaryocyte *n* large multinucleate bone marrow cell. Fragments break off to form non-nucleated platelets.

megaloblast *n* a large, nucleated, primitive red blood cell formed where there is a deficiency of vitamin B_{12} or folic acid. ⇒ anaemia — **megaloblastic** *adj.*

megalomania *n* delusion of grandeur, characteristic of GPI.

Meibomian cyst a cyst on the edge of the eyelid from retained secretion of the Meibomian glands.

Meibomian glands sebaceous glands lying in grooves on the inner surface of the eyelids, their ducts opening on the free margins of the lids.

Meigs syndrome a benign fibroma of the ovary associated with ascites and hydrothorax.

meiosis *n* the process which, through two successive cell divisions, leads to the formation of mature gametes, oocytes and spermatozoa. The process starts by the pairing of the partner chromosomes, which then separate from each other at the meiotic divisions, so that the diploid (2n) chromosome number of 23 pairs is halved to 23 chromosomes, only one member of each original pair; this set constitutes the haploid (n) complement. ⇒ mitosis.

Meissner's corpuscles n sensory receptors in the skin which detect light pressure.

Meissner's plexus n autonomic nerve fibres of the gastrointestinal tract. They facilitate communication between different parts and allow the tract to function as an integrated unit.

melaena n black, tar-like stools. Evidence of gastrointestinal bleeding.

melancholia n term reserved in psychiatry to mean severe forms of depression — **melancholic** adj.

melanin n a black or brown pigment found to varying degrees in hair, skin and the choroid of the eye. → melanocytes.

melanocytes npl cells of the basal layer of the skin that produce melanin when stimulated by melanocyte stimulating hormone (MSH) from the pituitary.

melanoma n a tumour arising from the melanocytes (pigment-producing cells of the skin) and less commonly in the pigment cells of the eye. malignant melanoma the most serious form of skin cancer. The incidence is rising worldwide, especially in fair-skinned people living near the equator, but is also increasing in more temperate areas, e.g. UK and USA. Exposure to sunlight is the most important cause. Prevention is important and involves: limiting exposure to sunlight, wearing protective clothing, such as hats, and use of an effective sunscreen — **melanomatous** adj.

melanosis n dark pigmentation of surfaces as in sunburn, Addison's disease, etc. melanosis coli black/brown pigmentation of the colonic mucosa. It may accompany the prolonged use of certain laxatives — **melanotic** adj.

melatonin n a hormone produced by the pineal body (gland) in response to the amount of light entering the eye. It appears to influence sexual maturation and is closely involved in reproductive function. Also involved in mood and various circadian rhythms, such as sleep, temperature and appetite. ⇒ jet lag.

melitensis n ⇒ brucellosis.

membrane n a thin lining or covering substance. basement membrane a thin layer beneath the epithelium of mucous surfaces. cell membrane thin, semipermeable membrane surrounding the cytoplasm of cells. hyaloid membrane the transparent capsule surrounding the vitreous humor of the eye. mucous membrane contains glands which secrete mucus. It lines the cavities and passages that communicate with the exterior of the body. serous membrane a lubricating membrane lining the closed cavities, and reflected over their enclosed organs. synovial membrane the membrane lining the intra-articular parts of bones and ligaments. It does not cover the articular surfaces. tympanic membrane the eardrum — **membranous** adj.

memory the ability to retain and recall prior learning (information and events). It is a very complex process and includes different types of memory. ⇒ episodic memory. → long term memory. → procedural memory. ⇒ semantic memory. ⇒ short term memory. memory lapses many adults experience a memory loss and some time later retrieve the appropriate information. Many people experience these when under stress, and increasing incidents as they become older. ⇒ Alzheimer's disease. ⇒ dementia.

menaquinones npl a group of compounds with vitamin K activity that are synthesized by the intestinal bacteria.

menarche n commencement of menstrual cycles; the first menstrual period.

Mendel's laws the fundamental theory of heredity and its laws, evolved by an Austrian monk, Gregor Mendel. The laws determine the inheritance of different characters, particularly the interaction of dominant and recessive traits in cross-breeding, the maintenance of the purity of such characters during hereditary transmission and the independent segregation of genetically different characteristics (see Figure 40). ⇒ gene.

Mendelson's syndrome inhalation of regurgitated stomach contents, which can cause rapid death from anoxia, or it may produce pulmonary oedema, severe bronchospasm and respiratory distress.

Menière's disease distension of endolymphatic system (membranous labyrinth) of the inner ear from excess fluid. This causes distortion of the cochlear and semicircular canals and leads to fluctuating deafness, tinnitus and repeated attacks of vertigo, which may be accompanied by nausea and vomiting.

meninges *npl* the surrounding membranes of the brain and spinal cord. They are three in number: (a) the dura mater (outer); (b) arachnoid mater (middle); (c) pia mater (inner) — **meningeal** *adj*.

meningioma *n* a slowly growing fibrous tumour arising in the meninges — **meningiomatous** *adj*.

meningism, meningismus *n* a condition presenting with signs and symptoms of meningitis (e.g. neck stiffness); meningitis does not develop.

meningitis *n* inflammation of the meninges due to infection by micro-organisms. It may be viral or bacterial. *viral meningitis* is the commonest cause, e.g. coxsackievirus, echovirus and mumps virus. It is usually a mild illness. *bacterial meningitis*

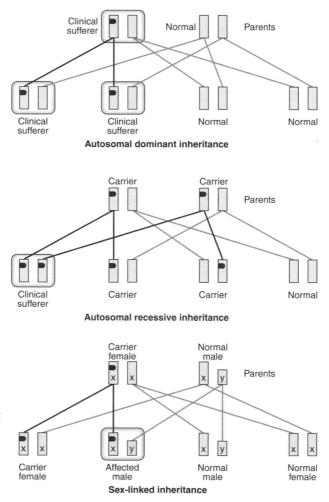

Figure 40 Mendelian laws of inheritance.

more severe illness with considerable morbidity and a high mortality rate. It may be caused by *Haemophilus influenzae, Streptococcus pneumoniae, Neissseria meningitidis* (meningococcal), Group B streptococci, Gram negative bacilli and less commonly *Listeria monocytogenes, Cryptococcus neoformans, Staphylococcus aureus* and *Mycobacterium tuberculosis* (where the onset is insidious). Acute infections are characterized by a vague 'flu-like' illness, headache, fever, neck stiffness, photophobia, vomiting, altered consciousness, convulsions, a positive Kernig's sign and changes in the CSF on lumbar puncture. In infants and small children the signs may be less specific with irritability and poor feeding. Patients with meningococcal septicaemia will also have a dark purple/red petechial rash that does not disappear when pressure is applied. Management involves the administration of the appropriate antimicrobial drugs, supportive treatment, such as mechanical ventilation, and skilled nursing care and observation. → group C meningococcal disease. ⇒ leptomeningitis. ⇒ pachymeningitis — **meningitides** *pl.*

meningocele *n* protrusion of the meninges through a bony defect in the skull or spine, usually in the thoraco-lumbar region. It forms a cyst filled with cerebrospinal fluid. → hydrocephalus. → spina bifida.

meningococcus *n Neisseria meningitidis* — **meningococcal** *adj* pertaining to the meningococcus. *meningococcal septicaemia* ⇒ group C meningococcal disease. ⇒ meningitis.

meningoencephalitis *n* inflammation of the brain and the meninges — **meningoencephalitic** *adj.*

meningomyelocele *n* (*syn* myelomeningocele) protrusion of a portion of the spinal cord and its enclosing membranes (meninges) through a bony defect in the spinal canal, usually in the thoracolumbar region. ⇒ spina bifida.

meniscectomy *n* the removal of a semilunar cartilage of the knee joint, following injury and displacement. The medial cartilage is damaged most commonly.

meniscus *n* 1. semilunar cartilage, particularly in the knee joint. 2. the curved upper surface of a column of liquid — **menisci** *pl.*

menopause *n* the cessation of menstruation. A single event occurring during the climacteric. It normally occurs between the ages of 45 and 55 years, the mean age in the UK is 51 years. *artificial menopause* an earlier menopause induced by radiotherapy or surgery for some pathological condition — **menopausal** *adj.*

menorrhagia *n* an excessive regular menstrual flow. May be associated with IUD, fibroids or systemic disease. → endometrial destruction.

menses *n* the sanguineous fluid discharged from the uterus during menstruation; menstrual flow.

menstrual *adj* relating to the menses. *menstrual or uterine cycle* the cyclical changes occurring in the uterus as the endometrium responds to ovarian hormones. It corresponds to the ovarian cycle and is repeated every 28 days or so (range 21–35), except during pregnancy, from the menarche to the menopause. It has three phases: proliferative, secretory, and menstrual in which bleeding (menstrual flow) occurs for approximately 5 days.

menstruation *n* the flow of blood and endometrial debris from the uterus once a month in the female. It commences about the age of 12–13 years in developed countries, and ceases about 51 years.

mental *adj* 1. pertaining to the mind. *mental age* the age of a person with regard to his/her intellectual development which can be determined by intelligence tests. If a person aged 30 years can only pass the tests normally achieved by a child of 12 years, the person's mental age is said to be 12 years. *mental illness/disorder* the definition in the English Mental Health Act is that 'mental illness, arrested or incomplete development of mind, psychopathic disorder and any other disorder or disability of mind, and "mentally disordered" shall be construed accordingly'. A patient can be detained in hospital only if, as one condition, they can be said to suffer from a 'mental disorder' in relation to this definition. The broader definition of mental distress includes any illness, developmental abnormality or personality disorder mentioned in the major classifications of mental distress. ⇒ learning disability. *Mental Health Acts* various acts of parliament which regulate and control the rights, admission, treatment and subsequent stay in hospital for certain patients with mental health disorders. ⇒ detained patient. *Mental Health Commission* a body whose function is concerned with the care and welfare of those individuals detained under the provisions of the relevant part of the Mental Health Act. *Mental Health Review Tribunal* a body set up in each Regional Health Administration area to deal with patients' applications for discharge or alteration of their conditions of detention in hospital (in England and Wales, with a separate, similar system in Northern Ireland). In Scotland, the same function is performed by requests for review of detention to the Mental Welfare Commission, or appeal to the sheriff. *Mental Health Welfare Officer* an approved social worker (ASW) appointed by the Local Health Authority to deal with: (a) applications for compulsory or emergency admission to hospital, or for conveyance of patients there; (b) applications concerning guardianship, the functions of the nearest relative, or acting as nearest relative if so appointed; (c) returning patients absent without leave, or apprehending patients escaped from legal custody. In addition the ASW may have a wide range of functions in the care and aftercare of the mentally disordered in the community. This includes home visiting, training centres, clubs and general supervision of the discharged patient. The Scottish equivalent is the Mental Health Officer (MHO). The MHO is also a social worker with special experience in mental disorder (mental distress is the preferred term). MHOs can make application for admission of a patient under the Mental Health (Scotland) Act 1984, or for guardianship under the same Act. They have a duty to provide reports on the social circumstances of patients who are detained in hospital and of certain other functions under the Act. 2. an anatomical term that pertains to the chin.

mental defence mechanisms (MDM) unconscious defence mechanism by which individuals attempt to cope with stressful, difficult or threatening emotions. ⇒ compensation. ⇒ conversion. ⇒ denial. ⇒ displacement. ⇒ fantasy. ⇒ identification. ⇒ intellectualization. ⇒ projection. ⇒ rationalization. ⇒ regression. ⇒ repression. ⇒ sublimation. ⇒ suppression. ⇒ withdrawal.

mental handicap ⇒ learning disability.

mental health a sense of well-being in the emotional, personal, spiritual and social domains of people's lives. *mental health nursing* a branch of nursing which is concerned with helping people to enhance, maintain or improve their emotional, personal, spiritual and social lives. It is an area of care that was first called 'mental nursing' and then 'psychiatric nursing'. Mental health nurses, increasingly, care for people in the community as the UK government's policy of community care continues. Mental health nursing concentrates, particularly, on the enhancement or maintenance of mental health, and one of the aims of mental health nursing is to prevent the onset of breakdown or illness, where this is possible. The skills of a mental health nurse include a range of interpersonal and therapeutic skills, such as listening, responding, problem-solving, crisis management and enabling the release of emotion. The Butterworth report (Department of Health 1994) highlighted the need for a flexible response to future mental health needs. Its recommendations included: greater understanding of racial and cultural needs; more research; the representation and participation of service users; links with the criminal justice system; a focus on severe mental illness; availability of mental health nursing skills to the primary care team; clinical supervision and the development of a framework for good practice. Mental health nursing skills are important in achieving the mental illness target of reducing deaths from suicide and undetermined injury by at least a fifth by 2010, set out in the government report (Department of Health (1999) *Saving Lives. Our Healthier Nation*. London: The Stationery Office). ⇒ specialist community practitioner.

menthol *n* mild analgesic obtained from oil of peppermint. Used in liniments and ointments, and as an inhalation or drops for nasal catarrh.

mentoanterior *adj* forward position of the fetal chin in the maternal pelvis in a face presentation.

mentoposterior *adj* backward position of the fetal chin in the maternal pelvis in a face presentation.

mentorship *n* a system which provides support to students during their training. A mentor – a qualified and experienced nurse – works with the student on clinical placements, ensuring he or she receives the appropriate experience. ⇒ preceptorship.

menu in computing a screen showing the options available with certain programs.

mercurialism *n* chronic poisoning with mercury, occurring in people whose work involves contact with the metal or through foods, such as fish, which may contain high levels. It is characterized by paraesthesia, ataxia, visual and hearing problems, stomatitis, loosening of teeth, gastrointestinal problems and possible renal damage.

mercury (Hg) *n* the only common metal that is liquid at room temperature. Used in measuring instruments such as thermometers and sphygmomanometers. Forms two series of salts: mercurous ones are univalent, and mercuric ones are bivalent. *mercury poisoning* mercury is toxic and local safety protocols should be followed in the event of accidental spillage. ⇒ mercurialism.

meridians *n* conceptual channels running through and across the body through which Qi energy flows. Treatment along the meridians is by means of pressing or inserting needles at key points (tsubos) at which the energy is most responsive to stimulus. ⇒ acupuncture. ⇒ shiatsu.

meritocracy a process whereby position or job are allocated on merit.

mesarteritis *n* inflammation of the middle coat of an artery.

mesencephalon *n* the midbrain.

mesenchyme *n* embryonic connective tissue that develops from mesoderm. It gives rise to all connective tissues.

mesentery *n* a large sling-like fold of peritoneum which enfolds the small intestine and secures it to the posterior abdominal wall, containing blood vessels, nerves and lymphatics (see Figure 48) — **mesenteric** *adj*.

mesocolon *n* double fold of peritoneum which secures the transverse colon to the abdominal wall (see Figure 48).

mesoderm *n* the middle of the three primary germ layers of the early embryo. From it are derived bone, muscles, blood, cardiovascular system, dermis of the skin, lymphatic system (spleen and cells), pleura, pericardium, peritoneum, urogenital tract, gonads and the adrenal cortex. ⇒ ectoderm. ⇒ endoderm.

mesophile *n* a bacterium that grows and multiplies within the range 25–40°C. Most human pathogens are mesophiles, thriving best at 37°C — **mesophilic** *adj*.

mesothelioma *n* a tumour of serous membranes: pleura and peritoneum. *malignant mesothelioma* a rapidly growing tumour of pleura or peritoneum which is usually associated with exposure to asbestos, especially blue asbestos, at work or within buildings. Patients have pleural effusion or ascites and pain. Treatment is palliative only.

mesovarian *n* peritoneal fold connecting the ovary to the broad ligament.

messenger RNA (mRNA) *n* → ribonucleic acid.

meta-analysis a statistical summary of many research studies using complex analysis of the primary data.

metabolic *adj* pertaining to metabolism. *basal metabolic rate (BMR)* the expression of basal metabolism in terms of kJ per m^2 of body surface per hour. *metabolic acidosis* ⇒ acidosis. *metabolic alkalosis* → alkalosis — **metabolically** *adv*.

metabolism *n* the continuous series of chemical reactions in the living body by which life is maintained. Food and tissues are broken down (catabolism), new substances are created for growth and rebuilding (anabolism), and energy is released in anabolism and utilized in catabolism and heat production. ⇒ adenosine diphosphate. ⇒ adenosine triphosphate. *basal metabolism* the minimum energy expended in the maintenance of respiration, circulation, peristalsis, muscle tonus, body temperature and other vegetative functions of the body.

metabolite *n* by-product of metabolism. An *essential metabolite* is a substance which is necessary for normal metabolism, e.g. vitamins.

metacarpophalangeal *adj* pertaining to the metacarpus and the phalanges.

metacarpus *n* the five bones which form that part of the hand between the wrist and fingers — **metacarpal** *adj*.

metaphase the second stage of mitosis and meiosis.

metaplasia *n* the change of cells to another type (usually less specialized – a reverse of differentiation). May occur in response to chronic inflammation; it is generally reversible but can progress to malignant changes.

metastasis *n* the spread of tumour cells from one part of the body to another, usually via the blood or lymph, but cancer cells may spread across serous membranes and may be 'seeded' to other areas during surgery. A secondary growth — **metastasize** *vi.*

metastatic *adj* pertaining to a metastasis or secondary growth.

metatarsalgia *n* pain under the metatarsal heads. *Morton's metatarsalgia* neuralgia caused by a neuroma on the digital nerve, most commonly that supplying the third toe cleft.

metatarsophalangeal *adj* pertaining to the metatarsus and the phalanges.

metatarsus *n* the five bones of the foot between the ankle and the toes — **metatarsal** *adj.*

meteorism *n* ⇒ tympanites.

methadone *n* a synthetic opioid used to relieve unpleasant symptoms in people undertaking heroin withdrawal programmes.

methaemoglobin *n* a form of haemoglobin in which the iron is oxidized to the ferric state. This pigment is unable to transport oxygen and may result in cyanosis. It is present normally in very small amounts, but may be formed abnormally following the administration of a wide variety of drugs, including the sulphonamides.

methaemoglobinaemia *n* methaemoglobin in the blood — **methaemoglobinaemic** *adj.*

methaemoglobinuria *n* methaemoglobin in the urine — **methaemoglobinuric** *adj.*

methane *n* CH_4, a colourless, odourless, inflammable gas produced as a result of putrefaction and fermentation of organic matter.

methicillin-resistant *Staphylococcus aureus* (MRSA) strains of *Staphylococcus aureus* that are resistant to most antibiotics, including methicillin (not used clinically) and flucloxacillin. Causes serious and sometimes fatal infections in hospitals, and patients with the micro-organism are increasingly encountered in community settings. Treatment involves vancomycin or teicoplanin, or various combinations of rifampicin, sodium fusidate and ciprofloxacin. Topical mupirocin is used to eliminate nasal or skin carriage. Infection control measures, such as strict adherence to hand washing policies, proper environmental cleaning and isolation or patient cohorting, are vital in the control of MRSA.

methionine *n* one of the essential (indispensable) sulphur-containing amino acids. Used in the management of paracetamol overdose to restore glutathione levels in order to prevent liver damage.

methylcellulose *n* ⇒ laxatives.

metre (m) *n* a measurement of length. One of the seven base units of the International System of Units (SI). One thousand millimetres.

metritis *n* inflammation of the uterus.

metrorrhagia *n* uterine bleeding, at a time other than during menstruation. It may follow coitus or examination and should always be investigated to exclude serious pathology. ⇒ postmenopausal bleeding.

MHC *abbr* major histocompatibility complex.

micelle *n* minute globules of fat and bile salts formed during the digestion of fats. They transport fatty acids and glycerol into the enterocytes (intestinal cells) and leave the bile salts within the lumen of the bowel.

Michel's clips small metal clips used instead of sutures for the closure of a wound.

Michigan Alcoholism Screening Test (MAST) an assessment designed to detect problematic alcohol use by rating its effect on an individual's physical and social circumstances.

microangiopathy *n* disease affecting small blood vessels. There is thickening of the basement membrane in capillaries. It occurs in diabetes mellitus and leads to kidney failure from diabetic nephropathy. ⇒ Kimmelstiel-Wilson syndrome.

microbe *n* ⇒ micro-organism — **microbial, microbic** *adj.*

microbiology *n* the science that studies micro-organisms — **microbiologically** *adv.*

microcephaly *adj* a congenital condition where the head is abnormally small in relation to the rest of the body and the brain is underdeveloped. There are numerous causes including: an abnormal gene, chromosomal abnormalities, intrauterine exposure to toxins or certain infections. Affected individuals have some degree of learning disability — **microcephalic** *adj* pertaining to an abnormally small head.

microcirculation *n* blood flow throughout the system of smaller vessels of the body, i.e. arterioles, blood capillaries and venules.

Micrococcus *n* a genus of Gram-positive cocci. They are part of the skin flora and are generally nonpathogenic.

microcyte *n* an undersized red blood cell found especially in iron deficiency anaemia. ⇒ anaemia — **microcytic** *adj* relating to microcytes. *microcytic anaemia* ⇒ anaemia.

microcytosis an increased number of microcytes.

microenvironment *n* the environment at the microscopic or cellular level immediately surrounding the body.

microfilaria *n* immature Filaria. ⇒ filariasis.

microglial cells *n* a type of macrophage found in the central nervous system. ⇒ neuroglia.

micrognathia *n* small jaw, especially the lower one; associated with Pierre Robin syndrome.

microgram (μg) *n* one millionth of a gram.

micrometre (μm) *n* one millionth of a metre. Often still known as a micron.

micron *n* a millionth part of a metre. ⇒ micrometre.

micronutrients *npl* nutrients, such as vitamins and minerals, required by the body in relatively small amounts. ⇒ macronutrients. ⇒ minerals. ⇒ trace elements. ⇒ vitamins.

micro-organism *n* (*syn* microbe) any microscopic plant or animal cell. Often synonymous with bacterium but includes: rickettsia, chlamydia, fungus, protozoon and virus.

microscopic *adj* extremely small; visible only with the aid of a microscope. ⇒ macroscopic *ant*.

Microsporum *n* a genus of fungi. Parasitic, living in keratin-containing tissues of humans and animals. *Microsporum audouini* is the commonest cause of scalp ringworm.

microsurgery *n* use of the binocular operating microscope during the performance of operations, such as that required to join vessels and nerves — **microsurgical** *adj*.

microvascular *adj* capillary vessels which are too small to be seen by the naked eye.

microvascular surgery surgery carried out on blood vessels using a binocular operating microscope.

microvilli *npl* microscopic projections from the free surface of cell membranes whose purpose is to increase the exposed surface of the cell for absorption, e.g. cells of proximal convoluted tubules, intestinal epithelium.

micturating cystogram after intravenous injection of a contrast medium (or, more commonly, after contrast is introduced via a urinary catheter until micturating begins), sequential X-rays are taken during the act of passing urine. Can be part of an investigation into urinary incontinence.

micturition *n* (*syn* urination) the act of passing urine.

midbrain part of the brainstem between the diencephalon and pons varolii.

middle ear (tympanum) an air-containing cavity bounded by the tympanic membrane on the outer side and the internal ear (cochlea) on the inner side. ⇒ ear. ⇒ glue ear. ⇒ grommet.

midriff *n* the diaphragm.

midwife *n* (mid=with; wife=woman) a person, usually a woman, who has undergone specific role preparation and who attends an expectant mother in childbirth; she also teaches and supports women during pregnancy and after the birth. In the UK, a person professionally qualified and registered with the regulatory body. They take responsibility for the conduct and supervision of normal pregnancy, labour and puerperium. Midwives work within the community, in hospital and as independent practitioners.

migraine *n* characterized by severe periodic localized (typically unilateral) headaches, which are often associated with vomiting and visual and sensory disturbances (the aura) and other neurological manifestations. It is caused by reduced cerebral blood flow and changes in the extracranial arteries that appear to be linked to changes in the amount of 5-hydroxytryptamine in the blood. Migraine attacks may be triggered by bright lights, stress, certain foods (cheese and chocolate), alcohol, hormonal changes during the menstrual cycle and some people have migraines at the weekends — **migrainous** *adj*.

milestone *n* a developmental 'norm' against which the physical, social and psychological development of an individual child is assessed. Used especially by health visitors, paediatric nurses in hospitals and the community, and school nurses.

milia *npl* small white cysts of the epidermis of the face and neck. Result from obstruction of a sebaceous gland duct. May be associated with seborrhoea. *milia neonatorum* those occurring in the newborn. They disappear within a few weeks as the top layers of skin are shed and replaced.

miliaria *n* prickly heat common in hot climates, and affects waistline, cubital fossae and chest. Vesicular and erythematous eruption, caused by blocking of sweat ducts and their subsequent rupture, or their infection by fungi or bacteria.

miliary *adj* resembling a millet seed. *miliary tuberculosis* ⇒ tuberculosis.

milieu the environment or setting. *milieu interieur* the physical and chemical environment experienced by individual cells, e.g. the pH of the fluid surrounding the cells. ⇒ homeostasis.

milk *n* secretion of the mammary glands. Provided that the mother is taking an adequate diet, human milk contains all the essential nutrients required by the newborn in the correct proportions. It contains IgA and lactoferrin which increases the newborn infant's resistance to infection. Cow's milk is not recommended as a main drink for infants under one year of age. *milk sugar* lactose.

Miller-Abbot tube a double lumen tube used for intestinal suction. The second channel leads to a balloon near the tip of the tube. This balloon is inflated when the tube reaches the duodenum and it is then carried down the intestine by peristaltic activity.

milligram (mg) one thousandth part of a gram.

millilitre (mL) one thousandth part of a litre. Equal to a cubic centimetre.

millimetre (mm) one thousandth part of a metre.

millimole (mmol) one thousandth part of a mole.

millisecond (ms) one thousandth part of a second.

Milwaukee brace a body splint which is worn at all times during the treatment period for correction of spinal curvature (scoliosis). It applies fixed traction between the occiput and the pelvis.

mineralocorticoids *npl* a group of steroid hormones secreted by the adrenal cortex, the most important being aldosterone. They regulate electrolyte and water balance by causing the renal tubules to reabsorb more sodium and water. ⇒ angiotensin. ⇒ renin.

minerals *npl* inorganic elements that play a vital role in body structure and functions. They are: calcium, chloride, iron, magnesium, phosphorus, potassium, sodium and zinc, and the trace elements: cobalt, chromium, copper, fluoride, iodine, manganese, molybdenum and selenium.

miner's anaemia hookworm disease. ⇒ ancylostomiasis.

minimally invasive surgery minimal access surgery. Techniques that utilize tiny incisions and endoscopic equipment to perform a variety of surgical procedures, such as cholecystectomy. ⇒ laparoscopy.

minute volume *n* ⇒ pulmonary ventilation.

miosis (myosis) *n* constriction of the pupil of the eye.

miotic (myotic) *adj* pertaining to or producing miosis (pupil constriction); usually refers to a drug, e.g. pilocarpine, used in the treatment of glaucoma.

miscarriage *n* spontaneous loss of pregnancy during the first or second trimester. ⇒ abortion.

missed abortion ⇒ abortion.

Misuse of Drugs Act (1971, Regulations 1985) in the UK. Controls the possession, supply, storage, prescription and administration of certain groups of habit-forming drugs that are liable to misuse. They are available to the public by medical prescription only; heavy penalties may follow any illegal possession or supply. The substances are known as controlled drugs and include the opioids, synthetic narcotics, cocaine, hallucinogens and barbiturates (with exceptions). They include: morphine, diamorphine, methadone, pethidine etc.

mitochondrion *n* membrane-bound subcellular organelles situated in the cytoplasm. They are the principal sites of ATP production from the oxidation of fuel molecules. They contain nucleic acids (DNA and RNA) and ribosomes, replicate independently, and synthesize some of their own proteins. They are particularly numerous in metabolically active cells, such as liver and muscle — **mitochondria** *pl.*

mitosis *n* the process of nuclear division (usually followed by cytokinesis) whereby somatic cells replicate themselves. It is preceded by the precise replication of chromosomes and results in two genetically identical 'daughter' cells that retain the diploid chromosome number (46). ⇒ meiosis — **mitotic** *adj.*

mitral *adj* mitre-shaped, as the valve between the left atrium and ventricle of the heart (bicuspid valve). *mitral incompetence* a defect in the closure of the mitral valve whereby blood tends to flow backwards into the left atrium from the left ventricle. *mitral stenosis* narrowing of the mitral orifice, usually due to rheumatic fever. *mitral valvulotomy (valvotomy)* an operation for splitting the cusps of a stenosed mitral valve.

mittelschmerz middle pain. Abdominal pain midway between menstrual periods, at time of ovulation.

mixed venous oxygen saturation *n* measured with a fibreoptic pulmonary artery catheter and shows the relationship between cardiac output, oxygen delivery and oxygen consumption. The normal is 73% and abnormal values can inform treatment and diagnosis.

MLNS *abbr* mucocutaneous lymph node syndrome.

MMR vaccine *abbr* measles, mumps and rubella vaccine. An injectable vaccine offered to children aged 12–15 months.

MMV *abbr* mandatory minute volume.

mnemonic a memory aid that helps an individual to remember information through a variety of cues.

mobility *n* in a nursing context, refers to a person's ability to walk, rise from and return to a bed, chair, lavatory and so on, as well as movements of the upper limbs. It is included in an assessment of a patient's activities of living in order to plan individualized nursing care.

mobilizations, mobilisations manual manipulations of spinal and peripheral (limb) joints to free them to move more normally. Physiotherapists use several methods named for their developers, e.g. Maitland mobilizations and Cyriax mobilizations. See Box – Spinal and peripheral joint mobilization (mobilisation).

mobilize, mobilise make ready for movement. *mobilize a person* locomotion. *mobilize joints and soft tissues* free them to move more normally.

mode the most common (frequent) value in a series of scores. ⇒ central tendency statistic.

modelling in psychology, the way we learn from watching and copying the behaviour of others.

modem *abbr* for MOdulator/DEModulator. A peripheral device used to transmit data from one computer to another via the telephone system.

MODS *abbr* multiple organ dysfunction syndrome.

moist wound healing achieved by application of an occlusive, semipermeable dressing which permits the exudate to collect under the film to carry out its bactericidal functions. ⇒ wound dressings.

molality the concentration of a solution expressed as the number of moles of solute (substance) per kilogram of solvent.

Spinal and peripheral joint mobilization (mobilisation)

Mobilization (mobilisation) of joints is an art that stretches back to prehistoric times and has been developed during the 20th century. Osteopathy was founded by Still of Kirksville, Missouri and chiropractic by Palmer of Ohio. Development of physiotherapeutic mobilization (mobilisation) of peripheral and spinal joints owes a great deal to British physicians like Mennell and Cyriax in the first half of the 20th century and physiotherapists like Grieve and Maitland during the second half. David Butler, Gwen Jull and Louis Gifford are among the influential leaders of the modern movement in physiotherapeutic mobilizations (mobilisations). Whereas osteopaths and chiropractors mobilize (mobilise) joints in order to restore function, physiotherapists also mobilize (mobilise) nerves, muscles and other soft tissues in order to relieve pain and restore freedom of movement.

molar describes a solution containing one mole of solute (substance) per litre of solution.

molar teeth the teeth 4th and 5th in the deciduous dentition (teeth) and 6th, 7th and 8th in the permanent dentition (teeth), used for grinding food.

molarity the concentration of a solution expressed as the number of moles of solute (substance) per litre of solution (mol/L).

mole (mol) *n* **1.** a measurement of amount of substance. One of the seven base units of the International System of Units (SI). One mole of any substance will contain the same number of particles (atoms or molecules): 6.02×10^{23} (also known as Avogadro's number). **2.** a pigmented area on the skin, usually brown. Some moles are flat, some are raised and occasionally have hairs growing from them. Malignant changes can occur in them, characterized by changes in colour, size and shape. ⇒ naevus.

molecule *n* a combination of two or more atoms from the same or different elements, joined by a chemical bond — **molecular** *adj* pertaining to molecules. *molecular weight* the total of the atomic weights of atoms in a molecule. ⇒ mole.

mollities *n* softness.

molluscum *n* a soft tumour. *molluscum contagiosum* an infectious condition common in infants caused by a virus. Tiny translucent papules with a central depression are formed.

monarticular *adj* relating to one joint.

Mönckeberg's sclerosis sclerosis of the muscle layer (tunica media) with calcium deposition in medium-sized arteries. It gives rise to the 'pipe-stem' arteries of old age.

monetarism a financial policy that prevailed in the early 1980s where the government tried to prevent inflation by controlling the rate of growth of the money supply. The economy was 'squeezed' to control the amount of money and credit generated in the economy.

Monilia *n* ⇒ Candida.

moniliasis *n* ⇒ candidiasis.

Monitor *n* an anglicized version of the US Rush Medicus quality assurance programme for use in hospitals. ⇒ quality assurance.

monitoring *n* sequential recording. Term is also used to describe the automatic visual display of such measurements as temperature, pulse, respiration and blood pressure.

monoamine *n* organic molecules containing one amine (NH_2), such as dopamine. ⇒ amines.

monoamine oxidase an enzyme which causes the breakdown of monoamines, such as 5-hydroxytryptamine (serotonin), dopamine and noradrenaline (norepinephrine) in the brain. *monoamine oxidase inhibitors (MAOIs)* drugs which inhibit this enzyme action are used as antidepressants, e.g. phenelzine. They were largely superseded by other antidepressants with fewer side-effects and greater clinical efficacy, but newer selective MAOIs, such as moclobemide, act more rapidly. ⇒ selective serotonin re-uptake inhibitors. ⇒ tricyclic antidepressants. Patients receiving MAOIs should avoid certain drugs e.g. adrenaline (epinephrine), noradrenaline (norepinephrine), pethidine and amfetamine (amphetamine), and alcohol. Foods containing tyramine (monoamine precursor), e.g. cheese, broad beans and yeast extract, are avoided to prevent the build-up of substances normally broken down by monoamine oxidase, leading to serious hypertensive crisis. Selective MAOIs are also used in the management of parkinsonism.

monoclonal *adj* derived from a single cell. *monoclonal antibodies* are produced by a single cell, and on cell division its clones continue to make the single identical antibody. Widely used for production of highly specific antibodies for research, diagnostic and therapeutic uses.

monocular *adj* pertaining to one eye.

monocyte *n* a large phagocytic white blood cell. Moves into the tissues to become a macrophage. Part of the monocyte-macrophage system (reticuloendothelial) — **monocytic** *adj*.

monocyte-macrophage system *n* a widely scattered system of specialized phagocytic cells in the liver, lymph nodes, spleen, bone marrow and other tissues. They break down blood cells and haemoglobin, forming bile pigment, dispose of cell breakdown products and have an important defensive role against infection. Also known as the reticuloendothelial system.

monomania *n* obsession with a single idea.

mononuclear *adj* with a single nucleus.

mononucleosis *n* an increase in the number of circulating monocytes (mononuclear cells) in the blood. ⇒ infectious mononucleosis.

monoplegia *n* paralysis of only one limb — **monoplegic** *adj*.

monorchid, monorchis having only one testis.

monosaccharide *n* a simple sugar carbohydrate with the general formula CH_2O. The basic unit from which other carbohydrates are formed. Examples are glucose, fructose and galactose (the 6-carbon sugars or hexoses), and ribose and deoxyribose (5-carbon sugars or pentoses). ⇒ disaccharides. ⇒ polysaccharides.

monosodium glutamate a chemical which can be added to food as a flavour enhancer. Often found in Chinese cooking and in many prepared meals.

monosomy *n* state resulting from the absence of a chromosome from an otherwise diploid chromosome complement (45 rather than 46), such as Turner's syndrome.

monounsaturated fatty acid describes a fatty acid with one double bond. ⇒ polyunsaturated fatty acid. ⇒ saturated fatty acid.

monovular *adj* ⇒ uniovular.

monozygotic pertaining to a single zygote. Describes twins arising from one zygote which splits into two identical embryos. ⇒ dizygotic.

mons veneris the eminence formed by the pad of fat which lies over the pubic bone in the female and covered by pubic hair after puberty.

Montgomery's glands *n* sebaceous glands of the breast areola. They enlarge during pregnancy and lactation.

mood *n* an involuntary state of mind or feeling. Variations in mood are normal, but frequent swings from depression to over-excitement may be considered abnormal. ⇒ cyclothymia. ⇒ depression. ⇒ mania.

moon face *n* a rounded face characteristic of Cushing's disease or syndrome.

Mooren's ulcer a gutter-like excoriation of the peripheral cornea with a tendency to spread.

morbidity *n* the state of being diseased. *standardized morbidity ratio (SMBR)* the amount of self-reported limiting long-term illness indirectly standardized for variations in age and sex.

morbilli *n* ⇒ measles.

morbilliform *adj* describes a rash resembling that of measles.

moribund *adj* in a dying state.

morning dip *n* an early morning decline in respiratory function, especially peak expiratory flow, seen in some types of asthma.

Moro reflex (startle reflex) a reflex normally present in the newborn. On being startled, the baby throws out its arms, then brings them together in an embracing movement. An asymmetrical response may indicate nerve damage or a fracture of the arm or clavicle. (See Figure 41).

morphoea ⇒ scleroderma.

morphology *n* the science which deals with the form and structure of living things - **morphologically** *adv*.

mortality *n* being mortal and subject to death. *death rate* the annual death rate is expressed as the number of deaths × 1000 and divided by the mid-year population. Specialized mortality rates and ratios include: *childhood mortality* the number of deaths in children aged 1–14 years in a defined area per 100 000 resident children of that age. *infant mortality* the number of infant deaths in the first year of life per 1000 related live births. *maternal mortality* the number of women who die from causes associated with pregnancy and childbirth per 1000 total births, *neonatal mortality* the number of deaths in the first four weeks of life per 1000 related live births. *perinatal mortality* the number of stillbirths plus deaths in the first week of life per 1000 total births. *postneonatal mortality* the number of deaths in infants aged from twenty eight days to one year per 1000 live births. *standardized mortality rate* number of deaths per 1000 population standardized

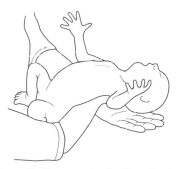

Figure 41 Moro or startle reflex. (Reproduced from Brooker 1996 with permission.)

for age. *standardized mortality ratio (SMR)* allows comparisons to be made between the death rates in populations with different sex and age structures. It involves the application of national age-specific mortality rates to local populations so that a ratio of expected deaths to actual deaths can be calculated. The figure obtained is multiplied by 100 to give the local SMR. The comparative national figure is, by convention, 100 and, for example, a local figure of 108 means there is an increased risk of 8% and, conversely, a local figure of 92 indicates a risk 8% lower. *stillbirth rate* the number of stillbirths per 1000 total births to women in that area.

mortification *n* death of tissue. ⇒ gangrene. ⇒ necrosis.

Morton's metatarsalgia ⇒ metatarsalgia.

morula *n* a pre-embryonic stage prior to implantation. The zygote formed from the fertilized ovum divides by mitosis (cleavage) to produce a mass of cells termed the morula.

mosquito-transmitted haemorrhagic fevers infections which occur mainly in a tropical climate: they include: chikungunya, dengue, Rift valley fever and yellow fever.

motile *adj* capable of spontaneous movement — **motility** *n.*

motion *n* an evacuation of the bowel. *motion sickness* nausea and vomiting associated with the motion of a car, plane or ship.

motivate *v* provision of an incentive or purpose for ensuing action.

motive *n* that which induces a person to act, examples being circumstance, desire, fear.

motor *adj* pertaining to action or movement. *motor end plate* communication between the axon terminal and muscle fibre. ⇒ neuromuscular junction. *motor unit* a group of muscle fibres innervated by a particular lower motor neuron axon. ⇒ neuron(e).

motor neuron disease a progressive degenerative disease of unknown origin that affects the motor neurons in the spinal cord, brainstem and cortex. It occurs in middle age, usually after 50 years of age, and results in increasing muscle weakness and wasting, leading to dys-phagia, dysarthria and immobility. Death usually occurs within 3–5 years from respiratory failure or infection, or problems associated with dysphagia and immobility.

mould *n* a multicellular fungus. Often used synonymously with fungus (excluding the yeasts). A member of the plant kingdom with no differentation into root, stem or leaf, and without chlorophyll. Structurally it consists of filaments or hyphae,which aggregate into a mycelium. Propagation is by means of spores. Occurs in infinite variety, as common saprophytes contaminating foodstuffs, and more rarely as pathogens.

moulding *n* the change in size and/or shape of the fetal head as it is forced through the pelvis during labour. The skull bones may overlap at the fibrous sutures.

mountain sickness symptoms of sickness, tachycardia, rapid respiration and headache caused by the reduced partial pressure of oxygen at high altitude. It occurs prior to physiological acclimatization to increased altitude.

mourning response that assists the individual to adjust to a loss. ⇒ bereavement. ⇒ grieving process.

mouth *n* a cavity bounded by the closed lips and facial muscles, the hard and soft palate, and lower jaw. It contains the teeth and the tongue and receives saliva. ⇒ salivary glands. *mouth care* (oral hygiene) the measures taken to keep the mouth clean and healthy. They include: assessment, adequate hydration, especially oral fluids, cleaning the teeth and oral surfaces, lip creams and mouth washes.

MRI *abbr* magnetic resonance imaging.

MRSA *abbr* methicillin-resistant *Staphylococcus aureus*.

MS *abbr* ⇒ multiple sclerosis.

MSH *abbr* melanocyte stimulating hormone.

MSP *abbr* Munchausen syndrome by proxy.

mucilage *n* the solution of a gum in water — **mucilaginous** *adj.*

mucin *n* a glycoprotein, found in mucus. It is present in mucus-secreting glands — **mucinous** *adj.*

mucinase *n* a specific mucin-dissolving substance contained in some aerosols. Useful in cystic fibrosis.

mucinolysis *n* dissolution of mucin — **mucinolytic** *adj.*

mucocele *n* distension of a cavity with mucus, such as the gallbladder.

mucociliary *adj* pertaining to the clearance of mucus and debris, by the ciliated mucosa, from the respiratory tract. The adequacy of mucociliary clearance by the nose can be investigated by: (a) the saccharin test – a small piece of saccharin is sited on the inferior turbinate bone and the time taken for the person to taste the saccharin is noted. If function is normal the cilia should take about 10–20 min to move the saccharin into the pharynx, where it is tasted; (b) a biopsy of the nasal mucosa is examined microscopically. ⇒ Kartagener's syndrome. ⇒ Young's syndrome.

mucocutaneous *adj* pertaining to mucous membrane and skin. *mucocutaneous lymph node syndrome* (MLNS) a disease affecting mainly babies and children, first noticed in Japan in the late 1960s. Characterized by fever, dry lips, red mouth and strawberry-like tongue. A rash in a glove-and-stocking distribution (i.e. on hands and legs) is followed by desquamation. There is cervical lymphadenopathy, polymorphonuclear leucocytosis and a raised ESR. Also called Kawasaki disease.

mucoid *adj* resembling mucus.

mucolytics *npl* drugs which reduce viscosity of secretion from the respiratory tract, e.g. acetylcysteine, used in the management of cystic fibrosis.

mucopolysaccharide a group of complex connective tissue polysaccharides. → mucopolysaccharidoses.

mucopolysaccharidoses *npl* a group of inherited neurometabolic conditions in which genetically determined specific enzyme defects lead to accumulation of abnormal amounts of mucopolysaccharides. ⇒ gargoylism. ⇒ Hunter's syndrome. ⇒ Hurler's syndrome.

mucoprotein *n* ⇒ glycoprotein.

mucopurulent *adj* containing mucus and pus.

mucosa *n* a mucous membrane — **mucosal** *adj*.

mucositis *n* inflammation of a mucous membrane, such as the lining of the mouth and throat.

mucous *adj* pertaining to or containing mucus. *mucous membrane* ⇒ membrane.

mucoviscidosis *n* ⇒ cystic fibrosis.

mucus *n* the viscid fluid secreted by mucous glands — **mucous, mucoid** *adj*.

mullerian ducts *npl* primitive embryonic ducts which give rise to the internal genitalia in a genetically female embryo. ⇒ wolffian ducts.

multicellular *adj* constructed of many cells.

multidisciplinary team within the healthcare system, a varying number of professionals are working towards the same objective – optimal independence of the patient/client, according to his or her circumstances and available resources.

multigravida *n* a woman who has had more than one pregnancy — **multigravidae** *pl*.

multi-infarct dementia *n* dementia caused by several ischaemic events that produce a build-up of cerebral infarcts.

multilobular *adj* possessing many lobes.

multilocular *adj* possessing many small cysts, loculi or pockets.

multinuclear *adj* possessing many nuclei, such as skeletal muscle cells — **multinucleate** *adj*.

multipara *n* a woman who has had more than one birth — **multiparae** *pl*.

multiple myeloma *n* myelomatosis. A malignant disease affecting plasma cells (derived from B lymphocytes) in which an abnormal immunoglobulin is produced. There is infiltration of the bone marrow with plasma cells, leading to anaemia, leucopenia and thrombocytopenia with bone pain and hypercalcaemia. Treatment includes chemotherapy, radiotherapy and supportive measures. ⇒ Bence-Jones protein.

multiple organ dysfunction syndrome (MODS) *n* describes a situation where the functions of interdependent organ systems, such as the kidneys, respiratory system, coagulation and gastrointesinal tract, are so compromised as to lead to metabolic derangement. It requires organ support, e.g. haemofiltration and mechanical ventilation. ⇒ acute respiratory distress syndrome. ⇒ disseminated intravascular coagulation. ⇒ renal failure. ⇒ tubular necrosis. See Box – Systemic inflammatory response syndrome/multiple organ dysfunction syndrome.

multiple sclerosis (MS) a condition of unknown aetiology where there is demyelination in the central nervous system. The clinical presentation depends on the site and the extent of lesions but includes: weakness or loss of control in a limb, muscle pain, extreme tiredness, ataxia, urinary symptoms including incontinence, sensory problems and visual defects, such as diplopia. A characteristic of the disease is its tendency to relapse and remit. The management includes: corticosteroids, interferon-β and symptomatic relief, e.g. drugs to reduce muscle spasm. Previously known as disseminated sclerosis.

multivariate statistics analysis of three or more variables at the same time. Used to elucidate the association of two variables after allowing for other variables.

mumps *n* (*syn* infectious parotitis) an acute, specific inflammation of the parotid glands, caused by a paramyxovirus. It is spread by droplets and mainly affects children and young adults. The incubation period is around 18 days. It is characterized by fever, malaise, swelling of the parotid salivary glands and pain. It can be complicated by orchitis, oophoritis, pancreatitis and meningitis. Active immunization is offered as part of the routine programme, in conjunction with protection against measles and rubella (MMR).

Munchausen syndrome patients consistently produce false stories so they receive needless medical investigations, operations and treatments. *Munchausen*

syndrome by proxy (MSP) is the term used when a parent, usually the mother, or both parents, or other carers produce false stories for the child and falsify signs and symptoms. See Box – Munchausen syndrome by proxy.

mural *adj* pertaining to the wall of a cavity, organ or vessel.

murmur *n* (*syn* bruit) abnormal sound heard on auscultation of heart or great vessels. *presystolic murmur* characteristic of mitral stenosis in regular rhythm.

Musca *n* genus of the common house-fly, capable of transmitting many enteric infections.

muscarinic *adj* describes a type of cholinergic receptor where muscarine would, if present, bind instead of the neurotransmitter acetylcholine. ⇒ nicotinic.

muscarinic agonist *n* drugs that mimic or stimulate parasympathetic activity, e.g. pilocarpine, used in glaucoma. They are structurally related to the neurotransmitter acetylcholine.

muscarinic antagonists (antimuscarinic drugs) *npl* drugs that inhibit cholinergic nerve transmission by preventing acetylcholine acting at the muscarinic receptors, e.g. atropine, hyoscine, ipratropium bromide etc. Their uses include: inhibition of bronchial secretions, treatment of bradycardia, dilatation of the pupil, relieving bronchospasm, motion sickness etc.

muscle *n* one of four basic body tissues. Specialized contractile tissue formed from excitable cells. There are three types: (a) skeletal muscle that is voluntary, striated

---

Munchausen syndrome by proxy

Munchausen syndrome by proxy (MSP) was first described by Sir Roy Meadow in 1977. He recognized this potentially fatal form of child abuse in which carers feign or create illnesses in children and, as a result, subject them to extensive and unnecessary medical investigation and treatment.

MSP usually meets 4 criteria:
- The child's illness has been fabricated by the parent;
- The child is persistently presented for medical care which results in multiple investigative procedures;
- The perpetrator denies the cause of the child's illness;

- The acute features of the child's illness are not present in the absence of the perpetrator.

Nurses are in a good position to observe family relationships and the care of the child, and careful record keeping is vital in any suspected case of MSP. Covert videoing has been used to observe parents in hospital but this method of observation has raised concerns about invasion of privacy, breach of trust and possible compromise of the role of the health professionals involved.

Further reading
Crouse K 1992 Munchausen syndrome by proxy: recognizing the victim. Paediatric Nursing. 18 (3) 349–352.

and innervated by the peripheral nerves; (b) smooth or involuntary muscle that is nonstriated. It is visceral and innervated by autonomic nerves; (c) cardiac muscle makes up the middle layer of the heart and has features of both striated and smooth muscle. It is innervated by autonomic nerves. ⇒ myocardium — **muscular** *adj*.

muscular dystrophies a group of genetically transmitted diseases; they are all characterized by progressive atrophy of different groups of muscles with loss of strength and increasing disability and deformity. Pseudohypertrophic or Duchenne type is the most severe. Presents in early childhood. ⇒ Duchenne muscular dystrophy.

musculature *n* the muscular system, or any part of it, such as an individual muscle.

musculocutaneous *adj* pertaining to muscle and skin.

musculoskeletal *adj* pertaining to the muscular and skeletal systems. ⇒ skeletomuscular.

music therapy may be used as an aid to socialization and expression or to help people with physical or learning disabilities to keep moving, listening and thinking.

mutagen *n* an agent which induces gene or chromosome mutation.

mutagenesis *n* the production of mutations — **mutagenetically** *adv*.

mutagenicity *n* the capacity to produce gene mutations or chromosome aberrations.

mutant *n* a cell (or individual) which carries a genetic change or mutation.

mutation *n* an alteration in genes or chromosomes of a living cell gives rise to genetic change, as a result of which the characters of the cell alter. The change is heritable. *induced mutation* a gene mutation or change produced by known agents outside the cell that interact with and affect the chromosomal DNA and may alter chromosome structure or number, e.g. ionizing radiation and mutagenic chemicals, ultraviolet radiation, etc. *spontaneous mutation* a genetic mutation taking place without apparent influence from outside the cell.

mute *adj* unable to speak.

mutilation *n* the removal of a limb or other part of the body. It results in a change of body image, to which there has to be considerable physical, psychological and social adjustment for a successful outcome.

mutism *n* (*syn* dumbness) inability or refusal to speak. It may be due to congenital causes, the most common being deafness; it may be the result of physical disease, the most common being a stroke, and it can be a manifestation of some mental health problems.

myalgia *n* pain in the muscles. *epidemic myalgia* ⇒ Bornholm disease — **myalgic** *adj*.

myalgic encephalomyelitis (ME) debilitating illness which is difficult to diagnose and which can last for years. Its many symptoms include malaise, exhaustion, myalgia, inability to concentrate, headache, digestive problems, memory loss and depression. Also called chronic fatigue syndrome or post-viral syndrome. Some affected individuals have serum antibodies to Epstein-Barr or coxsackie-B viruses.

myasthenia *n* muscular weakness. *myasthenia gravis* a disorder characterized by an inability to sustain contraction in striated muscle and extreme fatigue. Autoantibodies block receptor sites in the neuromuscular junctions and prevent the proper functioning of the neurotransmitter acetylcholine. In many cases there is an abnormality of the thymus gland. Patients may present with muscle fatigue especially after strenuous activity, ptosis, muscle weakness affecting the shoulder girdle, problems with speaking, chewing and swallowing and breathing difficulties if the respiratory muscles are affected. The management may include: anticholinesterase drugs, e.g. pyridostigmine, thymectomy, corticosteroids, immunosuppressant drugs, such as azathioprine, and plasma exchange to remove autoantibodies. ⇒ edrophonium test — **myasthenic** *adj* pertaining to myasthenia. *myasthenic crisis* a sudden exacerbation of myasthenia gravis affecting the respiratory muscles. Respiratory support and mechanical ventilation may be required as life saving measures.

mycelium *n* a mass of branching filaments (hyphae) of moulds or fungi, such as can be seen on mouldy food — **mycelial** *adj*.

mycetoma *n* (*syn* madura foot) chronic fungal disease affecting soft tissues and bones of the limbs (usually the foot), but it may occur in other sites. It is caused by several species of Actinomycetes and other fungi. It is characterized by swelling, nodules and sinus formation.

Mycobacterium *n* a genus of Gram-positive acid-fast bacteria. *Mycobacterium avium intracellulare (MAI)* atypical mycobacterium that causes infection in humans. *Mycobacterium bovis* causes tuberculosis in cattle. It can be transmitted to humans. *Mycobacterium kansasii* atypical mycobacterium that causes infection in humans. *Mycobacterium leprae* causes leprosy and *Mycobacterium tuberculosis* causes tuberculosis.

mycologist *n* a person who has expert knowledge of mycology and the methods used to study it.

mycology *n* the study of fungi — **mycologically** *adv*.

mycophyta group (division) of simple organisms. ⇒ fungi.

Mycoplasma *n* a genus of very small micro-organisms. They have features in common with bacteria, but lack a cell wall. Some are parasites, some are saprophytes and others are pathogens, e.g. *Mycoplasma pneumoniae* causes primary atypical pneumonia. It may occur in institutions and mainly affects children and young adults. Treatment is with antibiotics, e.g. tetracycline or erythromycin.

mycosis *n* disease caused by any fungus — **mycotic** *adj*.

mycotoxins *npl* the secondary metabolites of moulds or microfungi. Many chemical substances have been identified as mycotoxins, many capable of causing cancer as well as other diseases — **mycotoxic** *adj*.

mydriasis *n* dilation of the pupil of the eye. Can also relate to an abnormal dilation.

mydriatics *npl* drugs which cause mydriasis (pupil dilatation), e.g. atropine.

myelin *n* the white, fatty insulating material covering some nerve fibres. See Box – Myelin.

myelitis *n* inflammation of the spinal cord.

myeloblasts *npl* early precursor cells of the polymorphonuclear series of granulocytic white blood cells — **myeloblastic** *adj*.

myelocele *n* a spina bifida defect, commonly in the lumbar region, wherein development of the spinal cord itself has been arrested, and the central canal of the cord opens on the skin surface, exposing the meninges and discharging cerebrospinal fluid.

myelocytes *npl* precursor cells of the polymorphonuclear series of granulocytic white blood cells — **myelocytic** *adj*.

myelofibrosis *n* formation of fibrous tissue within the bone marrow cavity. Interferes with the formation of blood cells. A myeloproliferative disorder.

myelogenous *adj* produced in or by the bone marrow.

myelography *n* radiographic examination of the spinal canal by injection of a contrast medium into the subarachnoid space — **myelographically** *adv*.

Myelin

Myelin is a lipid and protein substance which forms in rings round many peripheral and central neurones. It is formed by the Schwann cells in the peripheral nervous system and the oligodendrocytes in the central nervous system. The ring-like structure of myelin arises because the myelin grows in a spiral fashion around the neurones forming a sheath with many hundreds of layers. Neurones with myelin sheaths are said to be myelinated. The purpose of myelin is to insulate the neurones and to speed up the conduction of nerve impulses along the neurones. The myelin covering is not complete and there are gaps along the neurones called the nodes of Ranvier. The nerve impulses are accelerated, compared with unmyelinated neurones because they jump from one node to the next by virtue of the myelin sheath. In a condition known as multiple sclerosis there is deterioration of the myelin sheaths of myelinated neurones (demyelination). This leads to short circuiting of the nerve impulses and they also slow down. This leads to symptoms of weakness, unusual sensations and double vision. The cause of multiple sclerosis is not known but there is evidence for the involvement of a virus.

myeloid *adj* 1. pertaining to the bone marrow. 2. pertaining to the granulocyte precursor cells; myeloblasts and myelocytes in the bone marrow. *myeloid leukaemia* ⇒ leukaemia. 3. pertaining to the spinal cord.

myeloma *n* ⇒ multiple myeloma — **myelomatous** *adj*.

myelomatosis *n* ⇒ multiple myeloma.

myelomeningocele *n* ⇒ meningomyelocele.

myelopathy *n* disease of the spinal cord. Can be a serious complication of cervical spondylosis — **myelopathic** *adj*.

myeloproliferative disorders *npl* any condition (premalignant or malignant) characterized by a proliferation of one or more of the cellular components of the bone marrow. They include: myelosclerosis (myelofibrosis), primary polycythaemia and thrombocythaemia. ⇒ leukaemia. ⇒ polycythaemia.

myelosclerosis ⇒ myelofibrosis.

myocardial infarction death of a part of the myocardium from deprivation of blood following coronary artery occlusion, for example from thrombosis. The patient experiences a 'heart attack' with sudden intense chest pain which may radiate to arms and jaws. Management includes: aspirin, pain relief, antiemetics, fibrinolytic (thrombolytic) therapy, oxygen therapy, bed rest, observations including continous ECG and later mobilization and cardiac rehabilitation. Patients should be nursed in a coronary care unit because of the risk of life threatening arrhythmias and the need for skilled staff to monitor the effects of fibrinolytic therapy. ⇒ angina pectoris. ⇒ cardiac enzymes. ⇒ ischaemic heart disease.

myocarditis *n* inflammation of the myocardium, such as that resulting from viral infections, bacterial toxins, or following rheumatic fever. ⇒ cardiomyopathy.

myocardium *n* the middle layer of the heart wall. Consisting of highly specialized cardiac muscle tissue. ⇒ muscle — **myocardial** *adj*.

myocele *n* protrusion of a muscle through its ruptured sheath.

myoclonus *n* clonic contractions of individual or groups of muscles.

myoelectric *adj* pertaining to the electrical properties of muscle.

myofibril *n* bundle of fibres contained in a muscle fibre. They are formed from filaments of contractile proteins. ⇒ actin. ⇒ myosin. ⇒ tropomyosin. ⇒ troponin.

myofibroblasts *npl* type of fibroblast that contains contractile protein filaments. They are responsible for the wound contraction that decreases wound size during healing.

myofibrosis *n* excessive connective tissue in muscle. Leads to inadequate functioning of part — **myofibroses** *pl*.

myogenic *adj* originating in or starting from muscle.

myoglobin a haem containing protein molecule found in skeletal muscle. It combines with the oxygen released by the red blood cells, stores it and transports it to the muscle cell mitochondria where energy is generated for synthesis and heat production. Also known as myohaemoglobin.

myoglobinuria *n* (*syn* myohaemoglobinuria) excretion of myoglobin in the urine as in the massive muscle damage of the crush syndrome. Leads to renal damage.

myohaemoglobin ⇒ myoglobin.

myohaemoglobinuria ⇒ myoglobinuria.

myokymia *n* muscle twitching. In the lower eyelid it is benign. ⇒ dyskinesia.

myoma *n* any tumour composed of muscle tissue — **myomatous** *pl*.

myomalacia *n* softening of muscle, as occurs in the myocardium after infarction.

myomectomy *n* removal of a myoma. Usually refers to the removal of uterine fibroid(s).

myometrium *n* the thick specialized muscular wall of the uterus.

myoneural *adj* pertaining to muscle and nerve.

myopathy *n* any disease of the muscles — **myopathic** *adj*.

myope *n* a shortsighted person — **myopic** *adj*.

myopia *n* short/near sightedness. The light rays entering the eye are over-refracted and distant objects are focused in front of, instead of on, the retina. It is corrected by use of a divergent biconcave lens. (See Figure 42) – **myopic** *adj*.

Myopia – short sight

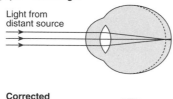

Light from distant source

Corrected

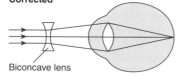

Biconcave lens

Figure 42 Myopia. (Reproduced from Brooker 1998 with permission.)

myoplasty *n* plastic surgery on muscle, in which portions of partly detached muscle are utilized to repair defects or deformities — **myoplastic** *adj*.

myosarcoma *n* a malignant tumour derived from muscle — **myosarcomatous** *adj*.

myosin *n* a contractile protein, one of the component filaments of a muscle myofibril. Reacts with actin during muscle contraction.

myosis *n* ⇒ miosis — **myotic** *adj*.

myositis *n* inflammation of a muscle. *myositis ossificans* a condition where muscle cells are replaced by bone cells.

myotomy *n* cutting or dissection of muscle tissue.

myotonia *n* a condition in which there is prolonged contraction of muscle fibres (tonic spasm of muscle). *myotonia congenita* a rare form of congenital muscular spasticity, usually presenting in infancy. It is characterized by hypertropy and stiffness — **myotonic** *adj*.

myringitis *n* inflammation of the tympanic membrane (ear drum).

myringoplasty *n* operation designed to close a defect in the tympanic membrane — **myringoplastic** *adj*.

myringotomy *n* incision into the tympanic membrane (ear drum). Performed for the drainage of pus or fluid from the middle ear. Middle ear ventilation maintained by insertion of a grommet or Teflon tube.

myxoedema *n* ⇒ hypothyroidism. *myxoedema coma* a rare but serious emergency characterized by altered consciousness and hypothermia, usually in an older person with hypothyroidism. There is a high mortality, and treatment involves the administration of parenteral thyroid hormone and supportive measures. *pretibial myxoedema* pink/purple indurated areas of skin, usually on anterior aspect of the leg and dorsum of the foot. It is a feature of Graves' disease. The skin may be itchy and coarse hair is present — **myxoedematous** *adj*.

myxoma *n* a connective tissue tumour composed largely of mucoid material — **myxomatous** *adj*.

myxosarcoma *n* a malignant myxoma.

myxoviruses *npl* two families of RNA viruses (orthomyxoviruses and paramyxoviruses) that include the influenza viruses, respiratory syncytial virus, measles virus and the mumps virus.

N

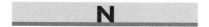

nabothian follicles small cysts arising in the chronically inflamed mucus-secreting glands of the uterine cervix, where the duct of the gland has become obliterated by a healing epithelial covering and the normal mucus cannot escape.

NAD *abbr* nicotinamide adenine dinucleotide.

NADP *abbr* nicotinamide dinucleotide phosphate.

naevoid amentia ⇒ Sturge-Weber syndrome.

naevus *n* a pigmented congenital lesion of the skin. It may arise from the pigment-producing cells (melanocytes) or be due to a developmental abnormality of blood vessels (angioma). Also called a mole or birthmark. ⇒ haemangioma — **naevoid** *adj*.

Nägele's obliquity tilting of the fetal head to one or other side to decrease the transverse diameter presented to the pelvic brim.

NAI *abbr* nonaccidental injury.

nails *npl* keratinized sheets derived from epidermal tissue that covers and protects the dorsal surface of the terminal phalanges, differentially called toe and finger nails. *nail bed* the epidermis underlying a nail. *hang nail* a break in the continuity of cuticle surrounding a nail. *ingrowing toe nail* penetration of the nail edge into soft tissue and can be the site of painful inflammatory reaction and superimposed infection. ⇒ onychocryptosis.

named nurse a concept introduced in the UK in the *Patient's Charter* of 1991, which promised that: 'Each patient will be told the name of the qualified nurse or midwife who will be responsible for his or her nursing/midwifery care when admitted to hospital, or midwife, community nurse or health visitor when in need of care in the community.' One qualified nurse, midwife or health visitor is accountable for the care of each patient or client and, wherever possible, the same nurse should care for, or supervise care for, the same patient during the time that person needs nursing, midwifery or health visiting care. The named nurse concept can be operated within primary nursing, team nursing, or patient allocation model.

nanogram (ng) *n* 10^{-9} of a gram. One thousandth part of a microgram.

nanometre (nm) *n* 10^{-9} of a metre. One thousandth part of a micrometre.

nape *n* the back of the neck, the nucha.

napkin (nappy) rash an erythema of the napkin area. It can vary from a simple erythema on the buttocks and labia/scrotum, to excoriation and maceration of the total napkin area. Usual causes are: ammonia from the decomposition of urine, thrush, infantile psoriasis, allergy to detergents, excoriation from diarrhoea. Secondary infection may occur.

narcissism *n* self-love. In psychiatry, the narcissistic type of personality is one where the sexual love-object is the self.

narcoanalysis *n* a technique used in psychotherapy. After the administration of a narcotic drug to produce a relaxed state, the individual is encouraged to talk freely and, in doing so, repressed thoughts may enter the consciousness — **narcoanalytically** *adv*.

narcolepsy *n* an irresistible tendency to go to sleep. It is more usual to speak of the narcolepsies rather than of narcolepsy, for sudden, repetitive attacks of sleep occurring in the daytime arise in diverse clinical conditions — **narcoleptic** *adj*.

narcosis *n* unconsciousness produced by a drug. *carbon dioxide narcosis* full bounding pulse, muscular twitchings, mental confusion and eventual coma due to increased $PaCO_2$. ⇒ hypercapnia. *continuous narcosis* treatment by prolonged sleep by spaced administration of narcotics.

narcosynthesis *n* the building up of a clearer mental picture of an incident involving the patient by reviving memories of it, after the administration of narcotic drugs, so that both patient and the therapist can examine the incident in clearer perspective.

narcotic *n, adj* describes a drug which produces abnormally deep sleep. Strong analgesic narcotics, e.g. opioids such as morphine, may cause profound respiratory depression which is reversible by the use of the narcotic antagonist, naloxone. → hypnotic. ⇒ sedative.

nares *npl* (*syn* choanae) the nostrils. *anterior nares* the pair of openings from the exterior into the nasal cavities. *posterior nares* the pair of openings from the nasal cavities into the nasopharynx — **naris** *sing*.

nasal *adj* pertaining to the nose. *nasal cannula* tube used to administer oxygen via the nose. *nasal cautery* a treatment for epistaxis. When the bleeding point can be seen it is cauterized with silver nitrate or an electrocautery. *nasal conchae* ⇒ turbinate. *nasal packs* a treatment for epistaxis where the bleeding point cannot be visualized or is impossible to reach. The pack may consist of specially produced gauze (bismuth iodoform paraffin paste) or an inflatable balloon.

nasendoscope *n* an endoscope for viewing the nasal passages and postnasal space and larynx.

nasoduodenal *adj* pertaining to the nose and duodenum. *nasoduodenal tube* a fine bore tube passed via the nose into the duodenum for enteral feeding. ⇒ enteral.

nasogastric *adj* pertaining to the nose and stomach. *nasogastric tube* a tube passed via the nose into the stomach, usually for aspirating gastric contents or feeding.

nasojejunal *adj* pertaining to the nose and jejunum, usually referring to a tube passed via the nose into the jejunum for feeding. ⇒ enteral.

nasolacrimal *adj* pertaining to the nose and lacrimal apparatus.

naso-oesophageal *adj* pertaining to the nose and the oesophagus, as passing a tube via this route.

nasopharynx *n* the portion of the pharynx above the soft palate — **nasopharyngeal** *adj*.

National Confidential Enquiries four national enquiries that investigate clinical practice in specific areas: Maternal Deaths, Perioperative Deaths, Stillbirths and Deaths in Infancy, and Suicide and Homicide by People with Mental Illness.

National Framework for Assessing Performance a framework that includes six areas for the assessment of NHS performance: effective delivery of appropriate health care; efficiency; fair access; health improvement; health outcomes and the patient/carer experience. ⇒ Performance Indicators.

National Institute for Clinical Excellence (NICE) a Special Health Authority set up to generate and distribute clinical guidance based on evidence of clinical and cost effectiveness. Functions include: identify health interventions for consideration; gather evidence via systematic approach, and produce protocols for practice (evidence – based). These protocols are disseminated by NICE to appropriate bodies.

National Service Frameworks (NSFs) evidence-based frameworks for major care areas and particular groups of disease, e.g. mental health and CHD, that state what patients/clients can presume to receive from the NHS.

National Survey of Patient and User Experience annual survey to elicit the views of patients on the care offered by the NHS.

National Vocational Qualifications (NVQs)/Scottish Vocational Qualifications (SVQs) *npl* in the UK. Work-based qualifications available in many fields and areas of work, e.g. health care, catering, construction industry etc. Credits are earned from the successful completion of various assessments of skills undertaken in the work setting. NVQs are available at several levels of attainment and are recognized nationally.

natural flora ⇒ normal flora.

natural killer (NK) cells *n* form part of the nonspecific body defences. They are non-phagocytic cells that belong to a group of large granular lymphocytes. NK cells destroy virus-infected cells and cancer cells by chemical lysis. ⇒ interferons.

naturopathy *n* a multidisciplinary approach to health care which includes all aspects of one's lifestyle, based upon the belief in the power of the body to heal itself — **naturopathic** *adj*.

nausea *n* a feeling of impending vomiting. Often accompanied by excess production of watery saliva, pallor and sweating — **nauseous** *adj*.

navel *n* ⇒ umbilicus.

navicular *adj* shaped like a canoe (as in bone of the foot).

nebula *n* a cloud or mist. Term applied to a greyish, corneal opacity.

nebulizer *n* a device that converts a liquid into a fine spray. It can contain medicaments for application to the skin or respiratory tract. Widely used in the treatment of asthma.

NEC *abbr* necrotizing enterocolitis.

Necator *n* a genus of nematode hookworms. ⇒ Ancylostoma.

necropsy *n* the examination of the body after death.

necrosis *n* localized death of tissue — **necrotic** *adj*.

necrotizing enterocolitis (NEC) a condition occurring primarily in preterm or low birthweight neonates. Caused by hypoxia, leading to acute ischaemia of the bowel. Parts of the bowel wall become necrotic with the development of obstruction, gangrene and peritonitis. The condition is especially associated with respiratory distress syndrome and congenital heart defects in low birthweight neonates.

necrotizing fasciitis *n* rare infection caused by some strains of group A *Streptococcus pyogenes*. It leads to very severe inflammation of the muscle sheath and massive soft tissue destruction. Patients may require amputation or radical excision of affected areas. The mortality rate is high.

needle phobia see Box – Needle phobia.

needlestick injury occupational hazard of healthcare workers (clinical and nonclinical staff) where the accidental injury with contaminated needles or other items may infect them with various hepatitis viruses or, more rarely, with HIV. All healthcare settings should have a risk assessment, staff training, and policies and procedures in place for protective clothing, proper disposal of equipment and action to be taken should injury occur. ⇒ accident form. ⇒ inoculation. ⇒ acquired immune deficiency syndrome.

needs *n* ⇒ human needs. ⇒ Maslow's hierarchy of human needs.

needs assessment the various means by which a community is supported and enabled to express their needs. It may take the form of a questionnaire survey, focus groups and interviews (structured and unstructured). ⇒ community development.

negative feedback ⇒ feedback.

negative symptoms of schizophrenia *npl* describes a group of symptoms associated with certain types of schizophrenia. They include: blunted affect, poverty of thought/speech, loss of drive etc. ⇒ alogia. ⇒ anhendonia. ⇒ avolition. ⇒ inattention. ⇒ neuroleptics. ⇒ Positive and Negative Syndrome Scale. ⇒ Schedule for the Assessment of Negative Symptoms.

negativism *n* active refusal to co-operate, usually shown by the patient consistently doing the exact opposite of what he is asked. Common in schizophrenia.

neglect see Box – Neglect. ⇒ abuse.

negligence *n* one form of professional malpractice which includes the omission of acts that a prudent professional nurse would have done or the commission of acts which a prudent professional

---

Needle phobia

Many children and young people who require medical intervention are most concerned about needles. Some of these children will develop an extreme fear or phobia. These children can develop manifestations of neurogenic shock when exposed to needles and this reaction can spread so that the child also fears objects or situations associated with needles. Smalley (1999) believes that there is a need for all children to be prepared effectively for any procedure involving needles to prevent the development of the phobia.

Preparation involves physical and psychological interventions:

- Topical anaesthetic cream can be used to numb the site for most needle procedures. It is most effective when used in conjunction with psychological preparation, as the fright-

ened child's fear will not be allayed merely by numbness of this site;

- Giving information to the child and family about the procedure. The child should be told honestly about the physical and sensory effects of the procedure in an appropriate age-related way;
- Providing a supportive environment by allowing parental presence in child-friendly surroundings with staff who are empathetic;
- Helping the child to cope by using distraction, play therapy, relaxation or guided imagery techniques during the procedure;
- Providing positive reinforcement to the child after the procedure with the use of bravery certificates or stickers, as well as verbal encouragement of their coping skills.

Further reading
Smalley A 1999 Needle Phobia. Paediatric Nursing 11 (3) 17–20.

Neglect

The persistent or severe neglect of a child or the failure to protect a child from exposure to any kind of danger including cold and starvation, or extreme failure to carry out important aspects of care resulting in the significant impairment of the child's health or development including non-organic failure to thrive (DoH 1999). Approximately 25% of children on child protection registers in the UK are registered under this category of child abuse.

Neglect is often caused by ignorance of child care and early education of caregivers about chil-

dren's fundamental physical and emotional needs can help to prevent this abuse. Nurses can help to identify problems by a thorough nursing assessment which includes finding out about children's usual routines and activities. Manifestations of neglect include physical and behavioural signs such as malnutrition, poor personal hygienic, inactivity and passivity.

Reference
Department of Health 1999 Working Together: A guide to interagency co-operation for the protection of children from abuse. The Stationery Office, London

nurse would not do. It can become the basis of litigation for damages. ⇒ Bolam test. ⇒ duty of care. See Box – Negligence.

Neisseria *n* a genus of bacteria. Gram-negative cocci, usually arranged in pairs, which are found as commensals of humans and animals, e.g. *Neisseria catarrhalis*, or pathogens to humans. *Neisseria gonorrhoeae* causes gonorrhoea and *Neisseria meningitidis* causes meningitis.

Nelaton's line an imaginary line joining the anterior superior iliac spine to the ischial tuberosity. The great trochanter of the femur normally lies on or below this line.

Nelson's syndrome the syndrome linked with a pituitary tumour, hypersecretion of adrenocorticotrophic hormone and skin pigmentation. It can occur in patients with Cushing's disease who are treated by bilateral adrenalectomy. The problem is avoided by irradiating the pituitary in addition to adrenal surgery.

Negligence

Negligence is used to describe an action which is careless and can be an element in a criminal act or the basis of a civil action. Gross negligence which results in the death of a person can be the basis of a charge of manslaughter (qv murder).

As an action brought in the civil courts for compensation, negligence forms one of a group of civil wrongs known as 'torts'. To succeed in an action for negligence, the claimant must establish that a duty of care was owed to him or her by the defendant or the defendant's employees; that there has been a breach of this duty of care and as a reasonably foreseeable consequence of this breach of duty the claimant has suffered harm. A duty of care exists in law where it can be reasonably foreseen that unless reasonable care is taken, harm could occur. Thus a nurse has a duty of care to her patients, a driver has a duty of care to other road users. The law does not require a person voluntarily to assume a duty of care: thus there is no duty in law to go to the assistance of a person involved in a road accident, caused by others. The UKCC does however consider that all its registered practitioners, though not under a legal duty to offer assistance, would have a professional duty under the Code of Professional Conduct. (See Guidelines for Professional Practice UKCC 1995). If a volunteer does assist, then a duty of care is assumed and all reasonable care is required from the volunteer.

The standard of care required by those under a duty of care is to act in accordance with a practice accepted as proper by a responsible body of professionals skilled in that particular art. This standard was laid down in the case of Bolam v. Friern Hospital Management Committee ([1957] 2 All ER 118) and is known as the Bolam Test. Experts are required to give evidence to the court over what would be regarded as the reasonable standard of care in the circumstances of the case and whether what actually took place

was in accordance with that standard. It is accepted that there may exist different bodies of competent professional opinion over what is reasonable practice in the circumstances. (Maynard v. West Midlands RHA [1984] 1 WLR 634) The House of Lords has emphasized that experts must give evidence of opinion which is reasonable, responsible and respectable and has a logical basis. (Bolitho v. City and Hackney HA [1997] 4 All ER 771)

The claimant must show on a balance of probabilities that there has been a failure to provide a reasonable standard of care and that this failure was a reasonably foreseeable cause of the harm which has been suffered. In a case where the casualty officer failed to examine a man suffering with severe vomiting, the widow failed in her claim against the hospital, since the man, who had been poisoned by arsenic, would have died even if he had been properly examined, such was the speed of arsenic poisoning. (Barnett v. Chelsea and Kensington Hospital Management Committee [1968] 1 All ER 1068) The House of Lords ordered a retrial of a case on the issue of causation, where there was clear breach of the duty of care by the Senior Registrar who failed , when asked for his observations, to note that a junior doctor had placed a catheter to monitor oxygen levels in a premature baby, in a vein rather than in an artery. The parents had failed to provide evidence that this failure had caused the retrolental fibroplasia from which the baby suffered. (Wilsher v. Essex Area Health Authority [1988] 1 All ER 871)

The claimant must also establish that he or she has suffered harm to obtain compensation in an action for negligence. This could include personal injury, pain and suffering, loss of amenity, and also loss or damage to property. Where the loss is loss of life, the action can be brought by the personal representatives of the deceased on behalf of the estate, and by dependents upon the deceased.

nematodes *npl* (roundworms) parasitic worms that can be divided into three groups: (a) those that mainly live in the intestine, e.g. *Ascaris lumbricoides* (roundworm), *Enterobius vermicularis* (threadworm), *Ancylostoma duodenale* (hookworm), *Strongyloides stercoralis* and *Trichuris trichiura* (whipworms); (b) those that are mainly tissue parasites, e.g. *Dracunculus medinensis* (guinea worm) and the filarial worms that include *Loa loa* and *Onchocerca volvulus*; (c) those from other species (zoonotic), e.g. *Toxocara canis* and *Trichinella spiralis*.

neoadjuvant therapy chemotherapy given prior to surgery or radiation to reduce the size of the tumour.

neologism *n* a specially coined word, often nonsensical; may express a thought disorder.

neonatal pertaining to the first 28 days of life. The period during which an infant adjusts to an extrauterine environment. It is the most hazardous time for any infant. *neonatal herpes* may be acquired during vaginal delivery where the woman has a primary genital herpes infection and is actively shedding herpes simplex virus type 2 (HSV 2) particles. Delivery in these circumstances should be by caesarean section. It is a devastating illness with a high mortality rate from encephalitis and a high incidence of severe neurological sequelae among survivors. ⇒ mortality. ⇒ neonatal respiratory distress syndrome.

neonatal hearing screening hearing screening can be performed by otoacoustic emission testing (OAE), using a small probe linked to a computer. Where OAE is not available, a less reliable distraction test using simple sounds can be performed in infants.

neonatal intensive care unit (NICU) unit that provides dedicated intensive care for neonates, especially low birthweight and preterm infants. It is staffed by healthcare professionals with the necessary qualifications, skills and experience to meet the highly specialized needs of preterm and seriously ill neonates.

neonatal respiratory distress syndrome (NRDS) due to a failure of secretion of the protein-lipid complex (pulmonary surfactant) by type II pneumocytes. It occurs most frequently in preterm infants

– the more immature the greater the risk of this condition, which may be fatal. The deficiency in surfactant leads to atelectasis and hypoxia, that necessitates assisted ventilation and the intratracheal administration of surfactant in seriously affected infants. Clinical features include severe retraction of the chest wall with every breath, cyanosis, and increased respiratory rate and an expiratory grunt. Formerly called hyaline membrane disease. ⇒ lecithins. ⇒ surfactant.

neonate *n* newborn. An infant during the first 28 days of life. *neonatal mortality* ⇒ mortality. ⇒ neonatal.

neonatology *n* the scientific study of the newborn. The branch of medicine dealing with the newborn.

neonatorum *adj* pertaining to the newborn.

neoplasia *n* literally, the formation of new tissue. By custom refers to the pathological process in tumour formation. Neoplasia is the end of a pathological process that starts with reversible cell changes and progresses through stages where cells become more and more abnormal. The cellular changes may be triggered by: ionizing radiation, viruses, e.g. human papilloma virus, chronic irritation, tobacco smoking and chewing, chemicals, alcohol and drugs etc. ⇒ dysplasia. ⇒ hyperplasia. ⇒ metaplasia — **neoplastic** *adj*.

neoplasm *n* a new growth; a tumour which is either cancerous or noncancerous — **neoplastic** *adj*.

nephralgia *n* pain in the kidney.

nephrectomy *n* surgical removal of a kidney.

nephritis *n* inflammation of the kidney. A general term that covers a diverse group of disorders affecting the kidneys. ⇒ glomerulonephritis. ⇒ glomerulosclerosis. ⇒ nephrotic syndrome. ⇒ renal failure — **nephritic** *adj*.

nephroblastoma *n* Wilms' tumour. A highly malignant kidney tumour arising from embryonic tissue. A common cancer of children, and usually presents during early childhood. Characterized by abdominal enlargement and haematuria. Early diagnosis with surgical treatment, radiotherapy and cytotoxic drugs offers the best chance of cure. Prognosis depends upon the stage of the disease and the child's age at diagnosis.

nephrocalcinosis *n* multiple areas of calcification with deposition of calcium within the renal tubules. It may occur in damaged tissue, such as in chronic pyelonephritis or as a result of renal tubular acidosis, hyperparathyroidism, hypervitaminosis D and malignancy.

nephrocapsulectomy *n* surgical removal of the kidney capsule. Occasionally done for polycystic kidney disease. ⇒ polycystic.

nephrogenic *adj* arising in or produced by the kidney.

nephrography *n* the technique of imaging renal shadow following injection of contrast medium — **nephrographically** *adv.*

nephrolithiasis *n* the presence of stones in the kidney.

nephrolithotomy *n* surgical removal of a stone from the kidney. Now also accomplished by extracorporeal shock-wave lithotripsy (ESWL). ⇒ Dornier lithotriptor. *percutaneous nephrolithotomy* a minimally invasive technique where the kidney pelvis is punctured under X-ray control, and a guide wire inserted through which, using a nephroscope (endoscope), the stone is removed. Hospital stay is substantially reduced.

nephrology *n* special study of the kidneys and the disorders affecting them.

nephroma *n* a renal tumour.

nephron *n* the microscopic functional unit of the kidney. It comprises a glomerulus and renal tubule. The renal tubule is divided into Bowman's capsule, proximal convoluted tubule, loop of Henle, distal convoluted tubules and a collecting duct which drains urine from several nephrons (see Figure 43).

nephropathy *n* kidney disease — **nephropathic** *adj.*

nephropexy *n* operation to fix a movable kidney.

nephroplasty *n* any plastic operation on the kidney, especially for large aberrant renal vessels that are dissected off the urinary tract and the kidney folded laterally upon itself. ⇒ hydronephrosis.

nephropyelolithotomy *n* ⇒ pyelolithotomy.

nephropyeloplasty *n* ⇒ pyeloplasty.

nephropyosis *n* pus formation in the kidney.

nephrosclerosis *n* renal insufficiency from hypertensive vascular disease, developing into a clinical picture identical with that of chronic nephritis. ⇒ renal failure — **nephrosclerotic** *adj.*

nephroscope *n* an endoscope for viewing kidney tissue. It can be designed to create a continuous flow of irrigating fluid and provide an exit for the fluid and accompanying debris — **nephroscopic** *adj.*

nephrosis *n* any degenerative, noninflammatory change in the kidney — **nephrotic** *adj.*

nephrostomy *n* a surgically established fistula from the pelvis of the kidney to the body surface.

nephrotic syndrome characterized by heavy proteinuria, hypoproteinuria and gross generalized oedema, usually with hyperlipaemia. There are minimal histological changes in the kidneys. It may occur in other conditions, such as amyloidosis (amyloid disease) and glomerulosclerosis complicating diabetes mellitus.

nephrotomogram *n* a tomograph of the kidney.

nephrotomy *n* an incision into the kidney substance.

nephrotoxic *adj* any substance which inhibits or prevents the functions of kidney cells, or causes their destruction. Includes certain drugs, e.g. gentamicin, captopril — **nephrotoxin** *n.*

nephroureterectomy *n* removal of the kidney along with a part or the whole of the ureter.

nerve *n* an elongated bundle of fibres which serves for the transmission of impulses between the periphery and the nerve centres. *afferent nerve* conveys impulses from the tissues to the nerve centres; also known as sensory nerves. *efferent nerve* conveys impulses outwards from the brain and spinal cord to muscles and glands; also known as motor nerves. *nerve growth factor (NGF)* a protein vital for the growth of nerves during embryonic growth and its later maintenance. *nerve impulse* ⇒ impulse.

nervous *adj* 1. relating to nerves or nerve tissue. 2. referring to a state of restlessness or timidity. *nervous breakdown* a euphemistic term for mental illness. There is some controversy about an exact meaning for 'mental illness' but it is generally conceded that the psychoses and neuroses

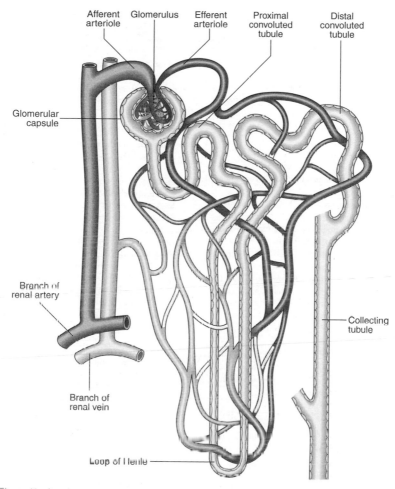

Afferent arteriole
Glomerulus
Efferent arteriole
Proximal convoluted tubule
Distal convoluted tubule
Glomerular capsule
Branch of renal artery
Collecting tubule
Branch of renal vein

Loop of Henle

Figure 43 A nephron.

are included. *nervous system* the structures controlling the actions and functions of the body; it comprises the brain and spinal cord, and the peripheral nerve fibres and ganglia. ⇒ autonomic nervous system. ⇒ central nervous system. ⇒ parasympathetic nervous system. ⇒ peripheral nervous system. ⇒ sympathetic nervous system.

nettlerash *n* ⇒ urticaria.

network *n* connecting computers together to allow sharing of files and resources. ⇒ intranet. ⇒ LAN. ⇒ WAN.

neural *adj* pertaining to nerves. *neural canal* ⇒ vertebral column. *neural tube*

formed from fusion of the neural folds early in embryonic development from which the brain and spinal cord arise. *neural tube defect* any of a group of congenital malformations involving the neural tube, including anencephaly, hydrocephalus and spina bifida. ⇒ folic acid.

neuralgia *n* pain in the distribution of a nerve. ⇒ trigeminal neuralgia — **neuralgic** *adj*.

neurapraxia *n* temporary loss of function in peripheral nerve fibres. Most commonly due to crushing or prolonged pressure. ⇒ axonotmesis.

295

neurasthenia *n* a frequently misused term, the precise meaning of which is an uncommon nervous condition consisting of lassitude, inertia, fatigue and loss of initiative. Restless fidgeting, oversensitivity and undue irritability are also present — **neurasthenic** *adj*.

neurectomy *n* excision of part of a nerve.

neurilemma *n* the thin membranous outer covering of a nerve fibre surrounding the myelin sheath.

neuritis *n* inflammation of a nerve — **neuritic** *adj*.

neuroblast *n* a primitive embryonic nerve cell.

neuroblastoma *n* malignant tumour arising in the adrenal medulla or sympathetic ganglia from embryonic nervous tissue — **neuroblastomatous** *adj*.

neurodermatitis *n* (*syn* lichen simplex) leathery, thickened patches of skin secondary to pruritus and scratching. As the skin thickens, irritation increases, scratching causes further thickening and so a vicious circle is set up. The appearance of the patch develops characteristically as a thickened sheet dissected into small, shiny, flat-topped papules. It may be a manifestation of atopic eczema.

neurofibrillary tangles *npl* common pathological change occurring in the brain of people with Alzheimer's disease. The cytoplasm of the affected neurons is filled with filaments arranged in a paired helical pattern. These abnormal neurons form clusters of tangles.

neurofibroma *n* a tumour arising from the connective tissue of nerves — **neurofibromatous** *adj*.

neurofibromatosis *n* an inherited condition where there are multiple neurofibroma on peripheral and cranial nerves. ⇒ von Recklinghausen's disease.

neurogenic *adj* originating within or forming nervous tissue. *neurogenic bladder* interference with the nerve control of the urinary bladder, such as with multiple sclerosis, diabetes mellitus or following spinal cord injury. It causes either retention of urine, which presents as overflow incontinence, or continuous dribbling without retention. When necessary, the bladder is emptied by exerting manual pressure on the anterior abdominal wall.

neurogenic shock a type of shock caused by the sudden cessation of sympathetic nerve impulses controlling the capacity of the peripheral vascular system. This results in pooling of blood and poor venous return to the heart.

neuroglia *n* (*syn* glia) the supporting tissue of the brain and cord. ⇒ astrocytes. ⇒ ependymal cells. ⇒ microglial cells. ⇒ oligodendrocytes. ⇒ Schwann cells — **neuroglial** *adj*.

neurohypophysis ⇒ pituitary gland.

neuroleptics *npl* (*syn* antipsychotics) drugs acting on the nervous system. They are used in the management of schizophrenia, affective disorders, e.g. depression, and organic psychoses, e.g. in alcohol misuse. Basically they all act as antagonists of dopamine receptors (mainly D_2-receptors) and other receptors, e.g. the 5-HT_2. They can be classified as either typical or atypical neuroleptics. The typical neuroleptics include: the phenothiazines, e.g. chlorpromazine, fluphenazine; the butyrophenones, e.g. haloperidol; the thioxanthines, e.g. flupentixol (flupentixol). Typical neuroleptics, especially the phenothiazines, give rise to extrapyramidal side-effects, e.g. tremor, rigidity etc. ⇒ parkinsonism. ⇒ tardive dyskinesia. Atypical drugs include: the benzamides, e.g. sulpiride; dibenzodiazepines, e.g. clozapine; the diphenylbutylpiperazines, e.g. pimozide. These drugs tend to cause less extrapyramidal effects. Atypical drugs such as risperidone (a benzisoxazole derivative) are effective against both positive (e.g. delusions) and negative (e.g. alogia) symptoms in patients with schizophrenia. *depot neuroleptic* a neuroleptic drug given as a depot injection to a client who is failing to take medication regularly, e.g. fluphenazine and flupentixol (flupenthixol).

neurological *adj* pertaining to neurology. *neurological assessment/observations* used to assess neurological status, for example following head injury or brain surgery. They include colour, respiration, blood pressure, pulse, temperature, level of consciousness, limb movement and pupil size and reaction. ⇒ Glasgow coma scale. *neurological physiotherapy* a clinical specialty in physiotherapy practice. See Box – Neurological physiotherapy.

neurologist *n* a specialist in neurology.

neurology *n* the science and study of the nervous system; structure, function and pathology — **neurological** *adj*.

Neurological physiotherapy
Successful neurological rehabilitation depends on members of multidisciplinary teams recognizing and respecting each other's expertise and the patient's right to determine the most effective way of dealing with his or her disability. Physiotherapists alleviate disorders of movement, posture and balance. Their ability to solve patients' problems depends on extensive knowledge of normal movement and impairments of the central nervous system that cause disturbances of muscle tone, such as spasticity, hypotonicity and rigidity, performance, such as intention tremor and bradykinesia, and equilibrium, which are often more subtle but no less complex. Additionally, they weigh the advantages and disadvantages of different interventions for an individual patient. For example, while a tripod might appear to offer a stroke patient assistance to walk, it might not only prevent recovery of lost function in the hemiplegic side but also increase spasticity. Treatment, therefore, is a balance between re-education of more normal patterns of movement and necessary compensation commensurate with the age and lifestyle of a patient. Neurological rehabilitation is a clinical speciality in physiotherapy and practitioners may subscribe to different approaches to treatment such as the Bobath concept and motor relearning theory.

Further reading
Edwards S 1996 Neurological physiotherapy: A problem-solving approach. Edinburgh: Churchill Livingstone.

---

neuromuscular *adj* pertaining to nerves and muscles. *neuromuscular junction* or motor end plate. The communication of an axon with a muscle fibre. ⇒ synapse.

neuron(e) *n* a nerve cell. Highly differentiated excitable cells capable of transmitting an action potential. The basic units of the nervous system comprising several short branching processes (dendrites) which convey impulses to the nerve cell; the nerve cell body, and a long process or fibre (axon) which conveys impulses from the cell (see Figure 44). Types include Interneuron, motor and sensory. *lower motor neuron* that part of the descending pyramidal motor tract from the anterior horn of the spinal cord to the neuromuscular junction of the voluntary muscle fibre. *upper motor neuron* that part of the descending pyramidal motor tract from the Betz or pyramidal cell in the motor cortex to the anterior horn of the spinal cord. ⇒ motor neuron disease — **neuronal, neural** *adj*.

neuronotmesis *n* ⇒ axonotmesis.

neuropathology *n* a branch of medicine dealing with diseases of the nervous system — **neuropathological** *adj*.

neuropathy *n* any disease of the nervous system — **neuropathic** *adj*.

neuropeptides *npl* a large group of neurotransmitters. They include the endorphins, somatostatin and enkephalins.

neuropharmacology *n* the branch of pharmacology dealing with drugs which affect the nervous system — **neuropharmacological** *adj*.

Myelinated neuron

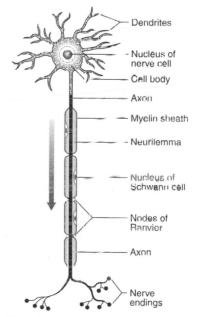

Figure 44 A neuron (arrow shows the direction of impulse transmission)

neuroplasticity *n* the capacity of nerve cells to regenerate.

neuroplasty *n* surgical repair of nerves — **neuroplastic** *adj*.

neuropsychiatry *n* the combination of neurology and psychiatry. Speciality dealing with organic and functional disease — **neuropsychiatric** *adj*.

neurorrhaphy *n* suturing the ends of a divided nerve.

neurosis *n* (*syn* psychoneurosis) a mental health problem where the person retains some insight into their condition and may function normally in some areas of his or her life. A neurosis may be associated with anxiety, stress and interpersonal problems. The symptoms of a neurosis differ from normal experience only in degree, e.g. someone suffering from an anxiety neurosis has symptoms indistinguishable from normal anxiety but out of context, or more severely than the situation warrants. People usually know that their experiences are abnormal, even though they might not be able to do anything about them. Other neuroses include obsessive compulsive disorders (OCD) and phobias. ⇒ psychosis, for comparison — **neurotic** *adj*.

neurosurgery *n* surgery of the nervous system — **neurosurgical** *adj*.

neurosyphilis *n* infection of the central nervous system by *Treponema pallidum*. The variety of clinical pictures produced is large, but the two common syndromes encountered are tabes dorsalis and GPI. The basic pathology is disease of the blood vessels, with later development of pathological changes in the meninges and the underlying nervous tissue. Very often symptoms of the disease do not arise until 20 years or more after the date of primary infection. ⇒ Argyll Robertson pupil. ⇒ Charcot's joints — **neurosyphilitic** *adj*.

neuroticism the emotional instability-stability part of Eysenck Personality Inventory (EPI). The scale has maladjusted, anxious people at the unstable end with well-adjusted individuals at the stable end.

neurotmesis *n* ⇒ axonotmesis.

neurotomy *n* surgical cutting of a nerve.

neurotoxic *adj* toxic or destructive to nervous tissue — **neurotoxin** *n*.

neurotropic *adj* with predilection for the nervous system. *Treponema pallidum* often produces neurosyphilitic complications. Neurotropic viruses (rabies, poliomyelitis, etc) make their major attack on cells of the nervous system.

neutron *n* subatomic particle without an electrical charge.

neutropenia *n* a deficiency of neutrophils in the peripheral blood. See Box – Neutropenia — **neutropenic** *adj*.

neutrophil *n* a phagocytic polymorphonuclear leucocyte (white blood cell) that contains granules. It forms the majority of white cells. ⇒ granulocyte.

newton (N) a derived SI unit (International System of Units) for force.

next friend a person who brings a court action on behalf of a minor.

next of kin an item frequently requested on the document used for recording data collected at the initial assessment of a patient. Great tact is required when acquiring information, as a spouse may be the legal next of kin, but may be estranged from the patient. ⇒ significant other.

NGU *abbr* nongonococcal urethritis.

NHL *abbr* nonHodgkin's lymphoma.

NHS *abbr* National Health Service.

Neutropenia

Neutropenia is a reduction in the number of circulating neutrophils to less than 1×10^9/L (Hawkins 1997). In the patient with cancer the most common cause is bone marrow depression arising from chemotherapy/radiotherapy treatment. Neutrophils are responsible for phagocytosis so the patient with neutropenia is at high risk of potentially fatal overwhelming infection. Patients with a neutrophil count of 0.5×10^9/L or less are nursed in a protective isolation environment until their count recovers. Potential sites of infection include the blood, lungs, urine and the skin, especially when venous access devices are in use. The nursing role in neutropenia is monitoring and prompt treatment of identified infections. Notably, patients who have neutropenia commonly fail to exhibit the signs of infection that present in people with a normal neutrophil count. The inflammatory response is altered so that pus is not produced and redness and inflammation may be absent. Furthermore, the infiltrates associated with pulmonary infection may be absent on radiograph (Hawkins 1997). Typical signs and symptoms of infection in the neutropenic patient include fever, erythema and increased warmth of the skin, cough, dysuria and pain at any site. Febrile patients are treated as if they have an infection until proven otherwise.

Reference
Hawkins R 1997 Patient evaluation. In: Gates R A, and Fink R M (eds) Oncology Nursing Secrets. Hanley and Belfus Inc., Philadelphia, 389–394

NHS Executive that part of the Department of Health that provides policy leadership and several management functions for the NHS.

NHS Guide introduced by the UK Government in 2001, telling the public what they can expect from the NHS. It covers patients' rights and responsibilities, the standards and service that can be expected, accessing advice and treatment and the procedures for voicing concerns or when things go wrong. It replaces the Patient's Charter.

NHS Information strategy a UK NHS white paper published in 1998 which sets out a strategy to utilize information technology in order to increase quality and efficiency. The strategy covers the period 1998–2005. ⇒ informatics.

NHS Trusts *npl* public accountable bodies that provide NHS health care to the population, either as a hospital or community trust.

niacin generic term that includes nicotinamide and nicotinic acid.

NICE *acr* National Institute for Clinical Excellence.

nicotinamide part of the vitamin B complex. It is obtained from food, formed from nicotinic acid or synthesized from the amino acid tryptophan. Required for the coenzymes NAD and NADP involved in glycolysis and oxidative phosphorylation. ⇒ niacin. ⇒ pellagra.

nicotinic *adj* describes a type of cholinergic receptor where nicotine would, if present, bind instead of the neurotransmitter acetylcholine. ⇒ muscarinic.

nicotinic acid part of the vitamin B complex. Has a direct vasodilatory action and is used therapeutically in the treatment of peripheral vascular disease. ⇒ niacin. ⇒ nicotinamide. ⇒ pellagra.

NICU *abbr* neonatal intensive care unit.

nidation *n* implantation of the early embryo in the uterine mucosa.

NIDDM *abbr* noninsulin dependent diabetes mellitus.

nidus *n* the focus of an infection. A septic focus.

Niemann-Pick disease an inherited lipid storage disease where there is an abnormal accumulation of sphingomyelin in the liver, spleen and lymph nodes. It occurs predominantly in Jewish people. The disorder causes an enlarged liver and spleen, lymphadenopathy, anaemia and learning disability. There is no effective treatment and it is usually fatal within a few years of the onset.

night blindness (*syn* nyctalopia) a state that causes vision to be worse at night. May be due to vitamin A deficiency and is a maladaptation of vision to darkness.

night cry a shrill noise, uttered during sleep. May be of significance in hip disease when pain occurs in the relaxed joint.

night sweat profuse sweating, usually during sleep; typical of tuberculosis.

Nightingale ward a rectangular ward housing as many as 36 patients, whose beds are arranged along the walls between the windows.

nihilistic *adj* involving delusions and ideas of unreality; of not existing.

Nikolsky's sign slight pressure on the skin causes 'slipping' of apparently normal epidermis, in the way that a rubber glove can be moved on a wet hand. Characteristic of pemphigus.

nipple *n* the conical eminence in the centre of each breast, containing the outlets of the milk ducts. Stimulation can cause erection of the nipple in both men and women. *inverted nipple* concavity of the nipple which may be a factor in unsuccessful breastfeeding.

NIPPV *abbr* noninvasive positive pressure ventilation.

Nissen's fundoplication *n* ⇒ fundoplication.

nit *n* the egg of the head louse (*Pediculus capitis*). It is firmly cemented to the hair.

nitrates *npl* drugs used as coronary vasodilators in people with angina, e.g. glyceryl trinitrate, isosorbide dinitrate. They provide rapid symptom relief and increase exercise tolerance. They may be given as tablets to be chewed, or dissolved under the tongue (sublingually) or between the gum and top lip, as a sublingual aerosol spray, or transdermally via a gel or skin patch. Sustained release and parenteral preparations are available.

nitric oxide (NO) *n* a naturally occurring chemical neuromodulator, which has different features to neurotransmitters, but similar actions. It is thought to be involved in areas such as learning, memory, nociception, gastric emptying, and penile erection.

In pathological conditions, excess production is involved with hypotension in some types of shock, and, because it also acts as a free radical, it is implicated in the brain tissue damage associated with a stroke. Nitric oxide may be used therapeutically in acute respiratory distress syndrome, and substances that donate nitric oxide are used as vasodilators, such as the organic nitrates, e.g. glyceryl trinitrate.

nitrogen (N) *n* a colourless gaseous element that forms 78–79% of the atmosphere. It is an important constituent of many complements of living cells, e.g. protein and nucleic acids. Atmospheric nitrogen cannot be utilized directly, however, certain bacteria in the soil and roots of legumes are capable of nitrogen fixation. Nitrogen is an essential constituent of protein foods. Nitrogen is excreted mainly as urea in the urine; creatinine and uric acid account for a further small amount. Some nitrogen is excreted via sweat and in faeces. *nitrogen balance* is when a person's daily intake of nitrogen from proteins equals the daily excretion of nitrogen; a positive balance exists where nitrogen intake exceeds the amount excreted and a negative balance occurs when excretion of nitrogen exceeds the daily intake. ⇒ catabolic state. ⇒ hypercatabolic — **nitrogenous** *adj* pertaining to nitrogen. *nitrogenous foods* those containing nitrogen, such as amino acids. *nitrogenous waste* urea, creatinine and uric acid.

nitrous oxide gas used in combination with intravenous agents for induction and maintenance of anaesthesia. ⇒ inhalation anaesthetic.

NK *abbr* natural killer.

NMC *abbr* Nursing and Midwifery Council.

NMET *abbr* Nonmedical Education and Training. ⇒ education consortia.

NMR *abbr* nuclear magnetic resonance.

no fault liability recognition that compensation is payable without the necessity of proving failures in fulfilling the duty of care.

nociceptors *npl* sensory receptors that respond to stimuli that are harmful to tissue and cause pain, such as inflammatory chemicals and trauma.

nocturia *n* the arousal from sleep to pass urine. A feature of increasing age as the kidneys lose their ability to produce concentrated urine.

nocturnal *adj* nightly; during the night. ⇒ enuresis.

node *n* a protuberance or swelling. A constriction. *node of Ranvier* the constriction in the neurilemma of a myelinated nerve fibre. They represent the boundaries between individual Schwann cells and assist in rapid transmission of impulses. ⇒ atrioventricular node. ⇒ Heberden's node. ⇒ sinoatrial node.

nodule *n* a small node — **nodular** *adj*.

noise induced hearing loss occupational deafness. Substantial sensorineural hearing loss caused by occupational noise. The average of pure tone losses measured by audiometry over the 1, 2 and 3 kHz frequencies. Employers are required by law to do proper risk assessment, offer proper protection, offer regular hearing tests as required and endeavour to reduce noise in the workplace. ⇒ health and safety law.

noma ⇒ cancrum oris.

nominal data categorical data where the classes have no particular value or order, such as colours or place names. ⇒ ordinal data.

nomogram graph with several variables used to determine another related variable, e.g. body surface area from height and weight.

nonaccidental injury (NAI) physical maltreatment, usually of children by their parents, other adults and sometimes other children. The injuries cannot be explained by natural disease or simple accident. The lesions are frequently multiple and typically include bruising, shaking injuries, fractures and burns, and involve the head, soft tissues, long bones and the thoracic cage. There may be evidence of neglect and usually there is accompanying psychological damage. ⇒ abuse.

noncompliance *n* a term used to describe a failure by patients to follow the advice of healthcare professionals, in relation to lifestyle changes and taking medication.

nongonococcal urethritis (NGU) (*syn* nonspecific urethritis, NSU) a common sexually transmitted infection. About half the cases are caused by *Chlamydia*; other causatory organisms are *Ureaplasma*, *Trichomonas vaginalis*, *Herpes simplex* and *Mycoplasma genitalium*.

nonHodgkin's lymphoma (NHL) ⇒ lymphoma.

noninsulin dependent diabetes mellitus (NIDDM) ⇒ diabetes mellitus.

noninvasive *adj* describes any diagnostic or therapeutic technique which does not require penetration of the skin or of any cavity or organ.

noninvasive blood pressure *n* the recording of arterial blood pressure using a sphygmomanometer and stethoscope, or an automatic device with a cuff. ⇒ arterial cannula.

noninvasive positive pressure ventilation a mode of mechanical ventilation that uses a nasal or full-face mask rather than an endotracheal or tracheostomy tube.

nonmaleficence ethical principle of doing no harm. ⇒ beneficence.

Nonmedical Education and Training (NMET) budget the budget used for pre and postregistration education and training for health professionals other than doctors and dentists. ⇒ education consortia.

nonmilk extrinsic sugars *npl* extrinsic sugars except milk sugar (lactose).

non-nursing duties duties, such as serving meals or doing clerical, administrative and domestic work, which, it may be argued, detract from direct clinical care and could equally well be done by others. However, there are implications for nursing care with activities perceived to be non-nursing, such as whether the nutritional needs of patients are being met and the adequacy of domestic work in control of infection.

nonparametric tests statistical test that makes no assumption about the distribution of data. See Box – Parametric and nonparametric tests.

nonpolar a molecule that is electrically balanced such as carbon dioxide.

nonprotein nitrogen (NPN) nitrogen derived from all nitrogenous substances other than protein, i.e. urea, uric acid, creatinine, creatine and ammonia.

nonsense syndrome Ganser syndrome.

nonspecific urethritis nongonococcal urethritis.

nonstarch polysaccharides (NSP) *npl* polysaccharides, other than starch, found in plant cell walls. In the diet they provide most of the dietary fibre and the term NSP should now be used in place of 'dietary fibre'. There are many different types of NSP, found in differing amounts in all plant structures – in cell walls and within the cells of roots, leaves, stems, seeds and fruits. NSP may be insoluble, such as the cellulose found in wheat, rice and maize, or soluble pectins and gums found in fruit, vegetables, oats, rye and barley. The NSPs have many functions that include: preventing constipation by adding bulk to faeces, reducing colonic transit time and increasing the frequency of defaecation; they help to prevent sudden increases in blood sugar after meals; some soluble NSPs can help to reduce blood cholesterol levels; they create a feeling of satiety and can be useful in weight reduction. Inadequate dietary intake has been linked with conditions that include: chronic constipation, haemorrhoids, diverticular disease and bowel cancer. The incidence of non-insulin dependent diabetes mellitus is higher where traditional diets are rich in refined, sugary foods (NSP is removed from a carbohydrate food when it is refined). Phytates present in NSPs can prevent the absorption of iron, calcium, copper and zinc. Small children may not receive sufficient energy if energy-containing foods are replaced by foods rich in NSP. ⇒ bran.

nonsteroidal anti-inflammatory drugs (NSAIDs) *npl* large group of drugs with variable anti-inflammatory, analgesic and antipyretic properties, e.g. naproxen. They act by inhibiting enzymes required for prostaglandin and thromboxane synthesis. Some drugs in the group have other properties, such as aspirin which reduces platelet stickiness. NSAIDs are used to treat minor aches and pains, e.g. headache, but are also useful in inflammatory joint diseases such as rheumatoid arthritis. They can produce peptic ulceration with perforation and bleeding from the gastrointestinal tract, headaches, liver and kidney toxicity, bone marrow depression, haemolytic anaemia, and may cause hypersensitivity and may worsen the symptoms of asthma. ⇒ acetic acids. ⇒ fenamates.⇒ oxicams. ⇒ paracetamol. ⇒ propionic acids. ⇒ pyrazolones. ⇒ salicylates.

nonverbal communication ⇒ body language.

noradrenaline (norepinephrine) *n* a catecholamine hormone produced by the adrenal medulla and a neurotransmitter functioning in the sympathetic division of the autonomic nervous system. Its physiological effects include: vasoconstriction and a rise in blood pressure. ⇒ adrenaline (epinephrine). ⇒ catecholamines.

norm *n* a measure of a phenomenon, against which other measures of the phenomenon can be measured, i.e. a standard against which values are measured.

normal distribution curve in statistics. When scores are plotted they form a bell-shaped curve that is symmetrical and has the mean, median and mode in the centre. ⇒ skewed distribution.

normal flora *n* the micro-organisms that normally colonize various parts of the body, e.g. *Escherichia coli, Staphylococcus epidermidis*. They are in most instances nonpathogenic, but in particular circumstances can become pathogenic.

normal saline ⇒ isotonic saline. ⇒ saline.

normalization *n* the philosophy underpinning learning disability nursing and service delivery. Programmes of learning and individualized goal setting can help in acquiring the skills of daily living and maximum levels of independence.

normoblast *n* a normal-sized nucleated red blood cell, the precursor of the erythrocyte — **normoblastic** *adj*.

normocyte *n* a red blood cell of normal size — **normocytic** *adj*.

normoglycaemic *adj* a normal amount of glucose in the blood — **normoglycaemia** *n*.

normotension *n* normal tension, by custom alluding to blood pressure — **normotensive** *adj*.

normothermia *n* normal body temperature, as opposed to hyperthermia and hypothermia — **normothermic** *adj*.

normotonic *adj* normal strength, tension, tone, by current custom referring to muscle tissue — **normotonicity** *n*.

Norton scale a numerical scale devised by Norton, McLaren and Exton-Smith for assessing the risk of developing pressure ulcers. The criteria used are physical condition, mental state, activity, mobility and incontinence. The total possible score is 20 and people scoring 14 or less are considered to be at risk. ⇒ Braden scale. ⇒ Waterlow scale.

Norwalk virus *n* RNA virus responsible for outbreaks of winter gastroenteritis. It is spread by the faecal-oral route and by droplets. It occurs in settings such as schools and hospitals.

nosocomial *adj* pertaining to a hospital. ⇒ infection.

nostalgia *n* homesickness; a longing to return to a 'place' to which, and where, one may be emotionally bound — **nostalgic** *adj*.

nostrils *npl* the anterior openings in the nose; the anterior nares; choanae.

notifiable diseases, incidents or occurrences that must by law be made known to the appropriate agency. Diseases such as food poisoning, diphtheria and measles must be reported to the relevant health authority/department.

NPF *abbr* nurse prescribers' formulary.

NRDS *abbr* neonatal respiratory distress syndrome.

NREM sleep *abbr* nonrapid eye movement sleep. Sometimes called orthodox sleep. ⇒ sleep.

NSAIDs *abbr* nonsteroidal anti-inflammatory drugs. ⇒ corticosteroids.

NSFs *abbr* National Service Frameworks.

NSP *abbr* nonstarch polysaccharides.

NSU *abbr* ⇒ nonspecific urethritis.

nucha *n* the nape of the neck — **nuchal** *adj*.

nuclear family the conventional family group in western societies, consisting of two married parents and their dependent offspring. ⇒ family.

nuclear medicine *n* radionuclide techniques used for diagnosis, treatment and study of disease.

nucleated *adj* possessing one or more nuclei.

nucleic acids *npl* long-chain organic macromolecules formed from many subunits called nucleotides. ⇒ deoxyribonuleic acid. ⇒ ribonucleic acid.

nucleolus *n* structure containing both nucleic acids (DNA, RNA) situated within the nuclear membrane. Usually two in number, they are involved in nuclear division.

nucleoplasm ⇒ protoplasm.

nucleoproteins *npl* proteins found in the nuclei of cells, consisting of a protein conjugated with nucleic acid. An end product of nucleoprotein metabolism is uric acid which is excreted in the urine. ⇒ gout.

nucleoside *n* a compound of a sugar (ribose or deoxyribose) and a nitrogenous base (a purine or pyrimidine).

nucleotides *npl* the subunits of nucleic acids. Consist of many nucleosides (sugars and nitrogenous bases) and phosphate groups.

nucleotoxic *adj* poisonous to cell nuclei. The term may be applied to chemicals and viruses — **nucleotoxin** *n*.

nucleus *n* **1.** the central part. *cell nucleus* the membrane-bound structure containing the genetic material. *nucleus pulposus* the soft core of an intervertebral disc which can prolapse into the spinal cord and cause back pain. **2.** circumscribed accumulations of nerve cells in the central nervous system associated with a particular function, e.g. basal nuclei. **3.** the combination of atoms forming the central element or basic framework of the molecules of a specific compound or class of compounds. **4.** the dense core of an atom, called the atomic nucleus — **nuclear** *adj* pertaining to the nucleus. *nuclear division* part of cell division. *nuclear family* ⇒ nuclear family. *nuclear magnetic resonance (NMR)* ⇒ magnetic resonance imaging. *nuclear medicine* the use of radionuclide imaging techniques for diagnosis, treatment and study of disease.

null cells ⇒ large granular lymphocytes.

null hypothesis a statement that declares there to be no relationship between the dependent and independent variables.

nullipara *n* a woman who has not borne a child — **nulliparity** *n*.

numbers needed to treat a way of stating the benefits of an intervention. The number of subjects who need to receive treatment before one subject has a positive outcome.

nummular *adj* coin-shaped; resembling rolls of coins, as the sputum in tuberculosis.

nurse consultant *n* new role for experienced clinical practitioners who have the necessary level of expertise in an area of practice; professional leadership and consultancy; education, training and development; and practice and service development, research and evaluation. Those appointed have considerable patient contact and work in diverse areas that include: critical care, mental health, continence care, dermatology, spinal injuries, stroke services, accident and emergency etc.

nurse practitioner a nurse who has undergone specific role preparation to enable him or her to function at an advanced level within a particular working environment. This may be within primary health care, in an accident and emergency setting, or working with certain client groups, such as homeless people. Nurse practitioners can offer a nurse-led service and invariably have highly developed skills in client assessment.

nurse prescribing in the UK limited drug prescribing by suitably registered health visitors and district nurses who have recorded their qualification with the UKCC. Individuals concerned have completed an appropriate course, demonstrated prescribing competence and are accountable for their prescribing from the Nurse Prescribers' Formulary. ⇒ formulary. See Box – Nurse prescribing.

Nurse prescribing

Nurse prescribing is not new and a number of groups have been allowed to prescribe from a nurse prescribers' formulary for a number of years, e.g. health visitors and district nurses. However, changes in health care, and greater expectations of patients have illustrated that products contained within this formulary are limited and potentially out of date, especially in the realms, for example, of wound care and stoma care products.

In March 1999, the final report of the *Review of prescribing, supply and administration of medicines*, commonly known as the 'Crown II report', was published. The report recommends the introduction of two new groups of prescribers – independent and dependent:

- Independent prescribers would make the initial clinical assessment, usually making a diagnosis, and then prescribe as appropriate;
- Dependent prescribers would not diagnose, but once diagnosis has been made, then prescription would be allowed using clinical guidelines.

However, the Crown Report still stipulates that prescribers should only be allowed to prescribe from a limited formulary relating to their specialist areas.

Reference
Department of Health. 1999 Review of Prescribing, Supply and Administration of Medicines: Final report (Crown II). Department of Health, London

Nursing and Midwifery Council (NMC) a smaller council established in 2001, for the regulation of nursing, midwifery and health visiting in the UK. The new body replaces the UKCC and the four National Boards.

nursing auxiliary ⇒ healthcare assistant.

nursing models frameworks that identify, describe and explain a range of nursing concepts; traditionally named after the writers who first propounded them, e.g. Roy's model, Rogers' model, Roper, Logan, Tierney model, etc. Nursing models may or may not be developed out of research.

nursing process a systematic approach to nursing care. It comprises four phases: assessing, planning, implementing and evaluating. Only for purposes of description can they be sequential; in reality, they overlap and occur and recur throughout the period a person is receiving nursing care.

nursing theory theory that explains, illuminates, or offers practical guidance about the field of nursing; generated by nursing research or, rationally, through the development of nursing ideas.

Nutritional Assessment

Nutritional assessment is used in a range of situations to determine whether an individual is likely to be suffering from a deficiency of a specific nutrient or general malnutrition. For example:

- to assess the population in famine relief so ensuring the appropriate type of food aid gets to the right people;
- on admission to hospital or during stay to ensure optimum recovery.

In many hospitals nutritional assessment on admission has become routine, particularly in the care of older people. This is because poor nutrition impairs wound healing, decreases resistance to infection and so increases recovery time and time spent in hospital.

Methods of assessing nutritional status

There are four methods of nutritional assessment which are usually used in conjunction with each other:

- clinical examination to identify medical conditions that impair nutrient intake and/or absorption and the specific signs of nutrient deficiency;
- anthropometric measurement of height, weight, body mass index, skinfold thickness, mid-arm circumference, and grip strength. Used to identify changes in body weight;
- diet history taken to obtain information about current dietary intake and any difficulties in the purchase and preparation of food;
- biochemical measurements such as the level of micronutrients in plasma or serum.

Nutritional support

Nutritional support is the prevention and treatment of malnutrition in patients who are unable to eat enough food or absorb sufficient nutrients to meet their nutritional needs. Nurses have an important role in the identification of patients at risk of malnutrition and the provision of nutritional support.

The type of nutritional support used depends on the underlying cause of the malnutrition:

- Dietary supplementation and food fortification – used for individuals who have a functioning gastrointestinal tract, but are unable to consume large volumes of food, e.g. those with a poor appetite. Nutritional support is provided as sip feeds, additional between-meal snacks and by fortifying foods such as soups to increase their energy and protein content.
- Enteral nutrition – used for those who have a functioning gastrointestinal tract, but are unable to swallow, e.g. unconscious patients. Nutritional requirements are met by the use of a liquid feed that is nutritionally complete. It

is usual to use a nasogastric tube for short term feeding and a gastrostomy tube for long term feeding.

- Parenteral feeding – which should only be used in patients whose gastrointestinal tract is non-functional. A sterile nutrient solution which does not need to be digested is delivered directly into the circulatory system via a central venous catheter or a catheter passed into a central vein via a peripheral vein. Hypertonic nutrient solutions should only be administered into a central vein where rapid transport occurs and blood flow is sufficient to dilute the solution. Infusing nutrient solutions into smaller peripheral veins can cause inflammation of the endothelial lining of the vein.

Further reading
Lennard-Jones J E (Ed) 1992 A positive approach to nutrition as treatment. London: King's Fund Centre.
Wood S, Creamer M 1996 Malnutrition in hospitals. The nurses' role in prevention. Nurs Times. 92 26: 67–70.

nutation *n* nodding; applied to uncontrollable head shaking.

nutrient *n, adj* a substance serving as or providing nourishment. ⇒ macronutrients. ⇒ micronutrients. *nutrient artery* one which enters a long bone. *nutrient foramen* hole in a long bone which admits the nutrient artery.

nutrition *n* **1.** the total process by which the living organism receives and utilizes the materials necessary for survival, growth and repair of worn-out tissues. **2.** the science of food and its utilization by the body.

nutritional *adj* relating to nutrition. *nutritional assessment* see Box – Nutritional assessment. *nutritional requirement* see Box – Dietary reference values (nutritional requirement). *nutritional support* see Box – Nutritional support.

NVQs *abbr* National Vocational Qualifications.

nyctalgia *n* pain occurring during the night.

nyctalopia *n* ⇒ night blindness.

nyctophobia *n* irrational fear of the night and darkness.

nymphomania *n* excessive sexual desire in a female — **nymphomaniac** *adj*.

nystagmus *n* involuntary and rhythmic oscillatory movements of the eyeball

May be caused by neurological disorders, vestibular apparatus problems, or as a side-effect of some drugs.

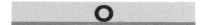

O

OAE *abbr* otoacoustic emission.

oat cell carcinoma a small cell bronchial cancer. Accounts for one quarter of lung cancers. It is characterized by ectopic hormone production where the cancer cells secrete hormones, such as ACTH and ADH. → bronchial cancer.

obesity *n* a common nutritional disorder in developed countries. It is characterized by the deposition of excessive fat around the body, particularly in the subcutaneous tissue. The intake of food is in excess of the body's energy requirements. ⇒ body mass index. See Box – Obesity.

objective *adj* pertaining to things external to one's self. ⇒ subjective *ant objective signs* those which the observer notes, as distinct from the symptoms of which the patient complains.

obligate *adj* characterized by the ability to survive only in a particular set of environmental conditions, e.g. an obligate parasite cannot exist other than as a parasite.

Obesity

Obesity is a condition in which the body fat stores are increased to a level that impairs health. It is the cause of preventable ill health including diabetes mellitus, coronary heart disease, hypertension, stroke (cerebrovascular accident), gallstones, osteoarthritis, reproductive disorders, sleep apnoea, some cancers and psychological disorders. Obesity is usually diagnosed from body mass index (BMI). Other methods of assessment include measurement of waist and hip circumference, bioelectrical impedance and skinfold thickness measurement. The incidence of obesity is increasing and differs with socioeconomic status and racial group. In the UK in 1995 15% of men and 16.5% of women aged 16–64 years had a BMI > 30.

Classification of obesity and overweight according to body mass index (WHO 1998)

Underweight – BMI < 18.5
Normal range – BMI 18.5–24.9
Overweight – BMI > 25
Pre-obese – BMI 25–29.9
Obese Class 1 – BMI 30–34.9
Obese Class 2 – BMI 35–39.9
Obese Class 3 – BMI > 40

Causes of obesity

The causes of obesity include: high fat diet, high sugar diet, physical inactivity, endocrine disorders, genetic make up, psychosocial factors etc.

Treatment

The treatment of obesity includes lifestyle changes such as dietary change and exercise. This usually needs to be accompanied by behaviour therapy to be successful. Surgery and drug treatments are considered as a last resort.

Further reading
British Nutrition Foundation. 1999 Obesity – the report of the British Nutrition Foundation task force. Blackwell Science, Oxford

Reference
WHO. 1998 Obesity: Preventing and Managing the Global Epidemic. World Health Organization, Geneva

OBS *abbr* organic brain syndrome. ⇒ dementia.

observational study research study where the researcher observes, listens and records the events of interest. *participant observational study* one where the researcher takes part and has a role. Used sometimes in qualitative social science research.

observations *npl* in a nursing context, the regular measurement of the patient's physiological status – blood pressure, temperature, pulse and respiration. ⇒ monitoring.

observing *v* one of the many complex skills required by nurses. Using the senses to assess a situation and to collect data required to plan individualized care.

obsessive compulsive disorder (OCD)/obsessional neurosis a neurosis characterized by obsessive thoughts that are recognized by the person as arising within themselves and/or repetitive physical actions that may, at first be resisted. The resistance may lead to considerable anxiety that is only relieved by performing the activity, although the person knows it to be unreasonable. The two distinct types recognized are: (a) obsessive-compulsive thoughts: constant preoccupation with a constantly recurring morbid thought which cannot be kept out of the mind, and enters against the wishes of the patient who tries to eliminate it. The thought is almost always painful and out of keeping with the person's normal personality; (b) obsessive compulsive actions: a feeling of compulsion to perform repeatedly a simple act, e.g. checking, handwashing, touching door knobs etc. Ideas of guilt frequently form the basis of an obsessional state. ⇒ neurosis.

obstetrician *n* a qualified doctor who practises the science and art of obstetrics.

obstetrics *n* the medical/surgical science dealing with the care of the pregnant woman during the antenatal, parturient and puerperal stages.

obstruction *n* any of the body's organs which are hollow tubes can be obstructed by something in the lumen, abnormality in the wall, or pressure from outside. Obstruction can occur as an emergency requiring immediate treatment or operation. ⇒ Heimlich manoeuvre.

obturator *n* that which closes an aperture. *obturator foramen* the opening in the innominate bone which is closed by muscles and fascia. *obturator internus* obturator nerve.

occipital *adj* pertaining to the back of the head. *occipital bone* forming the back of the cranium and part of the base of the skull. It contains a large hole through which the spinal cord passes. ⇒ foramen magnum.

occipitoanterior *adj* describes a position when the fetal occiput lies in the anterior half of the maternal pelvis.

occipitofrontal *adj* pertaining to the occiput and forehead.

occipitoposterior *adj* describes a position when the fetal occiput is in the posterior half of the maternal pelvis.

occiput *n* the posterior region of the skull.

occlusion *n* the closure of an opening, especially of ducts or blood vessels. *coronary occlusion* such as caused by a thrombosis in a coronary artery. *dental occlusion* the fit of the upper and lower teeth as the jaws meet — **occlusal** *adj*.

occult hidden, not visible. *occult blood* minute quantities of blood passed in the faeces that can only be demonstrated chemically.

occupation See Box – Occupation.

occupational disease ⇒ industrial disease.

Occupation

Occupation is the term used by occupational therapists to describe any productive and purposeful form of human endeavour. Occupations are developed across the lifespan and may include those related to work or recreation or activities connected with personal care or managing a home. (Activities of Daily Living; PADL, DADL, IADL). A person needs to have a balanced range of culturally appropriate occupations in order to maintain health and well-being. The act of participation in an occupation is referred to as occupational performance. The quality of occupational performance is affected by the nature of the occupation, the context of the environment and the knowledge, skills and attitudes of the individual. Occupational therapists take account of all three aspects when evaluating a client's performance problems or providing intervention.

occupational health assessment a one-to-one interaction between a client (the employee or prospective employee) and an occupational health professional, usually a doctor or a nurse, for the purposes of assessing the physical and/or mental health status of the client.

occupational health nursing client care offered by nurses specially educated to deliver care in the workplace. It includes examination of the workplace for accident/illness risk, preventive teaching, assessment of new workers, maintaining records, as well as running health promotion sessions or surgeries.

occupational therapy (OT) the treatment of physical and psychiatric conditions through specific activities in order to help people reach their maximum level of function and independence in all aspects of daily life. See Box – Occupational therapy. *occupational therapy assessment* see Box – Occupational therapy assessment.

OCD *abbr* obsessive compulsive disorder.

ocular *adj* pertaining to the eye. *ocular motility* eye movements.

oculist *n* a medically qualified person who treats eye disease.

oculogenital *adj* pertaining to the eye and genital region. ⇒ *Chlamydia trachomatis*. ⇒ gonorrhoea. ⇒ ophthalmia.

oculogyric making the eyes roll. *oculogyric cris* when the eyes are held in a fixed position for some time.

oculomotor *n* the third pair of cranial nerves. They innervate the four extrinsic muscles which move the eye and the muscle which raises the upper eyelid. They alter pupil size and the shape of the lens.

odds ratio ⇒ risk.

odontalgia *n* toothache.

odontic *adj* pertaining to the teeth.

odontoid *adj* resembling a tooth. *odontoid process* peg-like projection of the second cervical vertebra.

odontology *n* dentistry.

Occupational therapy

Occupational therapy (OT) relates to both the profession and the process used by occupational therapists to provide intervention.

Occupational therapists provide services to individuals who experience problems in occupational performance. They work with people of all ages in a variety of clinical and community settings. OT is founded on a set of assumptions concerning the importance of human occupations in maintaining health and well-being.

Occupational therapy involves active participation by the patient or client. Initially, using various techniques, the complex interactions between the individual, his occupations and his environment are explored. ⇒ occupational therapy assessment. On the basis of agreed goals and priorities, and through engagement in selected purposeful activities, skills are gained, knowledge is expanded, and attitudes to self and others can be explored. Through adaptation and analysis of activities, and adaptation and analysis of environments, barriers to performance can be removed. By means of these processes individuals are enabled to do more of the things they want and need to do in the course of their daily lives. In the environments which they use.

Occupational therapy assessment

Several kinds of assessment procedures are used by occupational therapists to discover the nature and extent of the occupational performance problems experienced by an individual. The results of assessment are used to set goals, measure changes in performance, predict performance capabilities, and provide outcome measures.

Assessment typically involves structured observation of actual performances in real or simulated environments. Problems may arise in the areas of work, leisure or self-care. ⇒ Activities of Daily Living (PADL, DADL, IADL). Measurement of physical function, cognitive, perceptual, social or intrapersonal skills may be included. The occupational therapist may also explore patterns of engagement over a period of time. Assessment may also be focused on the environment used by the individual in order to identify ways in which the physical or social environment can be enhanced or adapted to improve occupational performance.

A home assessment is undertaken by a hospital-based therapist who takes a patient to his or her home to assess performance, ascertain the need for environmental alterations, adaptive equipment or support services, and evaluate risk. Following return to hospital recommendations concerning suitability for discharge can be made, and action taken to provide the adaptations and services which are needed before discharge. Similar assessments are carried out by community-based occupational therapists.

odontoma *n* a tumour developing from or containing tooth structures — **odontomatous** *adj*.

odontotherapy *n* the treatment of diseases of the teeth.

oedema *n* swelling due to excess fluid in the tissue (interstitial) spaces and serous cavities. Causes include: (a) increased capillary permeability, e.g. release of inflammatory chemicals; (b) reduced osmotic pressure due to hypoproteinaemia, e.g. liver failure; (c) lymphatic obstruction, e.g. with malignancy; (d) increased venous hydrostatic pressure, e.g. heart failure. ⇒ anasarca. ⇒ angio-oedema. ⇒ ascites. ⇒ effusion. ⇒ lymphoedema. ⇒ pulmonary oedema — **oedematous** *adj*.

Oedipus complex an unconscious attachment of a son to his mother, resulting in a feeling of jealousy towards the father and then guilt, producing emotional conflict. This process was described by Freud as part of his theory of infantile sexuality and he considered it to be normal in male infants.

oesophageal *adj* pertaining to the oesophagus. *oesophageal atresia* congenital defect where the oesophagus ends in a blind pouch. It may be associated with a tracheo-oesophageal fistula. *oesophageal speech* a patient who has undergone a laryngectomy may learn to use this method of speech production, producing a pseudovoice using the top of the oesophagus. *oesophageal ulcer* ulceration of the oesophagus due to gastro-oesophageal reflux caused by hiatus hernia. *oesophageal varices* varicosity of the veins in the lower oesophagus due to hepatic portal hypertension; they often extend below the cardia into the stomach. These varices can bleed and cause a massive haematemesis. ⇒ Sengstaken tube.

oesophagectasis *n* a dilated oesophagus.

oesophagectomy *n* excision of part or the whole of the oesophagus.

oesophagitis *n* inflammation of the oesophagus, especially that caused by the reflux of acidic gastric contents due to hiatus hernia.

oesophagogastrectomy *n* excision of part of the oesophagus and the stomach.

oesophagogastroduodenoscopy (OGD) *n* endoscopic examination of the upper alimentary canal/tract.

oesophagoscope *n* an endoscope for passage into the oesophagus. Usually a flexible fibreoptic endoscope is used, but rigid metal instruments may be used occasionally — **oesophagoscopic** *adj*.

oesophagostomy *n* a surgically established fistula between the oesophagus and the skin in the root of the neck. Used temporarily for feeding after excision of the pharynx for malignant disease.

oesophagotomy *n* an incision into the oesophagus.

oesophagus *n* the muscular, membranous canal, 23 cm in length, extending from the pharynx to the stomach — **oesophageal** *adj*.

oestradiol (estradiol) *n* the principal endogenous oestrogen. It is produced by the corpus luteum during the second part of the menstrual cycle.

oestriol (estriol) *n* an endogenous oestrogen. Oestriol levels in maternal blood or urine have been used as an indicator of placental function and fetal well-being.

oestrogens (estrogens) *npl* a group of steroid hormones that includes: oestriol, oestrone and oestradiol. They are produced by the ovaries, the placenta, the testes and, to a lesser extent, the adrenal cortex in both sexes. They are responsible for female secondary sexual characteristics and the development and proper functioning of the female genital organs. Used therapeutically in the combined oral contraceptive and as hormone replacement — **oestrogenic** *adj*.

oestrone (estrone) *n* an endogenous oestrogen.

OGD *abbr* oesophagogastroduodenoscopy.

old age mental illness a term increasingly applied to the mental health problems of older people, instead of elderly mentally ill (EMI). The mental disorders most commonly associated with older people are acute or chronic confusional states, depression and dementia.

olecranon process the large process at the upper end of the ulna; it forms the tip of the elbow when the arm is flexed. *olecranon bursitis* ⇒ bursitis.

olfaction *n* the sense of smell — **olfactory** *adj* pertaining to the sense of smell. *olfactory nerve* the first pair of cranial nerves. They transmit impulses from the olfactory epithelium in the nose to the olfactory cortex of the brain. *olfactory organ* the nose.

olfactometry tests used to assess olfaction. The person is asked to distinguish between substances, such as menthol, cinnamon, coffee and vanilla.

oligodendrocyte *n* a neuroglial cell of the central nervous system. ⇒ neuroglia.

oligohydramnios *n* deficient amniotic fluid.

oligomenorrhoea *n* infrequent or sparse menstruation; normal cycle is prolonged beyond 35 days.

oligospermia *n* reduced number of spermatozoa in semen.

oliguria a reduction in the production of urine. ⇒ anuria.

ombudsman *n* a commissioner (e.g. health, local government) appointed by government to hear complaints in situations where it has not been possible to reach a satisfactory resolution at local level.

omentum *n* a fold of peritoneum. The omentum supports and protects organs, limits the spread of infection and stores fat. *greater omentum* is suspended from the greater curvature of the stomach and hangs in front of the intestine. *lesser omentum* passes from the lesser curvature of the stomach to the transverse fissure of the liver (see Figure 48) — **omental** *adj*.

omphalitis *n* inflammation of the umbilicus.

omphalocele *n* ⇒ hernia.

Onchocerca *n* a genus of parasitic filarial nematode worms, e.g. *Onchocerca volulus.* ⇒ filariasis. ⇒ onchocerciasis.

onchocerciasis *n* infestation of the skin, soft tissues and the eye by the filarial worm *Onchocerca volulus.* Adult worms encapsulated in subcutaneous connective tissue. Can cause 'river blindness' if the larvae migrate to the eyes. Treatment is with anthelmintics: diethylcarbamazine, albendazole.

oncogene *n* an abnormal gene that stimulates cells to grow in an uncontrolled way and become malignant. ⇒ proto-oncogene.

oncogenic *adj* capable of tumour production.

oncology *n* the scientific and medical study of tumours and their treatment — **oncologically** *adv*.

onychia *n* acute inflammation of the nail matrix; suppuration may spread beneath the nail, causing it to become detached and fall off.

onychocryptosis *n* ingrowing of the nail.

onychogryphosis, oncogryposis *n* a ridged, thickened deformity of the nails, especially of the great toe in older adults.

onycholysis *n* loosening of toe or finger nail from the nail bed — **onycholytic** *adj*.

onychomycosis *n* a fungal infection of the nails.

o'nyong-nyong fever disease caused by a togavirus transmitted by mosquitoes in East Africa.

oocyte *n* an immature ovum. A female gamete prior to its penetration by a spermatozoon.

oogenesis *n* the production of oocytes in the ovary. ⇒ gametogenesis. ⇒ spermatogenesis — **oogenetic** *adj*.

oophorectomy *n* (*syn* ovariectomy, ovariotomy) removal of an ovary.

oophoritis *n* (*syn* ovaritis) inflammation of an ovary.

opacity *n* nontransparency; cloudiness; an opaque spot, as on the cornea or lens.

operant conditioning ⇒ conditioning.

operating microscope an illuminated binocular microscope enabling surgery to be carried out on delicate tissues such as nerves and blood vessels. Some models incorporate a beam splitter and a second set of eyepieces to enable a second person to view the operation site.

operating system a program that a computer loads automatically before it can run any other programs, e.g. MS DOS and UNIX.

operation *n* surgical procedure upon a part of the body.

operational management the management of the day to day activities (operations) of an organization such as a district general hospital. ⇒ strategic management.

operculum *n* plug of mucus that occludes the cervical canal during pregnancy. Discharged as the 'show' when labour starts.

ophthalmia *n* (*syn* ophthalmitis) inflammation of the eye. *ophthalmia neonatorum* purulent inflammation of the eyes of a newborn. It occurs as the infant passes through the vagina. It is a notifiable condition. May be caused by chlamydial or gonococcal infections. *sympathetic ophthalmia* inflammation of the uveal tract (uvea) in a normal eye that follows injury or disease of the other eye.

ophthalmic *adj* pertaining to the eye.

ophthalmitis *n* ⇒ ophthalmia.

ophthalmologist *n* a doctor specializing in the treatment of eye diseases.

ophthalmology *n* the study of the structure, function and diseases of the eye — **ophthalmologically** *adv.*

ophthalmoplegia *n* paralysis of one or more muscles which move the eye. ⇒ extraocular — **ophthalmoplegic** *adj.*

ophthalmoscope *n* an instrument fitted with a lens and illumination for examining the interior of the eye — **ophthalmoscopic** *adj.*

opiate ⇒ opioids.

opioids *npl* a group of morphine-like drugs, that produce the same effects as morphine and can be reversed by antagonists such as naloxone. It includes: morphine analogues, e.g. morphine, diamorphine, codeine, naloxone; synthetic derivatives, e.g. pethidine, fentanyl, methadone, dextropropoxyphene, pentazocine, buprenorphine etc.

opisthotonos *n* extreme extension of the body with arching of the back, occurring in tetanic spasm. Patients may be supported on their heels and head alone. ⇒ tetanus — **opisthotonic** *adj.*

opium *n* the dried juice of opium poppy. Contains morphine and several other morphine-related alkaloids.

opportunistic infection ⇒ infection.

opportunity cost when a resource is used in a particular way, the opportunity to use it for another purpose is lost. This includes money, time and the activities which cannot be undertaken. An example in health care would be the budget allocation for an expensive drug leading to a lost opportunity to spend the money for another service.

opsins the protein component of the visual pigments present in the rods and cones.

opsonic index a measurement of the ability of phagocytes to ingest and destroy foreign bodies such as bacteria.

opsonin *n* antibodies or complement proteins which coat invading particles, such as bacteria, to render them more susceptible to phagocytosis. ⇒ immunoglobulins — **opsonic** *adj.*

opsonization process by which bacteria are rendered more susceptible to destruction by phagocytosis.

optic *adj* pertaining to sight. *optic chiasma* the meeting of the optic nerves; where the fibres from the medial or nasal half of each retina cross the midline to join the optic tract of the opposite side. *optic disc* the point where the optic nerve enters the eyeball. ⇒ blind spot. *optic nerves* second pair of cranial nerves. They carry impulses from photoreceptors in the retina to the visual cortex. *optic tracts* two bands of optic nerve fibres that run backwards from the optic chiasma.

optical *adj* pertaining to sight. *optical density* the light absorbed by a solution. Used to determine the concentration of substances.

optical aberration imperfect focus of light rays by a lens.

optician *n* a person qualified to make or prescribe spectacles and contact lenses to correct refractive errors.

optics *n* the branch of physics which deals with the properties of light.

optimum *adj* most favourable. *optimum position* that which will be least awkward and most useful should a limb remain permanently paralysed.

optometrist *n* a person qualified to practise optometry.

optometry *n* measurement of visual acuity.

oral *adj* pertaining to the mouth. *oral hygiene* ⇒ mouth care. *oral phase. oral rehydration solution (ORS)* a solution of glucose and electrolytes used in oral rehydration. *oral rehydration therapy (ORT)* the use of ORS to correct dehydration caused by diarrhoea — **orally** *adv.*

oral contraceptive commonly referred to as 'the pill'. *combined oral contraceptive* many different brands are available; each contains varying concentrations of the two hormones oestrogen and progestogen. ⇒ contraceptive. ⇒ progestogen only pill.

oral stage the first stage of psychosexual development, characterized by the child's sensual interest in the mouth and lips, especially suckling at the breast.

orbicular *adj* resembling a globe; spherical or circular.

orbicularis *n* a muscle which encircles an orifice, e.g. orbicularis oris around the mouth.

orbit *n* the bony socket containing the eyeball and its appendages — **orbital** *adj*.

orchidectomy *n* excision of a testis.

orchidopexy *n* the operation of bringing an undescended testis into the scrotum, and fixing it in this position.

orchis *n* the testis.

orchitis *n* inflammation of a testis.

ordinal data categorical data that can be ordered or ranked, e.g. size in general terms, as in 'bigger than', or general condition – good, moderate or bad. ⇒ nominal data.

orf *n* skin lesions caused by a virus transmitted from sheep and goats.

organ *n* a grouping together of different tissues to form a discrete functional unit. Organs may be compact, such as the liver, or hollow like the stomach. *organ transplantation* ⇒ transplant.

organ of Corti *n* situated in the inner ear. It contains the auditory receptor cells of the cochlear branch of the vestibulo cochlear (VIIth) nerve in the cochlea.

organelles *npl* tiny subcellular structures with specific functions within the cell, such as the mitochondria and ribosomes.

organic *adj* pertaining to an organ. Associated with life. *organic brain syndrome* ⇒ dementia. *organic compounds* chemical compounds that contain carbon and hydrogen in their structure, e.g. glucose. Include the large biological molecules, such as proteins and carbohydrates. *organic disease* one in which there is structural change. ⇒ functional *ant*.

organism *n* a living cell or group of cells differentiated into functionally distinct parts which are interdependent.

organogenesis *n* the formation and development of body organs from embryonic tissue.

organophosphorus compounds *npl* a group of highly toxic compounds used as agricultural insecticides.

orgasm *n* the climax of sexual excitement.

oriental sore (*syn* Delhi boil) a form of cutaneous leishmaniasis producing papular, crusted, granulomatous eruptions of the skin. A disease of the tropics and subtropics (old world).

orientation *n* clear awareness of one's position relative to the environment. In mental conditions, orientation 'in space and time' means that the patient knows where he is and recognizes the passage of time, i.e. can give the correct date. ⇒ reality orientation.

orifice *n* a mouth or opening.

origin *n* the commencement or source of anything. *origin of a muscle* the end that remains relatively fixed during contraction of the muscle.

ornithine an amino acid derived from arginine during the reactions of the urea cycle in the liver.

ornithosis *n* human illness resulting from disease of birds, such as psittacosis. ⇒ Chlamydia.

orogenital *adj* pertaining to the mouth and the external genital area.

oropharyngeal *adj* pertaining to the mouth and pharynx.

oropharynx *n* that portion of the pharynx which is below the level of the soft palate and above the level of the hyoid bone.

ORS *abbr* oral rehydration solution.

ORT *abbr* oral rehydration therapy.

orthodontics *n* a branch of dentistry dealing with prevention and correction of irregularities of the teeth.

orthodox sleep *n* (*syn* NREM sleep) ⇒ sleep.

orthopaedics *n* formerly a specialty devoted to the correction of deformities in children. It is now a branch of surgery dealing with all conditions affecting the locomotor system.

orthopnoea *n* breathlessness necessitating an upright, sitting position for its relief — **orthopnoeic** *adj*.

orthoptics *n* the diagnosis and nonsurgical correction of visual abnormalities, such as strabismus, by exercises.

orthosis *n* a device which can be applied to or around the body in the care of physical impairment or disability. ⇒ prosthesis — **orthotic** *adj*.

orthostatic *adj* pertaining to or caused by the upright stance. *orthostatic albuminuria* occurs in some healthy subjects only when they adopt the upright position.

orthotics *n* the scientific study and manufacture of devices which can be applied to or around the body in the care of physical impairment or disability.

orthotist *n* a person who practises orthotics.

Ortolani's sign/test a test performed, by an experienced clinician, shortly after birth for the diagnosis of developmental dysplasia of the hip (congenital dislocation of the hip). Often used in conjunction with Barlow's sign/test.

os *n* a mouth or opening. *external os* the opening of the cervix into the vagina. *internal os* the opening of the cervix into the uterine cavity — **ora** *pl*.

oscillation *n* a swinging or moving to and fro; a vibration.

oscillometry *n* measurement of vibration, using a special apparatus (oscillometer). Measures the magnitude of the pulse wave more precisely than palpation.

oscilloscope *n* a device which uses the fluorescent screen of a cathode ray tube to display various electrical waveforms such as that produced by the heart. ⇒ electrocardiogram (ECG).

Osgood-Schlatter's disease ⇒ Schlatter's disease.

Osler's nodes small painful areas in pulp of fingers or toes, or palms and soles, caused by emboli and occurring in subacute bacterial endocarditis.

osmolality *n* the osmotic pressure expressed as the number of osmoles (or milliosmoles) per kilogram of solution.

osmolarity *n* the osmotic pressure exerted by a given concentration of osmotically active solute in aqueous solution, defined in terms of the number of active particles per unit volume. The number of osmoles (or milliosmoles) per litre of solution.

osmole *n* the standard unit of osmotic pressure which is equal to the molecular weight in grams of a solute divided by the number of particles or ions into which it dissociates in solution. In low concentration solutions a smaller unit, the milliosmole, is used.

osmosis *n* the passage of water across a selectively permeable membrane under the influence of osmotic pressure (see Figure 45). The movement of a dilute solution (lower solute concentration) into a more concentrated solution with a higher solute concentration.

osmotic *adj* pertaining to osmosis. *osmotic pressure* the pressure with which solvent molecules are drawn across a selectively permeable membrane separating two concentrations of solute (such as sodium chloride or urea) dissolved in the same solvent, when the membrane is impermeable to the solute but permeable to the solvent. Important in fluid homeostasis.

osmotic diuretics *npl* pharmacologically inert substances such as mannitol, a sugar. They are given intravenously to reduce cerebral oedema or raised intraocular pressure in glaucoma or produce a diuresis after drug overdose. The diuresis occurs through the osmotic 'pull' created by the inert sugar (which is filtered by the kidney, but not reabsorbed) during its excretion.

osseous *adj* pertaining to or resembling bone.

ossicles *npl* small bones, particularly those contained in the middle ear: the malleus, incus and stapes.

ossiculoplasty *n* surgical replacement of part or all of the chain of ossicles.

ossification *n* the formation of bone, either from cartilage and membrane in the fetus and secondary ossification after birth, or bone growth during childhood and adolescence. Also known as osteogenesis — **ossify** *vt, vi*.

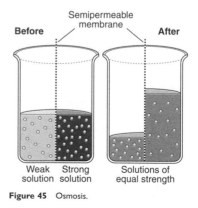

Figure 45 Osmosis.

osteitis *n* inflammation of bone. *osteitis deformans* ⇒ Paget's disease. *osteitis fibrosa cystica* ⇒ von Recklinghausen's disease.

osteoarthritis *n* also known as osteoarthrosis. A degenerative arthritis; may be primary, or may follow injury or disease involving the articular surfaces of synovial joints. The articular cartilage becomes worn, osteophytes form at the periphery of the joint surface and loose bodies may result. The joints most commonly affected are the knees, hips, spine and hands. There is pain, joint disruption and loss of mobility. Management includes: activity modification, physiotherapy to improve muscle strength, hydrotherapy, analgesia, NSAIDs, weight loss as appropriate, mobility aids, intra-articular injections of a corticosteroid and surgery. ⇒ arthropathy. ⇒ arthroplasty. ⇒ osteotomy — **osteoarthritic** *adj*.

osteoarthrosis *n* ⇒ osteoarthritis.

osteoblast *n* immature bone-forming cell. ⇒ chondroblast. → fibroblast. ⇒ haemocytoblast — **osteoblastic** *adj*.

osteochondritis *n* originally an inflammation of bone cartilage. Usually applied to nonseptic conditions, especially avascular necrosis involving joint surfaces, e.g. osteochondritis dissecans, in which a portion of joint surface may separate to form a loose body in the joint. ⇒ Scheuermann's disease. ⇒ Schlatter's disease.

osteochondroma *n* a benign tumour of bone and cartilage.

osteoclasis *n* the therapeutic fracture of a bone.

osteoclast *n* bone destroyer; the cell which dissolves or removes unwanted bone during periods of growth, for remodelling and following injury.

osteoclastoma *n* a tumour of the osteoclasts. May be benign, locally recurrent, or frankly malignant.

osteocyte *n* a bone cell.

osteodystrophy *n* faulty growth of bone.

osteogenesis *n* ⇒ ossification. ⇒ osteogenesis imperfecta.

osteogenesis imperfecta a hereditary disorder usually transmitted by an autosomal dominant gene. The disorder may be present at birth or develop during childhood. The congenital form is much more severe and may lead to early death. The bones are extremely fragile and may fracture after the mildest trauma.

osteogenic *adj* bone-producing. *osteogenic sarcoma* malignant tumour originating in cells which normally produce bone.

osteoid *n* organic matrix of bone comprising collagen and other complex molecules.

osteolytic *adj* destructive of bone, e.g. osteolytic malignant deposits in bone.

osteoma *n* a benign tumour of bone which may arise in the compact tissue *(ivory osteoma)* or in the cancellous tissue. May be single or multiple.

osteomalacia *n* softening of the bone with pain and eventual deformity. There is a failure to mineralize the osteoid. It is caused by lack of vitamin D (dietary or lack of exposure to sunlight). Sometimes known as adult rickets.

osteomyelitis *n* inflammation commencing in the marrow of bone, usually due to acute or chronic bacterial infection — **osteomyelitic** *adj*.

osteon *n* a haversian system, the basic structural unit of bone.

osteopath *n* one who practises osteopathy.

osteopathy *n* a clinical discipline and established system of assessment, diagnosis and treatment. Osteopathy is concerned with the inter-relationship between structure and function of the body. It is known to be effective for the relief or improvement of a wide variety of conditions, such as 'glue ear' and some digestive disorders, as well as mechanical problems of the body. Osteopathy is one of only a few complementary therapies to have achieved statutory self-regulation on a par with medicine (Osteopaths Act 1993) — **osteopathic** *adj*.

osteopetrosis (*syn* Albers-Schönberg disease, marble bone disease) inherited bone disease characterized by increasing bone density with loss of medullary space. The bones become extremely hard but brittle, which results in fractures. Loss of haemopoietic marrow leads to problems with blood cell formation.

osteophyte *n* a bony outgrowth or spur, usually at the margins of joint surfaces, e.g. in osteoarthritis — **osteophytic** *adj*.

osteoplasty *n* reconstructive operation on bone — **osteoplastic** *adj.*

osteoporosis *n* loss of bone mass due to reabsorption without the usual balance of bone deposition. The bones, which retain their normal composition, are lighter and weaker. They deform and fracture more easily, and fractures of the wrist, neck of femur and vertebrae (with a reduction in height) are especially common. Causes include: ageing in both sexes, nutritional deficiencies, immobility, hormonal, e.g. postmenopausal decline in oestrogens, Cushing's disease and corticosteroid therapy. Early detection may be through measuring bone density. Management includes: prevention through achievement of peak bone mass, weight-bearing exercise and replacement of oestrogens in postmenopausal women and ensuring adequate calcium and vitamin D intake (possibly as supplements) throughout the lifespan. The treatment of established disease includes the above plus biphosphonates to inhibit bone absorption, and fluorides, PTH and anabolic steroids to stimulate bone deposition — **osteoporotic** *adj.*

osteosarcoma *n* a malignant tumour of bone arising in osteoblasts — **osteosarcomatous** *adj.*

osteosclerosis *n* increased density or hardness of bone — **osteosclerotic** *adj.*

osteotome *n* an instrument for cutting bone; it is similar to a chisel, but it is bevelled on both sides of its cutting edge.

osteotomy *n* division of bone followed by realignment of the ends to encourage union by healing. Usually performed for the relief or cure of bony deformities. ⇒ McMurray's osteotomy.

ostium *n* the opening or mouth of any tubular passage — **ostial** *adj.*

OT *abbr* 1. occupational therapy. 2. operating theatre.

otalgia *n* earache.

OTC *abbr* over-the-counter drugs/medicines.

otitis *n* inflammation of the ear. *otitis externa* inflammation of the skin of the external auditory canal. *malignant otitis externa* is not a cancer, but occurs in immunocompromised individuals and diabetics. A severe otitis externa that exposes the bone in the external auditory canal and erosion and infection of part of the temporal bone. It can lead to various cranial nerve palsies. *otitis media* inflammation of the middle ear cavity. The effusion tends to be serous, mucoid or purulent. Nonpurulent effusions in children are often called glue ear. ⇒ grommet. *otitis interna* inflammation of the internal ear vestibular structures.

otoacoustic emission (OAE) a computer-linked hearing test used for screening infants soon after birth. ⇒ neonatal hearing screening.

otoliths tiny calcium deposits associated with the saccule and utricle of the internal ear.

otologist *n* a person who specializes in otology.

otology *n* the science which deals with the structure, function and diseases of the ear.

otorhinolaryngology *n* the science which deals with the structure, function and diseases of the ear, nose and throat; each of these three may be considered a specialty. ⇒ laryngology. ⇒ otology. ⇒ rhinology.

otorrhoea *n* a discharge from the external auditory meatus.

otosclerosis *n* a hereditary condition causing hearing impairment. It affects the ossicles, especially the stapes where changes to the bone of the ossicles alter their ability to conduct sound waves. It leads to progressive conductive hearing loss — **otosclerotic** *adj.*

otoscope *n* an instrument, usually incorporating both illumination and magnification. It is used to examine the external ear, tympanic membrane and, through the tympanic membrane, the middle ear ossicles. Also known as an auriscope.

otoscopy *n* the examination of the external ear and tympanic membrane using an otoscope.

ototoxic *adj* having a toxic action on the ear or vestibulocochlear nerves, such as aminoglycoside antibiotics and aspirin.

outcome *n* a word which can be used synonymously with patient goal or objective. It implies the measurable outcome which is expected from implementing the planned nursing intervention.

outflow obstruction usually refers to the passage of urine and may be caused by prostatic enlargement, urethral stenosis or stricture or bladder stone.

ovarian *adj* pertaining to the ovaries. *ovarian cyst* a tumour of the ovary, usually containing fluid; may be benign or malignant. It may reach a large size and can twist on its stalk creating an acute emergency surgical condition.

ovarian cycle *n* the events occurring in the ovary during follicular development and oogenesis. There are two phases: follicular, which includes ovulation (days 1–14), and the luteal phase (days 15–28). The cycle is controlled by the gonadotrophins: follicle stimulating hormone and luteinizing hormone. ⇒ menstrual cycle.

ovariectomy *n* ⇒ oophorectomy.

ovariotomy *n* literally means incision of an ovary, but usually applied to the removal of an ovary (oophorectomy).

ovaritis *n* ⇒ oophoritis.

ovary *n* a female gonad. One of two small oval structures situated on either side of the uterus on the posterior surface of the broad ligament. Under the cyclical influence of pituitary hormones they produce oocytes (ova) and ovarian hormones. *polycystic ovaries* ⇒ Stein-Leventhal syndrome. ⇒ oestrogens. ⇒ progesterones. ⇒ ovum — **ovaries** *pl*.

over-the-counter drugs/medicines (OTC) medicines which can be sold over-the-counter without a prescription. Countries vary as to which drugs are included in this category. ⇒ drug → general sales list.

overcompensation *n* describes any type of behaviour which a person adopts in order to cover up a deficiency. Thus a person who is afraid may react by becoming arrogant or boastful or quarrelsome.

overheads the cost of services that contribute to the general upkeep and running of the organization, e.g. grounds maintenance, that cannot be linked directly to the core activity of a department.

ovulation *n* the maturation and rupture of a Graafian follicle with the discharge of a secondary oocyte from the surface of the ovary.

ovum *n* the female gamete or reproductive cell. Strictly speaking, it is known as a secondary oocyte until penetration by a spermatozoon. *ovum donation* ova are retrieved from a donor following super-ovulation and donated to help another woman achieve a pregnancy, combined with IVF techniques — **ova** *pl*.

oxalates salts of oxalic acid.

oxalic acid poisonous organic acid found in rhubarb leaves and other plants. ⇒ oxalates.

oxaluria *n* the presence of oxalates in the urine. ⇒ hyperoxaluria.

Oxford grading system used for assessing pelvic floor strength for patients with genuine stress incontinence, prior to designing an individual pelvic floor exercise plan.

oxicams *npl* a group of nonsteroidal anti-inflammatory drugs, e.g. piroxicam.

oxidase *n* any enzyme which promotes oxidation.

oxidation *n* the act of oxidizing or state of being oxidized. It involves the addition of oxygen, such as the formation of oxides or the loss of electrons (an increase of positive charges on an atom or molecule) or the removal of hydrogen. Oxidation must be accompanied by reduction of an acceptor molecule. Part of the process of metabolism, resulting in the release of energy from fuel molecules. ⇒ reduction.

oxidative phosphorylation an energy-producing metabolic process occurring in the mitochondria, whereby a phosphate group is added to adenosine diphosphate (ADP) to produce adenosine triphosphate (ATP).

oximeter *n* a device for measuring haemoglobin oxygen saturation. ⇒ oxygenation. ⇒ pulse oximetry.

oxygen (O) *n* a colourless, odourless, gaseous element; necessary for life and supports combustion. Constitutes 20–21% of atmospheric air. Used medicinally as an inhalation, when precautions must be taken against fire. Usually supplied via a piped system and occasionally in cylinders (black with a white top) in which the gas is at a high pressure. *oxygen administration* used to increase blood oxygenation by various means including: mask, nasal cannulae and via a tracheostomy or endotracheal tube. ⇒ hyperbaric oxygen therapy. *oxygen concentrator* a device for removing nitrogen from the air to provide a high concentration of oxygen. Used in the community for patients requiring oxygen therapy for many hours per day. *oxygen debt*

315

or deficit occurs when the metabolic demand for oxygen exceeds supply, such as during strenuous exercise. The resultant anaerobic utilization of fuel molecules leads to an accumulation of metabolites including lactic acid which accounts for aching muscles after exercise.

oxygen consumption (VO$_2$) also called oxygen uptake. It is the rate at which the tissues are able to remove oxygen from the blood.

oxygen delivery (DO$_2$) the amount of oxygen delivered to the tissues which depends on the cardiac output, haemoglobin level and haemoglobin saturation.

oxygen dissociation *n* each of the four haem groups of a haemoglobin molecule has a different affinity for oxygen, which produces a sigmoid-shaped dissociation curve. It indicates the ease at which the haem groups give up their oxygen to the tissues, which also depends on temperature, pH and carbon dioxide tension. ⇒ Bohr effect.

oxygenation *n* the saturation of a substance (particularly of haemoglobin to form oxyhaemoglobin) with oxygen. Arterial oxygen tension (*P*aO$_2$) indicates degree of oxygenation; reference range 12–15 kPa. Arterial blood is normally >97% saturated. ⇒ pulse oximetry — **oxygenated** *adj.*

oxygenator *n* a device used to oxygenate the blood during open heart surgery, or to support critically ill patients. ⇒ cardiac bypass. ⇒ cardiopulmonary bypass.

oxyhaemoglobin *n* oxygenated haemoglobin, an unstable compound formed by the combination of haemoglobin and oxygen from exposure to alveolar air in the lungs.

oxyntic *adj* producing acid. *oxyntic cells* the cells in the gastric mucosa which produce hydrochloric acid and intrinsic factor. Also known as parietal cells.

oxytocic *adj, n* hastening parturition; an agent promoting uterine contractions, e.g. oxytocin, prostaglandins and ergometrine.

oxytocin *n* one of the posterior pituitary hormones. Causes contraction of uterine muscle. Synthetic preparation Syntocinon is used for the induction and augmentation of labour, often combined with ergometrine and used in the active man-

agement of the third stage of labour, and for the prevention and treatment of postpartum haemorrhage. Also causes contraction of the milk ducts and is part of the milk ejection reflex.

Oxyuris *n* a genus of nematodes (threadworms). Also called Enterobius.

ozone *n* a form of oxygen, O$_3$. Has powerful oxidizing properties and is therefore antiseptic and disinfectant. It is both irritating and toxic in the pulmonary system.

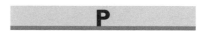

P

PAC *abbr* premature atrial contraction. ⇒ extrasystole.

pacemaker *n* the region of the heart which initiates atrial contraction and thus controls heart rate. The natural pacemaker is the sinoatrial node which is situated at the opening of the superior vena cava into the right atrium; the wave of contraction begins here, then spreads over the heart. *artificial pacemaker* ⇒ cardiac.

pachycephalia *n* a thick skull.

pachydermia *n* thick skin. ⇒ elephantiasis.

pachymeningitis *n* inflammation of the dura mater.

pacing occupational therapy techniques that help people to perform tasks in a pre-planned way, adhering to personal targets, using task analysis, activity and rest and different movements to achieve maximum performance and reduce adverse effects, such as pain, tiredness and joint stress.

packed cell volume (PCV) *n* the volume of red cells in the blood, expressed as a percentage of the total blood volume. Also known as the haematocrit.

PaCO$_2$ *abbr* the partial pressure or tension of carbon dioxide in arterial blood. The normal range is 4.4–6.1 kPa.

PACO$_2$ *abbr* the partial pressure of carbon dioxide in alveolar air.

PACT *abbr* Prescribing Analysis and Costs.

PADL *abbr* Personal Activities of Daily Living. ⇒ Activities of Daily Living.

paediatric advanced life support (PALS) ⇒ advanced life support. ⇒ Broselow paediatric resuscitation system.

paediatric intensive care unit (PICU) unit that provides dedicated intensive care for children. It is staffed by healthcare professionals with the necessary qualifications, skills and experience to meet the specialized needs of seriously ill children.

paediatrician *n* a specialist in children's diseases.

paediatrics *n* the branch of medicine dealing with children and their diseases — **paediatric** *adj*.

paedophilia *n* sexual attraction to children — **paedophiliac** *adj*. ⇒ abuse. ⇒ incest.

PAFC *abbr* pulmonary artery flotation catheter.

Paget's disease 1. (*syn* osteitis deformans) a disease of unknown aetiology with irregular softening and thickening of various bones, e.g. skull, pelvis, femur and tibia. There is bone resorption, rapid bone formation and high turnover with an excess of the enzyme alkaline phosphatase. There is loss of stature, crippling deformity, enlarged head, collapse of vertebrae and neurological complications can result. Sarcoma development may occur. **2.** inflammatory eczematous lesion of the nipple associated with breast cancer.

pain *n* distressing sensation felt when certain nerve endings (nociceptors) are stimulated. It is unique and subjective consisting of the physiological sensation and the emotional response. Pain varies in intensity from mild to agonizing, but individual responses are influenced by factors which include: knowledge about cause, location, age, associated conditions, whether acute or chronic and pain tolerance. *pain threshold* the lowest intensity at which a stimulus is felt as pain. It varies very little between individuals. *pain tolerance* the greatest intensity of pain that the individual is prepared to endure. This varies considerably between individuals. ⇒ gate control theory. ⇒ pain assessment. ⇒ pain management. ⇒ phantom pain. ⇒ referred pain.

pain assessment an important function of the nurse's role, and may be especially difficult with adults, children and infants who are unable to articulate their pain experience. Nurses should take account of the biological, psychological and social dimensions of pain. There are several pain assessment tools. Most of them include a longitudinal scale, at one end of which is 0 for 'no pain', and at the other 10 for 'the pain is as bad as it could possibly be'. The patient points to the number which equates with the current experience of pain. Several pain assessment tools have been developed for use with children of varying ages, e.g. 'faces scale', in which the child points to the facial expression corresponding to his pain experience. (See Figure 46).

pain management involves a multidisciplinary approach, and in some healthcare settings there is a nurse specialist or a designated pain team. Holistic management includes the consideration of the physical, psychological, emotional, spiritual and social aspects of pain. It requires staff education, a structured approach, adequate information and education for patients and regular assessment.

painful arc syndrome pain in the shoulder and upper arm as it is actively abducted.

painter's colic ⇒ colic.

PAL *acr* physical activity level.

palate *n* the roof of the mouth. *cleft palate* ⇒ cleft palate. *hard palate* the front part of the roof of the mouth formed by the two palatine bones. *soft palate* the posterior part of the palate consisting of muscle covered by mucous membrane. ⇒

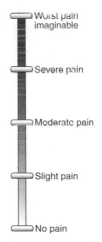

Worst pain imaginable

Severe pain

Moderate pain

Slight pain

No pain

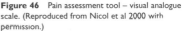

Figure 46 Pain assessment tool – visual analogue scale. (Reproduced from Nicol et al 2000 with permission.)

uvula — **palatal, palatine** *adj* pertaining to the palate. *palatine arches* the bilateral double pillars or arch-like folds formed by the descent of the soft palate as it meets the pharynx. *palatine bones* two bones of the face forming the hard palate and part of the nose and orbit. *palatine tonsils* paired masses of lymphoid tissue situated in the oropharynx. Form part of body defences.

palatoplegia *n* paralysis of the soft palate — **palatoplegic** *adj*.

palliative *adj, n* (describes) anything which serves to alleviate, but cannot cure, a disease. Palliative care may involve surgical procedures, such as stent insertion into the bile ducts, radiotherapy to reduce pain, and chemotherapy, as well as symptom control, e.g. drugs to manage pain and vomiting — **palliation** *n*.

pallidectomy *n* destruction of a predetermined section of globus pallidus. ⇒ chemopallidectomy. ⇒ stereotactic surgery.

palm *n* the anterior or flexor surface of the hand — **palmar** *adj* pertaining to the palm of the hand. *palmar arches* superficial and deep, are formed by the anastomosis of the radial and ulnar arteries.

palpable *adj* capable of being palpated or felt by manual examination.

palpation *n* the act of manual examination — **palpate** *vt*.

palpebra *n* an eyelid — **palpebral** *adj*.

palpitation *n* rapid forceful beating of the heart of which the patient is aware.

PALS *acr* paediatric advanced life support.

palsy *n* paralysis. A word which is only retained in compound forms – Bell's palsy, cerebral palsy and Erb's palsy.

panarteritis inflammation affecting all layers of an artery.

panarthritis *n* inflammation of all the structures of a joint.

pancarditis *n* inflammation of all the structures of the heart. ⇒ endocarditis. ⇒ myocarditis. ⇒ pericarditis.

pancreas *n* a dual purpose tongue-shaped glandular organ lying below and behind the stomach. It has a head encircled by the duodenum, a body and a tail. It is about 18 cm long and weighs about 100 g. In its endocrine role it secretes several hormones including insulin and glucagon which control blood sugar. The exocrine role involves producing an alkaline pancreatic juice which contains enzymes involved in the digestion of fats, proteins and carbohydrates in the small intestine. ⇒ islets of Langerhans.

pancreatectomy *n* excision of part or the whole of the pancreas.

pancreatic function test pancreatic exocrine function can be directly assessed via a double-lumen tube positioned in the stomach and the second part of the duodenum. Pancreatic secretions are collected after the administration of intravenous hormones (secretin–cholecystokinin test). Alternatively, a simple tube can be used to collect pancreatic secretions following a liquid meal of known composition.

pancreaticoduodenectomy *n* surgical excision of part of the pancreas and duodenum, carried out for cancer of the ampulla of Vater. ⇒ ampulla.

pancreatitis *n* inflammation of the pancreas. *acute pancreatitis* usually associated with biliary disease or alcohol misuse. Characterized by severe abdominal and back pain, nausea and vomiting, tachycardia, hypotension, tachypnoea, hypoxia and an elevated serum amylase. It is a serious illness with a mortality of 10–20% and is associated with complications, such as renal failure and shock. Management includes: pain relief, fluid replacement, careful monitoring and supportive measures, such as mechanical ventilation. Surgery may be required to deal with haemorrhage, abscess formation and where biliary problems exist. *chronic pancreatitis* chronic inflammation following acute attacks. Pancreatic failure can lead to diabetes mellitus and pancreatic exocrine insufficiency. Replacement of insulin and pancreatic enzymes will be required.

pancreatrophic *adj* having an affinity for or an influence on the pancreas.

pancreozymin *n* an intestinal hormone, identical to cholecystokinin (CCK) which is the name generally used. It stimulates pancreatic exocrine secretion.

pancytopenia *n* describes peripheral blood picture when red cells, granular white cells and platelets are reduced, as occurs in suppression of bone marrow function.

pandemic *n* an epidemic spreading over a wide area, such as a whole country or the world.

panic attacks sudden overwhelming attacks of extreme fear and anxiety. Associated with anxiety states and other mental health problems.

pannus *n* corneal vascularization, often associated with conjunctival irritation.

panophthalmia, panophthalmitis *n* generalized inflammation of the eyeball.

panosteitis *n* inflammation of all constituents of a bone – medulla, bony tissue and periosteum.

panproctocolectomy *n* ⇒ proctocolectomy.

PANSS *abbr* Positive and Negative Syndrome Scale.

pantothenic acid a constituent of the vitamin B complex. Needed as part of acetyl coenzyme A.

PaO₂ *abbr* the partial pressure or tension of oxygen in arterial blood. The normal range is 12–15 kPa.

PAO₂ *abbr* the partial pressure of oxygen in alveolar air.

Papanicolaou test Pap test. A smear of epithelial cells is taken from the cervix with a brush or spatula, stained and cytologically examined to detect abnormal cervical cells. ⇒ cervical intraepithelial neoplasia.

papilla *n* a minute nipple-shaped eminence. *dermal papilla* projection of the dermis into the epidermis. *optic papilla* ⇒ optic disc. *tongue papilla* projection on the tongue surface containing the taste buds — **papillary** *adj* pertaining to papilla. *papillary muscle* tiny muscles which, with the chordae tendineae, help to stabilize the atrioventricular valves of the heart.

papillitis *n* 1. inflammation of the optic disc. 2. inflammation of a papilla.

papilloedema *n* (*syn* choked disc) oedema of the optic disc; suggestive of increased intracranial pressure.

papilloma *n* a simple benign tumour arising from epithelial cells — **papillomatous** *pl*.

papillomatosis *n* the growth of benign papillomata on the skin or a mucous membrane. Removal by laser means fewer recurrences.

papovaviruses *npl* a family of DNA viruses that includes the papilloma viruses. ⇒ human papilloma virus.

papule *n* (*syn* pimple) a small circumscribed elevation of the skin — **papular** *adj*.

papulopustular *adj* pertaining to both papules and pustules, such as a rash containing both.

papulosquamous a skin condition characterized by papules and scales.

PAR *abbr* physical activity ratio.

para-aminobenzoic acid (PABA) 1. filters the ultraviolet rays from the sun, and in a cream or lotion protects the skin from sunburn or harmful exposure to sunlight. 2. an essential metabolite (part of the folic acid molecule) needed for the growth of many micro-organisms.

para-aortic *adj* near the aorta, such as lymph nodes.

paracentesis *n* ⇒ aspiration **paracenteses** *pl*.

paracetamol *n* a nonsteroidal anti-inflammatory drug with analgesic and antipyretic properties, but, having virtually no anti-inflammatory effects, it is of no value in rheumatoid joint disease. Does not cause indigestion or gastric bleeding. Overdose causes potentially life-threatening liver failure. The antidotes are acetylcysteine and methionine.

paracrines hormone like substances which have a local regulatory role, e.g. gastrin and gastric secretion.

paradigm an example, pattern, model or set of assumptions. *paradigm shift* the changes occurring as the accumulation of evidence causes a paradigm to be questioned and eventually discarded for a new set of ideas.

paradoxical respiration ⇒ respiration.

paradoxical sleep (*syn* REM sleep) ⇒ sleep.

paraesthesia *n* any abnormality of sensation, such as tingling and 'pins and needles'.

paraffin *n* medicinal paraffins are: *liquid paraffin* ⇒ laxative. *soft paraffin* the familiar ointment base. *hard paraffin* used in wax baths for rheumatic conditions.

paraffin gauze dressing a nonadhesive dressing for wounds. Gauze impregnated with soft paraffin and sterilized.

parainfluenzavirus *n* causes acute upper respiratory infection. One of the myxoviruses.

paralysis *n* complete or incomplete loss of nervous function to a part of the body. This may be sensory or motor or both. *flaccid paralysis* mainly due to lower motor neuron lesions; there is loss of muscle tone and tendon reflexes are absent. *spastic paralysis* affected muscles are rigid and tendon reflexes are exaggerated; usually results from an upper motor neuron lesion. ⇒ monoplegia. ⇒ paraplegia. ⇒ tetraplegia.

paralytic *adj* pertaining to paralysis. *paralytic ileus* paralysis of the intestinal muscle so that the bowel content cannot pass onwards even though there is no mechanical obstruction. ⇒ aperistalsis. ⇒ ileus.

paramedian *adj* near the middle.

paramedical *adj* allied to medicine.

paramenstruum *n* the four days before the start of menstruation and the first four days of the period itself.

parameter 1. statistical or mathematical measure of a population characteristic, e.g. mean, standard deviation. **2.** a numerically measurable property, e.g. blood sugar. **3.** general term meaning limits or constraints.

parametric tests statistical tests that assume the data are from a sample from a population that has a normal distribution curve. See Box – Parametric and nonparametric tests.

parametritis *n* inflammation of the cellular tissue adjacent to the uterus.

parametrium *n* the connective tissues immediately surrounding the uterus — **parametrial** *adj.*

paramyxoviruses subgroup of myxoviruses that cause diseases such as measles and mumps.

paranasal *adj* near the nasal cavity. *paranasal sinus* ⇒ sinus.

paranoia *n* a mental disorder characterized by the insidious onset of delusions of persecution — **paranoid** *adj.*

paranoid relating to paranoia. *paranoid behaviour* acts denoting suspicion of others. *paranoid personality* an individual who is mistrustful and abnormally sensitive to the reaction of others.

paranoid schizophrenia a form of schizophrenia dominated by delusions and, to a lesser extent, hallucinations.

paraoesophageal *adj* near the oesophagus.

paraphimosis *n* retraction of the prepuce behind the glans penis so that the tight ring of skin interferes with the blood flow in the glans. ⇒ circumcision.

paraphrenia *n* a mental illness affecting older people, characterized by well-circumscribed delusions, usually of a persecutory nature — **paraphrenic** *adj.*

paraplegia *n* paralysis of the lower limbs and trunk with motor and sensory loss. Depending on the level of the spinal lesion, it may include loss of bladder and bowel function. Causes include: trauma – sporting injuries, road traffic accidents, falls and diseases, such as tumours — **paraplegic** *adj.*

Parametric and nonparametric tests

Any statistical test makes some assumptions about the data. A group of tests, so called parametric tests, assume the data are normally distributed, i.e. the histogram of values shows a bell shaped curve, with most values lying close to the middle of the distribution, and increasingly extreme values seen with increasingly lower frequency. However, not all data are normally distributed, and then these tests should not be applied (in most cases), but an equivalent nonparametric test which does not assume a normal distribution is to be preferred. Parametric tests are more powerful than nonparametric tests, and if the data support them, parametric tests are preferred.

Example – the researcher wants to test the hypothesis that mental health branch students score lower than adult branch nursing students. They create a histogram and see the data appear normally distributed. The researcher chooses the parametric test Student's t test for independent groups, and finds that their hypothesis is rejected, i.e. they score significantly differently (higher say) than adult branch. If the data had not been normally distributed the researcher would have used the nonparametric test Mann Whitney, which does the same thing (tests whether two groups differ with respect to some, at least ordinal, measurement).

paraprax known as a 'Freudian slip'. It is a verbal error caused by unconscious conflicts.

parapsychology *n* the study of extrasensory perception, telepathy, psychokinesis and other psychic phenomena.

paraquat dichloride *n* chemical widely used as a herbicide. Exposure leads to local effects depending on the route, but include: skin blistering, epistaxis, or severe inflammation of the conjunctiva or cornea, damage to the mouth and oesophagus. Systemic effects that may be delayed are usually associated with ingestion and include damage to the lungs, myocardium, liver and kidneys.

pararectal *adj* near the rectum.

parasitaemia *n* parasites in the blood — **parasitaemic** *adj*.

parasite *n* an organism which obtains food or shelter from another organism, the 'host'. ⇒ commensals — **parasitic** *adj*.

parasiticide *n* an agent which will kill parasites, e.g. mebendazole.

parasomnias *npl* a broad class of disturbances around sleep; it includes behaviours such as sleepwalking, nightmares and bruxism.

parasuicide *n* also known as deliberate self-harm (DSH). A suicidal gesture; an act, such as self-mutilation or drug overdose, which may or may not be motivated by a genuine desire to die. It is common in young people who are distressed but not mentally ill. It may be associated with low self-esteem. ⇒ Samaritans.

parasympathetic nervous system *adj* part of the peripheral nervous system (PNS), it describes the division of the autonomic nervous system (ANS) having craniosacral outflow. Opposing the sympathetic nervous system, it is mainly concerned with 'normal' at rest processes such as digestion. ⇒ sympathetic nervous system.

parasympatholytic *adj* muscarinic antagonist. Describes an agent, usually a drug, that reduces or eliminates the effects of parasympathetic stimulation, e.g. atropine.

parasympathomimetic *adj* muscarinic agonist. Describes an agent, such as a drug, that produces the same effects as or causes parasympathetic activity.

parathion *n* an organophosphorus insecticide used in agriculture. Has a powerful and irreversible anticholinesterase action.

parathormone *n* ⇒ parathyroid hormone.

parathyroid glands *npl* four small endocrine glands lying close to or embedded in the posterior surface of the thyroid gland. They secrete a hormone, parathyroid hormone (PTH), which helps to maintain a normal serum calcium level in association with calcitonin and vitamin D.

parathyroid hormone (PTH) *n* the protein hormone secreted by the parathyroid glands. It is vital in the regulation of calcium and phosphate homeostasis and is released when serum calcium level falls. It raises serum calcium and reduces phosphate levels in several ways: (a) by stimulating the reabsorption of calcium and phosphate from bone; (b) by causing the kidney to reabsorb more calcium and excrete phosphates; (c) increasing calcium absorption in the bowel. ⇒ calcitonin.

parathyroidectomy *n* excision of one or more parathyroid glands.

paratracheal *adj* near the trachea.

paratyphoid fever an infectious enteric fever caused by the bacterium *Salmonella paratyphi* A and B which usually originates from animals. Transmission is by the faecal-oral route and humans may become infected by direct contact with animals, such as poultry, or indirectly via contaminated food, water or milk. Food may become contaminated by food handlers who are carriers. It tends to be less severe and of shorter duration than typhoid fever. The presentation includes: fever, headaches, myalgia, acute enteritis with vomiting and diarrhoea and a rash. Intestinal complications are less common than with typhoid.

paraurethral *adj* near the urethra.

paravaginal *adj* near the vagina.

paraventricular nucleus *n* a hypothalamic nucleus with nerve fibres extending to the posterior pituitary gland. Together with the supraoptic nucleus it produces antidiuretic hormone and oxytocin.

paravertebral *adj* near the spinal column. *paravertebral block anaesthesia* (more correctly, 'analgesia') is induced by infiltration of local anaesthetic around the spinal nerve roots as they emerge from the intervertebral foramina. *paravertebral ganglia* ⇒ sympathetic chain. *paravertebral injection* of local anaesthetic into sympathetic chain; can be used as a test in ischaemic limbs to see if sympathectomy will be of value.

parenchyma *n* the parts of an organ concerned with its function, as distinct from its interstitial tissue — **parenchymal, parenchymatous** *adj*.

parenteral *adj* outside or apart from the alimentary canal/tract. Therapy such as drugs, fluids or nutrition administered by a route other than the alimentary canal/tract. *parenteral feeding* should only be used in situations where the enteral route is unsuitable. It can be used to provide total parenteral nutrition (TPN) or for supplemental nutrition. A special catheter is used to infuse various nutrient solutions into a central vein. Usually the catheter is sited centrally, through the subclavian vein into the superior vena cava. It is, however, possible to use peripherally inserted central catheters (PICC) which are inserted through the basilic vein (of the arm) to the superior vena cava via the right subclavian vein. A feeding regimen of nutrients is prescribed by the dietitian and administered using an infusion pump to regulate the flow rate. Nursing considerations include: recording accurate intake and output, strict adherence to aseptic technique, dressing the site and line flushing according to local policy, oral hygiene, proper storage of feeds, protecting feeds from sunlight to stop vitamin breakdown, ensuring that the line is only used to infuse feeds, observation for complications, such as infection and hyperglycaemia. Nurses can help patients and their families to manage parenteral feeding following discharge — **parenterally** *adv*.

paresis *n* partial or slight paralysis; weakness of a limb — **paretic** *adj*.

pareunia *n* coitus.

parietal *adj* pertaining to a wall. *parietal bones* the two bones which form the sides and vault of the skull. *parietal lobe* lobe of the cerebrum lying under the parietal bone.

parieto-occipital *adj* pertaining to the parietal bones and the occiput. Also applied to that part of the brain underlying the bones.

parity *n* status of a woman with regard to the number of children she has borne.

parkinsonism *n* a syndrome characterized by muscle rigidity, tremor and bradykinesia. It is linked to degeneration of the basal nuclei, or a deficiency of, or blockade of the neurotransmitter dopamine. There is a mask-like expression, 'pill-rolling' movements of the fingers, a shuffling gait, and patients have difficulty initiating a voluntary movement, turning and stopping. There is a distinction between idiopathic Parkinson's disease (paralysis agitans) and parkinsonism where the causes include: repeated trauma to the head (as in boxers), tumours, Wilson's disease, infection, e.g. viral encephalitis (encephalitis lethargica), various toxic agents, e.g. methyl-phenyl-tetrahydropyridine and drugs, such as phenothiazines. Management may include: anticholinergic drugs, e.g. trihexyphenidyl (benzhexol), levodopa (L-dopa), and dopamine receptor agonists such as pergolide. Patients also benefit from the interventions of a physiotherapist, speech and language therapist and occupational therapist. Surgery for tremor is sometimes helpful where drug therapy fails. Transplantation of dopamine producing tissues is being evaluated. ⇒ tardive dyskinesia.

Parkinson's disease ⇒ parkinsonism.

paronychia *n* (*syn* whitlow) inflammation around a fingernail which may be bacterial or fungal. The herpes simplex virus may also cause multiple vesicles over inflamed skin *herpetic paronychia*.

parosmia *n* disordered sense of smell; it may be hallucinatory.

parotid gland *n* the salivary gland situated in front of and below the ear on either side.

parotitis *n* inflammation of a parotid gland. *epidemic or infectious parotitis* mumps. *septic parotitis* refers to ascending infection from the mouth via the parotid duct, when a parotid abscess may result.

parous *adj* having borne a child or children.

paroxysm *n* a sudden, temporary attack.

paroxysmal *adj* coming on in attacks or paroxysms. *paroxysmal atrial tachycardia (PAT)* a period of atrial tachycardia

(150–200 beats per minute) that starts and stops suddenly. It is caused by an abnormal focus in the atrium. *paroxysmal nocturnal dyspnoea* occurs mostly at night in patients with cardiac disease. There is severe breathlessness due to pulmonary oedema resulting from left ventricular failure. *paroxysmal supraventricular tachycardia* ⇒ supraventricular tachycardia.

parrot disease ⇒ psittacosis.

partial agonist a drug that only stimulates a partial physiological effect, having less efficacy than a full agonist.

partial pressure pressure exerted by an individual gas in a mixture of gases. The pressure is directly related to its concentration and the pressure exerted by the total mixture. ⇒ Dalton's law.

partnership the working relationship between central government, local NHS, local government authority, and local communities. It enables greater co-ordination and co-operative multiagency/multi professional working that aims to improve health. ⇒ Health Action Zone ⇒ Healthy Living Centres.

parturient *adj* pertaining to childbirth.

parturition *n* labour and giving birth.

Pascal *n* a powerful computer language. ⇒ computer language.

pascal (Pa) *n* the derived SI unit (International System of Units) for pressure. The kilopascal (kPa) is increasingly used for measuring blood gases and would replace millimetres of mercury pressure (mmHg) for blood pressure.

passive *adj* inactive. ⇒ active *ant*. *passive hyperaemia* → hyperaemia. *passive immunity* ⇒ immunity. *passive movement* performed by the therapist, the patient being relaxed.

Pasteurella *n* ⇒ Yersinia.

pasteurization *n* a method that uses heat to destroy most pathogenic bacteria in milk and other fluids. *flash method of pasteurization* (HT, ST – high temperature, short time) the fluid is heated to 72°C, maintained at this temperature for 15s, then rapidly cooled. *holder method of pasteurization* the fluid is heated to 63–65.5°C, maintained at this temperature for 30 min, then rapidly cooled. Pasteurization, using moist heat, is also used to disinfect medical equipment, such as instruments.

PAT *abbr* paroxysmal atrial tachycardia.

Patau's syndrome trisomy 13. An abnormality affecting chromosomes in group D;13–15, the individual has a third chromosome 13 which results in them having 47 chromosomes. It is characterized by: central nervous system defects, learning disability, cataracts, cleft lip and palate. ⇒ trisomy.

patch test a skin test for identifying reaction to allergens which are incorporated in an adhesive patch applied to the skin. Allergy is apparent by redness and swelling.

patella *n* a triangular, sesamoid bone; the kneecap — **patellar** *adj*.

patellectomy *n* excision of the patella.

patent *adj* open, not closed or occluded. *patent ductus arteriosus* failure of ductus arteriosus to close soon after birth, so that an abnormal shunt between the pulmonary artery and the aorta is preserved. *patent foramen ovale* failure of closure of the foramen ovale, so that an opening between the right and left atria remains after birth — **patency** *n*.

paternalism restricting, over-protective, such as well-meaning rules and regulations that reduce individual autonomy.

pathogen *n* a disease-producing agent, usually restricted to a living agent — **pathogenicity** *n*.

pathogenesis *n* the origin and development of disease — **pathogenetic** *adj*.

pathogenic *adj* pertaining to an agent capable of producing disease.

pathogenicity *n* the capacity to produce disease.

pathognomonic *adj* characteristic of or peculiar to a disease.

pathology *n* the study of disease, particularly regarding the changes in tissues resulting from disease — **pathologically** *adj*.

pathophobia *n* a morbid dread of disease — **pathophobic** *adj*.

pathophysiology *n* the science which deals with the physical and biological features of disease and how these correlate with the abnormal functioning of the body — **pathophysiologically** *adv*.

patient *n* 1. designates a person whose name is on the list of a general practitioner, whether or not he or she is attending the doctor's surgery or health clinic. 2. designates a person who is attending a hospital outpatient clinic at intervals; or is being visited in his home by a district nurse; or is an inpatient in hospital. ⇒ client. ⇒ sickness certificate. ⇒ sick role. *patient advocate* this includes the notion that a nurse or other professional argues on behalf of a patient, e.g. when the patient does not want to take a prescribed drug or undergo a particular treatment. ⇒ advocacy. ⇒ ombudsman. *patient compliance or concordance* a term used for the situation when a patient follows correctly the prescribed treatment regimen. ⇒ noncompliance. *patient moving and handling* includes the safe-handling or no-lifting techniques, and encompasses many of the transfers with which nurses help patients move from one surface to another, and techniques to help patients get into and out of a bath etc, and equipment to help them with walking. ⇒ manual handling. ⇒ safe-handling or no-lifting policies. *patient participation* nurses are encouraged to interact with patients, especially in the initial assessment interview, to support, prompt, reflect and help them to give their perception of their current health problem. Identification of problems with everyday living, actual and anticipated, goal setting and interventions to achieve the goal, all require patient participation which is a criterion of good nursing practice. *patient problems* in a nursing context, those related to everyday living activities which are amenable to nurse-initiated intervention. Some other interventions to relieve a problem will be doctor prescribed and are therefore collaborative nursing interventions.

patient advocacy liaison service provides an advocacy service to patients in NHS and primary care trusts by representing their concerns and complaints to the relevant department within the trust. Depending on the necessary legislation being in place they will replace some of the functions of the CHC from 2002.

patient/client records *npl* a general term for all the health-related records held for a particular person, e.g. nursing care plan, primary care records, hospital notes. *patient held records* those health records held by individual patients. *multidisciplinary records* those health records used by several groups of health and social care professionals.

Patient's Charter introduced by the UK Government in 1991. It set out an indi-vidual's rights to treatment and national standards for care within the NHS. Now replaced by 'Your Guide to the NHS'. ⇒ named nurse. ⇒ NHS Guide.

patients' forum a statutory and independent body comprising patients. It is planned that the body will exist in every trust to represent the views of patients about how their local NHS services are run. Depending on the necessary legislation being in place they will replace some of the functions of the CHC from 2002.

patriarchy a community or family where the oldest male (father) dominates and is the highest authority.

Paul-Bunnell test a serological test used in the diagnosis of infectious mononucleosis.

Paul-Mikulicz operation a method for excision of a portion of the colon whereby the two cut ends of the bowel are kept out on the surface of the abdomen, and are joined at a later date without entering the peritoneal cavity.

Pavlov, Ivan Russian physiologist (1849–1936). ⇒ conditioned reflex. ⇒ conditioning.

PC *abbr* personal computer.

PCA(S) *abbr* patient controlled analgesia (system). ⇒ analgesia.

PCEA *abbr* patient controlled epidural analgesia. ⇒ analgesia. ⇒ epidural.

PCG *abbr* Primary Care Group.

PCM *abbr* protein-calorie malnutrition.

PCO$_2$ *abbr* the partial pressure of carbon dioxide, such as in atmospheric or expired air.

PCP *abbr* *Pneumocystis carinii* pneumonia.

PCT *abbr* Primary Care Trust.

PCV *abbr* packed cell volume.

PDP *abbr* Personal Development Plan.

peak bone density (PBD) or mass (PBM) *n* the greatest bone density, typically reached in the 30s. Affected by many factors that include: calcium intake, vitamin D, exercise, hormones, drugs and smoking.

peak expiratory flow rate (PEFR) a respiratory function test. The flow of air is measured during a forced expiration using a peak-flow meter. Used to indicate presence, severity and response to treatment of respiratory disease, especially asthma. (See Figure 47). ⇒ morning dip.

peau d'orange orange-skin appearance. A term describing the appearance of the skin of the breast in acute inflammation or in some cancers.

pectins *npl* soluble nonstarch polysaccharides (NSPs) found in some root vegetables, e.g. turnips and in fruit, such as apples. It and other soluble NSPs help to reduce the blood cholesterol level. Used for setting jam.

pectoral *adj* pertaining to the breast. *pectoral girdle* the shoulder girdle comprising the clavicles and scapulae. *pectoral muscles* on the anterior surface of the chest. The pectoralis major and pectoralis minor.

pectus *n* the chest. *pectus carinatum* ⇒ pigeon chest. *pectus excavatum* ⇒ funnel chest.

pedal *adj* pertaining to the foot. *pedal pulse* palpation of the dorsalis pedis artery on the dorsum of the foot.

pedicle *n* the stalk of an organ or tumour. Describes a type of skin graft. ⇒ flap.

pediculosis *n* infestation with lice (pediculi).

Pediculus *n* a genus of parasitic insects (lice) important as vectors of disease. *Pediculus capitis* the head louse. *Pediculus corporis* the body louse. *Pediculus* (more correctly, *Phthirius*) *pubis* the pubic or crab louse. In some parts of the world, body lice are involved in transmitting relapsing fever and typhus.

pedopompholyx *n* ⇒ cheiropompholyx.

peduncle *n* a stalk-like structure, often acting as a support. *cerebral peduncle* bulging structures of the midbrain containing the descending voluntary motor

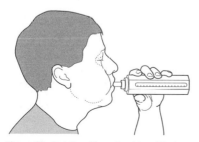

Figure 47 Peak flow. (Reproduced from Nicol et al 2000 with permission.)

tracts. *cerebellar peduncles* structures containg nerve tracts, that connect the cerebellum to the midbrain — **peduncular, pedunculated** *adj*.

peeling *n* desquamation.

PEEP *abbr* positive end expiratory pressure.

peer support support from other members of a group to which one belongs, either temporarily or permanently. It is known for instance that new patients perceive established patients as providing support. Likewise, nurses and other health professionals use their peer groups to gain and provide support, particularly in stressful circumstances.

PEFR *abbr* peak expiratory flow rate.

PEG *acr* percutaneous endoscopic gastrostomy. ⇒ gastrostomy.

Pel-Ebstein fever *n* an intermittent fever that may occur in Hodgkin's disease (lymphoma).

pellagra *n* a deficiency disease caused by lack of the B vitamin niacin and the amino acid tryptophan. It is characterized by anorexia, stomatitis, glossitis, dysphagia, diarrhoea, dermatitis (initially resembling sunburn), delirium and dementia. Management involves oral nicotinamide, nutritional assessment and the provision of a nutritious diet containing high levels of protein and B vitamins and iron.

pellet *n* a little pill. → implants.

pelvic *adj* pertaining to the pelvis. *pelvic floor* the muscles and ligaments supporting the pelvic organs. Consists of a mainly muscular partition with the pelvic cavity above and the perineum below. In the female, weakening of these muscles, e.g. after childbirth, can contribute to urinary incontinence and uterine prolapse; they can be toned with pelvic floor exercises. *pelvic girdle* the bony pelvis comprising two innominate bones, the sacrum and coccyx.

pelvic floor repair ⇒ Manchester repair.

pelvic inflammatory disease (PID) inflammatory disease of the female internal genitalia. Usually due to bacterial infection, e.g. *Chlamydia* or gonorrhoea. It affects the uterine tubes and uterus, and can lead to reduced fertility and chronic pain if not treated at an early stage.

pelvic pain syndrome pelvic pain which occurs in women but for which no pathological cause is evident. Investigation can reveal congested pelvic blood vessels which may be treated with progestogens. Counselling is also beneficial.

pelvimetry *n* the measurement of the dimensions of the pelvis — **pelvimetric** *adj.*

pelvis *n* 1. a basin-shaped cavity, e.g. pelvis of the kidney. 2. the large bony basin-shaped cavity formed by the innominate bones and sacrum, containing and protecting the bladder, rectum and, in the female, the reproductive organs. *contracted pelvis* one in which one or more diameters are smaller than normal; this may result in difficulties in childbirth. *false pelvis* the wide expanded part of the pelvis above the brim. *true pelvis* that part of the pelvis below the brim — **pelvic** *adj.*

PEM *abbr* protein-energy malnutrition.

pemphigoid *n* allied to pemphigus. A bullous eruption of autoimmune aetiology occurring in later life. Histological examination of the base of a blister differentiates it from pemphigus.

pemphigus *n* skin conditions with bullous (blister) eruptions, but more correctly used to describe a group of dangerous diseases called pemphigus vulgaris, pemphigus vegetans and pemphigus erythematosus. The latter two are rare. *pemphigus neonatorum* (a) a misnomer; it is, in fact, a very serious acute staphylococcal impetigo occurring in newborns. May cause serious epidemics in hospital neonatal units; (b) bullous eruption seen in neonates born with congenital syphilis. *pemphigus vulgaris* a bullous disease of middle-age and later, of autoimmune aetiology. Oedema of the skin results in blister formation in the epidermis, with resulting secondary infection and rupture, so that large raw areas develop. Bullae develop also on mucous membranes. Death is from malnutrition or intercurrent disease.

pendulous *adj* hanging down. *pendulous abdomen* a relaxed condition of the anterior wall, allowing it to hang down over the pubis.

penetrating ulcer an ulcer which is locally invasive and may erode a blood vessel, such as a peptic ulcer causing haematemesis or melaena.

penetrating wound (*syn* puncture wound) caused by a sharp, usually slim object, or a missile, which passes through the skin into the tissues beneath.

penicillinase *n* ⇒ beta (β)-lactamase.

penicillins *npl* large group of antibiotics that contain a beta (β)-lactam ring in their structure, e.g. benzylpenicillin, amoxicillin (amoxycillin), flucloxacillin, piperacillin etc. Many have a wide spectrum of activity but they produce hypersensitivity reactions and some bacteria have developed resistance to penicillin. Some bacteria produce beta (β)-lactamase (penicillinase) enzymes that render the drug ineffective by destroying the beta (β)-lactam ring. Newer penicillins, such as flucloxacillin, are beta (β)-lactamase resistant.

Penicillium *n* a genus of moulds. The hyphae bear spores characteristically arranged like a brush. A common contaminant of food. *Penicillium chrysogenum* is now used for the commercial production of the antibiotic. *Penicillium notatum* is a species shown by Fleming (1928) to produce penicillin.

penis *n* the male organ of copulation and urination — **penile** *adj.*

pentose *n* a sugar containing five carbon atoms, such as ribose and deoxyribose.

pentosuria *n* pentose in the urine. Associated with an inherited error of metabolism — **pentosuric** *adj.*

pepsin *n* a proteolytic enzyme secreted by the stomach in the gastric juice. Breaks down proteins to polypeptides. It is stimulated by food and has an optimum pH of 1.5–2.0.

pepsinogen *n* a proenzyme secreted mainly by the chief (zymogen) cells in the gastric mucosa and converted into pepsin by contact with hydrochloric acid (gastric acid) or pepsin itself.

peptic *adj* pertaining to pepsin or to digestion generally. *peptic ulcer* a nonmalignant ulcer in those parts of the digestive tract which are exposed to the gastric secretions; hence usually in the stomach or duodenum but sometimes in the lower oesophagus, with a Meckel's diverticulum or in the jejunum following surgical anastomosis to the stomach.

peptidases *npl* enzymes that split proteins into amino acids. ⇒ aminopeptidases. ⇒ dipeptidases.

peptides *npl* low molecular weight organic compounds formed from two or more amino acids, e.g. dipeptides, tripeptides and polypeptides. *peptide bond* a chemical bond formed in a dehydration reaction between two amino acids to form peptides.

peptones *npl* large fragments produced when a proteolytic enzyme (e.g. pepsin) or an acid acts upon a protein during the first stage of protein digestion.

percept the mental product of a sensation; a sensation plus memories of similar sensations and their relationships.

perception *n* the reception of a conscious impression through the senses by which we distinguish objects one from another and recognize their qualities according to the different sensations they produce.

percolation *n* the process by which fluid slowly passes through a hard but porous substance.

percussion *n* a diagnostic method. Tapping to determine the resonance or dullness of the area examined. Normally a finger of the left hand is laid on the patient's skin and the middle finger of the right hand is used to strike the left finger.

percutaneous *adj* through the skin. *percutaneous endoscopic gastrostomy (PEG)* a gastroscope is used to aid the insertion of a feeding tube into the stomach which exits via the abdominal wall. *percutaneous myocardial revascularization* a treatment for angina. A catheter with laser energy source is introduced into the heart via the femoral artery. The laser is used to produce channels through to the myocardium, thus allowing more oxygenated blood to reach the heart muscle. *percutaneous nephrolithotomy* ⇒ nephrolithotomy. *percutaneous transhepatic cholangiography* ⇒ cholangiography.

perforation *n* a hole in an intact sheet of tissue. Used in reference to perforation of the tympanic membrane, or the wall of the stomach or gut (perforating ulcer), constituting a surgical emergency.

Performance Indicators (PIs) quantitative measures of the activities and resources used in delivering health care. High level performance indicators, e.g. deaths from all causes (people aged 15–64), early detection of cancer, cost-effective prescribing, day case rate, can-

celled operations, conceptions under age 16 etc, and clinical indicators, e.g. deaths in hospital after surgery, a heart attack or hip fracture etc, are used to assess the six areas of the National Framework for Assessing Performance.

performance skills those skills needed for the successful performance of the social and occupational roles that individuals have assumed.

perfusion the flow of blood through a tissue or organ, e.g. lung, kidney etc.

perianal *adj* surrounding the anus.

periarterial *adj* surrounding an artery.

periarteritis *n* inflammation of the outer sheath of an artery and the periarterial tissue. *periarteritis nodosa* ⇒ polyarteritis.

periarthritis *n* inflammation of the structures surrounding a joint. Sometimes applied to frozen shoulder.

periarticular *adj* surrounding a joint.

pericardectomy *n* surgical removal of the pericardium.

pericardiocentesis *n* aspiration of the pericardial sac.

pericarditis *n* acute or chronic inflammation of the pericardium. It may or may not be accompanied by an effusion and formation of adhesions between the two layers. Causes include: myocardial infarction, viral or bacterial infection, rheumatic fever, malignancy, trauma and uraemia. ⇒ Broadbent's sign. → cardiac tamponade. ⇒ Dressler's syndrome. ⇒ pericardiocentesis.

pericardium *n* the double serous membrane which forms a sac that envelops the heart. There are two layers: an outer fibrous sac which is lined with serous membrane (parietal layer) and a visceral layer (also called the epicardium) which is part of the wall of the heart. Between the two is a potential space (pericardial cavity), which normally contains a small amount of serous fluid which prevents friction as the heart contracts. The fibrous layer protects the heart and prevents over-distension. ⇒ tamponade — **pericardial** *adj* pertaining to the pericardium. *pericardial adhesions* fibrosis following inflammation causes the two layers to adhere. *pericardial effusion* abnormal collection of fluid between the two layers.

pericardotomy *n* an opening into the pericardium.

perichondritis *n* condition affecting the pinna; can result in gross deformity of the ear. Caused by a pyogenic infection of the perichondrium or a progressive systemic condition in which elastic cartilage elsewhere in the body is affected.

perichondrium *n* the membranous covering of cartilage — **perichondrial** *adj*.

pericolic *adj* around the colon, such as local abscess formation, commonly associated with diverticulitis.

pericranium *n* the periosteal covering of the cranium — **pericranial** *adj*.

perifollicular *adj* around a follicle.

perilymph *n* the fluid contained in the internal ear, between the bony and membranous labyrinth.

perimetrium *n* the peritoneal covering of the uterus — **perimetrial** *adj*.

perimysium *n* fibrous connective tissue which encloses bundles of muscle fibres.

perinatal *adj* relating to the time around birth. The weeks before a birth, the birth and the week following birth. ⇒ mortality. ⇒ stillbirth.

perineal toilet the term usually applies to the female perineum. Girls from an early age should learn to cleanse the area from front to back so that faecal bacteria do not gain entry to the urinary bladder (via the short urethra), where they are pathogenic and cause infection. ⇒ cystitis. ⇒ urinary tract infection.

perineometer *n* a pressure gauge inserted into the vagina to register the strength of contraction in the pelvic floor muscles.

perineorrhaphy *n* an operation for the repair of a torn perineum.

perineotomy *n* episiotomy.

perinephric *adj* surrounding the kidney.

perineum *n* or perineal body. Wedge-shaped structure lying between the external genitalia and the rectum. Consists of muscle and connective tissue covered with skin — **perineal** *adj*.

perineurium *n* the sheath of connective tissue around a bundle of nerve fibres.

periodic breathing a period of apnoea in a newborn baby of 5–10 seconds, followed by a period of hyperventilation at a rate of 50–60 breaths a minute, for a period of 10–15 seconds. The overall respiratory rate remains between 30 and 40 breaths per minute. Apnoea occurs quite frequently in very low birthweight babies, often without definite cause. Attacks are only a problem if they are prolonged and do not respond to simple stimulation.

periodontal *adj* pertaining to the tissues around the teeth. *periodontal disease* an inflammatory disease of the periodontal tissues, resulting in the gradual loss of the supporting membrane and bone around the root of the tooth and a deepened gingival sulcus or periodontal pocket. ⇒ pyorrhoea. *periodontal membrane (ligament)* fibrous tissue attaching the tooth to the socket.

perionychia *n* red and painful swelling around nail fold. Common in hands that are much in water or have poor circulation. Due to infection from the fungus *Candida*. More common now because of the use of antibiotics which subdue organisms that previously curtailed the activity of *Candida*. Secondary infection can occur.

perioperative *adj* refers to the period during which a surgical operation is carried out, as well as to the pre and post-operative periods.

perioral *adj* around the mouth.

periorbital *adj* area around the eye socket.

periosteum *n* the membrane which covers a bone. In long bones only the shaft as far as the epiphyses is covered. It is protective and essential for regeneration — **periosteal** *adj*.

periostitis *n* inflammation of the periosteum. *diffuse periostitis* that involving the periosteum of long bones. *haemorrhagic periostitis* that accompanied by bleeding between the periosteum and the bone.

peripheral *adj* pertaining to the outer parts of an organ or of the body. *peripheral nervous system (PNS)* a general term for that part of the nervous system outside the brain and spinal cord. Usually reserved for those nerves which supply the musculoskeletal system and surrounding tissues to differentiate from the autonomic nervous system. *peripheral resistance* the force exerted by the arteriolar walls which is an important factor in the control of normal blood pressure. *peripheral vascular disease (PVD)* any abnormal condition arising in the blood vessels outside the heart, the main one being atherosclerosis, which can lead to thrombosis and occlusion of the vessel resulting in gangrene. *peripheral vision* that surrounding the central field of vision.

periportal *adj* surrounding the hepatic portal vein.

periproctitis *n* inflammation around the rectum and anus.

perirenal *adj* around the kidney.

perisplenitis *n* inflammation of the peritoneal coat of the spleen and of the adjacent structures.

peristalsis *n* the rhythmic wave-like contraction and dilatation occurring in a hollow tube, such as the gastrointestinal tract and ureter. The characteristic movement of the intestines by which the contents (food and waste) are moved along the lumen. It consists of a wave of contraction preceded by a wave of relaxation — **peristaltic** *adj*.

peritoneoscopy ⇒ laparoscopy.

peritoneum *n* the delicate serous membrane which lines the abdominal and pelvic cavities and also covers the organs contained in them (see Figure 48). See Box – Peritoneum. ⇒ mesentery. ⇒ mesocolon. ⇒ omentum — **peritoneal** *adj* pertaining to the peritoneum. *peritoneal dialysis* ⇒ dialysis.

peritonitis *n* inflammation of the peritoneum which may be bacterial or chemical. Results from: a perforated organ, intestinal obstruction, visceral inflammation, penetrating abdominal wounds and blood-borne infections. It may be generalized or local with the formation of an abscess, e.g. pelvic or subphrenic.

peritonsillar abscess quinsy. Acute inflammation of the tonsil and surrounding loose tissue, with abscess formation. It is characterized by severe sore throat, fever, dysphagia, otalgia, voice changes and sometimes difficulty opening the mouth (trismus). ⇒ tonsillitis.

peritrichous *adj* applied to bacteria which possess flagella on all sides of the cell. ⇒ Bacillus.

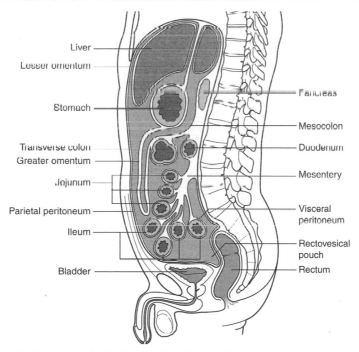

Figure 48 The peritoneum (male). (Reproduced from Brooker 1998 with permission.)

> **Peritoneum**
> The peritoneum is the largest serous membrane in the body. The visceral peritoneum covers the organs of the abdomen while the parietal peritoneum lines the abdominal wall. The potential space between the two layers of the peritoneum, the peritoneal cavity, contains peritoneal fluid. If the peritoneal fluid becomes infected this is called peritonitis which is an extremely painful and life threatening condition. It is possible to develop peritonitis after surgery and the nurse must observe patients postoperatively for the development of this condition. It is evident if the patient is in pain with a rapid pulse (tachycardia) and low blood pressure (hypotension), as in shock. There are four major divisions of the peritoneum in the body – these are the greater omentum, the lesser omentum, the mesocolon and the mesentery. These 'folds' of the peritoneum join certain parts of the digestive system together such as the stomach and the large intestine in the case of the greater omentum. Other folds of the peritoneum anchor parts of the digestive system in the abdomen, for example, the mesocolon holds the large intestine to the posterior abdominal wall while allowing it flexibility to expand and move as digested food passes along it.

perityphlitis *n* inflammation around the appendix and caecum.

periumbilical *adj* surrounding the umbilicus.

periurethral *adj* surrounding the urethra, as a periurethral abscess.

perivascular *adj* around a blood vessel.

perléche *n* dryness and cracking at the angles of the mouth with maceration, fissuring, or crust formation. May result from persistent lip licking or poorly fitting dentures, bacterial infection, fungal infection, vitamin B deficiency, drooling or thumb-sucking. ⇒ cheilosis.

permeability *n* in physiology, the extent to which substances dissolved in the body fluids are able to pass through the membranes of cells or layers of cells (e.g. the walls of capillary blood vessels, or secretory or absorptive tissues).

permeable *adj* pervious; permitting passage of a substance.

pernicious *adj* deadly, noxious. *pernicious anaemia* ⇒ anaemia.

perniosis *n* chronic chilblains. The smaller arterioles go into spasm readily from exposure to cold.

peromelia *n* a teratogenic malformation of a limb.

peroneal *adj* pertaining to the fibula or outer aspect of the leg. Applied to nerve and muscles of the lower leg.

peroral *adj* through the mouth.

peroxide *n* hydrogen peroxide.

perseveration *n* constant repetition of irrelevant words or phrases. It may be a characteristic of some mental health problems and of some types of dysphasia. ⇒ echolalia.

persistent generalized lymphadenopathy (PGL) palpable lymph node enlargement (>1 cm in diameter) at two distinct sites which persists for more than 3 months in the absence of an identifiable cause other than HIV infection. Patients are usually asymptomatic, but some may present with loss of weight and fever. ⇒ acquired immune deficiency syndrome.

persistent vegetative state (PVS) the totally dependent state occurring when the cerebral cortex is irreparably damaged, but the brainstem, which controls vital functions, continues to function. The individual, who appears awake, is unresponsive and unable to initiate any voluntary action.

persona *n* what one presents of one's 'self' to be perceived by others — **personae** *pl*.

personal development plan plan developed by nurses and other health professionals as a part of their lifelong learning commitment.

personal hygiene includes all those activities which have as their objective body cleanliness; they include washing, bathing, care of hair, nails, teeth and gums, as well as changes of clothing and bedding. ⇒ bed bath. ⇒ mouth care. ⇒ perineal toilet.

personal professional profile *n* see Box – Personal professional profile.

personal relationship the relationship of one person to another. In general, the term is taken to mean the interaction between two people, who have chosen to be in that relationship, and feel equal and comfortable in it. Currently, the providers of a professional service are encouraged to personalize, rather than dominate, the service to each client.

personality *n* the various mental attitudes and characteristics which distinguish a person. The sum total of the mental make-up. See Box – Personality. ⇒ anakastic personality disorder. ⇒ avoidant personality disorder. ⇒ histrionic personality disorder. ⇒ paranoid personality. ➡ psychopathic personality. ⇢ type A behaviours. ⇒ type B behaviours.

perspiration *n* the excretion from the sweat glands through the skin pores. *insensible perspiration* that water which is lost by evaporation through the skin

surface other than by sweating. It is greatly increased in inflamed skin. *sensible perspiration* the term used when there are visible drops of sweat on the skin.

Perthes' disease (*syn* pseudocoxalgia) avascular degeneration of the upper femoral epiphysis in children; revascularization occurs, but residual deformity of the femoral head may subsequently lead to arthritic changes.

pertussis *n* (*syn* whooping cough) a serious infectious respiratory disease, mainly occurring in children under 5 years. It is caused by the bacterium *Bordetella pertussis* and is spread by droplets. The incubation period is 7–14 days. Its effects include:

Personal professional profile

The UKCC define a profile as "a record of career progress and professional development". (UKCC 1997). The intention is that an individual will develop a profile which is indicative of their own development, and which will grow and develop as the individual gains more experience, expertise and knowledge. It can therefore be seen that a personal professional profile illustrates career development, continuing professional development and life long learning. It can also be seen that this profile can be used for a variety of needs, including the potential to demonstrate higher level practice. However, the UKCC (1997) stress that "your profile is your personal document. It does not belong to the UKCC or your employer ..." Nevertheless, how you use this document is

up to you, and you may chose to keep some sections as confidential entries, whilst opting to share other sections with selected personnel when and where appropriate.

It therefore appears logical that individuals begin to develop a personal professional profile at the point of registration, and indeed earlier, i.e. at the commencement of a pre-registration programme.

The UKCC state that a profile "is more than a record of achievement. It is based on a regular process of reflection and recording what you learn from every day experiences, as well as planned learning activity." (UKCC 1997)

Reference
UKCC 1997 PREP and you. UKCC, London

Personality

The study of personality is concerned with individual differences. However, it must be emphasized that in spite of individual differences, people will not respond differently in all situations. For example, the experience of fear and impending doom will affect both passengers and cabin crew of a plane heading for a crash.

Some psychologists have argued that personality and temperament have been defined in similar ways (Eisenberg et al 2000). On the other hand, trait theories associate differences in personality to the cognitive approaches used by individuals such as: thinking and feeling and how behaviour is subsequently influenced. The term temperament, however, refers to a person's emotional landscape, motor reaction and attention to personal management in response to subjective and external experiences.

Personality and temperament are inextricably linked and are seen to be part of our genetic inheritance (Rothbart et al 2000). For instance, individual differences in patients' responses to hospitalization, illhealth and surgery can be observed in clinical practice. Responses to pain, terminal illness, and mental illhealth will vary according to personality make up. Assessment of needs must be subsequently tailored according to individual differences.

References
Eisenberg N, Fabes R A, Guthrie I K, Reiser M 2000 Dispositional emotionality and regulation: the role in predicting quality of social functioning. Journal of Personality and Social Psychology 78(1):136–157
Rothbart M K, Evens D E, Ahadi S A 2000 Temperament and personality: origins and outcomes. Journal of Personality and Social Psychology 78(1):122–135

conjunctivitis, rhinitis, dry cough and later bouts of paroxysmal coughing with a 'whoop' and vomiting. It may be complicated by pneumonia, bronchiectasis and convulsions. Active immunization, as part of the DTPer triple vaccine (diphtheria, tetanus and pertussis), is available as part of the routine immunization programme in infancy. Prophylactic vaccination is responsible for a decrease in case incidence.

pes *n* a foot or foot-like structure. *pes cavus* ⇒ claw-foot. *pes planus* ⇒ flat-foot.

pessary *n* **1.** a device inserted into the vagina to correct uterine displacements. A *ring* or *shelf pessary* is used to support a prolapse. A *Hodge pessary* is used to correct a retroversion. **2.** a medicated suppository used to treat vaginal infections, or as a contraceptive.

pesticides *npl* substances which kill pests, such as insects.

PET *acr* positron emission tomography.

petechia *n* a small, red or purple haemorrhagic spot — **petechial** *adj*.

petit mal ⇒ epilepsy.

pétrissage *n* rhythmical massage manipulations of muscle and other soft tissues, using pressure to assist venous and lymphatic drainage and to mobilize skin and connective tissue; brisk to invigorate; slow and deep to induce relaxation and reduce spasm; may be performed with both hands working alternately or one hand alone. Includes *kneading* in which the muscles and subcutaneous tissues are pressed with the whole hand, moved and released in a circular movement in the direction of the heart, and *picking up* in which the tissues are grasped with the whole hand, lifted away from the bone, squeezed and released. Small areas may be manipulated with finger pads and thumb pads.

Peyer's patches submucosal aggregates of lymphoid tissue situated in the ileum. They help to prevent bacteria entering the blood but are the seat of infection in typhoid fever.

Peyronie's disease deformity and painful erection of penis due to fibrous tissue formation from unknown cause. Often associated with Dupuytren's contracture.

PFI *abbr* Private Finance Initiative.

PGL *abbr* persistent generalized lymphadenopathy.

pH *abbr* the concentration of hydrogen ions expressed as a negative logarithm. ⇒ hydrogen ion concentration.

phacoemulsification *n* ⇒ phakoemulsification.

phaeochromocytoma *n* a rare tumour of the adrenal medulla or of the sympathetic chain. It secretes the catecholamines noradrenaline (norepinephrine) and adrenaline (epinephrine), causing hypertension which may be paroxysmal, headache, sweating, anxiety and palpitations. Treatment is usually excision of the tumour or, where this is not possible, drugs that block both α and β adrenoceptors are used long-term.

phage typing a method of identifying bacterial strains by their bacteriophages.

phagocyte *n* a cell capable of engulfing bacteria and other particulate material, such as neutrophils and monocytes. ⇒ phagocytosis — **phagocytic** *adj*.

phagocytosis *n* the engulfment by phagocytes of bacteria or other particles (see Figure 49). ⇒ endocytosis. ⇒ exocytosis. ⇒ pinocytosis.

phakoemulsification, phacoemulsification *n* ultrasonic vibration is used to liquefy mature lens fibres. The liquid lens matter is then sucked out.

phalanges *npl* the small bones of the fingers and toes — **phalanx** *sing* — **phalangeal** *adj*.

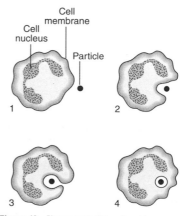

Figure 49 Phagocytosis. (Reproduced from Brooker 1998 with permission.)

phallic stage the third stage of psychosexual development, characterized by the child's sensual interest in the genitalia; the penis or clitoris, and attachment to the parent of the opposite sex.

phallus *n* the penis — **phallic** *adj*.

phantasy *n* ⇒ fantasy.

phantom pain/limb syndrome the sensation that a limb or part of the body is still attached to the body after it has been amputated. Phantom pain is experienced as coming from the amputated limb or body part.

phantom pregnancy ⇒ pseudocyesis. Signs and symptoms simulating those of early pregnancy; it may occur in a childless woman with an overwhelming desire to have a child.

pharmacist *n* a person qualified and registered to dispense medicines and advise the public and other healthcare professionals.

pharmacodynamics the study of drug action in living systems and how it changes cellular processes to have an effect.

pharmacokinetics *n* the study of drug action within the body. See Box – Pharmacokinetics.

pharmacology *n* the science dealing with drugs — **pharmacologically** *adv*.

pharmacopoeia *n* an authorized handbook of drugs available in a particular country, e.g. British pharmacopoeia (BP), United States pharmacopoeia. ⇒ formulary.

pharmacy 1. the science of preparing or mixing drugs. 2. the place where drugs are prepared and dispensed. *pharmacy*

only medicines (P) drugs that may be purchased by the public from a pharmacy, but only when a qualified pharmacist is present.

pharyngeal pouch pathological dilatation of the lower part of the pharynx.

pharyngectomy *n* surgical removal of part of the pharynx.

pharyngismus *n* spasm of the pharynx.

pharyngitis *n* inflammation of the pharynx.

pharyngolaryngeal *adj* pertaining to the pharynx and larynx.

pharyngolaryngectomy *n* surgical removal of the pharynx and larynx.

pharyngoplasty *n* any plastic operation to the pharynx.

pharyngotomy *n* the operation of opening into the pharynx.

pharyngotympanic *adj* pertaining to the pharynx and middle ear (tympanic cavity). *pharyngotympanic tube* a canal, partly bony, partly cartilaginous, measuring 40–50 mm in length, connecting the pharynx with the tympanic cavity. It allows air to pass into the middle ear, so that the air pressure is kept even on both sides of the eardrum. Also called the auditory tube and previously known as the eustachian tube. *pharyngotympanic catheter* an instrument used for insufflating the pharyngotympanic tube when it becomes blocked.

pharynx *n* the cavity at the back of the mouth. It is cone-shaped, varies in length (average 75 mm), and is lined with mucous membrane; at the lower end it opens into the oesophagus. The

---

Pharmacokinetics

Pharmacokinetics is the study of what the body does to a drug over time. It explores the processes of drug absorption, distribution, metabolism and excretion. Each of these processes occurs at a specific rate characteristic for that drug, and the overall action of the drug, (be it therapeutic or toxic), will be dependent on these processes.

A number of factors can affect the pharmacokinetics of a drug and so alter its effect on the body. For example, drug absorption is affected by the formulation of the drug, the gut contents, and gut motility. Drug distribution depends on blood flow to the tissues, obstacles such as the blood-brain barrier that make it difficult for drugs to enter the central nervous system, and plasma protein binding. Enzymes within the liver carry out drug metabolism, and as there is considerable genetic variation in hepatic enzymes, the ability to metabolize drugs can vary significantly from one person to another. The presence of other drugs can also affect the rate of metabolism, either speeding it up or slowing it down. Drugs are mainly eliminated by the kidneys and are particularly affected by glomerular filtration rate, which decreases with age and disease.

pharyngotympanic tubes pierce its lateral walls and the posterior nares pierce its anterior wall. The larynx lies immediately below it and in front of the oesophagus. It has three parts: nasopharynx, oropharynx and laryngopharynx — **pharyngeal** *adj*.

PHC *abbr* primary health care.

phenol *n* (*syn* carbolic acid) a disinfectant. Phenolic compounds are used for environmental disinfectants.

phenomenology the study of occurrences as they form part of human experience.

phenothiazines *npl* a group of typical neuroleptics, e.g. chlorpromazine, fluphenazine. ⇒ parkinsonism. ⇒ tardive dyskinesia.

phenotype *n* the physical characteristics that result from genetic inheritance and environmental factors.

phenylalanine *n* an essential (indispensable) amino acid. ⇒ phenylketonuria.

phenylketonuria (PKU) *n* a metabolic disorder inherited as an autosomal recessive condition. The enzyme phenylalanine hydroxylase, which converts phenylalanine to tyrosine, is absent or deficient. Toxic metabolites of phenylalanine, such as phenylketones derived from phenylpyruvate, accumulate in the blood and are excreted in the urine (phenylketonuria). Untreated, it leads to individuals with severe learning disability who have very fair hair and skin (lack of tyrosine needed for the pigment melanin). A routine screening blood test during the first few days of life ensures early diagnosis and a treatment regimen which includes reducing phenylalanine intake and monitoring for toxic metabolites. The special dietary regimen is required until brain development is complete, but is recommenced when females with phenylketonuria plan to become pregnant. ⇒ Guthrie test — **phenylketonuric** *adj*.

pheromone *n* chemicals with a specific odour secreted by an organism. In humans they are present in the sweat produced by the apocrine sweat glands. They may be involved in the communication between individuals and an influence on sexual behaviour.

Philadelphia chromosome (Ph) an anomaly affecting chromosome 22. Present in the blood cells of most individuals with chronic myeloid leukaemia.

phimosis *n* tightness of the prepuce so that it cannot be retracted over the glans penis. It makes hygiene more difficult and increases the risk of balanitis. ⇒ circumcision.

phlebectomy *n* excision of a vein. *multiple cosmetic phlebectomy* removal of varicose veins through little stab incisions which heal with minimal scarring.

phlebitis *n* inflammation of a vein. May be associated with thrombosis. ⇒ thrombophlebitis — **phlebitic** *adj*.

phlebography ⇒ venography.

phlebolith *n* a concretion which forms in a vein.

phlebothrombosis *n* thrombosis in a vein. ⇒ deep vein thrombosis. ⇒ embolism. ⇒ pulmonary embolism.

phlebotomist *n* a technician who is trained to carry out phlebotomy.

phlebotomy *n* venotomy. ⇒ venesection.

phlegm *n* sputum. The secretion of mucus expectorated from the bronchi.

phlegmasia alba dolens ⇒ white leg.

phlegmatic *adj* describes an emotionally stable person.

phlyctenule *n* a minute blister (vesicle), usually occurring on the conjunctiva or cornea — **phlyctenular** *adj*.

phobia *n* irrational focused fear, either of an event, or of an object or state, that causes the individual to experience anxiety. A phobia may seriously interfere with normal life if it is encountered frequently. ⇒ agoraphobia. ⇒ claustrophobia. ⇒ needle phobia. ⇒ nyctophobia — **phobic** *adj*.

phobic anxiety ⇒ anxiety. ⇒ phobia.

phocomelia (seal limbs) *n* a deficiency of long bones, with relatively good development of hands and feet attached at or near the shoulders or hips. Most reduction deformities are associated with primary defects of development. Prosthetic devices are fitted whenever possible and at the earliest possible stage of development. (A series of severe limb abnormalities in the 1960s was associated with women who had taken the drug thalidomide during pregnancy.)

phonation *n* the production of voice by vibration of the vocal cords.

phosphatases *npl* group of enzymes involved in the reactions concerning phosphate esters, such as phospholipids and nucleotides. ⇒ acid phosphatase. ⇒ alkaline phosphatase.

phosphate *n* a salt or ester of phosphoric acid.

phospholipids *npl* organic molecules consisting of a lipid (two hydrocarbon chains and a glycerol molecule) plus nitrogen and phosphate groups, important in the formation of the plasma membrane of cells.

phosphonecrosis *n* 'fossy-jaw'. An industrial disease previously occurring in workers engaged in the manufacture of matches made with white phosphorus; necrosis of the jaw with loosening of the teeth.

phosphorus (P) *n* a poisonous nonmetallic element. Present in the body (as phosphates), forming an important constituent of nucleic acids, bone, teeth and all cells.

phosphorus-32 (^{32}P) *n* a radioactive isotope of phosphorus used in the management of primary proliferative polycythaemia and essential thrombocythaemia. ⇒ myeloproliferative disorders. → polycythaemia. ⇒ thrombocythaemia.

phosphorylases *npl* enzymes that catalyse the addition of phosphate groups to other molecules, such as hexokinase and phosphofructokinase involved in glucose metabolism.

photalgia *n* pain in the eyes from exposure to intense light.

photochemotherapy *n* the effect of the administered drug is enhanced by exposing the patient to ultraviolet light.

photocoagulation *n* burning of the tissues with a powerful, focused light source. ⇒ Laser.

photoendoscope *n* an endoscope to which a camera is attached for the purpose of making a permanent record — **photoendoscopically** *adv*.

photophobia *n* abnormal intolerance of light, such as with inflammatory conditions of the eye or conditions of the nervous system, e.g. meningitis — **photophobic** *adj*.

photoreceptors receptors that respond to light energy. ⇒ cones. ⇒ rods.

photorefractive keratectomy (PRK) surgical reshaping of the cornea, using a laser, in order to correct refractive error, usually myopia and/or astigmatism.

photosensitive sensitive to light, as the pigments in the retina.

photosensitivity abnormally sensitive to sunlight, such as the skin.

phototherapy *n* therapeutic use of light, such as the exposure to artificial blue light used in the treatment of mild hyperbilirubinaemia in neonates.

phren *n* pertaining to the diaphragm — **phrenic** *adj* *phrenic nerves* innervate the diaphragm.

phrenicotomy *n* division of the phrenic nerve to paralyse one-half of the diaphragm.

phrenoplegia *n* paralysis of the diaphragm — **phrenoplegic** *adj*.

phylloquinone *n* a plant substance that has vitamin K activity.

phylum *n* a major group in the classification of animals.

physical relating to the body or the natural sciences. *physical activity level (PAL)* the ratio of overall energy used per 24 hours to the basal metabolic rate; varies between 1.4 and 1.9. *physical activity ratio (PAR)* the ratio of the energy expenditure of an activity per minute to the energy expenditure of the basal metabolic rate per minute. It varies according to the activity and individual lifestyles, e.g. sitting watching television 1.2, walking at 4–6 km/h 3.7, and playing tennis 6.9. *physical medicine* a branch of medicine which makes use of physiotherapy and occupational therapy. *physical therapy* ⇒ physiotherapy.

physical abuse ⇒ abuse. ⇒ nonaccidental injury.

physician *n* a qualified medical practitioner. One who practises medicine rather than surgery.

physicochemical *adj* pertaining to physics and chemistry.

physiological *adj* in accordance with natural processes of the body. Adjective often used to describe a normal process or structure, to distinguish it from an abnormal or pathological feature (e.g. the physiological level of calcium in the blood is from 2.1–2.6 mmol per litre; higher and lower levels are pathological and indicative of disease). *physiological solution* a solution having the same solute concentration and osmotic pressure as plasma, i.e. isotonic with the body fluids and containing similar salts.

physiological saline ⇒ isotonic saline. ⇒ physiological solution.

physiology *n* the science which deals with the normal functions of the body — **physiologically** *adv*.

physiotherapy *n* traditionally, treatment to ameliorate, restore and sometimes cure, using electrotherapy, manipulation and exercise therapy and rehabilitation following injury or disease. Contemporarily, it also includes assessment and diagnosis, health education, health promotion and prevention of disabling conditions. ⇒ extended scope physiotherapy practitioners (ESPs). ⇒ neurological physiotherapy.

phytates/phytic acid constituents of wholegrain cereals. In common with phosphates, they inhibit the intestinal absorption of some minerals. ⇒ nonstarch polysaccharides.

phyto-oestrogen *n* substances with oestrogenic properties found in plants, such as soya beans.

pia, pia mater *n* the innermost of the meninges; the vascular membrane which lies in close contact with the substance of the brain and spinal cord.

pica *n* a craving for extraordinary food or non-food items, a feature of some pregnancies and in some people with mental health problems.

PICC *abbr* peripherally inserted central catheter.

Pick's disease 1. syndrome of ascites, hepatic enlargement, oedema and pleural effusion occurring in constrictive pericarditis. 2. a type of cerebral atrophy which produces dementia in midlife.

picornavirus *n* from pico (very small) and RNA (ribonucleic acid). Small RNA viruses. The family includes the enteroviruses (poliovirus, coxsackie, echo and hepatitis A virus) and the rhinoviruses.

PICU *abbr* paediatric intensive care unit.

PID *abbr* 1. prolapse of an intervertebral disc. ⇒ prolapse. 2. pelvic inflammatory disease.

Pierre Robin syndrome an inherited condition characterized by micrognathia, cleft palate, cleft lip and glaucoma.

pigeon chest (*syn* pectus carinatum) a narrow chest, with an unusually prominent sternum.

pigeon-toed *adj* walking with the toes of one or both feet turned inwards.

pigment *n* any colouring matter of the body, such as melanin, haemoglobin, retinal pigments and bile pigments.

pigmentation *n* the deposit of pigment, especially when abnormal or excessive. ⇒ Addison's disease. ⇒ albinism. ⇒ vitiligo.

piles *n* ⇒ haemorrhoids.

pili *npl* hair-like appendages of many bacteria. Concerned with the transfer of genetic material during conjugation.

pilomotor nerves nerves attached to the hair follicle; innervation causes the hair to stand upright and give the appearance of 'goose flesh'.

pilonidal *adj* hair-containing. *pilonidal sinus* a sinus containing hairs which is usually found in hirsute people in the cleft between the buttocks. In this situation it is liable to infection and abscess formation.

pilosebaceous *adj* pertaining to the hair follicle and the sebaceous gland opening into it.

pilot study an initial smaller scale study used prior to the main research project to assess feasibility and to highlight deficiencies in the methodology.

pimple *n* ⇒ papule.

Pinard's stethoscope trumpet-shaped instrument enabling direct auscultation of the fetal heart through the abdominal wall.

pineal body (gland) a small reddish-grey conical structure on the dorsal surface of the midbrain. Its functions are not fully understood but there is evidence that it secretes various substances which include 5-hydroxytryptamine and melatonin. The release of melatonin is linked to the amount of light entering the eye. Melatonin levels rise at night and drop at dawn and appear to influence the secretion of gonadotrophins, processes which follow diurnal rhythms such as sleep and influence mood. ⇒ depression. ⇒ seasonal affective disorder.

pinguecula *n* a yellowish, slightly elevated thickening of the bulbar conjunctiva near the lid aperture. Associated with the aging eye.

pink-eye *n* a popular name for acute contagious conjunctivitis, which spreads rapidly in closed communities or institutions where children share facecloths.

pinna *n* that part of the ear which is external to the head; the auricle.

pinnaplasty *n* corrective surgery for bat ears.

pinocytosis *n* process by which the cell plasma membrane surrounds a minute water droplet, which is taken into the cell. → endocytosis. ⇒ exocytosis. → phagocytosis.

pinta *n* a treponemal disease of Central and South America caused by the spirochaete *Treponema carateum*. It affects the skin and spreads by contact within families. ⇒ bejel. ⇒ yaws.

PIs *abbr* Performance Indicators.

pisiform *n* one of the carpals or wrist bones.

pitting *n* 1. making an indentation in oedematous tissues. 2. depressed scar left on the skin at the sites of former pustules.

pituitary gland (*syn* hypophysis cerebri) a small oval endocrine gland lying in the pituitary fossa of the sphenoid bone. It is connected by a stalk to the hypothalamus. The anterior lobe (adenohypophysis) produces and secretes several hormones: growth hormone (GH), adrenocorticotrophic hormone (ACTH), thyroid stimulating hormone (TSH), luteinizing hormone (LH), follicle stimulating hormone (FSH), melanocyte stimulating hormone (MSH) and prolactin. The posterior lobe (neurohypophysis) stores and secretes oxytocin and antidiuretic hormone (ADH) (also known as vasopressin). Both these hormones are produced by the nerve fibres of two nuclei in the hypothalamus.

pityriasis *n* a group of dermatoses characterized by scaly (bran-like) lesions of the skin. *pityriasis alba* a common eruption in children characterized by scaly hypopigmented macules on the cheeks and upper arms. *pityriasis rosea* a slightly scaly eruption of ovoid erythematous lesions which are widespread over the trunk and proximal parts of the limbs. There may be mild itching. It is a self-limiting condition. *pityriasis rubra pilaris* a chronic skin disease characterized by tiny red papules of perifollicular distribution. *pityriasis versicolor* chronic condition associated with the yeast *Pityrosporum orbiculare*, usually seen on the upper trunk. The condition is characterized by itching and scaling with areas of hyperpigmentation.

Pityrosporum *n* genus of yeasts. *P. orbiculare* is associated with pityriasis versicolor.

PKU *abbr* phenylketonuria.

placebo *n* 1. a harmless substance given as medicine. In a randomized placebo controlled trial, an inert substance, identical in appearance with the material being tested, is used. When neither the researcher nor the patient knows which is which it is termed a double blind trial. *placebo effect* a therapeutic effect that occurs following the administration of a placebo, or some non-drug intervention, e.g. information in advance of surgery may reduce the need for pain relieving drugs. 2. in complementary medicine, a self-healing response.

placement *n* a period of time a student spends in a specific clinical area for explicit learning purposes.

placenta *n* the afterbirth. The temporary hormone-secreting vascular structure developed and functional by the third month of pregnancy and attached to the inner wall of the uterus. It facilitates the exchange of substances: oxygen, nutrients, antibodies, carbon dioxide and nitrogenous waste between maternal and fetal blood. In normal labour it is expelled from the uterus, with the fetal membranes, during the third stage of labour. When this does not occur it is termed a *retained placenta* and may be an *adherent placenta*. The placenta is usually attached to the upper segment of the uterus; when it lies in the lower uterine segment it is called a *placenta praevia* and usually causes painless antepartum haemorrhage.

placental abruption bleeding after the 24th week of pregnancy and before labour, caused by partial or complete separation of the placenta, it may be associated with abdominal pain and tenderness and shock. Bleeding may be concealed, or revealed via the vagina. ⇒ antepartum haemorrhage. ⇒ placenta praevia.

placental insufficiency inefficiency of the placenta for a variety of reasons. Can occur due to maternal disease, giving rise to a 'small-for-dates' baby, or to postmaturity of fetus.

placentography *n* radiographic examination of the placenta after injection of opaque substance.

plague *n* very contagious epidemic disease caused by the bacterium *Yersinia pestis*, and spread by infected rats. Transfer of infection from rat to human is through bites from rat fleas, but spread between humans may occur via droplets. Plague is still endemic in parts of Asia, Africa and South America, with occasional cases in the United States. The main clinical types are: *bubonic plague* where there is fever, headache and swelling of lymph nodes and surrounding tissue to form a bubo, *septicaemic plague* where there is no bubo formation, but patients may have meningitis and pneumonia, and *pneumonic plage* where there is rapid onset of cough and dyspnoea with cyanosis and frothy sputum.

plaintiff *n* ⇒ claimant.

planning *v* regarded as the second phase of the nursing process. After identification of the patient's actual and potential problems with everyday living activities, the patient participates in setting appropriate goals to be achieved by the selected nursing interventions. A date is set for evaluation of whether or not the goals have been achieved. ⇒ assessment. ⇒ implementing. ⇒ evaluating.

plantar *adj* pertaining to the sole of the foot. *plantar arch* the union of the plantar and dorsalis pedis arteries in the sole of the foot. *plantar flexion* downward movement of the big toe. *plantar reflex* after infancy there is normally plantar flexion of the great toe when the outer aspect of the sole is stroked. ⇒ Babinski's reflex.

plaque *n* 1. ⇒ dental plaque. 2. small raised circular area.

plasma *n* the fluid part of blood. *blood plasma* may be used for infusion, as in severe burns. *plasma cell* an immune cell derived from the B lymphocyte and concerned with the production of antibodies. ⇒ lymphocyte. *plasma thromboplastin antecedent (PTA)* factor XI in the blood coagulation cascade.

plasma membrane cell membrane.

plasmapheresis *n* ⇒ apheresis.

plasmid *n* DNA present in the cytoplasm of some bacteria. During sexual reproduction, the genetic material in the plasmid is transferred between bacteria, thus allowing genes for antibiotic-resistance to be exchanged.

plasmin *n* the proteolytic enzyme derived from the activation of plasminogen. It breaks down fibrin clots when healing is complete. Also called fibrinolysin. ⇒ fibrinolysis.

plasminogen *n* the inactive precursor of plasmin, produced by the liver. Release of activators, such as tissue plasminogen activator (t-PA), from damaged tissue promotes the conversion of plasminogen into plasmin. ⇒ fibrinolysis.

Plasmodium *n* a genus of protozoa. Parasites in the blood of warm-blooded animals which complete their sexual cycle in blood-sucking arthropods. Four species cause malaria in humans — **plasmodial** *adj*.

plaster of Paris ⇒ gypsum.

plastic *adj* capable of changing shape and taking a form or mould. *plastic surgery* reconstruction and refashioning of soft tissue to repair defects and deformities, and to restore and create form.

platelet *n* also known as thrombocyte. Disc-shaped cellular fragments playing an important role in blood coagulation. ⇒ platelet plug.

platelet plug *n* one of the four overlapping stages of haemostasis. Platelets adhere and aggregate at the site of blood vessel damage and form a temporary plug to close the defect. The platelets release substances, such as ADP, thromboxanes and 5-hydroxytryptamine which cause further aggregation and vasoconstriction. ⇒ coagulation. ⇒ fibrinolysis. ⇒ haemostasis.

platyhelminthes *npl* flat worms; includes the trematodes (flukes) and cestodes (tapeworms). ⇒ Echinococcus. ⇒ schistosomiasis. ⇒ Taenia.

play spontaneous or planned activities vital to normal social, physical, emotional and intellectual development during childhood. *play group* organized play and appropriate learning activities for a group of preschool children. *play therapist* a qualified person who uses play constructively to help children to come to terms with their illness or to prepare for various aspects of treatment. Other staff may be employed to play with children in hospital under the direction of the play therapist.

pleomorphism *n* denotes a wide range in shape and size of individuals in a bacterial population — **pleomorphic** *adj*.

plethysmograph *n* an instrument used to measure the volume or size of an organ or extremity by accurately measuring the blood flow — **plethysmographic** *adj*.

pleura *n* the serous membrane covering the surface of the lung (visceral pleura), the diaphragm, the mediastinum and the chest wall (parietal pleura) enclosing a potential space, the pleural cavity, to allow frictionless movement during respiration — **pleural** *adj* pertaining to the pleura. *pleural effusion* excess fluid between the layers of pleura. → hydrothorax.

pleurectomy *n* stripping off parietal pleura to obliterate pleural space and prevent recurrence of pneumothoraces.

pleurisy, pleuritis *n* inflammation of the pleura. May be fibrinous (dry), be associated with an effusion (wet), or be complicated by empyema — **pleuritic** *adj*.

pleurodesis *n* adherence of the visceral to the parietal pleura. Can be achieved therapeutically to treat recurrent pleural effusion by instilling a sclerosing substance.

pleurodynia *n* intercostal myalgia or muscular rheumatism (fibrositis). It is a feature of Bornholm disease.

pleuropulmonary *adj* pertaining to the pleura and lung.

plexus *n* a network of vessels or nerves.

plication *n* a surgical procedure of making tucks or folds to decrease the size of an organ — **plicate** *adj*, *vt*.

plumbism *n* ⇒ lead poisoning.

Plummer-Vinson syndrome (*syn* Kelly-Paterson syndrome) rare condition characterized by dysphagia due to changes in the pharynx and oesophagus (post-cricoid 'web'), it is associated with severe glossitis and iron deficiency anaemia. Iron taken orally usually leads to complete recovery. Also called sideropenic dysphagia.

pluriglandular *adj* pertaining to several glands, as cystic fibrosis.

pluripotent stem cells *npl* uncommitted bone marrow cell that has the potential to develop into many types of mature cell, including: erythrocytes, lymphocytes, granulocytes and thrombocytes.

PMB *abbr* postmenopausal bleeding.

PMS *abbr* premenstrual syndrome.

pneumaturia *n* the passage of flatus with urine, usually as a result of a vesicocolic (bladder-bowel) fistula.

pneumococcus *n* *Streptococcus pneumoniae*. A Gram-positive diplococcus. It causes pneumonia, otitis media and meningitis — **pneumococcal** *adj*.

pneumoconiosis *n* an occupational lung disease characterized by pulmonary fibrosis, caused by the inhalation of inorganic dusts, e.g. anthracosis, asbestosis, siderosis and silicosis — **pneumoconioses** *pl*.

Pneumocystis carinii an opportunistic micro-organism causing pneumonia in individuals who are immunologically compromized, e.g. with AIDS, after immunosuppression, severely debilitated patients or infants; mortality is high.

pneumocytes *npl* special cells which line the alveolar walls in the lungs. Type I are flat, Type II are cuboidal and secrete surfactant.

pneumoencephalography *n* radiographic examination of cerebral ventricles after injection of air by means of a lumbar or cisternal puncture — **pneumoencephalogram** *n*.

pneumogastric *adj* pertaining to the lungs and stomach. ⇒ vagus nerve.

pneumomycosis *n* fungus infection of the lung such as aspergillosis, actinomycosis, candidiasis — **pneumomycotic** *adj*.

pneumonectomy *n* total or part excision of a lung.

pneumonia *n* traditionally used for inflammation of the lung; when resulting from allergic reaction it is often referred to as alveolitis; that which is due to physical agents is pneumonitis, the word 'pneumonia' being reserved for invasion by microorganisms. ⇒ bronchopneumonia. ⇒ lobar pneumonia.

pneumonic plague *n* ⇒ plague.

pneumonitis *n* inflammation of lung tissue.

pneumoperitoneum *n* air or gas in the peritoneal cavity. Can be introduced for diagnostic or therapeutic purposes.

pneumotaxic centre *n* a respiratory centre in the brain that ensures a smooth respiratory rhythm. ⇒ apneustic centre.

pneumothorax *n* air or gas in the pleural cavity separating the visceral from the parietal pleura so that lung tissue is compressed. Caused by either rupture of the visceral pleura or the perforation of the chest wall. A pneumothorax can be secondary to asthma, carcinoma of bronchus, chronic bronchitis, congenital cysts, emphysema, pneumonia, tuberculosis, mechanical ventilation or trauma. Management involves the insertion of a cannula into the chest and connecting it either to a nonreturn valve or an underwater-seal drainage system. The underlying disease or injury is also appropriately treated. *artificial pneumothorax* deliberate introduction of air/gas into the pleural space to collapse the lung for therapeutic purposes. *spontaneous pneumothorax* occurs when an overdilated pulmonary air sac ruptures, permitting communication of respiratory passages and pleural cavity. *tension pneumothorax* occurs when a valve-like wound allows air to enter the pleural cavity at each inspiration but not to escape on expiration, thus progressively increasing intrathoracic pressure that leads to mediastinal shift and lung collapse. It constitutes an acute medical emergency requiring immediate treatment. ⇒ underwater seal — **pneumothoraces** *pl*.

PNI *abbr* psychoneuroimmunology.

PO₂ *abbr* the partial pressure of oxygen, such as in atmospheric or expired air.

podalic version ⇒ version.

podiatrist *n* (*syn* chiropodist) a healthcare professional qualified in the diagnosis, care and treatment of disorders of the feet.

podiatry *n* (*syn* chiropody) the theory and practice relating to the maintenance of feet in a healthy condition and the treatment of disease and disability.

podopompholyx *n* pompholyx on the feet.

poikilocytosis *n* a marked variation in the shape of red blood cells. It is always accompanied by anisocytosis.

polar describes a molecule without electrical balance, such as water. ⇒ nonpolar.

polar body *n* one of two small haploid bodies formed during the reduction divisions (meiosis) of oogenesis.

polarized describes the resting state of the plasma membrane of an excitable cell in which no impulse transmission is occurring. The inside of the membrane is electrically negative relative to the outside. ⇒ depolarization.

polioencephalitis *n* inflammation of the cerebral grey matter — **polioencephalitic** *adj*.

poliomyelitis *n* (*syn* infantile paralysis) an epidemic infection caused by three polioviruses. It attacks the motor neurons of the anterior horns in the brainstem (*bulbar poliomyelitis*) and spinal cord to cause inflammation. An attack may or may not lead to paralysis of the lower motor neuron type with loss of muscular power and flaccidity. Immunization, using oral vaccine, is available as part of the routine immunization programme during infancy with pre-school and school leaving boosters. Cases of poliomyelitis have followed immunization and people are advised to wash their hands after defaecation or contact with recently vaccinated babies, especially after changing napkins. ⇒ Sabin vaccine. ⇒ Salk vaccine.

polioviruses three related enteroviruses that cause poliomyelitis. ⇒ picornaviruses. ⇒ virus.

Politzer's bag a rubber bag for inflation of the pharyngotympanic tube.

pollenosis *n* an allergic condition arising from sensitization to pollen.

pollicization *n* a surgical procedure whereby the index finger is rotated and shortened to produce apposition as a thumb.

pollution *n* diminished purity or quality. *air pollution* from industrial processes, vehicle exhaust, tobacco etc. Air pollution has been linked to general poor health, development problems and serious diseases, e.g. asthma and cancers. *noise pollution* excessive environmental noise is linked to hearing loss, poor concentration, insufficient sleep and mental health problems. *water pollution* natural lakes, rivers and seas can become polluted from chemicals in land seepage, accidental chemical spillage and untreated sewage, rendering them unfit for swimming and poisoning fish which are rendered unsafe for human consumption.

polyarteritis *n* inflammation of many arteries. In *polyarteritis nodosa (syn* periarteritis nodosa) aneurysmal swellings and thrombosis occur in the affected vessels. Further damage may lead to haemorrhage and the clinical picture presented depends upon the site affected. → collagen.

polyarthralgia *n* pain in several joints.

polyarthritis *n* inflammation of several joints at the same time. ⇒ Still's disease.

Polya's operation partial gastrectomy.

polycystic *adj* composed of many cysts. *polycystic kidneys* genetic condition that results in enlarged, spongy kidneys; it is also associated with cysts in the liver and other organs. There are several varieties of the disease: a rare infantile form and adult polycystic kidney diseases (APKD). The adult form is characterized by abdominal or loin discomfort and acute pain if bleeding occurs, hypertension, urinary tract infection, uraemia and chronic renal failure.

polycythaemia *n* increase in the number of circulating red blood cells. ⇒ erythrocythaemia. ⇒ erythrocytosis. *primary proliferative polycythaemia (polycythaemia vera)* an idiopathic myeloproliferative disorder characterized by an abnormal increase in red cells causing increased blood viscosity. The patient complains of headache and lassitude, and there is danger of thrombosis and haemorrhage. *secondary polycythaemia* an increase in red cells that may result from dehydration or in response to a low oxygen tension such as at high altitude or with chronic respiratory disease. It may occur in conditions where there is inappropriate secretion of erythropoietin.

polydactyly, polydactylism *n* having more than the normal number of fingers or toes.

polydipsia *n* excessive thirst.

polygene inheritance occurs where physical characteristics, such as skin or hair colour, are determined by the influence of a group of paired genes at different locations acting together.

polygraph *n* instrument which records several variables simultaneously.

polyhydramnios *n* an excessive amount of amniotic fluid.

polymer *n* a molecule formed from the combination of many smaller molecules or subunits, such as glycogen which is a polymer of glucose subunits.

polymorphonuclear *adj* having a many-shaped or lobulated nucleus. *polymorphonuclear leucocytes (white cells)* the series of white cells: neutrophils, basophils and eosinophils.

polymyalgia rheumatica a syndrome occurring in older people comprising of a sometimes crippling ache in the shoulders, pelvic girdle muscles and spine, with pronounced morning stiffness and a raised ESR. There is an association with giant cell (temporal) arteritis. → arthritis.

polymyositis *n* manifests as muscle weakness, most commonly in middle age. Microscopic examination of muscle reveals inflammatory changes, they respond to corticosteroid drugs. ⇒ dermatomyositis.

polyneuritis *n* multiple neuritis usually affecting several peripheral nerves at the same time. Also known as polyneuropathy — **polyneuritic** *adj.*

polyneuropathy *n* generalized disease affecting the peripheral nerves. Varied aetiology, e.g. vitamin B deficiency and after viral or bacterial infection etc.

polyopia seeing multiple images of the same object.

polyp, polypus a pedunculated tumour arising from any mucous surface, e.g. cervical, endometrial, intestinal, nasal, etc. Usually benign but may become malignant — **polypous** *adj.*

polypectomy *n* surgical removal of a polyp.

polypeptides *npl* several amino acids joined by peptide bonds. Intermediate in size between a peptide and a protein.

polypharmacy *n* a word used when multiple drugs are prescribed for the same person, usually inappropriately. Substantially increases the risk of adverse effects. See Box – Polypharmacy.

polyploidy a chromosome number that is a multiple of the normal haploid (23) number, other than the normal diploid (46) number, such as 69, which is not compatible with life. ⇒ triploid.

Polypharmacy

Polypharmacy is the administration of multiple medications to an individual client, with the implication that more drugs are being given than is clinically justified. This phenomenon is frequently seen in older people and commonly involves the 'prescribing cascade', in which a drug is prescribed that causes a side effect, another drug is prescribed to combat the side effect, and the second drug causes further side effects, and so on. Polypharmacy often also involves use of duplicate medications in the same drug category, prescription of drugs with no apparent indication or that are contraindicated for use among older people, the use of inappropriate dosages, and concurrent use of interacting medications. The problem is also augmented by use of over the counter medications, including conventional drugs and complementary therapies. When discussing medications with a patient it is important to identify what drugs they are taking and the sources. Discontinuation of all or most of the drugs usually results in improvement of the patient's clinical condition.

---

polypoid *adj* resembling a polyp(us).

polyposis *n* a condition in which there are numerous polypi in an organ. *polyposis coli* inherited as an autosomal dominant condition. There are polypi throughout the large bowel which eventually become malignant. Affected individuals are monitored carefully by colonoscopy and polyps are removed, but proctocolectomy may eventually be performed to prevent cancer of the colon.

polysaccharide *n* complex carbohydrate formed from many monosaccharide units. They are important as energy storage and structural molecules and include: starch, inulin, glycogen, dextrin and cellulose.

polyserositis *n* inflammation of several serous membranes.

polyunsaturated fatty acid (PUFA) describes a fatty acid with two or more double bonds in its structure. ⇒ essential fatty acids. ⇒ monounsaturated fatty acid.

polyuria *n* excretion of an excessive amount of urine, such as with diabetes insipidus — **polyuric** *adj*.

POM *abbr* prescription only medicine.

pompholyx *n* also known as dyshidrotic eczema. ⇒ eczema. ⇒ cheiropompholyx.

pons *n* a bridge; a process of tissue joining two sections of an organ. *pons varolii* part of the brainstem between the midbrain and medulla. Contains fibres which form a bridge between the cerebellar hemispheres and connect the brain to the spinal cord. It forms part of the fourth ventricle and contains several cranial nerve nuclei and a respiratory centre — **pontine** *adj*.

Pontiac fever ⇒ *Legionella pneumophilia.* ⇒ Legionnaires' disease.

POP *acr* progestogen only pill.

popliteal *adj* pertaining to the popliteus. *popliteal space* the diamond-shaped depression at the back of the knee joint, bounded by the muscles and containing the popliteal nerve and vessels.

popliteus *n* a muscle in the popliteal space which flexes the leg and aids it in rotating.

pore *n* a minute surface opening. One of the mouths of the ducts (leading from the sweat glands) on the skin surface; they are controlled by fine muscles, contracting and closing in the cold and dilating in the presence of heat.

porphyrias *npl* a group of rare inherited or acquired enzyme abnormalities that cause defective haem biosynthesis leading to the accumulation of intermediate porphyrins. The effects vary with the type of porphyria, but include: abdominal pain, vomiting. liver dysfunction, hypertension, polyneuropathy, mental illness, severe skin reactions to sunlight, urine that turns red-brown on standing, blindness etc. Excess porphyrins or precursors are found in the urine (porphyrinuria) or stools or both. In some cases attacks are precipitated by certain drugs, e.g. barbiturates, oestrogens and alcohol. Prognosis is good if diagnosed early, if attention is given to management of fluids and diet, and avoidance of contraindicated drugs.

porphyrins *npl* a group of organic pyrrole compounds synthesized from amino acids. They form the basis of respiratory pigments, including haemoglobin and cytochromes. ⇒ porphyria.

porphyrinuria presence of porphyrins in the urine.

port *n* a computer interface or socket for plugging in other devices. *parallel port* a socket used to connect the computer to other devices with a parallel port such as a printer. These ports carry information by a faster method than that used by a serial port. Often called a Centronics port. *serial port* a socket used to connect the computer to other devices with a serial port, e.g. modem or mouse They transmit information more slowly than parallel ports. Also known as RS232.

porta *n* the depression (hilum) of an organ at which the vessels enter and leave. *porta hepatis* the transverse fissure through which the hepatic portal vein, hepatic artery and bile ducts pass on the undersurface of the liver.

portacaval, portocaval *adj* pertaining to the hepatic portal vein and inferior vena cava. *portacaval anastomosis/shunt* the hepatic portal vein is joined to the inferior vena cava so that some blood bypasses the liver; used to reduce the pressure within the hepatic portal vein in cases of hepatic portal hypertension, such as with cirrhosis of the liver.

Portage system based on behaviour modification techniques which are used by family members and a home visitor who work together to help children with a physical or learning disability to develop and acquire skills required for everyday living. The kit includes a checklist, box of teaching cards, an activity chart and a system for monitoring progress.

portahepatitis *n* inflammation around the transverse fissure of the liver.

portal circulation *n* ⇒ hepatic portal circulation.

portal hypertension ⇒ hepatic portal hypertension.

portal vein *n* ⇒ hepatic portal vein.

portfolio *n* a personal and private collection of evidence, which demonstrates the owner's continuing professional and personal development. It documents the acquisition of knowledge, skills, attitudes, understanding and achievements; in recording these events, it deals with the past. It contains reflections on current practice and progress, and in doing this it deals with the present. However, it also contains an action plan for future career and personal development, and in this it looks to the future. It does not simply record outcomes, but rather it documents the journey taken *en route* to the outcomes. As such it is a valuable tool in continuing professional development. A portfolio should allow the practitioner to select profiles for a number of different purposes. ⇒ Personal Professional Profile.

position *n* posture.

Positive and Negative Syndrome Scale (PANSS) a scale used by mental health practitioners to rate positive and negative symptoms. It is a thirty item scale; seven items address negative symptoms, seven address positive symptoms and the remaining sixteen focus on general psychopathology. It uses a Likert scale (0–6 with 6 most severe) to rate each item.

positive end expiratory pressure (PEEP) *n* during mechanical ventilation the pressure at the end of expiration is kept high enough to prevent alveolar collapse, by maintaining partial lung inflation.

positive feedback *n* → feedback.

positive pressure ventilation (PPV) ⇒ mechanical ventilation.

positive symptoms of schizophrenia *npl* describes a group of symptoms associated with certain types of schizophrenia. They include: hallucinations, delusions, thought disorder etc. ⇒ neuroleptics. ⇒ Positive and Negative Syndrome Scale.

positron emission tomography (PET) uses cyclotron produced isotopes of extremely short half life that emit positrons. PET scanning is used to evaluate physiological function of organs, e.g. the brain.

positrons *npl* positively charged particles that combine with negatively charged electrons, causing gamma rays to be emitted.

posseting *n* regurgitation of small amounts of milk in infants, usually after feeding; associated with swallowing air during the feed.

POSSUM *acr* Patient-Operated Selector Mechanism. A device that can be operated by a slight touch, or by suction using the mouth if no other muscle movement is possible. It may transmit messages or be adapted for computing, telephoning and other activities.

postabsorptive state the fasted state. Metabolic state that exists between meals, such as late morning, late afternoon and during the night. Fuel molecules are in short supply and catabolic processes predominate as the body strives to maintain blood glucose by glycogenolysis, lipolysis and later the breakdown of body protein. ⇒ absorptive state.

postanal *adj* behind the anus.

postcoital *adj* after sexual intercourse. *postcoital contraception* oestrogen and progesterone (or progesterone alone) hormones administered within 72 hours of unprotected intercourse, or the insertion of an intrauterine contraceptive device.

postconcussional syndrome the association of headaches, giddiness and a feeling of faintness, which may persist for a considerable time after a head injury.

postdiphtheritic *adj* following an attack of diphtheria. Refers especially to the paralysis of limbs and palate.

postencephalitic *adj* following encephalitis lethargica. The adjective is commonly used to describe the syndrome of parkinsonism, which often results from an attack of this type of encephalitis.

postepileptic *adj* following an epileptic seizure. *postepileptic automatism* is a fugue state, following on a fit, when the patient may undertake a course of action, even involving violence, without having any memory of this (amnesia).

posterior *adj* situated at the back. ⇒ anterior *ant.* *posterior chamber of the eye* the space between the anterior surface of the lens and the posterior surface of the iris. ⇒ aqueous.

postganglionic *adj* situated after (distal) a collection of nerve cells (ganglion) as in postganglionic nerve fibre.

posthepatic *adj* behind the liver.

postherpetic *adj* after shingles.

posthitis *adj* inflammation of the prepuce.

posthumous *adj* occurring after death. *posthumous birth* delivery of a baby by caesarian section after the mother's death, or birth occurring after the death of the father.

postmature *adj* past the expected date of delivery. A baby is postmature when labour is delayed beyond the usual 40

weeks. Intervention is now often delayed to 42 or 43 weeks, provided the maternal and fetal well-being is monitored and gives no cause for concern — **postmaturity** *n.*

postmenopausal *adj* relating to the time after the menopause. *postmenopausal bleeding (PMB)* vaginal bleeding after the menopause. It may indicate serious pathology, such as endometrial cancer, and should always be fully investigated.

postmortem *adj* after death, usually implying dissection of the body. ⇒ antemortem *ant.* ⇒ autopsy.

postmyocardial infarction syndrome Dressler's syndrome. Pyrexia and chest pain associated with pericarditis and pleurisy occurring some weeks after a myocardial infarction. Possibly due to an autoimmune reaction to substances released from the necrotic myocardium.

postnasal *adj* situated behind the nose and in the nasopharynx — **postnasally** *adv.*

postnatal *adj* after birth or delivery. ⇒ antenatal *ant.* *postnatal (postpartum) blues* describes emotional lability and or a low mood experienced by some women for a few days following the birth of a baby; sometimes called 'fourth-day blues'. Less severe than *postnatal depression* ⇒ puerperal psychosis. *postnatal examination* routine examination 6 weeks after delivery. Includes general physical and mental health, involution of the uterus, the pelvic floor and perineal healing. *postnatal period* a period of time of at least 10 days and no more than 28 days, during which the attendance of a midwife on mother and infant is mandatory.

postoperative *adj* after surgical operation — **postoperatively** *adv.*

postpartum *adj* after a birth (parturition). *postpartum haemorrhage* excessive vaginal bleeding after the birth of the baby. Causes include: incomplete separation of the placenta during the third stage of labour, or later infection caused by a small part of the placenta being retained. *postpartum pituitary necrosis* ⇒ Sheehan's syndrome.

postprandial *adj* following a meal.

Postregistration Education and Practice see Box – PREP – Postregistration Education and Practice.

post-traumatic stress disorder (PTSD)
anxiety, with nightmares, irritability, poor
memory and concentration, headaches,
flashbacks and depression, that may
occur after involvement in any traumatic
situation such as: serious road accidents;
crimes, e.g. rape; fire; explosion; war;
natural disasters etc. The condition may
affect the professionals involved, the victims and people who witness the event.

postural *adj* pertaining to posture. *postural
albuminuria* ⇒ orthostatic albuminuria.
postural drainage using gravity and position to drain secretions from the respiratory tract. The airways of infected lung
lobes or segments are positioned as vertically as possible. Also known as tipping
because the lower lobes need to be raised
higher than the mouth for secretions to
drain into the trachea to stimulate the
cough reflex. Apical segments of the
upper lobe drain in sitting. The chest is
percussed with clapping and vibrated and
sputum coughed into a disposable carton
or removed by suctioning. Children with
cystic fibrosis need to have this treatment
at home and the family members learn to
do it. Small children can be tipped across
their parents' thighs. Older children and
adults are usually tipped by elevating the
foot of the bed, or over a roll or special
frame. ⇒ tapôtement. *postural hypotension* orthostatic hypotension. A fall in
blood pressure when the individual
adopts an upright posture from lying or
sitting. *postural reflex* any one of many
reflexes associated in establishing or
maintaining the posture of an individual,
particularly against the pull of gravity.

posture *n* the way in which the body is
held in lying, sitting, standing and walking; a particular position or attitude of
the body. *hemiplegic posture* the position
of the head, neck, trunk and limbs following a stroke. *opisthotonic posture* the
arched position of total extension of the
head, spine and limbs seen in severe
meningeal irritation and other severe
neurological conditions. ⇒ opisthotonos.

post-viral syndrome *n* ⇒ myalgic
encephalomyelitis.

potassium (K) *n* a metallic element. A
major intracellular cation. It is required
for normal neuromuscular function. ⇒
hyperkalaemia ⇒ hypokalaemia. *potassium chlorate* a mild antiseptic used in

mouthwashes and gargles. Distinguish
from potassium chloride. *potassium chloride* used in potassium replacement solutions, and as a supplement in thiazide
diuretic therapy. *potassium permanganate*
purple crystals with powerful disinfectant
and deodorizing properties.

potassium deficiency ⇒ hypokalaemia.

potassium sparing diuretics *npl* diuretic
drugs that cause a diuresis without loss of
potassium in the urine. They include:
spironalactone which is an aldosterone
antagonist and competes with its tubular
receptor sites in the nephron, resulting in
retention of potassium and increased
excretion of water and sodium. It also
potentiates the action of thiazide and loop
diuretics. Other potassium sparing diuretics include amiloride, which acts on the
collecting ducts to reduce sodium reabsorption and potassium excretion by
blocking the sodium channels through
which aldosterone operates. They are
used with potassium-losing diuretics and
to treat the oedema of liver cirrhosis.

potter's rot one of the many popular names
for silicosis arising in workers in the pot-
tery industry.

Pott's disease spondylitis; spinal caries;
spinal tuberculosis. The resultant necrosis
of the vertebrae causes kyphosis.

Pott's fracture a fracture dislocation of the
ankle joint. A fracture of the lower end of
the tibia and fibula, 75 mm above the
ankle joint, and a fracture of the medial
malleolus of the tibia.

pouch *n* a pocket or recess. *pouch of
Douglas* the rectouterine pouch.

Poupart's ligament inguinal ligament.
Stretching from the anterior superior
spine of the ilium to the pubis.

poverty it may be defined as *absolute
poverty* where individuals lack sufficient
resources to maintain physical health,
such as not receiving sufficient nutrition,
or *relative poverty* when a person's living
standards are less than those that generally exist in a particular population. The
defining level for relative poverty shows
variation between different populations
and the same populations over time.

power calculation a measure of statistical
power. The likelihood of the study to produce statistically significant results.

powerlessness *n* a feeling that one is trapped and unable to control or influence circumstances. People may feel powerless in their dealings with healthcare professionals and healthcare systems.

poxviruses *npl* a family of DNA viruses that include those causing orf, vaccinia and variola.

PPD *abbr* purified protein derivative. ⇒ Heaf test. ⇒ Mantoux reaction.

PPLO *abbr* pleuropneumonia-like organism. ⇒ Mycoplasma.

PPV *abbr* positive pressure ventilation.

PQRST complex *n* the letters used to denote the five deflection waves of the typical waveform produced during a cardiac cycle. The P wave represents atrial depolarization as the impulse is conducted across the atria. The PR interval is the time taken for impulse conduction from the sinoatrial node, across the atria, to the atrioventricular node and to the ventricles. The next three waves are close together and are known collectively as the QRS complex and represent ventricular depolarization which immediately precedes contraction. The T wave represents ventricular repolarization. The period from the start of ventricular depolarization through contraction to repolarization is termed the QT interval. The ST segment represents a short period of inactivity and ventricular depolarization following the QRS complex. (See Figure 50). ⇒ electrocardiogram.

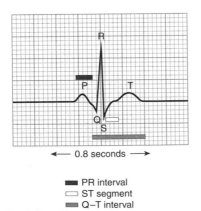

← 0.8 seconds →

■ PR interval
▢ ST segment
▨ Q–T interval

Figure 50 PQRST complex. (Reproduced from Brooker 1998 with permission.)

PR *abbr* per rectum; describes the route used for examination of the rectum, or introduction of substances into the body.

practice nurses registered nurses who are employed by general practitioners to carry out minor procedures, run nurse-led services and clinics, e.g. asthma clinics, advise on health problems and offer health checks. As members of the primary healthcare team, they are also responsible for the clinical nursing care of the practice population together with the community nursing team. ⇒ community nurse. ⇒ specialist community practitioner.

practitioner *n* in a nursing context, a clinician. In a wider health context, any professional who works with patients/clients. ⇒ general practitioner. ⇒ nurse practitioner.

Prader-Willi syndrome an inherited condition that arises from mutations in the paternal chromosome 15 during gametogenesis. It is characterized by learning disability, hypotonia, short stature and obesity. ⇒ Angleman syndrome. ⇒ genetic imprinting.

praecordial *adj* ⇒ precordial.

prana one of several terms used in complementary medicine to describe the individual's innate energy. ⇒ Qi energy.

precancerous *adj* obsolete term. ⇒ carcinoma-in-situ.

precedent a decision that may have to be followed in a subsequent court hearing.

preceptorship *n* a system to help the newly qualified nurse achieve confidence in the early months of registered practice, under the guidance of a preceptor.

precipitin *n* an antibody which is capable of forming an immune complex with an antigen and becoming insoluble – a precipitate. This reaction forms the basis of many delicate diagnostic serological tests for the identification of antigens in serum and other fluids. ⇒ immunoglobulins.

preconceptual *adj* before conception. Preconception care refers to the physical and mental preparation for childbearing of both parents before pregnancy. Attention to an adequate diet, e.g. ensuring sufficient folic acid, avoidance of alcohol, drugs (prescribed, over the counter and illegal) and smoking in the months before a couple decide to have a baby, reduces the risk of fetal problems and maternal complications during pregnancy and labour.

preconscious information in the subconscious mind that can be assessed and brought into the conscious mind if we so wish.

precordial, praecordial *adj* pertaining to the area of the chest immediately over the heart. *precordial thump* direct blow with closed fist over precordium. Sometimes used in the initial stages of resuscitation, where the cardiac arrest is witnessed, to shock the heart into sinus rhythm.

precordium area of the chest over the heart.

precursor *adj* forerunner. Often describes an inactive hormone or enzyme.

prediabetes *n* potential predisposition to diabetes mellitus — **prediabetic** *adj, n.*

predisposition *n* a natural tendency to develop or contract certain diseases.

pre-eclampsia *n* a very serious condition of pregnancy characterized by albuminuria, hypertension and oedema, arising usually in the latter part of pregnancy and endangering the health of both mother and fetus. ⇒ eclampsia — **pre-eclamptic** *adj.*

prefrontal *adj* situated in the anterior portion of the frontal lobe of the cerebrum, such as the precentral motor area of the cortex.

preganglionic *adj* preceding or in front of a collection of nerve cells (ganglia), as a preganglionic nerve fibre.

pregnancy *n* being with child, i.e. gestation from last menstrual period to parturition, normally 40 weeks or 280 days. ⇒ ectopic pregnancy. → pseudocyesis. *pregnancy test* confirmation of pregnancy denoted by the presence of the hormone chorionic gonadotrophin in the blood or urine. Some sophisticated techniques can confirm pregnancy before the first menstrual period has been missed. Self-test kits are available for use after the period is 2 weeks overdue.

pregnanediol *n* a urinary excretion product from progesterone.

prehensile *adj* equipped for grasping.

prejudice *n* a preconceived opinion or bias which can be negative or positive. It can be for or against members of particular groups and may lead to discrimination, racism, sexism or intolerance.

preload the degree of stretch present in the myocardial muscle fibres at the end of diastole. It depends on the end diastolic volume (EDV). In situations where venous return is reduced, such as shock, there is a reduction in the degree of stretch or preload. ⇒ afterload. ⇒ Starling's law of the heart. ⇒ stroke volume.

premature *adj* occurring before the proper time. ⇒ preterm.

premedication *n* drugs given before the administration of another drug, such as those given before an anaesthetic. The use of premedication has decreased with the development of daycase surgery. When given they may be: (a) sedative or anxiolytic, or (b) drugs which inhibit salivary and bronchial secretions.

premenstrual *adj* preceding menstruation. *premenstrual (cyclical) syndrome (PMS)* also known as premenstrual tension (PMT); a group of physical and mental changes which begin any time between 2 and 14 days before menstruation and which are relieved almost immediately the flow starts. The aetiology is unclear, but hormonal activity, deficiency of vitamin B_6 and of essential fatty acids have all been suggested as a possible cause. Its effects include: mood change, fluid retention with weight gain, lethargy, food cravings, breast discomfort, bruising and joint pains. Some women are treated successfully with pyridoxine (vitamin B_6), evening primrose oil, progestogens or oestrogens.

premolar teeth *npl* the teeth, also called bicuspids, situated 4th and 5th from the midline of the jaws, used with the molars for gripping and grinding food.

prenatal *adj* pertaining to the period between the last menstrual period and birth of the child, normally 40 weeks or 280 days — **prenatally** *adv.*

preoperative *adj* before operation. *preoperative assessment* often nurse-led clinics to assess general condition and suitability for day case surgery, order appropriate investigations, and give patients information and the opportunity to ask questions and discuss worries — **preoperatively** *adv.*

PREP *abbr* Postregistration Education and Practice. See Box – PREP – Postregistration Education and Practice.

PREP – Postregistration Education and Practice

In order for all nurses, health visitors and midwives to maintain their registered status with the UKCC they have to:

- Complete a notification of practice form at the point of re-registration every 3 years and/or when their area of professional practice changes to one where they will use a different registerable qualification;
- Demonstrate a minimum of 35 hours learning activity every 3 years;
- Maintain a personal professional profile containing details of professional development.

For individuals returning to practice, who have worked less than 750 hours in the preceding 5 years, they must undertake a 'return to practice' programme.

The area that causes most concern is continuing professional development, and the issues as to what exactly does '35 hours of learning activity' mean. The UKCC stress that they "do not approve any study days for PREP" (UKCC 1997). They state that "it is up to you to choose the most appropriate study for your professional development needs" and suggest that this can be as diverse as individual learning, for example reading up on new techniques, conditions and treatments; visiting areas of clinical expertise, shadowing other professionals, and attending study sessions. They stress that it is not purely undertaking an activity that fulfils your PREP needs, but your demonstration, through your profile and reflective practice, as to how your learning has affected your practice and therefore benefited patient/client care.

Reference
UKCC 1997 PREP and You. UKCC, London

---

preparalytic *adj* before the onset of paralysis, usually referring to the early stage of poliomyelitis.

prepatellar *adj* in front of the kneecap, as applied to a large bursa. ⇒ bursitis.

prepubertal *adj* relating to the time before puberty.

prepuce *n* the foreskin of the penis.

prerenal *adj* literally, before or in front of the kidney, but used to denote states in which, for instance, renal failure has arisen because of poor renal perfusion and reduced GFR. The cause being within the vascular fluid compartment, as in severe dehydration, or vasodilatation due to sepsis, or intravascular haemolysis.

presbycusis *n* sensorineural deafness occurring in older people.

presbyopia *n* longsightedness, due to failure of accommodation, typically commencing in those aged 45 years and over. It occurs as the lens becomes less elastic and affects near vision — **presbyope** *n*.

prescribed diseases a list of occupational diseases prescribed under the UK industrial injuries scheme. An advisory body advises the Secretary of State whether to accept or reject the arguments for prescription.

Prescribing Analysis and Costs (PACT) data sent to prescribers (general practitioners) regarding their prescribing.

prescription *n* a written formula, signed by the prescriber, directing the pharmacist to supply the required drugs.

prescription only medicines (POM) medicines which require a written prescription, except in an emergency when it may be dispensed by a pharmacist, providing certain criteria are met.

presenile dementia ⇒ dementia. ⇒ Alzheimer's disease.

presentation *n* the part of the fetus which first enters the pelvic brim; it may be vertex, face, brow, shoulder, breech or foot (footling).

pressor *n* a substance which raises the blood pressure.

pressure areas any area of the body subjected to pressure sufficient to compress the capillaries and disrupt the microcirculation. Usually occurs where tissues are compressed between a bone and a hard surface, e.g. trolley, bed, chair, splint etc, or where two skin surfaces are in contact. Pressure areas include: elbows, heels, ankles, hips, sacrum, spine, shoulders, head, buttocks and under breasts etc. ⇒ pressure ulcer.

pressure garment a garment for a particular part of the body. It is made of a strong, flesh-coloured Lycra material which produces firm, even pressure to the part. Often used in the treatment of varicose veins; and burns and scalds to prevent keloid scarring. ⇒ disfigurement.

pressure groups organizations that exist to put pressure on government (central and local) and advance the interests of certain groups, such as pensioners or people with disabilities.

pressure point a place at which an artery passes over a bone, against which it can be compressed to stop bleeding. (See Figure 51).

pressure sore ⇒ pressure ulcer.

pressure support ventilation (PSV) ⇒ mechanical ventilation.

pressure transducer *n* a transducer that converts pressure changes to an electrical trace, such as in the direct monitoring of blood pressure via an arterial cannula. ⇒ transducer.

pressure ulcer (*syn* pressure sore, decubitus ulcer). The European Pressure Ulcer Advisory Panel (EPUAP) defines a pressure ulcer as an area of localized damage to the skin and underlying tissue caused by pressure, shear, friction, or a combination of these factors. Pressure ulcers develop when any area of the body is subjected to unrelieved pressure that leads to tissue hypoxia, ischaemia and necrosis with inflammation and ulcer formation. Shearing forces also disrupt the microcirculation when they cause the skin layers to move against one another, such as a person slipping down the bed or being dragged instead of being moved correctly. Shearing injury damages the deeper tissues and can result in an extensive pressure

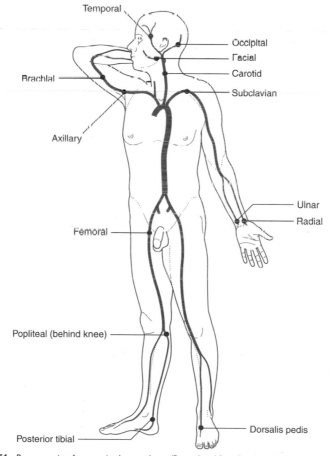

Figure 51 Pressure points for arresting haemorrhage. (Reproduced from Brooker 1996 with permission.)

ulcer. Friction from continual rubbing leads to blisters, abrasions and superficial pressure ulcers, and is exacerbated by the presence of moisture such as sweat or urine. Factors which predispose to pressure ulcer formation include: poor oxygenation, incontinence, age over 65–70, immobility, altered consciousness, dehydration and malnutrition. Assessment of the skin condition and the severity of existing pressure ulcers is an important part of the nursing assessment required for choosing the most appropriate interventions. There are several pressure ulcer grading scales, but the EPUAP recommends the use of a 4 point grading scale.

pressure ulcer prevention starts with assessment of skin condition and pressure areas using the most appropriate pressure ulcer risk scale on a regular basis. ⇒ Braden scale. ⇒ Norton scale. ⇒ Waterlow scale. Relief of pressure from the part is achieved by moving patients or encouraging them to move themselves, use of external aids such as special beds or mattresses, keeping the skin dry and clean, ensuring that fluid and nutritional needs are met, and avoiding shearing force and friction. ⇒ pressure areas. ⇒ pressure ulcer. ⇒ shearing force.

presystole *n* the period in the cardiac cycle preceding the systole or contraction of the heart muscle — **presystolic** *adj*.

preterm *adj* before term or premature. *preterm (premature) baby/birth* defined as the birth of a baby after 24 but before 37 weeks gestation. The baby is likely to be of low birthweight and possibly small-for-dates or dysmature through placental insufficiency.

prevalence *n* total number of cases of a disease existing in a population at a single point in time. *prevalence ratio* the number of cases of a disease existing in a population at a single point in time, expressed as a ratio of population size.

priapism *n* prolonged penile erection in the absence of sexual stimulation. May be a feature of spinal cord damage and some types of leukaemia.

prickle cells cells contained in the germinative layer of the epidermis.

prickly heat ⇒ miliaria.

prima facie at first sight, or sufficient evidence brought by one party to require the other party to provide a defence.

Primary Care Group in England, a grouping of primary healthcare professionals (family doctors, primary health teams and community nurses) and their services covering an area with a population of around 100 000. Working with the Health Authority, local authority and other relevant bodies, e.g. voluntary sector, they assess local health needs, plan and develop community and primary healthcare services and commission secondary services for the local population in order to improve health, and reduce inequalities in health and improve access to health care. In Scotland they are called Local Halth Co-operatives, and in Wales Local Health Groups (LHGs). ⇒ Primary Care Trust.

Primary Care Trust freestanding body developed from a PCG which, having autonomy, can respond more flexibly to local health needs. They may be a Level 3 PCT, which in addition to commissioning services may employ some staff, or a Level 4 PCT, which may, in addition, commission and provide community services, run community hospitals, own property and employ staff.

primary complex (*syn* Ghon focus) the initial tuberculous infection in a person, usually in the lung, and manifest as a small focus of infection in the lung tissue and enlarged caseous, hilar lymph nodes. It usually heals spontaneously.

primary health care health care that is provided outside of the hospital sector to individuals and families in their own homes or in the community. The World Health Organization declaration at Alma Ata in 1978 stated that such care should be acceptable, accessible, involve community participation and be available at a cost all families could afford. Most contacts that people have with health services are through primary care. ⇒ secondary care. ⇒ tertiary care. *primary healthcare team* an interdependent multiprofessional group of individuals who share a common purpose and responsibility, each member clearly understanding his or her own role, and those of other team members, in offering an effective primary healthcare service. The professionals involved may include: community nurses, counsellors, general practitioners, health visitors, midwives, occupational therapists, physiotherapists, podiatrists, practice nurses, speech and language therapists etc.

primary nursing a professional model of practice, based on a belief in the therapeutic value of the nurse-patient relationship. A qualified nurse (primary nurse) is responsible and accountable for the assessment, planning and implementation of all the nursing care of a particular patient or group of patients for the entire duration of their stay in a particular care setting. The nurse is supported in this role by an associate nurse who cares for the patient while the primary nurse is absent, according to the nursing plan drawn up by the primary nurse. Other nurses, including students and healthcare assistants, may also provide care for the patient, but this is always under the supervision and co-ordination of the primary nurse. Primary nursing is not the same as named nursing – it is simply one form of named nursing, although probably the most highly developed. ⇒ named nurse, ⇒ team nursing.

primary prevention ⇒ disease prevention.

primigravida *n* a woman who is pregnant for the first time   **primigravidae** *pl*.

primipara *n* a woman who has given birth to a child for the first time — **primiparous** *adj*.

primordial *adj* primitive, original; applied to the primitive cells formed during early embryonic development. *primordial follicles* ovarian follicles containing primary oocytes, present in the ovary at birth.

prion *n* an infectious agent consisting of protein, similar to viruses but containing no nucleic acids. Prions are responsible for the transmission of diseases which include: Creutzfeldt-Jakob disease in humans, and bovine spongiform encephalopathy and scrapie in animals.

priority setting see Box – Priority setting.

Private Finance Initiative (PFI) a collaboration between private and public sector where a facility, such as a hospital, is built using private as opposed to treasury finance. The building is then leased to the NHS. In some schemes, certain support services are also provided within the lease agreement.

privilege in relation to evidence, being able to refuse to disclose it in court.

proaccelerin ⇒ factor V. ⇒ labile factor.

proactive interference ⇒ interference.

proband *n* the original person presenting for investigation of a genetically-inherited disease, who forms the basis for genetic study.

probity dealing with matters with integrity and honesty.

problem-oriented records a multiprofessional system of patient records in which each patient's problem has a numbered page and entries are made using the SOAP formula: S=subjective, O=objective, A=analysis of the subjective and objective data, P=plan.

procedural memory that part of memory that stores information needed to do things, e.g. take a blood pressure or switch on your computer.

process *n* 1. a prominence or outgrowth of any part. 2. a series of sequential steps such as the nursing process.

procidentia *n* complete prolapse of the uterus, so that it lies within the vaginal sac but outside the contour of the body.

proconvertin ⇒ factor VII. ⇒ stable factor.

proctalgia *n* pain in the rectal region.

proctitis *n* inflammation of the rectum. Usually a feature of ulcerative colitis, ⇒ inflammatory bowel disease. *granular proctitis* acute proctitis, so called because of the granular appearance of the inflamed mucous membrane. May follow radiotherapy for abdominal cancers.

proctoclysis *n* the introduction of fluid into the rectum for absorption.

Priority setting

This activity seeks to arrive at a decision which will result in a particular client group or range of services being designated higher priority than others, and thus can receive a greater share of the NHS resource. These priorities are identified within national guidelines, and thus inform decisions locally throughout the UK. New funding may be offered to services deemed priority. Rationing of care is different from priority setting in that rationing seeks to award funding based on the evidence of effectiveness of the intervention. Priority setting tends to be based on overall social values of what is deemed to require significant resourcing from the NHS. Examples of priority services are cancer services and mental health services.

proctocolectomy *n* surgical excision of the rectum and colon resulting in a permanent colostomy. *restorative proctocolectomy* avoids a permanent stoma: an ileal reservoir is formed and ileoanal anastomosis carried out.

proctocolitis *n* inflammation of the rectum and colon; usually a feature of ulcerative colitis. ⇒ inflammatory bowel disease.

proctoscope *n* an instrument for examining the rectum. ⇒ endoscope — **proctoscopy** *n*.

proctosigmoiditis *n* inflammation of the rectum and sigmoid colon.

prodromal *adj* preceding. Relating to the period that elapses in an infectious disease between the first symptoms and the appearance of the rash. *prodromal rash* the transitory rash before the true rash of an infectious disease.

prodrug *n* a drug administered as an inactive form that is activated within the body, e.g. by enzymes in the liver, in the brain or by bacteria in the bowel. They are used for a variety of reasons that include: overcoming gastrointestinal side-effects and damage such as with the cytotoxic drug cyclophosphamide that is only activated in the liver; the antiviral drug zidovudine is activated by the reverse transcriptase enzymes present in HIV-infected cells, thus allowing it to act selectively; oral L-dopa (given for parkinsonism) can be absorbed and passes through the blood-brain barrier where it is converted to dopamine (whereas dopamine given parenterally acts upon renal blood vessels and does not cross the blood-brain barrier).

proenzyme *n* precursor or inactive form of an enzyme, such as pepsinogen. ⇒ zymogen.

professional disciplinary process nurses are required to be self-disciplined and to act responsibly while nursing, so that they are accountable for their actions. Complaints against nurses are made to the statutory regulatory body, where the professional conduct of a nurse is investigated and judged by peers. Where the complaint is upheld, the nurse may be cautioned, allowed to practise with conditions attached or their name removed from the professional register. ⇒ professional self-regulation.

professional judgement a complex skill, using cognition, intuition, a high level of professional education and experience to make a decision, often in emergency, without being conscious of using a logical process.

professional self-regulation the professional quality and continuing professional development standards set by various professional regulatory bodies for health professionals, e.g. GMC, UKCC (NMC), for professional practice, discipline and conduct. ⇒ professional disciplinary process.

profiling (community) process of creating a profile of a particular community. It includes information such as the age profile, existing facilities, networks and services etc. The profile may be produced by members of the community with varying degrees of support from the local authority, development agencies or health services. ⇒ community development.

progeria *n* a congenital condition characterized by premature aging occurring during childhood.

progestational agent that supports gestation (pregnancy), usually applied to progestogen hormones.

progesterone *n* gestation hormone. A steroid hormone produced by the corpus luteum, placenta and, to a limited extent, the adrenal glands. It influences the endometrium, myometrium, cervical mucus and breasts. It is important in preparing for and maintaining pregnancy. Therapeutic uses have included: threatened miscarriage, contraception and functional uterine bleeding. It is given by injection and has mostly been replaced by synthetic progestogens that are active by mouth.

progestogen *n* any natural or synthetic progestational hormone with a similar action to progesterone.

progestogen only pill *n* an oral contraceptive that only contains progestogen. It is taken continuously and at regular times in order to provide effective contraception; it is less reliable than the combined oral contraceptive.

proglottis *n* a sexually mature segment of tapeworm — **proglottides** *pl*.

prognosis *n* the expected course or outcome of a disease — **prognostic** *adj*.

program a set of coded numeric instructions that instruct the CPU to perform a specific task, e.g. word processing.

progress sheets a name used by some documentation systems for recording the implementation of planned nursing interventions, ongoing assessment and summative evaluation data.

Project 2000 a system of preregistration nurse education, launched by the UKCC in the late 1980s. Nurses were educated to diploma level through a common foundation programme of 18 months, followed by a chosen branch of nursing: care of the adult, the child, people with mental illness and people with a learning disability. Curricula were rooted in health promotion and primary health care. Major changes to preregistration nurse education are planned, and new curricula are being piloted in several sites, based on the two documents: Commission for Education (1999) *Fitness for Practice* London: UKCC and Department of Health (1999); *Making a difference* London: The Stationery Office. → Fitness for practice.

projectile vomiting forceful ejection of stomach contents. Occurs shortly after feeding in babies with pyloric stenosis, when peristaltic movement is visible on the upper abdomen. Characteristic of some cerebral conditions.

projection *n* a mental defence mechanism occurring in normal people unconsciously, and in exaggerated form in mental illness, especially paranoia, whereby the person fails to recognize certain motives and feelings in himself but attributes them to others.

projective techniques *npl* using creative media, such as music, art, writing and modelling, to encourage personal interpretation of the material to facilitate the exploration of experiences and feelings.

prokaryote *n* a cell where the genetic material is scattered within the cytoplasm, such as in many micro-organisms. There is no true nucleus. ⇒ eukaryote.

prolactin (PRL) *n* a hormone secreted by the anterior pituitary, concerned with lactation and reproduction. Also known as the lactogenic hormone. Increased levels are found in some pituitary tumours. ⇒ hyperprolactinaemia.

prolapse *n* descent; the falling of a structure. *prolapse of an intervertebral disc (PID)* protrusion of the disc nucleus into the spinal canal. Most common in the lumbar region where it causes low back pain and/or sciatica. ⇒ backache. *prolapse of the iris* iridocele. *prolapse of the rectum* the lower portion of the intestinal tract descends outside the external anal sphincter. *prolapse of the umbilical cord* the umbilical cord prolapses through the cervix after the membranes have ruptured during labour. It constitutes an obstetric emergency. *prolapse of the uterus* the uterus descends into the vagina and may be visible at the vaginal orifice. ⇒ procidentia.

proliferation *n* reproduction. Increase in cell division and growth, such as in tissue repair or cancer — **proliferative** *adj*.

proliferative phase *n* 1. the stage of the menstrual cycle that commences after bleeding has stopped and lasts until ovulation. It is charaterized by endometrial regeneration and corresponds to the follicular phase of the ovarian cycle. 2. phase of wound healing that includes: production of a collagen network and granulation tissue, epithelialization and wound contraction.

prolific *adj* fruitful, multiplying abundantly.

promontory *n* a projection; a prominent part.

pronate *vt* to place ventral surface downward, e.g. on the face; to turn (the palm of the hand) downwards. → supinate *ant* — **pronation** *n*.

pronator *n* that which pronates, usually applied to a muscle, such as the pronator teres in the arm. ⇒ supinator *ant*.

prone *adj* 1. lying on the anterior surface of the body with the face turned to one or other side. 2. of the hand, with the palm downwards. ⇒ supine *ant*.

pronephros *n* an early embryonic structure formed during the development of the urinary tract.

proof evidence that secures the establishment of the plaintiff's case or the prosecution's or defendant's case.

prophase the first stage of mitosis and meiosis.

prophylaxis *n* (attempted) prevention — **prophylactic** *adj* relating to prophylaxis or an agent that prevents disease, such as a drug or vaccine.

propionic acids *npl* a group of non-steroidal anti-inflammatory drugs, e.g. ibuprofen, naproxen.

proprietary name the brand name given to e.g. a drug by the pharmaceutical firm which produced it. The name should always be spelt with a capital letter to distinguish it from the approved (generic) name which can be used by any manufacturer. ⇒ approved name.

proprioception a nonvisual awareness of spatial orientation and the position of body parts. Transmission of sensory stimuli, such as those from pressure, position or stretch, arising within the body, to a proprioceptor, from which they are transmitted in the central nervous system to produce the necessary response to the stimulus.

proprioceptor *n* sensory end organ able to detect changes in the position of the body. They are located in the muscles, joints, tendons and the inner ear.

proptosis *n* forward protrusion, especially of the eyeball.

prosector's wart ⇒ verruca.

prosecution the pursuing of criminal cases in court.

prosody *n* a descriptive term for the phonological features of speech, including rate, stress, rhythm, loudness and pitch.

prospective study research that collects data in the future, moving forward in time. ⇒ retrospective study.

prostacyclin *n* a prostaglandin derivative. Formed by endothelial cells of blood vessel walls. It inhibits platelet aggregation and is a potent vasodilating agent. Important in preventing intravascular clotting.

prostaglandins *npl* a large group of regulatory lipds derived from arachidonic acid (fatty acid). They are present in most body tissues where they regulate many physiological functions that include; smooth muscle contraction, inflammation, gastric secretion, blood clotting and reproduction. Used therapeutically to: induce termination of pregnancy, induce labour, manage postpartum haemorrhage, prevent platelet aggregation during haemodialysis, and maintain a patent ductus arteriosus in neonates with impaired lung perfusion due to heart defects such as pulmonary stenosis prior to surgical correction. A synthetic analogue is used to prevent peptic ulceration.

prostate *n* a small structure consisting of several glands within a capsule. It surrounds the male bladder neck and urethra. It secretes an alkaline fluid containing enzymes into the semen prior to ejaculation. *prostate cancer* a common cancer, usually affecting older men. It is characterized by dysuria, cystitis or prostatitis, frequency, poor stream, hesitancy and retention of urine. Management may involve: observation only in some cases, radical prostatectomy, radiotherapy, or hormone therapy. Advanced disease causes weight loss and bone pain from metastases and patients may have signs of uraemia caused by obstruction of the ureters. ⇒ prostate specific antigen — **prostatic** *adj* pertaining to the prostate gland. *benign prostatic hyperplasia (BPH)* benign enlargement of the prostate gland occurring mainly in older men. Leads to urinary problems such as retention. *prostatic acid phosphatase* ⇒ acid phosphatase.

prostate specific antigen (PSA) *n* an antigen which, if found in the serum, acts as a tumour marker for prostate cancer. Levels may be raised in conditions other than cancer.

prostatectomy *n* surgical removal of the prostate gland. Most commonly, this is achieved by transurethral resection of the prostate (TURP or TUR), but in some cases, such as where the prostate is very large, it is not possible. In these cases it is necessary to remove the gland by opening the lower abdomen, either by a transvesical approach (*transvesical prostatectomy*) or by the retropubic operation (*retropubic* or *Millin's prostatectomy*).

prostatism *n* general condition produced by an enlarged prostate gland, such as with benign prostatic hyperplasia (BPH), occurring mainly in older men, prostate cancer, or chronic disease of the prostate gland. It is characterized by the obstructive symptoms of frequency, hesitancy, a poor stream, postmicturition dribbling, recurrent UTI and retention.

prostatitis *n* inflammation of the prostate gland.

prostatocystitis *n* inflammation of the prostate gland and male urinary bladder.

prosthesis *n* an artificial substitute for a body part, such as a limb, heart valve or breast — **prosthetic** *adj.*

prosthetics *n* the branch of surgery which deals with prostheses.

prosthokeratoplasty *n* keratoplasty in which the corneal implant is of some material other than human or animal tissue.

protease *n* any enzyme which digests protein: a proteolytic enzyme.

protective isolation reverse barrier nursing. Separation of immunocompromised individuals (through disease or treatment) to protect them from infection. This may be necessary when the patient has leukaemia or AIDS, and during treatment with immunosuppressant drugs for organ transplantation, chemotherapy or radiation or whenever the neutrophil count is low. ⇒ containment isolation. ⇒ source isolation.

protein-calorie malnutrition (PCM) → protein-energy malnutrition (PEM).

protein-energy malnutrition (PEM) *n* a form of malnutrition caused by an insufficient intake of protein and energy, such as in famine situations or anorexia. May occur in hospitalized individuals who develop a negative nitrogen balance because protein is primarily being used to produce energy. A negative balance is associated with starvation or any severe physiological stress which increases protein catabolism, e.g. burns, sepsis, major surgery and multiple injuries. → kwashiorkor. → marasmus.

proteins *npl* complex nitrogenous organic compounds formed from amino acids in different combinations and sequences. They are found in animal and vegetable tissues. Those from animal sources are generally of high biological value since they contain the essential amino acids. Those from vegetable sources have low biological value because they do not contain all the essential amino acids; for example, wheat and rice have low levels of lysine and legumes are low in methionine and tryptophan. It is important that people who eat little or no animal protein select a mixture of plant source proteins. Protein is a vital component of all living organisms and they are needed for cell division, growth and repair and to form functional proteins which include: enzymes, hormones and haemoglobin. Proteins are hydrolysed in the body to produce amino acids which are then used to build up new body proteins. ⇒ kilojoule.

proteinuria *n* protein in the urine. ⇒ albuminuria.

proteolysis *n* the hydrolysis of the peptide bonds of proteins with the formation of smaller polypeptides — **proteolytic** *adj.*

proteolytic enzymes enzymes that promote proteolysis; they are used as a desloughing agent for leg ulcers, e.g. streptokinase and streptodornase.

proteose *n* a mixture of products from the breakdown of proteins, between protein and peptone.

Proteus *n* a bacterial genus. Gram-negative motile bacilli. Found in damp surroundings. A commensal of the intestinal tract. Causes wound and urinary tract infection.

prothrombin *n* Factor II in blood coagulation. An inactive precursor of the enzyme thrombin formed in the liver. The *prothrombin time* tests the activity of the extrinsic coagulation pathway. It is the time taken for plasma to clot in a test tube after thromboplastin is added in the presence of calcium. It is inversely proportional to the amount of prothrombin present, a normal person's plasma being used as a standard of comparison. Prothrombin time is lengthened in certain haemorrhagic conditions and in a patient having anticoagulant drugs. ⇒ coagulation.

proto-oncogene *n* a gene that has the potential to become a cancer-causing oncogene if stimulated by mutagenic carcinogens. ⇒ oncogene.

proton *n* subatomic particle with a positive charge.

proton pump inhibitors *npl* a group of drugs that reduce gastric acid production by irreversibly blocking the proton pump (H^+/K^+-ATPase), e.g. omeprazole. Used in the management of peptic ulcer and oesophageal reflux.

protopathic *adj* describes the somatic sensations of fast localized pain; slow, poorly localized pain; and temperature. ⇒ epicritic.

protoplasm *n* the viscid, gel-like substance that forms the main part of a cell. It is enclosed by the cell (plasma) membrane and contains the subcellular organelles. Comprises a complex mix of molecules. The protoplasm contained in the nuclear membrane is called nucleoplasm and that in the rest of the cell is called cytoplasm — **protoplasmic** *adj*.

protozoa *npl* unicellular microscopic animals. They are usually harmless, but may be pathogenic. Some may infect immunocompromised individuals. The phylum includes the genera *Plasmodium*, *Leishmania* and *Entamoeba*. ⇒ amoebiasis. ⇒ giardiasis. ⇒ leishmaniasis. ⇒ malaria. ⇒ toxoplasmosis. ⇒ trichomoniasis — **protozoon** *sing* — **protozoal** *adj*.

proud flesh excessive granulation tissue.

provitamin *n* a precursor substance that can be converted to the active vitamin in the body, e.g. carotene into vitamin A and tryptophan into nicotinamide.

proxemics study of how space and spatial relationships affect behaviour, e.g. population density.

proximal *adj* nearest to the head or source. *proximal convoluted tubule* ⇒ nephron. ⇒ distal — **proximally** *adv*.

prune belly syndrome a rare condition found in male infants with obstructive uropathy and atrophy of the abdominal musculature. The term is descriptive. Various surgical measures are available for most types of bladder neck obstruction.

prurigo *n* any chronic, itching skin disease with papules.

pruritus *n* intense itching. Repeated scratching can lead to secondary infection. It may occur as a manifestation of a particular skin disease. Generalized pruritus may be a symptom of systemic disease as in infection, renal failure, diabetes, jaundice, thyroid disease, allergy and malignancy, such as Hodgkin's disease and other lymphomas. *pruritus ani* intense itching around the anus. Causes include: threadworm infestation, haemorrhoids, candidiasis and psychogenic illness. *pruritus vulvae* intense itching of the external genitalia. Causes include vaginitis due to candidiasis and trichomoniasis, glycosuria, malignancy and psychogenic illness. ⇒ leukoplakia — **pruritic** *adj*.

PSA *abbr* prostate specific antigen.

pseudoangina *n* false angina. Chest pain that may occur in anxious individuals. Usually there is no cardiac disease present. May be part of effort syndrome.

pseudoarthrosis *n* a false joint.

pseudobulbar paralysis gross disturbance in control of tongue, following on from a succession of 'strokes'.

pseudocoxalgia ⇒ Perthes' disease.

pseudocrisis *n* a rapid reduction of body temperature resembling a crisis, followed by further fever.

pseudocyesis false or phantom pregnancy. When there are signs and symptoms of pregnancy in a woman who believes she is pregnant, when she is not. ⇒ phantom pregnancy.

pseudohermaphrodite *n* a person in whom the gonads of one sex are present, whilst the external genitalia comprise those of the opposite sex.

pseudohermaphroditism ⇒ intersexuality.

pseudologia fantastica a tendency to tell, and defend, fantastic lies plausibly, found in some people suffering from a psychopathic personality.

pseudomembranous colitis *n* a condition caused by superinfection with *Clostridium difficile* in patients whose normal bowel flora has been destroyed by broad spectrum antibiotics. It is characterized by watery diarrhoea and can be life-threatening. Treatment is with antibiotics, e.g. metronidazole or vancomycin. ⇒ superinfection.

Pseudomonas *n* a bacterial genus. Gram-negative motile bacilli. Found in water and decomposing vegetable matter. *Pseudomonas aeruginosa* causes wound, urinary and respiratory infection in humans. It can cause superinfection where the normal commensals have been destroyed by broad spectrum antibiotics. Produces blue-green exudate or pus which has a characteristic musty odour. ⇒ superinfection.

pseudomucin *n* a gelatinous substance (not mucin) found in some ovarian cysts.

pseudoparalysis *n* a loss of muscular power not due to a lesion of the nervous system.

pseudophakia *n* presence of an artificial intraocular lens implant following cataract surgery.

pseudoplegia *n* paralysis mimicking that of organic nervous disorder but usually originating from a hysterical neurosis.

pseudopodia *npl* literally false legs; cytoplasmic projections of an amoeba or any mobile cell which help it to move. Not to be confused with cilia or microvilli which are nonretractile projections from the cell surface — **pseudopodium** *sing*.

pseudosyncytium a tissue where the boundaries between individual cells are poorly defined. ⇒ syncytium.

psittacosis *n* disease of parrots, pigeons and budgerigars which is occasionally responsible for atypical pneumonia with systemic illness in humans. Caused by *Chlamydia psittaci*. It behaves as a bacterium though multiplying intracellularly. Sensitive to tetracyclines and macrolide antibiotics, e.g. erythromycin.

psoas *n* muscles of the loin. *psoas abscess* a cold abscess in the psoas muscle, resulting from tuberculosis of the lower dorsal or lumbar vertebrae. Pressure in the abscess causes pus to track along the tough ligaments so that the abscess appears as a firm smooth swelling which does not show signs of inflammation, hence the adjective 'cold'.

psoriasis *n* a chronic inflammatory skin disease in which erythematous areas are covered with adherent scales. Although the condition may occur on any part of the body, the characteristic sites are extensor surfaces, especially over the knees and elbows. Factors implicated in its aetiology include: a genetic predisposition, immunological and biochemical factors. There are several types of psoriasis: (a) erythrodermic, which is characterized by red and scaly skin; (b) guttate in children where the rash develops quickly with small lesions; (c) the most common plaque type with well demarcated red lesions with silvery white scales; (d) pustular, which may be local or general pustule formation. Generalized pustular type is usually accompanied by systemic effects, such as fever. Some 3–5% of people develop an arthropathy that may be similar to rheumatoid arthritis — **psoriatic** *adj*.

PSV *abbr* pressure support ventilation.

psyche *n* the Greek term for 'life force', used to describe that which constitutes the mind and all its processes, and sometimes used to describe 'self'.

psychiatric nursing ⇒ mental health nursing.

psychiatry *n* the branch of medicine devoted to the diagnosis, treatment and care of people suffering from mental illness — **psychiatric** *adj*.

psychic *adj* of the mind.

psychoactive drugs and other substances that may alter the processes of the mind.

psychoanalysis *n* a method of psychotherapy in which the relationship between patient and therapist is analysed and traced back to the patient's earliest relationships. Concerned with unconscious feelings and attitudes — **psychoanalytic** *adj*.

psychochemotherapy *n* the use of drugs to improve or cure pathological changes in the emotional state. ⇒ antidepressants. ⇒ anxiolytics. ⇒ neuroleptics. ⇒ sedative. ⇒ tranquillizers — **psychochemotherapeutic** *adj*.

psychodrama *n* a method of psychotherapy whereby patients act out their personal problems by taking roles in spontaneous dramatic performances. Group discussion aims at giving the patients a greater awareness of the problems presented and possible methods of dealing with them.

psychodynamics *n* the science of the mental processes, especially of the causative factors in mental activity.

psychogenesis *n* the development of the mind.

psychogenic *adj* arising from the psyche or mind. *psychogenic symptom* originates in the mind rather than in the body.

psychogeriatric *adj* old-fashioned term, pertaining to psychology as applied to geriatrics. The phrase elderly mentally ill (EMI) has also been used.

psychokinesis describes how mental influences cause physical events in the absence of any physical forces. ⇒ parapsychology.

psychology *n* the scientific study of the behaviour of an organism and mental processes.

psychometry *n* the science of mental testing. ⇒ intelligence.

psychomotor *adj* pertaining to the motor effect of psychic or cerebral activity.

psychoneuroimmunology (PNI) *n* study of the integration of neural and immune response in relation to psychological state. Psychological distress/stress is linked with reduced immunological functioning.

psychoneurosis *n* ⇒ neurosis.

psychopath *n* one who has a psychopathic personality — **psychopathic** *adj*.

psychopathic personality a persistent disorder or disability of mind which results in abnormally aggressive or seriously irresponsible conduct. The person lacks the ability to feel a sense of guilt for the consequences of his or her actions. They often behave in a destructive and antisocial manner.

psychopathology *n* the pathology of abnormal mental processes — **psychopathological** *adj*.

psychopathy *n* any disease of the mind. The term is used by some people to denote a marked immaturity in emotional development — **psychopathic** *adj*.

psychopharmacology *n* the use of drugs which influence the affective and emotional state. The study of drugs in psychiatry.

psychophysics *n* a branch of experimental psychology dealing with the study of stimuli and sensations — **psychophysical** *adj*.

psychophysiological the physiological status determined by the current state of mind — **psychophysiology** *n*.

psychoprophylactic *adj* that which aims at preventing mental disease.

psychosexual pertaining to the mental aspects of sexuality. *psychosexual development* according to Freud's theory, development occurs through five stages (oral, anal, phallic, latent and genital). Each stage is characterized by a different area of pleasurable stimulation. ⇒ anal stage. ⇒ genital stage. ⇒ latency stage. ⇒ oral stage. ⇒ phallic stage.

psychosexual counselling usually sought by one or both members of a partnership because one or both is not experiencing emotional and sexual satisfaction within the relationship. Psychosexual counselling of otherwise 'healthy' people is provided by specialists and is rarely provided by the NHS in the UK. In a nursing context, nurses should be aware that patients whose treatment results in a negative change of body image need information to help them to adjust to changes in the emotional and sexual spheres of their living. Some of the conditions which may involve such a need are: arthritis and other musculoskeletal disorders; debilitating diseases such as cancer, especially during treatment with chemotherapy and radiotherapy; infections of the male and female reproductive and urinary tracts; mastectomy; cardiac disease; surgery on the female reproductive and male genitourinary systems; paraplegia; tetraplegia; postchildbirth due to tiredness and perineal soreness; poststroke; renal dialysis; stoma formation; mental health problems etc. Healthcare professionals need to be aware that any health disturbance may create actual or potential psychosexual problems. ⇒ sexual dysfunction.

psychosis *n* a major mental health disorder in which the individual lacks insight into their condition; they do not recognize that they are ill or that their experiences are part of illness. The symptoms of psychosis are qualitatively quite different from normal experience, e.g. hallucinations. It is usually characterized by loss of reality, hallucinations, delusions, impulses and disintegration of personality. ⇒ neurosis, for comparison. Various classifications exist, but broadly it may be: (a) organic: acute, as in delirium, e.g. electrolyte imbalance or alcohol etc; or chronic, as in dementia, which may be due to brain pathology, nutritional deficiencies, etc; (b) functional: conditions occurring without brain disease or impairment, e.g. schizophrenia, major depression and manic-depressive illness — **psychotic** *adj*.

psychosocial *adj* pertaining to both psychological and social factors, such as in a client assessment.

psychosocial family intervention see Box – Psychosocial family intervention.

psychosomatic *adj* relating to the mind and body. *psychosomatic disorder* a physical condition caused by a psychological factor, such as some types of peptic ulcer.

Psychosocial family intervention

Psychosocial family intervention assumes that schizophrenia has a defined genetic component and is exacerbated by stressful life events and emotional environments. The interventions are evidence based and were designed to promote low expressed emotion characteristics and address the problems faced by families after their family member has been discharged from hospital. The interventions used are psychosocial and educational in nature, because unlike traditional family 'therapy', they involve educating families about the diagnosis and treatment of schizophrenia, engaging them in the treatment process, teaching communication skills, problem solving and managing concerns in a nonblaming atmosphere (Barrowclough & Tarrier, 1992). The devised interventions draw from a cognitive behavioural model, a structured form of psychotherapy that incorporates problem-solving strategies. By mastering methods to objectively identify and eliminate the behaviours and thinking errors that cause them to feel upset, clients and their relatives are more likely to learn to cope with everyday burdens and feel more positive about the illness and its outcome.

Reference
Barrowclough C, Tarrier N 1995 Families of Schizophrenic Patients: Cognitive behaviour intervention. Chapman and Hall, London

---

psychosomimetics, psychotomimetics *npl* drugs which produce the symptoms of a psychosis.

psychosurgery surgical procedures, usually involving the brain, carried out for the relief of a mental health disorder. Rarely undertaken.

psychotherapy *n* a way of dealing with psychological and emotional problems by interaction between individuals or groups, usually by 'talking', but there are many different methods. Psychotherapists are not necessarily medically qualified. *group psychotherapy* also known as 'group therapy'. With a therapist, patients are encouraged to understand and analyse their own and one another's problems — **psychotherapeutic** *adj*.

psychotropic *adj* that which exerts its specific effect upon the brain cells, e.g. certain drugs.

psychrophile a bacterium that grows best at temperatures around 20°C, but some may grow slowly at temperatures as low as 4°C. They are responsible for spoiling food that has not been refrigerated properly — **psychrophilic** *adj*.

PTA *abbr* plasma thromboplastin antecedent.

pteroyl glutamic acid ⇒ folic acid.

pterygium *n* a wing-shaped degenerative condition of the conjunctiva which encroaches on the cornea — **pterygial** *adj*.

PTH *abbr* parathyroid hormone.

ptosis *n* a drooping, particularly that of the eyelid — **ptotic** *adj*.

PTSD *abbr* post traumatic stress disorder.

ptyalin *n* ⇒ amylase.

ptyalism *n* excessive salivation.

ptyalolith *n* a salivary calculus.

pubertas praecox premature (precocious) sexual development.

puberty *n* the period of time during which the reproductive organs become functional. It is associated with the appearance of the secondary sexual characteristics — **pubertal** *adj*.

pubes *n* the hairy region covering the pubic bone.

pubiotomy *n* rarely performed procedure whereby the pubic bone is cut to increase the pelvic diameter to facilitate the delivery of a live child. ⇒ symphisiotomy.

pubis *n* the pubic bone. The anterior part of the pelvis, the right and left pubic bones which meet at the symphysis pubis — **pubic** *adj*.

public health see Box - Public health.

public health nurse term used primarily to describe health visitors and school nurses although other community nurses have a public health role. ⇒ public health nursing. ⇒ specialist community practitioner.

public health nursing health visitors, school nurses, practice nurses and other community nurses who promote public health and work to prevent ill health in a variety of settings, e.g. schools, workplaces and communities.

pubocervical pertaining to the pubis and cervix.

pudendal block the rendering insensitive of the pudendum by the injection of local anaesthetic. Used mainly for episiotomy and instrumental delivery ⇒ transvaginal

---

Public health
Public health or the health of the population depends on many factors that are the remit of government such as transport, housing and the quality of the environment. The improvements in health in the nineteenth century owed more to policy interventions to ensure clean water, waste and sewage disposal, food hygiene and housing than they did to developments in clinical medicine. The new public health looks for the roots and causes of health and ill health. It does not isolate individual health within a medical perspective but puts it in a social and political context that includes wider factors that impede well-being such as poor housing, family breakdown, lack of employment. Public health work means working in partnership with other agencies, drawing attention to health issues in a community or society through needs assessments and profiling, developing services that are appropriate, accessible and acceptable to disadvantaged groups and finding ways to involve people in decisions affecting their health.

---

pudendum *n* the external genitalia, especially of the female — **pudendal** *adj* pertaining to the pudendum.

Pudenz-Hayer valve one-way valve implanted at operation for relief of hydrocephalus.

puerperal *adj* pertaining to childbirth. *puerperal psychosis* severe mental health disorder occurring after childbirth. *puerperal sepsis or fever* infection of the genital tract occurring within 21 days of abortion or childbirth.

puerperium *n* the period of 6–8 weeks following childbirth, in which the reproductive structures return to normal nonpregnant state in a process known as involution — **puerperia** *pl.*

PUFA *abbr* polyunsaturated fatty acid.

pulmonary *adj* pertaining to the lungs. *pulmonary circulation* deoxygenated blood leaves the right ventricle, flows through the lungs where it loses carbon dioxide and becomes oxygenated and returns to the left atrium of the heart. ⇒ circulation. *pulmonary embolism* an embolism which occurs in the pulmonary arterial system; most commonly as a result of phlebothrombosis and can be instantly fatal. Supervision of patients' deep breathing and foot exercises, early mobilization and the wearing of antithromboembolic stockings after surgery are preventive nursing interventions used in conjunction with the administration of prophylactic heparin in at-risk groups. *pulmonary emphysema* overdistention and subsequent destruction of alveoli and reduced gas exchange in the lungs. Linked to cigarette smoking, it is a form of chronic obstructive pulmonary disease (COPD). ⇒ bronchitis. *pulmonary function tests* series of tests used to assess lung function, e.g. spirometry, peak flow, blood gases. *pulmonary hypertension* raised blood pressure within the pulmonary circulation, due to increased resistance to blood flow within the pulmonary vessels. It is associated with increased pressure in the right cardiac ventricle, then the atrium. It may be due to disease of the left side of the heart or in the lung. In primary pulmonary hypertension the cause is not known. It usually leads to death from congestive heart failure in 2–10 years. *pulmonary infarction* necrosis of lung tissue resulting from an embolus. *pulmonary oedema* fluid within the alveoli. The lungs are 'waterlogged' and gas exchange is reduced, e.g. in left ventricular failure, mitral stenosis, fluid excess in renal failure, toxic gas inhalation. *pulmonary stenosis* narrowing of the pulmonary valve. *pulmonary tuberculosis* ⇒ tuberculosis. *pulmonary valve* semilunar valve situated between the pulmonary artery and right cardiac ventricle. *pulmonary ventilation* or minute volume. The amount of air moved in and out of the lungs in one minute.

pulmonary artery flotation catheter (PAFC) *n* catheter inserted into the pulmonary artery. Used in critical care situations to measure: pulmonary artery occlusion pressure (and indirectly the pressure on the left side of the heart). Modified PAFCs can be used to measure cardiac output from which the cardiac index, stroke volume, pulmonary vascular resistance and systemic vascular resistance can be calculated.

pulmonary artery occlusion pressure (PAOP) *n* also known as pulmonary artery wedge pressure.

pulmonary artery pressure *n* the pressure measured in the pulmonary artery (using a PAFC). The normal systolic is 15–25 mmHg, the diastolic is 8–15 mmHg and the mean is 10–20 mmHg.

pulmonary artery wedge pressure a method of measuring end diastolic left ventricular pressure by means of a catheter (e.g. Swan-Gantz) passed into a small pulmonary artery via the right side of the heart. At intervals a small balloon in the catheter tip is inflated to wedge it and block off the pulmonary artery behind. Now the pressure being recorded in the pulmonary capillaries will reflect that in the left atrium and ventricle.

pulmonary vascular resistance (PVR) *n* the resistance in the pulmonary vascular bed that the right ventricle must overcome in order to pump blood into the pulmonary circulation.

pulp *n* the soft, interior part of some organs and structures. *digital pulp* the tissue pad of the finger tip. Infection of this is referred to as 'pulp space infection'. ⇒ dental pulp.

pulsatile *adj* beating, throbbing.

pulsation *n* beating or throbbing, as of the heart or arteries.

pulse *n* the wave of expansion in an artery that corresponds to left ventricular contraction. It can be felt in a superficial artery, especially where it passes over a bone, e.g. radial artery at the wrist. The *pulse rate* is the number of beats per minute and is about 130 in the newborn infant, 70–80 in the adult and 60–70 in older people. The *pulse rhythm* is its regularity – it can be regular or irregular; the *pulse volume* is the amplitude of expansion of the arterial wall during the passage of the wave; the *pulse force* or tension is its strength, estimated by the force needed to obliterate it by pressure of the finger. *pulse deficit* the difference in rate of the heart (counted by stethoscope) and the pulse (counted at the wrist). It occurs when some of the ventricular contractions are too weak to open the aortic valve and hence produce a beat at the heart but not at the wrist, and occurs commonly in atrial fibrillation. *pulse pressure* is the difference between the systolic and diastolic blood pressures. ⇒ beat. ⇒ pulse oximetry.

pulse oximetry a noninvasive method of measuring haemoglobin oxygen saturation using an oximeter. Sensors can be attached to the ear lobe, finger or the nose (see Figure 52). It is used routinely in

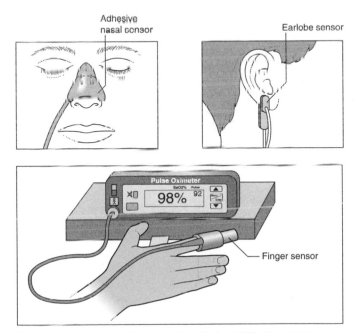

Adhesive nasal sensor

Earlobe sensor

Pulse Oximeter

98%

Finger sensor

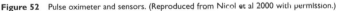

Figure 52 Pulse oximeter and sensors. (Reproduced from Nicol et al 2000 with permission.)

many situations including the perioperative period. Results of oxygen saturation can be misleading in some situations and must be interpreted carefully. ⇒ arterial blood gases. ⇒ oxygenation.

'pulseless' disease (*syn* Takayasu's disease) also called aortic arch syndrome. It is a chronic inflammatory panarteritis of the aortic arch and its major branches. It is characterized by nonspecific symptoms, such as fever, anaemia and weight loss, and various signs of vascular insufficiency that include angina, fainting, upper limb claudication and diminished or absent pulses in the neck and arms. Management involves oral corticosteroids and, occasionally, vascular surgery.

pulsus alternans a regular pulse with alternate beats of weak and strong amplitude; a sign of left ventricular disease.

pulsus bigeminus double pulse wave produced by interpolation of extrasystoles. A coupled beat. A heart rhythm often due to excessive digitalis administration of paired beats, each pair being followed by a prolonged pause. The second weaker beat of each pair may not be strong enough to open the aortic valve, in which case it does not produce a pulse beat and the type of rhythm can then only be detected by listening at the heart.

pulsus paradoxus an inconsistent pulse. *arterial pulsus paradoxus* an alteration of the volume of the arterial pulse sometimes found in pericardial effusion. The volume becomes greater with expiration. *venous pulsus paradoxus (Kussmaul's sign)* is an increase in the height of the venous pressure with inspiration, the reverse of normal. Sometimes found in pericardial or right ventricular disease.

pulvis *n* a powder.

punctate *adj* dotted or spotted, e.g. punctate basophilia describes the abnormal immature red cell in which there are droplets of blue-staining material in the cytoplasm. A feature of severe anaemia, lead poisoning and thalassaemia — **punctum** *n*.

puncture *n* a stab; a wound made with a sharp pointed hollow instrument for withdrawal or injection of fluid or other substance. *cisternal puncture* insertion of a special hollow needle with stylet through the atlanto-occipital ligament between the occiput and atlas, into the

cisterna magna. One method of obtaining cerebrospinal fluid. *lumbar puncture* insertion of a special hollow needle with stylet, either through the space between the third and fourth lumbar vertebrae or, lower, into the subarachnoid space to obtain cerebrospinal fluid. *puncture wound* ⇒ penetrating wound.

punishment in psychology, describes a negative reinforcer (aversive stimulus) used in operant conditioning to reduce unwanted responses to a stimulus.

PUO *abbr* pyrexia of unknown origin.

pupil *n* the opening in the centre of the iris of the eye to allow the passage of light.

pupillary *adj* pertaining to the pupil. *pupillary reflex* the reflex constriction and dilatation of the pupil in response to the amount of light entering the eye. It is controlled by the third cranial or oculomotor nerves.

purgative *n* a drug causing evacuation of fluid faeces. *drastic purgative* even more severe in action, when the fluid faeces may be passed involuntarily.

purines *npl* nitrogenous bases such as adenine and guanine, required in the formation of nucleosides, nucleotides and nucleic acids. Uric acid is a metabolite produced when purine is broken down, such as during the digestion of nucleoproteins. A high level of uric acid in the blood is associated with the disturbed metabolism and excretion of uric acid, and leads to the development of gout.

Purkinje's cells nerve cells found in the cerebellum.

Purkinje's fibres part of the cardiac conduction system. Specialized conducting fibres in the ventricles that carry the impulse from the right and left bundle branches to the ventricular muscle cells.

purpura *n* a disorder characterized by extravasation of blood from the capillaries into the skin, or into or from the mucous membranes. Manifest either by small red spots (petechiae) or large bruises (ecchymoses). It can be divided into non-thrombocytopenic causes that include: normal age changes that increase capillary fragility, Cushing's syndrome, infections, such as menigococcal septicaemia, or thrombocytopenic that may be a primary idiopathic disorder or secondary to drugs affecting the marrow or radiation etc. ⇒ Henoch-Schönlein (anaphylactoid) purpura. ⇒ idiopathic thrombocytopenic purpura (ITP). ⇒ thrombocytopenia.

purulent *adj* pertaining to or resembling pus.

pus *n* matter. A liquid, usually yellowish in colour, formed in pyogenic infections and composed of tissue fluid containing bacteria, cell debris and leucocytes. Various types of bacteria are associated with pus, having distinctive features, e.g. the faecal smell of pus due to *Escherichia coli*; the blue-green colour of pus with distinctive odour due to *Pseudomonas aeruginosa*.

pustule *n* a small inflammatory swelling containing pus. *malignant pustule* ⇒ anthrax — **pustular** *adj*.

putrefaction *n* the process of rotting; destruction of organic material by bacteria — **putrefactive** *adj*.

putrescible *adj* capable of undergoing putrefaction.

PUVA *abbr* psoralen (P), a naturally occurring photosensitive compound, with ultraviolet (UV) light of a (A) long wavelength. A systemic photochemotherapy used in the management of extensive psoriasis.

P value the symbol used to denote the probability of the results of a test occurring by chance. See Box - P value.

PVD *abbr* peripheral vascular disease.

PVR *abbr* pulmonary vascular resistance.

PVS *abbr* persistent vegetative state.

pyaemia *n* the circulation of septic emboli in the bloodstream causing multiple abscesses, such as in the liver, brain, kidneys and lungs — **pyaemic** *adj*.

pyarthrosis *n* pus in a joint cavity.

pyelitis *n* obsolete term for inflammation of the renal pelvis. ⇒ pyelonephritis.

pyelography *n* ⇒ urography — **pyelographically** *adv*.

pyelolithotomy *n* the operation for removal of a stone from the renal pelvis.

pyelonephritis *n* inflammation of the renal pelvis and renal parenchyma. It is caused by pyogenic micro-organisms that include: *Escherichia coli*, *Streptococcus faecalis* and *Pseudomonas aeruginosa* which usually spread upwards from a bladder infection, but can spread to the kidney in the blood. It is characterized by fever, rigors, vomiting, pain in the loins, iliac fossae and suprapubic region, and signs of cystitis, such as dysuria and cloudy urine containing blood, bacteria and pus. Treatment is with the appropriate antibiotic which may be given intravenously in severe cases. Patients are encouraged to take oral fluids but, where this is not possible, hydration is maintained with intravenous fluids. *chronic pyelonephritis* (or *interstitial nephritis*) may develop following acute urinary tract infection in the presence of vesicoureteric reflux. It may progress to chronic renal failure — **pyelonephritic** *adj*.

pyeloplasty a plastic operation on the renal pelvis to relieve obstruction. ⇒ hydronephrosis.

pyelostomy *n* surgical formation of an opening into the renal pelvis.

pyknolepsy *n* infrequently used term to describe repeated attacks of petit mal epilepsy seen in children. Attacks may number a hundred or more in a day.

P value

In all inferential statistics there is a P value given. This is the probability that the results found have occurred by chance alone. This is measured on a scale of 0–1, so a P value of P=0.05 means 5% or a one in twenty chance, and P=0.01 means a 1% or one in a hundred chance. A common error is to assume a high P value means the result is significant, a low value shows significance. So the probability of a test result occurring by chance is the P value. Lower case p is used for proportions.

It is always possible that the apparent relationships among your data came about by chance, so

the P value is always above zero. The interpretation of the P value is dependent upon:

- α value – the significance at which you say a test result is significant, by convention this is typically 0.05;
- 1-tailed or 2-tailed test – a test where you are only interested in results in one direction, e.g. a positive correlation rather than a positive or negative one is one-tailed. A test where you are interested in results in either direction, e.g. a positive correlation or a positive or negative one, is two-tailed.

pylephlebitis *n* inflammation of the veins of the hepato-portal system secondary to intra-abdominal sepsis.

pylethrombosis *n* an intravascular blood clot in the hepatic portal vein or any of its branches.

pylorectomy *n* excision of the pyloric end of the stomach.

pyloric stenosis narrowing of the pylorus. (a) congenital hypertrophic pyloric stenosis, in which there is thickening of the sphincter muscle between the pylorus of the stomach and the duodenum, occurs in the first few weeks of life and is characterized by projectile vomiting, dehydration, electrolyte imbalance, poor weight gain and palpable pylorus. Treatment is generally by pyloromyotomy (Ramstedt's operation) after correction of fluid and electrolyte imbalance; (b) in adults, it occurs secondary to tumours or peptic ulceration.

pyloroduodenal *adj* pertaining to the pyloric sphincter and the duodenum.

pyloromyotomy *n* (*syn* Ramstedt's operation) incision of the pyloric sphincter muscle as in pyloroplasty.

pyloroplasty *n* a plastic operation on the pylorus designed to widen the passage and improve drainage from the stomach.

pylorospasm *n* spasm of the pylorus and pyloric sphincter, such as in pyloric stenosis.

pylorus *n* the region containing the opening of the stomach into the duodenum, encircled by a sphincter muscle — **pyloric** *adj* pertaining to the pylorus. *pyloric sphincter* circular sphincter muscle between the stomach and duodenum. *pyloric stenosis* ⇒ pyloric stenosis.

pyocolpos *n* pus in the vagina.

pyodermia, pyoderma *n* any purulent disease of the skin, such as impetigo — **pyodermic** *adj*.

pyogenic *adj* pertaining to the formation of pus.

pyometra *n* pus retained in the uterus and unable to escape through the cervix, due to malignancy or atresia — **pyometric** *adj*.

pyonephrosis *n* distension of the renal pelvis with pus. May complicate chronic pyelonephritis and require nephrectomy — **pyonephrotic** *adj*.

pyopericarditis *n* pericarditis with purulent effusion.

pyopneumothorax *n* pus and gas or air within the pleural sac.

pyorrhoea *n* a flow of pus, usually referring to that caused by periodontal disease, *pyorrhoea alveolaris*.

pyosalpinx *n* a uterine tube containing pus.

pyothorax *n* empyema. Pus in the pleural cavity.

pyramidal *adj* applied to some conical eminences in the body. *pyramidal cells* nerve cells in the precentral motor area of the cerebral cortex, from which originate impulses to voluntary muscles. Also called Betz cells. *pyramidal tracts* the main motor pathways (tracts) in the brain and spinal cord which transmit the impulses arising from the pyramidal cells. Most decussate in the medulla. ⇒ extrapyramidal.

pyrazolones *npl* a group of nonsteroidal anti-inflammatory drugs, e.g. phenylbutazone, which, in the UK, is used only for ankylosing spondylitis due to its toxicity.

pyrexia *n* elevation of body temperature above normal. Usually applied to a temperature between 37.2°C and 40/41°C. *pyrexia of unknown origin (PUO)* where no reason for the elevation in temperature is immediately obvious. ⇒ fever. ⇒ hyperpyrexia. ⇒ hypothermia — **pyrexial** *adj*.

pyridoxine *n* vitamin B_6; a mixture of the phosphates of pyridoxine, pyridoxal and pyridoxamine, important as cofactors in glycogen and amino acid metabolism, e.g. conversion of tryptophan to nicotinamide. It is also required for the formation of haemoglobin. It occurs in many foods and deficiency is rare.

pyrimidines *npl* nitrogenous bases such as cytosine, thymine and uracil, required in the formation of nucleosides, nucleotides and nucleic acids.

pyrogen *n* a substance capable of producing fever — **pyrogenic** *adj*.

pyromania *n* an uncontrollable impulse to set fire to things. May occur on several occasions before apprehension — **pyromanic** *adj*.

pyrosis *n* (*syn* heartburn) eructation of acid gastric contents into the mouth, accompanied by a burning sensation felt behind the sternum.

pyrotherapy *n* production of fever by artificial means. ⇒ hyperthermia.

pyrroles *npl* substances forming part of the porphyrin which forms the organic part of a haem molecule.

pyruvate *n* the salt of pyruvic acid.

pyruvic acid *n* an important metabolic molecule produced by glycolysis. It is converted to acetyl CoA which is utilized in the Krebs' cycle, or to lactic acid when glucose metabolism is anaerobic.

pyuria *n* pus in the urine — **pyuric** *adj*.

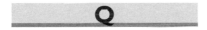

Q fever a febrile disease caused by *Coxiella burnetti*, a rickettsia-like organism. Human infection is transmitted from sheep and cattle via droplets or unpasteurized milk. It is characterized by fever, myalgia and headache. Other features include: atypical pneumonia, myocarditis, hepatitis and iritis.

QALYs *abbr* quality-adjusted life years.

Qi energy *n* in complementary medicine, the individual's innate energy directed towards maintaining health and well-being. An interruption to the flow, movement or existence of this energy may result in illness, physical, emotional or spiritual disharmony. The concept of this form of energy is fundamental to a number of complementary therapies, e.g. acupuncture, shiatsu, therapeutic touch, reflexology. In certain therapies, such as acupuncture or shiatsu, this energy is said to flow through meridian channels. In complementary therapies, energy may be referred to by different terms, such as chi, prana, aura and yin/yang.

quadriceps *n* having four heads. *quadriceps femoris* large four-part extensor muscle of the anterior thigh.

quadriplegia *n* ⇒ tetraplegia — **quadriplegic** *adj*.

qualitative *adj* pertaining to quality. *qualitative research* describes a research study based on observation and/or interviews to ascertain people's opinions, feelings or beliefs. ⇒ quantitative research.

quality-adjusted life years (QALYs) a method of evaluating healthcare outcomes by looking at quality of life, such

as the degree of dependency and levels of pain, as well as life expectancy (the extra years of life). They are used to inform decisions regarding the use of resources for particular interventions.

quality assurance systematic monitoring and evaluation of agreed levels of service provision which are followed by modifications in the light of the evaluation and or audit. It has both clinical and managerial inputs, involves audit and usually applies to all aspects of a healthcare service. ⇒ benchmarking. ⇒ clinical audit. ⇒ cost effectiveness analysis. ⇒ Monitor. ⇒ Performance Indicators. ⇒ quality circles. ⇒ Qualpacs.

quality circles an initiative to improve the quality of care in a specific area. The nurses and other health professionals in a clinical area are guided by a practitioner experienced in this process, to investigate a healthcare intervention systematically and relate it to good standards of practice.

quality of life the measure of the factors that allow individuals to cope successfully with every aspect of life and challenges encountered. *quality of life scales* conceptual or operational measurement. See Box – Quality of life.

Qualpacs *n* a quality assurance programme for nurses. Trained personnel observe for 2 h, up to five randomly selected patients. A further 1 h is also spent reviewing the nursing records and listening to handover reports. A numerical score is given for each of the 68 items in the schedule.

quantitative *adj* pertaining to quantity. *quantitative research* describes a research study based on gained facts and statistics. → qualitative research.

quarantine *n* a period of isolation of infected or potentially infected people in order to prevent spread to others. It is usually the same period as the longest incubation period for the specific disease.

quartan *adj* recurring every 72 h (fourth day), such as the intermittent fever of quartan malaria. ⇒ malaria.

Queckenstedt's test used to check the circulation of CSF. Performed during lumbar puncture. Compression on the internal jugular vein produces a rise in CSF pressure and normally causes the

---

Quality of life

Quality of life is a conceptual or operational measurement that is commonly used in the cancer setting as a means to assess the impact of chemotherapy and radiotherapy treatment on the person with cancer. Conceptual measurements include well-being, quality of survival, human values and satisfaction of needs, whilst operational measures record a person's ability to independently fulfill the tasks of daily living (Montazeri et al 1996). One major critique of quality of life scales is that they seek to get quantitative (statistical) data about an aspect of life that is fundamentally subjective and qualitative and individual patients may attribute different meanings to their responses. Only the patient can make a valid assessment of their quality of life, so they are required to complete questionnaires themselves, unless they are not in a position to do so because of their physical or psychological condition. It is notable that the outcome of any assessment of the patient's quality of life is dependent upon how they feel and what life circumstances are affecting them at that time. These aspects may not be directly related to the cancer and its treatment, therefore it is important to seek qualitative data to inform nursing interventions.

Reference
Montazeri A, Gillis C R, McEwen J 1996 Measuring quality of life in oncology: is it worthwhile? European Journal of Cancer Care 5:159–167

---

fluid level in the manometer to rise. If there is some obstruction to the free flow and circulation of CSF there will be little or no movement of the fluid level in the manometer.

quelling reaction swelling of the capsule of a bacterium when exposed to specific antisera. The test identifies the genera, species or subspecies of bacteria causing a disease.

quickening *n* the first perceptible fetal movements felt by the woman, usually around 16–18th week of gestation.

quicksilver *n* mercury.

quiescent *adj* becoming quiet. Used especially of a skin disease which is settling under treatment.

quinine *n* the chief alkaloid of cinchona, once the standard treatment for malaria. For routine use and prophylaxis, synthetic antimalarials are now preferred, but with the increasing risk of drug-resistant malaria, quinine is coming back into use in some areas. Used to reduce skeletal muscle spasm in 'night cramps'.

quininism *n* toxic effects from overdose or long-term use of quinine that include: headache, tinnitus, partial deafness, disturbed vision and nausea.

quinsy *n* ⇒ peritonsillar abscess.

quotient *n* a number obtained by division. *intelligence quotient* ⇒ intelligence. *respiratory quotient* the ratio between the volume of carbon dioxide given off to the volume of oxygen absorbed by the alveoli per unit of time.

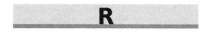

R

RA latex test for rheumatoid arthritis; discerns the presence in the blood of rheumatoid factor. ⇒ antinuclear antibodies. ⇒ SCAT.

rabid *adj* infected with rabies.

rabies *n* (*syn* hydrophobia) fatal infection in man caused by rabies virus. Transmission is via the saliva of infected animals and infection follows the bite of a rabid animal, e.g. dog, cat, fox, vampire bat. The virus attacks the central nervous system and has a very variable incubation period. It is characterized by severe muscle spasm, hydrophobia, paralysis, altered consciousness, delusions and hallucinations. Death usually occurs within seven days or so after the onset of symptoms. It is of worldwide distribution; vaccines are available for humans and susceptible animals.

race often linked to ethnicity, but race only applies to biological features, e.g. skin colour, hair type, facial features, that characterize a specific group. ⇒ ethnicity.

racemose *adj* resembling a bunch of grapes. *racemose gland* has cells arranged in saccules with numerous ducts leading into a main duct, such as a salivary gland.

rachitic pertaining to or caused by rickets.

racism a view of particular groups, based on race alone, that results in negative stereotyping, prejudice and discrimination. It may be overt, where individuals are subjected to oppressive acts, or covert, where a culture of institutional racism allows a section of society to oppress and subordinate other groups.

rad *n* old unit of measurement of absorbed dose of radiation. Now replaced by the SI unit (International System of Units), the gray.

radial keratectomy surgical reshaping of the cornea to correct refractive error, sometimes performed with a surgical blade but more commonly using lasers (photorefractive keratectomy).

radiation the emanation of radiant energy in the form of electromagnetic waves including: X-rays, infrared, gamma rays, ultraviolet rays and visible light rays. Subatomic particles, such as electrons or neutrons, may also be radiated. Radiation can be ionizing or nonionizing and has numerous diagnostic and therapeutic uses. ⇒ ionizing radiation. *radiation sickness* tissue damage from exposure to ionizing radiation results in diarrhoea, vomiting, anorexia and bone marrow failure.

radiation oncologist a medical specialist in the treatment of disease by X-rays and other forms of radiation.

radical *adj* pertaining to the root of a thing. *radical operation* usually extensive so that it is curative, not palliative.

radiculography *n* X-ray of the spinal nerve roots after rendering them radiopaque to locate the site and size of a prolapsed intervertebral disc — **radiculogram** *n*.

radioactive *adj* exhibiting radioactivity. Describes an unstable atomic nucleus which emits charged particles as it disintegrates. ⇒ isotopes. *radioactive decay* the spontaneous disintegration of radioactive atoms within a radioactive substance. ⇒ half life. *radioactive fallout* release of radioactive particles into the atmosphere. Results from industrial processes or accidents, and the testing or use of nuclear weapons.

radioactivity the emission of radiant energy in the form of alpha, beta or gamma radiation from an element as it undergoes spontaneous disintegration.

radioallergosorbent test (RAST) *n* an allergen-specific IgE measurement.

radiobiology *n* the study of the effects of radiation on living tissue — **radiobiologically** *adv*.

radiocarbon *n* a radioactive isotope of the element carbon, such as carbon-14 (^{14}C), used for investigations, e.g. absorption tests and research. ⇒ xylose absorption test.

radiodermatitis reddening of the skin occurring after exposure to ionizing radiation.

radiograph *n* a photographic image formed by exposure to X-rays; the correct term for an 'X-ray' — **radiographic** *adj*.

radiographer *n* there are two types of radiographer, diagnostic and therapeutic, they are health professionals qualified in the use of ionizing radiation and other techniques, either in diagnostic imaging or radiotherapy.

radiography *n* the use of imaging techniques to create images of the body from which medical diagnosis can be made (diagnostic radiography).

radioimmunoassay technique using radioactive substances to measure hormones, drugs and proteins in the blood.

radioimmunosorbent test (RIST) *n* a test that measures total serum IgE.

radioisotopes *npl* (*syn* radionuclide) heavy unstable isotopes of an element which have the same atomic number but different mass numbers, exhibiting the property of spontaneous nuclear disintegration. They emit radioactivity as the atomic nucleus disintegrates, e.g. radioactive iodine (^{131}I). They may occur naturally or be produced artificially for various industrial and medical purposes including research, diagnosis and treatment of disease. ⇒ radionuclide.

radiologist *n* a medical specialist in diagnosis by the use of X-rays and other allied imaging techniques. Some radiologists use imaging techniques to help them carry out interventions.

radiology *n* the branch of medical science dealing with the diagnosis of disease, using X-rays and other allied imaging techniques — **radiologically** *adv*.

radiolucent substance that permits the passage of X-rays.

radionuclide *n* a radioisotope such as technetium (^{99}MTc). *radionuclide imaging/scanning* the use of radionuclides, given orally, intravenousy or by inhalation, to scan and produce images of structures such as bone, liver, lung, thyroid and kidney. ⇒ radioisotope.

radiopaque describes a substance which does not allow the passage of X-rays. Often used as contrast medium, e.g. barium sulphate.

radioresistance the ability of normal tissues and some tumours to withstand the effects of radiation.

radiosensitive *adj* term applied to those normal tissues and tumours which are affected by radiation. In the case of tumours it can be enhanced by the use of radiosensitizing drugs.

radiotherapist *n* ⇒ radiation oncologist.

radiotherapy *n* the treatment of proliferative disease, especially cancer, by X-rays and other forms of ionizing radiation. See Box – Radiotherapy.

radium (Ra) *n* a radioactive element occurring in nature which results from the disintegration of uranium. It has a half life of 1690 years and produces both alpha and gamma radiation. It is rarely used in the treatment of malignant disease and has been replaced by other isotopes, e.g. caesium-137.

radius *n* the outer long bone of the forearm — **radial** *adj* pertaining to the radius; applied to the nerve, artery and vein. *radial pulse* ⇒ pulse.

RAI *abbr* Relatives Assessment Interview.

raised intracranial pressure (RIP) a dangerous situation where the intracranial pressure is raised. Causes include: tumours, intracranial haemorrhage, trauma causing oedema or haematoma and obstruction to the flow of cerebrospinal fluid. The features depend on the cause, but there may be headache, vomiting, papilloedema, fits, bradycardia, arterial hypertension and altered consciousness. ⇒ hypertension.

RAISSE *abbr* Relatives Assessment Interview for Schizophrenia in a secure environment.

rale *n* abnormal inspiratory sound heard on auscultation of lungs when fluid is present in the airways or alveoli.

RAM *acr* for Random Access Memory. The part of computer memory that holds data and programs whilst the CPU is working. Once the power supply is interrupted the RAM will lose its contents. ⇒ ROM.

Radiotherapy

Radiotherapy is the use of ionizing radiation in the treatment of malignant and certain non-malignant diseases. It may be used alone but is commonly used as an adjunct to surgery, chemotherapy, or hormone therapy and other treatment modalities with curative intent or as a palliative treatment to alleviate symptoms of advanced disease. The ionizing radiation disrupts DNA synthesis so that cellular replication is prevented, although several cell divisions may need to take place before cell death ultimately occurs.

The radiation may be applied by external beam methods (teletherapy) by employing the use of linear accelerators which emit megavoltage radiation in order to treat deeply seated tumours, and lower energy units such as orthovoltage or kilovoltage units for more superficial lesions. Treatment commonly takes a few minutes each day, extended over several weeks. Other radiotherapeutic modalities include the use of sealed and unsealed radiation sources (brachytherapy). This is the delivery of radiation close to the tumour source, via a radioactive source placed into the body, i.e. the Selectron therapy for gynaecological cancers. In systemic therapy, radioactive isotopes are administered orally or intravenously and are preferentially taken up by the target tissue.

The main aims of radiotherapy are to apply a homogeneous tumouricidal dose to a precisely localized area of the body, to avoid as much normal tissue as possible without compromising the outcome to treatment and to avoid any critical structures such as spinal cord or kidney which may be sensitive to radiation. Although radiation is unable to discriminate between normal and malignant tissues there is a differential effect and cancer cells are more sensitive to the effects of treatment. Because healthy cells surrounding the tumour are affected during treatment localized toxicity can develop. The nursing role is to provide information to the patient and their family, monitoring, proactive management of potential toxicity and support.

Further reading
Bomford C K, Kunklen I H, Sherriff S B 1993 Textbook of radiotherapy. Edinburgh: Churchill Livingstone.
Holmes S 1996 Radiotherapy: A guide for practice. 2nd Edn. Leatherhead: Asset Books.

Ramsay Hunt syndrome herpes zoster infection affecting the geniculate ganglion. It is characterized by vesicles on the ear lobe with ear pain, facial paralysis and loss of taste.

Ramstedt's operation ⇒ pyloromyotomy.

ramus *n* 1. a branch of a nerve or blood vessel. 2. a thin projection from a bone.

random sampling selection process whereby every individual in the population has an equal chance of being selected.

randomized controlled trial research using two or more randomly selected groups: experimental and control. Produces a high level of evidence for practice.

range a measure of the span of values (lowest to highest) observed in a sample.

ranula *n* a cystic swelling beneath the tongue due to blockage of a duct — **ranular** *adj*.

rape *n* unlawful sexual intercourse without consent which is achieved by force or deception. Full penetration of the vagina (or other orifice) by the penis and ejaculation of semen is not necessary to constitute rape. Most rapes include force and violence, but acquiescence because of verbal threats should not be interpreted as consent. Incidents of rape are underreported to the police because of the gruelling process of having to give evidence in court. If women are admitted to hospital, a police surgeon examines them and takes the necessary specimens in the presence of specially trained female police officers who then provide support throughout the interviews and subsequent investigation. Most police forces provide purpose built facilities for dealing with the examination and interview of alleged rape victims. There are voluntary agencies to assist rape victims to regain confidence and rebuild their lives. Male rape, the rape of a man by another man, is increasingly recognized.

raphe *n* a seam, suture, ridge or crease; the median furrow on the dorsal surface of the tongue.

rapid plasma reagin (RPR) *n* a nonspecific serological test for syphilis.

rapport *n* a sense of mutuality, understanding and respect for each other; it is an essential component of a nurse/patient relationship.

rarefaction *n* becoming less dense, as applied to diseased bone — **rarefied** *adj*.

RAS *abbr* reticular activating system.

rash *n* skin eruption. *nettle rash* ⇒ urticaria.

Rashkind's septostomy balloon septostomy. Performed to relieve heart failure by improving heart oxygenation in certain congenital heart defects. An artificial atrial septal communication is produced by passing an inflatable balloon-ended catheter through the foramen ovale, inflating the balloon and withdrawing the catheter. It allows some mixing of oxygenated blood from the lungs and systemic blood until corrective surgery can be undertaken.

RAST *abbr* radioallergosorbent test.

rat-bite fever a relapsing fever caused by *Spirillum minus* or by *Streptobacillus moniliformis*. Usually transmitted by rat bites, they also produce local inflammation, lymphadenitis and splenomegaly and rash.

ratio data measurement data with a numerical score, e.g. height, that has an absolute zero of 0. It is interval data with an absolute zero. ⇒ interval data.

rationalization *n* a mental defence mechanism whereby a person justifies his or her behaviour after the event, so that it appears more rational or socially acceptable.

rationing a limitation placed on the overall ability of a specific service, procedure or treatment, e.g. an expensive drug or assisted fertility treatment. The rationing may be explicit, via exclusions, or implicit, e.g. via waiting lists.

Raynaud's disease/phenomenon paroxysmal spasm of the digital arteries in response to cold, vibration, drugs and arterial disease. It is characterized by pallor or cyanosis of fingers or toes, and redness and pain when circulation returns. Occasionally it leads to ischaemic changes resulting in necrosis and gangrene. It is known as Raynaud's disease when it occurs in the absence of associated disease or cause and is more common in women. ⇒ hand-arm vibration syndrome.

RBC *abbr* red blood cell. ⇒ blood. ⇒ erythrocyte.

RCT *abbr* randomized controlled trial.

RDA *abbr* recommended daily allowance.

reaction *n* **1.** response to a stimulus. *reaction time* the time between the onset of the stimulus and the start of a noticeable response. **2.** a chemical change, e.g. acid or alkaline reaction to litmus paper. *allergic reaction* ⇒ allergy.

reaction formation mental defence mechanism where the person exhibits behaviour which is opposite to stressful emotions, drives and impulses which are repressed.

reagent *n* an agent capable of participating in a chemical reaction, so as to detect, measure, or produce other substances. *reagent strips* a strip is impregnated with particular chemicals to detect the presence of particular substances in, e.g. urine and faeces. One strip may test for several substances.

reality orientation (RO) a form of therapy useful for withdrawn, confused and depressed patients; they are frequently reminded of their name, the time, place, date and so on. Reinforcement is provided by clocks, calendars and signs prominently displayed in the environment.

reasonable doubt to secure a conviction in criminal proceedings, the prosecution must establish beyond reasonable doubt the guilt of the accused.

rebore *n* ⇒ disobliteration. ⇒ endarterectomy.

recalcitrant *adj* refractory. Describes medical conditions which are resistant to treatment.

recall *n* part of the process of memory.

recannulation *n* re-establishment of the patency of a vessel.

receptaculum *n* receptacle, often acting as a reservoir. *receptaculum chyli* ⇒ cisterna chyli.

receptive aphasia a type of aphasia characterized by problems in language comprehension, occurring with varying degrees of severity. Patients may also exhibit expressive language difficulties. ⇒ expressive aphasia.

receptor *n* **1.** sensory afferent nerve ending capable of receiving and transmitting stimuli. **2.** a protein molecule present on or in a cell membrane, or in the cell that reacts with hormones, specific antigens or other chemical mediators. Many drugs act by combining with cell receptors. See Box – Receptors and drugs.

recessive *adj* receding; having a tendency to disappear. *recessive trait* a genetically controlled character or trait which is expressed when the specific allele which determines it is present at both paired chromosomal loci (i.e. in the homozygous state). When the specific allele is present in single dose, the characteristic is not manifest as its presence is concealed by the dominant allele at the partner locus. The exception is for X-linked genes in males, in which the single recessive allele on the X-chromosome will express itself so that the character is manifest. ⇒ dominant. ⇒ Mendel's law.

recipient *n* a person who receives something from a donor, such as blood, bone marrow or an organ. ⇒ blood groups.

Receptors and drugs

Receptors are proteins found in the cell membrane or cytoplasm of a cell. They act as binding sites for endogenous molecules such as hormones and neurotransmitters. When a molecule binds to a receptor, the protein undergoes a conformational change that triggers a cascade of events within the cell leading to a response.

Drugs can interact with receptors in one of two main ways. Drugs can act as agonists and bind to the receptor causing a similar response to the endogenous molecule; for example, morphine acts on receptors which normally respond to the body's endorphins. Drugs can also act as antagonists and bind to receptors, preventing agonists from binding. For example, propranolol blocks the effect of noradrenaline (norepinephrine) at β adrenoceptors (adrenergic receptors), whilst naloxone blocks the effect of morphine at endorphin receptors and so acts as an antidote to morphine.

Receptors that respond to a particular endogenous chemical exist in different subtypes throughout the body. Scientists are identifying these subtypes and making selective drugs that target one receptor subtype and not the others. Histamine for example has three receptor subtypes, and H_2-blockers (antagonists) like cimetidine have been designed to only act as antagonists at those receptors found on the stomach. This selectivity minimizes drug side effects.

recliner's reflux syndrome this is due to severe disturbance of the antireflux mechanism which allows stomach contents to leak at any time whatever position the patient is in, although it is most likely to happen when the patient lies down or slumps in a low chair.

recombinant DNA DNA which is produced by deliberately piecing together (recombining chemically) of the DNA of two different organisms. It is used for the study of the structure and function of both normal and abnormal genes and so, of the molecular basis of human genetic disorders. Its practical applications are in diagnosis (including prenatal diagnosis) and in the production of agents, such as human insulin. Research continues into the development of organs that can be transplanted from one species to another without rejection.

recommended daily allowance (RDA) a standard for the intake of individual nutrients for groups of people. In the UK they were replaced in 1991 by dietary reference values.

Recommended International Nonproprietary Name (rINN) a new system by which drugs will have a recommended nonproprietary name that is used internationally. ⇒ approved name.

reconstituted family a family with stepparents resulting from divorce or remarriage. ⇒ family.

recovery a return to health or a normal state. It may be partial or total. *recovery position* a first aid measure where an unconscious casualty is placed in such a position as to maintain their airway and prevent aspiration of secretions or vomit.

recrudescence *n* the return of symptoms.

recruitment *n* apparent paradox seen in people with impaired hearing, with the person not hearing quiet sounds then, with increasing loudness of the sound, the patient suddenly hears it very loudly.

rectal varices haemorrhoids.

rectocele *n* prolapse of the rectum through the posterior vaginal wall. Repaired by a posterior colporrhaphy. ⇒ procidentia.

rectopexy *n* surgical fixation of a prolapsed rectum.

rectoscope *n* an instrument for examining the rectum, a proctoscope. ⇒ endoscope — **rectoscopic** *adj*.

rectosigmoid *adj* pertaining to the rectum and sigmoid portion of colon.

rectosigmoidectomy *n* surgical removal of the rectum and sigmoid colon.

rectouterine *adj* pertaining to the rectum and uterus. *rectouterine pouch* a peritoneal pouch between the rectum and the uterus/vagina.

rectovaginal *adj* pertaining to the rectum and vagina. *rectovaginal fistula* abnormal communication between the rectum and vagina.

rectovesical *adj* pertaining to the rectum and bladder. *rectovesical fistula* abnormal communication between the rectum and the bladder. *rectovesical pouch* peritoneal pouch between the rectum and bladder in the male.

rectum *n* the lower part of the large intestine between the sigmoid flexure and anal canal. ⇒ bowel — **rectal** *adj* pertaining to the rectum. *rectal examination* digital examination of the rectum. *rectal reflex* defaecation reflex. Urge to defaecate when the rectum (which is normally empty) fills with faeces.

recumbent *adj* lying or reclining. *recumbent position* lying on the back with the head supported on a pillow; the knees are flexed and parted to facilitate inspection of the perineum — **recumbency** *n*.

recurrent abortion ⇒ abortion.

recurring costs regular and ongoing costs, such as planned maintenance and staff salaries.

reduction 1. the act of reducing or state of being reduced. It involves the removal of oxygen or the addition of hydrogen or electrons (increasing the negative charge on an atom or molecule) to a substance. ⇒ oxidation. 2. replacing in the normal position, such as following dislocation or fracture and hernia.

REF *n* renal erythropoietic factor.

reference nutrient intake (RNI) *n* a dietary reference value. See Box – Dietary reference values (nutritional requirement).

referred pain pain occurring at a distance from its source, e.g. pain felt in the upper limbs from angina pectoris; that from the gallbladder felt in the scapular region.

reflection *n* consciously and systematically thinking about personal actions. The ability to review, analyse and evaluate situations, during or after events — **reflective**

adj pertaining to reflection. *reflective practice* a means of monitoring professional and personal competence by consciously thinking about actions during or after events. See Box – Reflective practice.

reflex literally, reflected or thrown back; involuntary, not able to be controlled by the will. A reflex action is an instantaneous involuntary physiological response (motor or secretory) to a stimulus that operates through a simple nerve pathway. Reflexes are protective or postural and include: sneezing, blinking, coughing, tendon stretch, accommodation, corneal, plantar, abdominal and swallowing. Various primitive reflexes are present in newborns and are used to assess their development, e.g. Moro, stepping, grasp and rooting. Reflexes may be innate or conditioned. The testing of various reflexes provides valuable information in the localization and diagnosis of diseases involving the nervous system. *accommodation reflex* constriction of the pupils and convergence of the eyes for near vision. *conditioned reflex* a reaction acquired by repetition or practice. *corneal reflex* a reaction of blinking when the cornea is touched. *reflex arc* the sensory, connector and motor neurons through which some reflexes operate (see Figure 53). *reflex zone therapy* ⇒ reflexology.

reflexology *n* a complementary therapy based upon the premise that the internal organs of the body are mapped out on the soles of the feet and palms of the hands. It is believed that gentle pressure upon the areas relating to specific organs can initiate a therapeutic response.

reflux *n* backward flow. ⇒ gastro-oesophageal reflux. ⇒ vesicoureteric reflux.

refraction *n* the bending of light rays as they pass through media of different densities. In normal vision, the light rays are so bent that they meet on the retina. *errors of refraction* ⇒ astigmatism. ⇒ hypermetropia. ⇒ myopia — **refractive** *adj*.

refractory *adj* resistant to treatment; stubborn, unmanageable; rebellious.

regeneration *n* renewal of injured tissue.

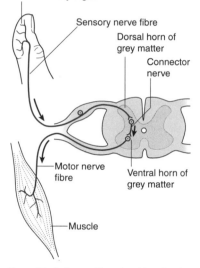

Figure 53 Reflex arc. (Reproduced from Brooker 1996 with permission.)

Reflective practice

Boyd and Fales (1983) define reflective practice as "the process of creating and clarifying the meaning of experience in terms of self in relation to both self and the world. The outcome of this process is changed conceptual perspectives." In the world of work, and in particular nursing, this simply means looking back at recent experiences, analysing the event, including personal actions and individual and collective outcomes, and learning from the experience. The outcome might be that the event went well and could not have been improved upon, or that there were instances which could have been handled differently, and therefore practice will be changed next time the situation arises.

Such examples can be entered in individual portfolios or profiles, and form some sort of formal or informal learning contract. The whole process then fits into the concept of 'life long learning', indicating and confirming that learning is never static, and self development is on-going.

Street (1992) sums this up by stating "The confrontation with experience through reflection and of the meanings and assumptions that surround it, can form a foundation upon which to make choices about future actions based on chosen value systems and new ways of thinking about and understanding nursing practice."

References
Boyd E M, Fales A W 1983 Reflective learning; key to learning from experience. Journal of Humanistic Psychology 23(2):99–117
Street A F 1992 Inside Nursing: A critical ethnography of clinical nursing. Suny, New York

Regional Cancer Centres *npl* in the UK. Regional centres with facilities to support the site-specific treatment of common and rarer cancers, e.g. endometrial, cervical and ovarian cancers.

regional ileitis Crohn's disease. ⇒ inflammatory bowel disease.

registered nurse *n* a term protected by law in many countries including the UK. Only those whose name appears on the central register, after having successfully undergone the prescribed educational programme, can legally be called a registered nurse. ⇒ named nurse.

regression *n* a mental defence mechanism. In psychiatry, reversion to an earlier stage of development, becoming more childish. Occurs in dementia, especially that occurring in old age, or in childhood itself, e.g. following the birth of a sibling.

regression techniques *npl* several analytical techniques used in multivariate statistics. Used to predict dependent variable(s) from independent variable(s).

regurgitation *n* backward flow, e.g. of stomach contents into, or through, the mouth, or the back flow of blood through a defective heart valve (semilunar or atrioventricular).

REHAB *acr* ⇒ Rehabilitation Evaluation of Hall and Baker.

rehabilitation *n* a planned programme in which the convalescent or disabled person progresses towards, or maintains, the maximum degree of physical and psychological independence of which he or she is capable. ⇒ habilitation.

Rehabilitation Evaluation of Hall and Baker (REHAB) a broad assessment system developed by two psychologists; can be used by nurses. Information is requested about everyday living skills, work skills and any disturbed or deviant behaviour.

rehearsal in memory memory processing depends on two forms of rehearsal of facts: *maintenance rehearsal* where information re-enters short term memory (STM) by repetition (such as repeating a telephone number); each time the information enters STM appears to increase its chance of being stored in long term memory (LTM); and *elaborative rehearsal* processing information in STM so that it can be coded for storage in LTM. It may use sensory characteristics, such as

sound, or focus on the meaning of the information.

reinforcement in psychology, the processes used during conditioning to increase the probability and strength of a response.

Reiter protein complement fixation (RPCF) a serological test previously used for the diagnosis of syphilis.

Reiter's syndrome a syndrome characterized by arthritis, conjunctivitis and nonspecific urethritis. It may follow exposure to a sexually transmitted infection or bacterial dysentery.

rejection *n* 1. the act of excluding or denying affection to another person. 2. an immune reaction against grafted tissue or organs, leading to the destruction of implanted grafts.

relapsing fever louse-borne or tick-borne infection caused by spirochaetes of the genus *Borrelia*. Prevalent in many parts of the world. Characterized by a febrile period of a week or so, with apparent recovery, followed by a further bout of fever.

relationship *n* the state of being related. In the case of people, it can be a family relationship decreed by custom, the quality of which is mainly determined by the emotional bonding between the people in the relationship. The degree of emotional involvement is shown by using such words as 'acquaintanceship', 'friendship', or 'close friendship'. → personal relationship.

Relatives Assessment Interview (RAI) based on the Camberwell family interview, but modified for clinical use. ⇒ expressed emotion. Used by mental health nurses and others to obtain essential information that helps to direct family intervention work. It covers seven main areas which are summarized as: client's family background and contact time; chronological history of the illness; current problems' symptoms; irritability; relatives' relationship with client; and the effects of the illness on relatives.

Relatives Assessment Interview for Schizophrenia in a secure environment (RAISSE) an adaptation of RAI for use in secure environments. The assessment is based on a semistructured interview where three areas are covered: schizophrenia; admission; and visits.

relaxant *n* any agent, drug or technique that reduces tension.

relaxation a state of altered consciousness characterized by the release of muscle tension, anxiety and stress. *relaxation techniques* these are being incorporated into health care and health education programmes. They include progressive muscle relaxation, visual guided imagery, yoga and meditation. ⇒ autogenic therapy. ⇒ biofeedback. ⇒ hypnosis.

relaxin *n* a hormone secreted by the ovaries and placenta that softens the cervix and loosens the pelvic ligaments in preparation for labour.

releaser/releasing mechanism describes a stimulus that initiates a cycle of instinctive behaviour.

reliability in research, consistency of results. The likelihood of producing the same findings using the same research conditions over a period of time or with different researchers. See Box – Reliability.

relief of pressure ⇒ pressure ulcer prevention.

REM sleep *abbr* rapid eye movement sleep. Sometimes called paradoxical sleep. ⇒ sleep.

reminiscence therapy the use of objects from the past, such as photographs, film/video, music, food, clothes and household equipment, with people with dementia and very old people to trigger discussion and reflection. It facilitates the sharing and validation of personal memories, histories and experiences. Also known as nostalgia therapy.

remission *n* period when a disease subsides and has no signs or symptoms.

remittent *adj* increasing and decreasing at periodic intervals, such as a fever.

remote afterloading a method of delivering brachytherapy radiation to treat cancer without radiation exposure risk to staff. ⇒ Selectron.

renal *adj* pertaining to the kidney. *renal adenocarcinoma* cancer of the kidney. *renal calculus* stone in the kidney. *renal colic* intense pain caused by the movement of a stone within the kidney or ureter. *renal cortex* the pale outer region of the kidney under the capsule. *renal erythropoietic factor (REF)* a substance released by the kidneys in response to renal hypoxia. It acts upon a plasma protein to form active erythropoietin prior to its release. *renal failure* may be classified as acute or chronic. Acute renal failure (ARF) occurs when previously healthy kidneys suddenly fail because of a variety of problems affecting the kidney and its perfusion with blood. This condition is potentially reversible. Patients with ARF are usually treated by haemofiltration or haemodiafiltration until renal function improves. Chronic renal failure (CRF) occurs when irreversible and progressive pathological destruction of the kidney leads to terminal or end stage renal disease (ESRD). This process usually takes several years but once ESRD is reached, death will follow unless the patient is treated with renal replacement therapy, such as dialysis or a kidney transplant. ⇒ crush syndrome. ⇒ glomerulonephritis. ⇒ multiple organ dysfunction syndrome. ⇒ tubular necrosis. ⇒ uraemia. *renal function tests* a variety of tests that include: routine urine testing, urine concentration/dilution tests,

---

Reliability

Reliability is a measure of how repeatable are the data that are captured, i.e. if a researcher does this experiment again will they get the same value, or if the researcher interviews the same person twice will their answers be similar on both occasions.

It is possible to get highly repeatable results that are inaccurate, for example a blood glucose device may always give a result 1 mmol too high, but gives near identical results on successive testing of the same blood sample.

If a measure is repeatable then we should get the same result when we measure the same thing

twice (say). Reliability measures give a quantitative value for repeatability. It may be used for example to assess how repeatable a machine is, or to what extent two humans give the same value.

Various measures of reliability exist:

- Stability – 'test-retest' tests whether a measuring device gives the same result when the measurement is repeated.
- Equivalence – comparing two forms of test, or two observers. For example, do two nurses allocate the same Waterlow score to a patient?

serum urea and electrolytes, serum creatinine and renal clearance to estimate GFR. *renal glycosuria* occurs in patients with a normal blood sugar and a lowered renal threshold for sugar. *renal medulla* darker inner region of the kidney containing the renal pyramids. *renal rickets* ⇒ rickets. *renal threshold* the level of a substance in the blood at which it is excreted in the urine, e.g. glucose. *renal transplant* kidney transplant. *renal tuberculosis* tuberculosis affecting the kidney. It is usually secondary to TB in another site. Characterized by haematuria and dysuria and general signs of TB, such as weight loss and high temperature. *renal tubule* ⇒ nephron. ⇒ tubule.

renin *n* an enzyme released into the blood by the juxtaglomerular apparatus in response to low serum sodium or low blood pressure. It initiates the angiotensin-aldosterone response. Angiotensinogen (a plasma protein) is activated to produce angiotensin I, which in turn is converted into angiotensin II by an enzyme in the lungs. Excessive production of renin results in hypertensive kidney disease.

rennin *n* milk curdling enzyme found in the gastric juice of human infants and ruminants. It converts caseinogen into casein, which, in the presence of calcium ions, is converted to an insoluble curd.

reovirus *n* a family of RNA viruses that include the rotovirus which causes gastroenteritis.

repetitive strain injury (RSI) (*syn* work related upper limb disorder) the definition of this condition is controversial. It usually refers to pain and discomfort in the upper limbs as a result of repetitive movements or constrained posture. It encompasses a variety of symptoms, including tenderness, tingling and numbness, swelling, etc. Some clinicians include similar signs and symptoms in lower limbs.

replogle tube a double lumen aspiration catheter, attached to low pressure suction apparatus.

repolarization the stage of an action potential during which the membrane potential returns from the depolarized state to its polarized resting (negative) state.

repression *n* a mental defence mechanism whereby unacceptable thoughts, impulses and painful experiences are forced into, and remain in, the unconscious.

reproductive system the organs and tissues necessary for reproduction. In the male it includes the testes, vas deferens, prostate gland, seminal vesicles, urethra and penis. In the female it includes the ovaries, uterine tubes, uterus, vagina and vulva (see Figure 54).

RES *abbr* reticuloendothelial system ⇒ monocyte-macrophage system.

research *n* systematic investigation of data, reports and observations to establish facts or principles. See Box – Research. See Box – Research and informed consent.

research design *n* how a research study is to be undertaken. Covers aspects such as data collection method, need for a control group, statistical analysis etc.

research methods *npl* the various ways that data can be collected, e.g. observation, postal survey, interviews, using records etc.

resection *n* surgical excision, such as bowel resection. ⇒ submucous resection.

resectoscope *n* an instrument passed along the urethra; it permits resection of tissue from the base of the bladder and prostate under direct vision. ⇒ prostatectomy.

resectotome *n* an instrument used for resection.

reservoirs of infection micro-organisms colonize humans and animals and form reservoirs. In humans, the skin, respiratory tract and bowel are colonized by bacteria and fungi which form the normal flora. Under certain circumstances these micro-organisms can become pathogenic. Animal reservoirs of potential infection in humans include *Salmonella* which colonizes the gut of poultry.

residential care a term used for provision of care for frail older people. It can be provided in a variety of settings, such as independent homes for older people. See Box – Residential care.

residual *adj* remaining. *residual air* the air remaining in the lung after forced expiration. *residual urine* urine remaining in the bladder after micturition.

residual volume (RV) *n* amount of air left in the lungs after a maximal expiratory effort. ⇒ respiratory function tests.

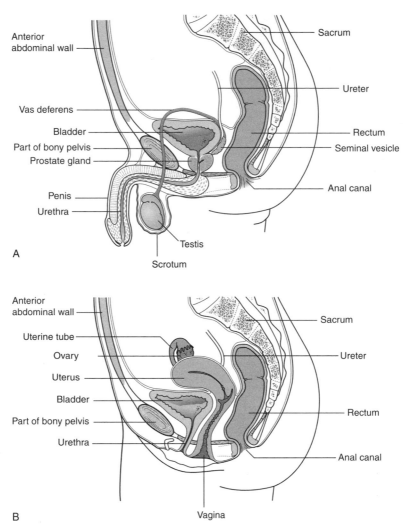

Figure 54 Reproductive system. A Male. B Female. (Reproduced from Brooker 1996 with permission.)

resistance *n* power of resisting. In psychology, the name given to the force which prevents repressed thoughts from re-entering the conscious mind from the unconscious. *resistance to infection* the capacity to withstand infection. ⇒ immunity. *peripheral resistance* ⇒ peripheral.

resolution *n* the subsidence of inflammation; describes the earliest indications of a return to normal, as when, in lobar pneumonia, the consolidation begins to liquefy.

resonance *n* the musical quality elicited on percussing a cavity which contains air. *vocal resonance* is the reverberating note heard through the stethoscope when the patient is asked to say 'one, one, one' or '99'.

resorption *n* the act of absorbing again, e.g. absorption of (a) callus following bone fracture; (b) roots of the deciduous teeth; (c) blood from a haematoma.

respiration *n* the process whereby there is gaseous exchange between a cell and its environment. Atmospheric oxygen is sup-

Research

Research is the purposeful, systematic, and rigorous collection of data, which are analysed and interpreted to gain new knowledge. Its purpose is to produce organized scientific knowledge.

In nursing we use both quantitative and qualitative research methods. In quantitative research one defines the variables to be collected, and these are translated into numerical values. The data are analysed to either describe the data (descriptive statistics) or to test whether there are relationships among the data (inferential statistics). In qualitative research typically one is not sure what data are relevant, and predefining the data to collect makes little sense. Qualitative research tends to use smaller samples, but collect more data on each subject, typically by observing them, or interviewing them.

In either case one needs a research question or a hypothesis. A research question is a concise statement of what the research is attempting to find out. A hypothesis is a statement which is testable, such that one may state the hypothesis to be accepted (true) or rejected (false). A hypothesis is needed in all cases where inferential statistics are used, otherwise a research question is required.

Typically one uses the null hypothesis which means that there is no difference between two groups, or no correlation between two variables, etc.

Concrete examples:

- A researcher wants to know the level of professional training for health care assistants (HCAs). A questionnaire is sent to a random sample of HCAs, with tick box items to determine the types of training they have had. The data are summarized in tables and charts to describe the situation, this is descriptive quantitative research.
- A researcher wants to determine if female HCAs are more or less likely to receive professional training. Their hypothesis is that there is no difference between the two genders. They apply a statistical test, and decide that the null hypothesis is not rejected, i.e. there appears to be little or no difference between the genders. This is inferential quantitative research.
- A researcher wants to discover how HCAs feel about their professional development. A series of interviews with HCAs are arranged where the researcher asks a set of questions, tapes their responses, and develops themes from the transcripts. This is qualitative research.

Research and informed consent

Consent needs to be informed. An information sheet for the research subjects, written in language they can understand, in a font size they can read, and laid out professionally, should address what the study is about, what will the subject have to do, what are the benefits, what are the risks, what are the alternatives, what if the subject does not want to take part, what happens to the information, who else is taking part, what if something goes wrong, what happens at the end of the study, what if the subject has more questions or does not understand something, what happens if the subject decides to take part, what happens if the subject changes their mind during the study. A contact name and telephone number, and where appropriate an

e mail address, should be given for further information.

A suitably worded, user friendly, consent form should be included. This should preferably not contain any technical terms which the patients may have difficulty understanding. The patients should not feel coerced in any way and it must be clear to the patients that they may decline to take part, or withdraw at any time, without affecting any future treatment or care. There should be a place for the patients to sign and date that they have understood fully what will be involved. There should also be a place for a witness to sign and date. The form should include the full title of the study. Children should be given the opportunity to give consent and a suitably worded consent form should be included.

plied to the tissues for cellular metabolism and waste carbon dioxide is removed. It consists of three processes: (a) ventilation which involves inspiration and expiration; (b) *external respiration* involves gaseous exchange between alveolar air and pulmonary capillary blood. Oxygen in the alveolar air passes into the blood, and carbon dioxide passes from the blood in the lung capillaries into the air in the lungs to be excreted; (c) *internal* or *tissue respira-* *tion* is the reverse process occurring at the tissues, whereby oxygen passes from the blood, via the tissue fluid, to the cells, and carbon dioxide from the cells passes into the blood for onward transport to the lungs. *paradoxical respiration* occurs when the ribs on one side are fractured in two places, such as in flail chest. The injured side of the chest moves in (i.e. deflates) on inspiration and vice versa, resulting in inadequate oxygenation of blood. ⇒

abdominal breathing. ⇒ anaerobic. ⇒ Cheyne-Stokes respiration. ⇒ Kussmaul respiration. ⇒ resuscitation — **respiratory** *adj* pertaining to respiration. *respiratory acidosis* ⇒ acidosis. *respiratory alkalosis* ⇒ alkalosis. *respiratory centres* specialized centres in the medulla and pons which control the rate, depth and rhythm of breathing. They receive inputs from chemoreceptors (which respond to carbon dioxide, pH and oxygen levels of the blood), stretch receptors, higher centres and the hypothalamus. ⇒ apneustic centre. ⇒ pneumotaxic centre. *respiratory distress syndrome* ⇒ acute respiratory distress syndrome. *respiratory quotient* ⇒ quotient.

respirator *n* **1.** an appliance worn over the nose and mouth and designed to purify the air breathed through it. **2.** a device used to maintain adequate respiration when the normal mechanisms are impaired. It may work on the principle of positive or negative pressure. ⇒ mechanical ventilation.

respiratory failure a term used to denote failure of the lungs to oxygenate the blood adequately or remove carbon dioxide. It may be classified as either type I where there is hypoxia, or type II (also known as asphyxia) which is characterized by both hypoxia and hypercapnia. Both type I and II may be acute or chronic. Causes include: ARDS, asthma, chest trauma, pneumothorax, pneumonia, pulmonary oedema, pulmonary fibrosis, retained secretions, pulmonary embolism, COPD, depression of the respiratory centres, e.g. by narcotic drugs. The management depends on the type, cause and severity, but includes: oxygen therapy, mechanical ventilation, supportive measures and treatment of the underlying cause. (See Figure 55). ⇒ acute respiratory distress syndrome.

Residential care

The expression residential care is applied generically to care for older people provided by social services, private nursing homes and NHS continuing care wards but is also applied uniquely to social service provision in order to distinguish it from the other two long-term care environments. Older people admitted to social services residential care do not require continuing nursing care and tend to be less dependent than older people in either continuing care or nursing homes. However, with the increased proportion of older people in the UK the distinctions between the three care environments has become blurred. UK government policies, aimed at promoting care in the community, have changed the profile of provision of residential care. Since the late 1980s there has been an increase in the places available for older people in private nursing homes and this has arisen partly as a result of the increased proportion of older people and the closure of NHS continuing care wards. The number of places in nursing homes and social services residential care was approximately equal in the 1980s, but the amount of social service provision has remained constant while the amount of private nursing home provision has increased by an order of magnitude.

Type I
Usually acute but may be chronic

The blood gases show:

Hypoxaemia – PaO_2 is low (<8.0 kPa) without hypercapnia and the $PaCO_2$ is normal or reduced (<6.6 kPa)

It occurs in conditions that damage lung tissue, e.g. pneumonia, pulmonary oedema, acute respiratory distress syndrome, pulmonary fibrosis, etc.

Type II
May be chronic or acute (acute type II respiratory failure is also known as asphyxia)

The blood gases show:

Hypoxaemia – PaO_2 is low (<8.0 kPa)
Hypercapnia – $PaCO_2$ is high (>6.6 kPa)

It occurs in situations where alveolar ventilation is inadequate to excrete the waste CO_2 generated by cell metabolism, e.g. inhaled foreign body, narcotic drugs, chronic obstructive pulmonary disease.

Figure 55 Respiratory failure – types I and II.

respiratory function tests also known as lung or pulmonary function tests. A series of tests employed to determine the efficiency of ventilation within the lungs and the presence of disease and response to treatment. Measurement of lung volumes and capacities; these include: peak expiratory flow rate, tidal volume, vital capacity (VC), total lung capacity (TLC), functional residual capacity (FRC), inspiratory capacity (IC), expiratory reserve volume (ERV), residual volume (RV), forced vital capacity (FVC) and forced expiratory volume in one second (FEV_1). Other tests used include: gas transfer tests and exercise tolerance tests. ⇒ arterial blood gases. ⇒ pulse oximetry. ⇒ spirometer.

respiratory syncytial virus (RSV) *n* a myxovirus responsible for bronchiolitis and pneumonia in infants and small children. May be very severe in infants under six months.

respiratory system the organs and structures involved with breathing and gaseous exchange. Comprises the nose, nasopharynx, larynx, trachea, bronchi, lungs and alveoli.

respite care short-term or temporary care provided within a health or social care facility to allow relief for family and other home carers. May be provided on a daily or residential basis.

resting potential *n* the difference in electrical charge between the inside and outside of the plasma membrane of an excitable cell in the resting state, the inside of the membrane being negative relative to the outside.

restless leg syndrome restless legs characterized by paraesthesiae like creeping, crawling, itching and prickling.

restlessness *n* inability to keep still. Often accompanies a raised body temperature, disordered body chemistry or a state of anxiety.

restrictive respiratory disease *n* one characterized by a limited ability to expand the lungs and chest, such as with the presence of fibrosis.

resuscitation *n* ⇒ advanced life support. ⇒ basic life support. ⇒ cardiopulmonary resuscitation — **resuscitative** *adj*.

retardation *n* 1. the slowing of a process which has already been carried out at a quicker rate or higher level. 2. arrested growth or function from any cause.

retching *n* ineffectual efforts to vomit.

retention *n* 1. retaining of facts in the mind. 2. holding back. Accumulation of that which is normally excreted. *retention cyst* a cyst caused by blocking of a duct. ⇒ ranula. *retention of urine* an inability to void urine which accumulates within the bladder. It has a variety of causes that include: problems affecting the nerve supply, obstruction, such as an enlarged prostate gland, or psychological factors.

reticular *adj* resembling a net. Applied to tissues.

reticular activating system (RAS) *n* functional area of the brainstem. It is concerned with the state of cortical arousal, conscious level and the modification of sensory inputs helps to prevent sensory overload. ⇒ sleep.

reticulocyte *n* an immature circulating red blood cell which still contains traces of the nucleus and endoplasmic reticulum which were present in the cell when developing in the bone marrow. They form up to 2% of circulating red cells.

reticulocytosis *n* an increase in the number of reticulocytes in the blood, indicating over-active red blood cell formation in the marrow, such as occurs in severe anaemia.

reticuloendothelial system (RES) ⇒ monocyte-macrophage system.

retina *n* the light-sensitive inner part of the eye. It consists of a multiple-layer complex of pigment cells, rods and cones (photoreceptors) and other neurons. The photoreceptors receive the light entering the eye and convert it chemically to nerve impulses which leave the eye via the optic nerve. *detached retina* a condition where the layers of the retina become torn. Lasers are often used to repair the tear before vision is permanently impaired. ⇒ cones. ⇒ eye. ⇒ rods — **retinal** *adj* pertaining to the retina.

retinitis *n* inflammation of the retina. *retinitis pigmentosa* a noninflammatory, familial, degenerative condition which progresses to night blindness, tunnel vision and blindness. The term retinopathy is becoming more widely used.

retinoblastoma *n* a malignant tumour arising from cells in the retina, occurring in children. Some cases are inherited.

retinoids *npl* vitamin A derivatives, e.g. tretinoin, used in the treatment of acne and with cytotoxic chemotherapy for some acute leukaemias, and etretinate, used for severe psoriasis. Retinoids are teratogenic and are not used during pregnancy. Patients are advised regarding effective contraception during treatment and the necessity with some retinoids to avoid pregnancy for at least 2 years after treatment as the drug stays in body fat.

retinol *n* a light-absorbing molecule derived from vitamin A. It combines with an opsin (protein) to form the visual pigment rhodopsin. Also called retinene. ⇒ rhodopsin. ⇒ vitamin A.

retinopathy *n* any noninflammatory disease of the retina, such as that affecting people with diabetes mellitus or hypertension. ⇒ retinitis. *retinopathy of prematurity (ROP)* retinal disease affecting premature infants. ⇒ fibroplasia.

retinoscope *n* instrument for measuring refractive errors in order to prescribe spectacles.

retinoscopy an examination to determine the refractive errors of the eye.

retinotoxic *adj* toxic to the retina.

retractile *adj* capable of being drawn back, i.e. retracted.

retractor *n* a surgical instrument for holding apart the edges of a wound to reveal underlying structures.

retrieval the recovery of information from stored memory.

retroactive interference ⇒ interference.

retrobulbar *adj* pertaining to the back of the eyeball. *retrobulbar neuritis* inflammation of that portion of the optic nerve behind the eyeball.

retrocaecal *adj* behind the caecum, e.g. a retrocaecal appendix.

retroflexion *n* the state of being bent backwards, especially of the uterus. ⇒ anteflexion *ant*.

retrograde *adj* going backward. *retrograde amnesia* ⇒ amnesia. *retrograde ejaculation* discharge of semen into the urinary bladder. *retrograde urography/pyelography* ⇒ urography. ⇒ anterograde *ant*.

retrolental behind the lens of the eye. ⇒ fibroplasia.

retro-ocular *adj* behind the eye.

retroperitoneal *adj* behind the peritoneum, such as the kidneys. *retroperitoneal fibroplasia* fibrous tissue behind the peritoneum. May be a side-effect of some drugs.

retropharyngeal *adj* behind the pharynx. *retropharyngeal abscess* collection of pus between the pharynx and the cervical vertebrae.

retroplacental *adj* behind the placenta, such as a blood clot.

retropubic *adj* behind the pubis.

retrospection *n* morbid dwelling on the past.

retrospective audit a type of nursing audit where the nursing charts and records are examined and the outcomes assessed after the care has been completed or the person discharged. ⇒ audit.

retrospective study research that collects data from the past, moving backwards in time. ⇒ prospective study.

retrosternal *adj* behind the sternum.

retrotracheal *adj* behind the trachea.

retroversion *n* turning backward. ⇒ anteversion *ant*. *retroversion of the uterus* tilting of the whole of the uterus backward with the cervix pointing forward — **retroverted** *adj*.

retroviruses *npl* a family of RNA viruses that include the human immunodeficiency viruses (HIV 1 and 2) and the human T-cell lymphotropic viruses (HTLV 1 and 2).

Rett's syndrome a very rare genetic defect caused by a sporadic mutation of a gene on the X chromosome. It is almost always seen in girls and is characterized by normal development during the first year, followed by gradual deterioration in motor and intellectual ability. Affected children have severe learning and physical disability, and are prone to epilepsy and abnormal breathing patterns, breath holding and hyperventilation.

revascularization *n* the regrowth of blood vessel into a tissue or organ after deprivation of its normal blood supply. ⇒ percutaneous myocardial revascularization.

revenue budget the allocation of money for day to day running costs, e.g. salaries, consumables, telephone, lighting, heating and drugs etc. ⇒ capital budget.

reverse barrier nursing used to protect immunosuppressed individuals from infection. ⇒ protective isolation.

reverse transcriptase inhibitors *npl* drugs that inhibit viral reverse transcriptase enzymes. Examples include: didanosine and zalcitabine, used in the management of HIV infection.

Reye's syndrome rare condition characterized by encephalopathy and cerebral oedema with acute fatty degeneration of the liver, occurring in children after a viral infection. Associated with the administration of salicylates in some cases, which has led to the recommendation that children under the age of 12 do not receive products containing aspirin, except in some cases of juvenile arthritis. The condition presents with vomiting, progressing to impaired consciousness and jaundice. The condition is often fatal, although full recovery may follow early diagnosis.

Rh *abbr* Rhesus factor. ⇒ blood groups.

rhabdomyolysis *n* breakdown of skeletal muscle. The release of myoglobin into the blood can lead to renal failure. ⇒ crush syndrome.

rhabdoviruses *npl* a family of RNA viruses that include the rabies virus.

rhagades *npl* superficial elongated scars radiating from the nostrils or angles of the mouth, found in congenital syphilis.

Rhesus factor (Rh) antigen on red blood cell surface. ⇒ blood groups.

Rhesus incompatability, isoimmunization arises when a Rhesus negative person is transfused with Rhesus positive blood or is pregnant with a Rhesus positive fetus. During labour, abortion, trauma and antepartum haemorrhage there is mixing of fetal and maternal bloods. The mother's body then develops anti-D antibodies against the Rhesus positive blood. If a subsequent fetus is also Rhesus positive, maternal antibodies will attack the fetal blood supply, causing severe haemolysis. ⇒ anti-D. ⇒ blood groups. ⇒ haemolytic disease of the newborn.

rheumatic *adj* pertaining to rheumatism. *rheumatic diseases* a diverse group of diseases affecting connective tissue, joints and bones. They include: inflammatory joint disease, e.g. rheumatoid arthritis; connective tissue disease, e.g. systemic lupus erythematosus; septic arthritis; osteoarthritis; crystal deposition disorders, e.g. gout; nonarticular/soft tissue rheumatism, e.g. fibrositis etc. *rheumatic heart disease* chronic cardiac disease with valve damage resulting from rheumatic fever.

rheumatic fever (*syn* acute rheumatism) a disorder, tending to recur but initially commonest in childhood, classically presenting as fleeting polyarthritis of the larger joints with swelling and pain, tachycardia, pyrexia, rash and pancarditis of varying severity within 3 weeks following a streptococcal throat infection. Atypically, but not infrequently, the symptoms are trivial and ignored, but carditis may be severe and result in permanent cardiac damage, particularly of heart valves. It may also cause neurological manifestations. ⇒ chorea. → rheumatism.

rheumatism *n* a nonspecific term embracing a diverse group of diseases and syndromes which have, in common, disorder or diseases of connective tissue and hence usually present with pain, or stiffness, or swelling of muscles and joints. Used colloquially to describe ill-defined aches and pains. ⇒ rheumatic diseases. *nonarticular/soft tissue rheumatism* involves the soft tissues and includes fibrositis etc.

rheumatoid *adj* resembling rheumatism. *rheumatoid arthritis* an inflammatory condition of connective tissue characterized by polyarthritis mainly affecting small peripheral joints that progresses to joint destruction with pain, swelling, muscle wastage, deformity and eventual loss of function. Its systemic effects include: general ill health, fever, weight loss, fatigue, eye damage, pericarditis, myocarditis, endocarditis and damage to heart valves, aortitis, vasculitis, anaemia and lung changes, e.g. alveolitis. There is a genetic predisposition to the condition which has an autoimmune aetiology. Management depends on severity and presentation but includes: rest, both general and for specific joints with splints; good positioning and posture with expert physiotherapy; warmth; drugs (NSAIDs, oral and intra-articular corticosteroids, antimalarial drugs, e.g. chloroquine, gold, cytotoxic drugs, immunosuppressants, etc); immunotherapy, e.g. anti-tumour necrosis factor (TNF) monoclonal antibody and surgery. ⇒ Felty's syndrome. ⇒ juvenile chronic arthritis. ⇒ Still's disease. *rheumatoid factors* immunoglobulins that can be detected in the serum of patients with rheumatic and other diseases, e.g. liver cirrhosis. ⇒ antinuclear antibodies. ⇒ RA latex test. ⇒ SCAT.

rheumatologist *n* a doctor who specializes in the management of rheumatic diseases.

rheumatology *n* the science or the study of the rheumatic diseases.

rhinitis *n* inflammation of the nasal mucous membrane. The cause may be: allergic, infective, atrophic or vasomotor.

rhinology *n* the study of diseases affecting the nose — **rhinologist** *n*.

rhinomanometry *n* test used to assess the patency of the nasal airway and measure the nasal airflow and pressure during breathing.

rhinophyma *n* nodular enlargement of the skin of the nose.

rhinoplasty *n* plastic operation to correct nasal deformity caused by disease or injury.

rhinorrhoea *n* nasal discharge. May be clear, mucoid, bloodstained or purulent. It is important to note that a clear discharge may be leakage of cerebro-spinal fluid following skull fracture.

rhinoscopy *n* inspection of the interior of the nose. *anterior rhinoscopy* uses a nasal speculum. Allows the anterior septum, middle and inferior turbinate bones to be examined. *posterior rhinoscopy* uses either a nasopharyngeal mirror or a nasendoscope to examine the posterior nasal cavity — **rhinoscopic** *adj*.

rhinosinusitis *n* inflammation of the nose and adjacent sinuses.

rhinovirus *n* a group of picornaviruses that cause the common cold. ⇒ coryza.

rhizotomy *n* surgical division of a root; usually the dorsal (posterior) root of a spinal nerve to relieve pain. *chemical rhizotomy* accomplished by injection of a chemical.

rhodopsin *n* the visual purple (pigment) contained in the retinal rods. Its colour is preserved in darkness, bleached by daylight and is needed for vision in low intensity light. Its formation is dependent on vitamin A.

rhomboid *adj* diamond-shaped.

rhonchus *n* abnormal sound heard on auscultation of the lung. Passage of air through bronchi obstructed by oedema or exudate produces a rumbling/rattling sound.

riboflavin *n* part of the vitamin B complex. Also known as riboflavine. It is required by the body for the formation of coenzymes important in all oxidation reactions that release energy from nutrients. It occurs in many foods, but most is found in food of animal origin, such as offal. In the UK the most important source is milk and milk products. Riboflavin is destroyed by sunlight. Deficiency is rare and is characterized by angular stomatitis. It may occur in vegans and others who do not have milk.

ribonuclease *n* an enzyme that degrades ribonucleic acid.

ribonucleic acid (RNA) *n* nucleic acids found in the nucleus, ribosomes and cytoplasm of cells. They consist of a single chain of nucleotides containing phosphate, ribose (a 5-carbon sugar) and the nitrogenous bases: adenine (A), guanine (G), cytosine (C) and uracil (U). There are three types: messenger (mRNA), ribosomal (rRNA) and transfer (tRNA), which perform specific roles during protein synthesis. ⇒ deoxyribonucleic acid. ⇒ transcription. ⇒ translation.

ribosomal RNA (rRNA) *n* ⇒ ribonucleic acid.

ribosome *n* very small subcellular organelle found in the cytoplasm or associated with the rough endoplasmic reticulum. They consist of protein and RNA and are involved in protein synthesis.

ribs *npl* the 12 pairs of curved bones which articulate with the 12 thoracic vertebrae posteriorly and form the walls of the thorax. The upper seven pairs are *true ribs* and are attached to the sternum anteriorly by separate costal cartilages. The remaining five pairs are the *false ribs*; the first three pairs of these are attached indirectly to the sternum by their costal cartilage joining to the costal cartilage above. The lower two pairs are the *floating ribs* which have no anterior articulation. *cervical ribs* are formed by an extension of the transverse process of the 7th cervical vertebra in the form of bone or a fibrous tissue band; this causes an upward displacement of the subclavian artery. A congenital abnormality.

RICE *acr* rest, ice, compression and elevation. Treatment for strains and sprains.

rice-water stool the watery stools that occur in cholera. The 'rice grains' are small pieces of desquamated epithelium from the intestine.

rickets *n* bone disease due to a lack of vitamin D during infancy and childhood (prior to ossification of the epiphyses) which results from a low dietary intake or insufficient exposure to sunlight. This leads to abnormal calcium and phosphate metabolism with faulty ossification and poor bone growth. It is characterized by features that include: muscle weakness, anaemia, respiratory infections, bone tenderness and pain and hypocalcaemia. There is delay in: motor development such as walking, eruption of teeth and closure of the fontanelles. Later there may be bony deformities such as bow legs. Rickets may be secondary to malabsorption of vitamin D, e.g. in coeliac disease, or defective metabolism, such as with certain drugs and chronic renal failure. Treatment is with vitamin D and sufficient calcium. Some types of inherited rickets are resistant to treatment. In adults the same condition is called osteomalacia.

Rickettsia *n* small pleomorphic parasitic Gram-negative micro-organisms that have characteristics of both viruses and bacteria. They are smaller in size than bacteria and larger than the viruses. Many of their physiological characteristics resemble the bacteria, but, like the viruses, they are obligate intracellular parasites. They are parasitic in the gut of ticks, fleas, lice and mites; transmission to humans is by bites from these arthropods. They cause diseases of the typhus group and Rocky mountain spotted fever. ⇒ rickettsial fevers. ⇒ spotted fever.

rickettsial fevers *npl* a group of rickettsial fevers transmitted by ticks, lice, mites and fleas. They are associated with overcrowding and poor hygiene, such as might occur in refugee camps and after natural disasters. It is only sporadic in Britain. Types include: epidemic typhus caused by *Rickettsia prowazekii*, endemic

typhus caused by *R. mooseri*, scrub typhus caused by *R.tsutsugamushi* and Rocky Mountain spotted fever caused by *R. rickettsii*. The diseases are characterized by fever, headache and petechial rash. Mortality depends upon the type, but may be up to 40% in epidemic typhus.

rickety rosary a series of protuberances (bossing) at junction of ribs and costal cartilages in children suffering from rickets.

Riedel's thyroiditis a rare chronic fibrosis of the thyroid gland. It is characterized by a gland which is hard and irregular, and involvement of nearby structures. There are pressure symptoms and eventually hypothyroidism and hypoparathyroidism.

Rift valley fever one of the mosquito-transmitted haemorrhagic fevers.

right occipitoanterior used to describe the position where the fetal occiput is against the right anterior part of the maternal pelvis.

right occipitoposterior used to describe the position where the fetal occiput is against the right posterior part of the maternal pelvis.

rights the recognition in law that certain inalienable rights, such as the right to life, should be respected, e.g. Human Rights Act 1998.

rigor *n* an attack of shivering occurring when the heat-regulating centre malfunctions. This causes a sudden increase in body temperature which may remain elevated or fall as profuse sweating takes place. *rigor mortis* the contraction of muscle fibres due to chemical changes after death. Causes stiffness of the body which lasts for a variable period dependent on several factors.

Ringer's solution *n* isotonic intravenous solution containing sodium chloride with potassium and calcium salts. *lactated Ringer's solution* one that contains lactate.

ringworm *n* (*syn* tinea) generic term used to describe contagious infection of the skin by a fungus, because the common manifestations are circular (circinate) scaly patches. ⇒ dermatophytes.

rINN *abbr* Recommended International Nonproprietary Name.

Rinne's test a tuning fork (512 Hz) is used to test the conduction of sound through air and bone. The struck tuning fork is held by the external auditory meatus and placed on the mastoid bone. Used to differentiate between conductive and sensorineural hearing loss. ⇒ Weber's test.

RIP *acr* raised intracranial pressure.

risk a potential hazard. *attributable risk* describes the disease rate in people exposed to the risk factor minus the occurrence in unexposed people. *relative risk* the ratio of disease rate in exposed people to those who have not been exposed. It is related to the odds ratio, which is the odds (as in betting) of disease occurring in an exposed person divided by the odds of the disease occurring in an unexposed person. ⇒ risk assessment. ⇒ risk factor.

risk assessment a structured assessment of risk carried out for a particular area or activity. ⇒ risk management. See Box – Risk assessment.

risk factor any factor which causes a person or a group of people to be more vulnerable to disease, injury or complications. Risk factors for health include the main behavioural risk factors, e.g. smoking, habitual excessive intake of alcohol, lack of physical activity, high fat and refined carbohydrate diet, lack of vegetables and fruit, and drugs misuse etc. Factors such as obesity, hypertension and hypercholesterolaemia are risk factors that may be detected during screening programmes. ⇒ well man clinic. ⇒ well woman clinic. Social risk factors, such as job control and sense of security and environmental factors such as particulate air pollution, are cited in the National Service Framework for CHD.

risk management see Box – Risk management.

RIST *abbr* radioimmunosorbent test.

risus sardonicus the abnormal grin produced by facial muscle contraction, seen in tetanus.

rite of passage a customary ritual enacted to confirm that a person has been accepted into a particular group. It may be a ceremony or event which marks a specific age or life event of some importance, such as reaching puberty.

river blindness a form of onchocerciasis.

RNA *abbr* ribonucleic acid.

RNA viruses *npl* several families of viruses that contain RNA as their nucleic acid, e.g. picornavirus, retrovirus etc.

RNI *abbr* reference nutrient intake.

RO *abbr* reality orientation.

ROA *abbr* right occipitoanterior.

Risk Assessment

Assessing risk means being aware of the problem areas (RCN 1999). This assessment then enables decisions to be made about problems, actual and potential. Decisions may be based upon a number of criteria, such as placing people at risk, and this may then be sub-divided into patients, staff and others. Other criteria may be the frequency of the problem, and whether incidents are likely to cause major injury or contribute to cumulative strain.

However, risk assessments are useless and likely to become simply 'paper exercises' unless the identified problems are acted upon. Changes may be relatively simple, immediately applicable and cost-free, e.g. making space before patient handling takes place; or major, costing large amounts of money, and taking time to implement, e.g. altering the layout of a whole department to minimize risk.

Risk assessments must be carried out because:

- Regulations require it, e.g. The manual handling operations regulations 1992 require risk assessments to be carried out if the employer cannot avoid the need for a manual handling action which involves risk of injury;
- Assessment is a logical method of reducing accidents and ill health;
- Assessments increase awareness;
- They are needed for use when something goes wrong. All risk assessments must be documented and may be used if something goes wrong. (RCN 1999)

The commonest example of the uses of risk assessment is patient handling, but the principles can and must be applied to all cases where risk is actual or potential.

Reference
Royal College of Nursing 1999 Manual Handling Assessments in Hospitals and the Community — RCN Guide; Working well initiative. RCN, London. (Revised)

Risk management

Risk management was introduced in the NHS following the establishment of Trusts, which resulted in:
(a) the removal of crown immunity from prosecution for non- compliance with statutory health and safety policy and (b) the requirement that Trusts meet their own financial liabilities.

Identifying the risk

This is a data gathering exercise to establish the kinds of risks likely to occur, and to make judgements about their frequency.

Analysing the risk

This is a complex process, which involves understanding the risks identified, and examining them within a framework of incidence, causes and impact on the organization. A range of management tools such as flowcharts, pathway charts and cause and effect diagrams are useful processes to use to analyse the material gathered.

Controlling the risk

Phase one involves introducing a range of focused activities which may include physical safety features, e.g. handrails, or organizational controls in the form of protocols or guidelines. Phase two is to decide whether the Trust will retain the responsibility for the risk – i.e. will it deal with the financial consequences of any mishaps, or will it seek to transfer the risk to some form of insurance.

Rocky Mountain spotted fever *n* ⇒ rickettsial fevers. ⇒ spotted fever.

rodent ulcer ⇒ basal cell carcinoma.

rods *npl* photoreceptors within the retina that contain rhodopsin. Rods are concerned with peripheral and low light intensity vision. → cones.

Rogerian counselling a humanistic client-centred approach to counselling and psychotherapy, introduced by Carl Rogers in the 1950s.

Rogers, Carl American psychologist (1902–1987). ⇒ Rogerian counselling.

role *n* the characteristic social behaviour of a person in relation to others in the group, e.g. the role of the nurse vis-à-vis that of the doctor. *role conflict* a person can experience conflict when enacting various roles, e.g. the role of being a parent may conflict at times with that of being a nurse. *role model* a person who acts as a model for another person's behaviour in a particular role. It is important for both childhood and professional development. *role playing* can be used in an educational programme when a student assumes the role of a patient/client so that other students may practise a particular skill, such as communication. It can be used therapeutically, e.g. in mental health nursing, to help patients see themselves as others see them and to understand intrapsychic conflict.

ROM *abbr* for Read-only Memory. The part of the computer memory that stores the fixed contents installed at manufacture. It can be read by the CPU but not altered in any way. This information remains even when the power supply is switched off. ⇒ RAM.

Romberg's sign a sign of ataxia. Inability to stand erect (without swaying) when the eyes are closed and the feet together.

rooting reflex primitive reflex seen in newborns. When the cheek is touched the infant will turn his or her head to that side.

ROP *abbr* right occipitoposterior.

rosacea *n* a skin disease which shows on flush areas of the face, such as the cheeks and forehead. In areas affected there is chronic dilation of superficial capillaries, redness and hypertrophy of sebaceous follicles, often complicated by a papulopustular eruption.

roseola *n* any rose-coloured skin rash. An early manifestation of secondary syphilis.

rotator *n* a muscle having the action of turning a part.

rotavirus *n* RNA virus responsible for outbreaks of winter gastroenteritis, but it occurs at other times. It is spread by direct contact, especially the hands. Mainly affects infants and children.

Roth spots round white spots in the retina. A rare clinical feature of infective endocarditis.

roughage *n* an obsolete term that does not describe fibre adequately and should not be used. 'Nonstarch polysaccharides' better describes the complex mixture of substances which have a wide range of effects on the gastrointestinal tract. ⇒ nonstarch polysaccharides.

rouleaux *n* a row of red blood cells which, when aggregated, resemble a stack of coins. Seen in disorders such as inflammatory diseases and multiple myeloma.

round ligaments fibrous uterine supports that run from each uterine cornu through the inguinal canal to the labium majora.

roundworm *n* (*Ascaris lumbricoides*) belong to a larger group of intestinal nematodes. Worldwide distribution. Parasitic to man. Eggs passed in stools; ingested; hatch in bowel; migrate through tissues, lungs and bronchi before returning to the bowel as mature worms. During migration worms can be coughed up, which is unpleasant and frightening. Heavy infections can produce pneumonia. They cause abdominal discomfort and may be vomited or passed per rectum. A tangled mass can cause intestinal obstruction or appendicitis. Adult worms can obstruct pancreatic and bile ducts. Drug treatment is with anthelmintics, such as piperazine and pyrantel. ⇒ Toxocara.

Roux-en-Y operation originally, the distal end of divided jejunum was anastomosed to the stomach, and the proximal jejunum containing the duodenal and pancreatic juices was anastomosed to the jejunum about 75 mm below the first anastomosis. The term is now used to include joining of the distal jejunum to a divided bile duct, oesophagus or pancreas, in major surgery of these structures.

Rovsing's sign pressure in the left iliac fossa causes pain in the right iliac fossa in appendicitis.

RPCF *abbr* Reiter protein complement fixation.

RPR *abbr* rapid plasma reagin.

RSI *abbr* repetitive strain injury.

RSV *abbr* respiratory syncytial virus.

rubefacients *npl* substances which, when applied to the skin, cause redness (hyperaemia).

rubella *n* (*syn* German measles) an acute, infectious disease, with an incubation period of 14–21 days. Caused by a virus and spread by droplet infection. There is mild fever, a pink, maculopapular rash and enlarged occipital and posterior cervical lymph nodes. Complications are rare, except when contracted in the first trimester of pregnancy, when it may produce fetal abnormalities, such as heart defects, deafness, cataracts and brain damage. Immunization is available as part of the routine programme, in conjunction with protection against measles and mumps (MMR), and subsequently to individuals who did not receive MMR or any nonpregnant woman of childbearing age with insufficient immunity.

Rubenstein-Taybi syndrome a constellation of abnormal findings first described in 1963. It includes learning disability, motor retardation, broad thumbs and toes, growth retardation, susceptibility to infection in the early years and characteristic facial features.

rubor *n* redness; usually used in the context of being one of the four classical signs of inflammation, the others being calor, dolor, tumor.

rugae *npl* folds or creases, such as those in the mucosa of the stomach and vagina.

RV *abbr* residual volume.

Ryle's tube a narrow-bore plastic nasogastric tube with a weighted tip which is passed via the nose into the stomach. It is used to aspirate (intermittent or continuous) stomach contents, such as following gastrointestinal surgery, or occasionally for feeding. Nursing management includes: full explanation and psychological support, oral hygiene, skin care and monitoring for soreness around the tube, managing hydration, which is often by intravenous infusion, and careful observation and recording of aspirate (amount, time, colour and odour) on an intake and output chart.

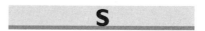

S

Sabin vaccine *n* live attenuated, oral poliomyelitis vaccine. Used in the routine immunization programme.

saccharides *npl* one of the three main classes of carbohydrates: monosaccharides, disaccharides and polysaccharides.

sacculation *n* appearance of several saccules.

saccule *n* a minute sac. A fluid-filled sac in the internal ear. Part of the vestibular apparatus, it contains the hair cells and otoliths: the receptors for static equilibrium that respond to head position relative to gravity and to linear changes in speed and direction. ⇒ utricle — **saccular, sacculated** adj.

sacral adj pertaining to the sacrum.

sacroanterior adj describes a breech presentation in midwifery. The fetal sacrum is directed to one or other acetabulum of the mother — **sacroanteriorly** adv.

sacrococcygeal adj pertaining to the sacrum and the coccyx.

sacroiliac adj pertaining to the sacrum and the ilium or the joint between the two bones.

sacroiliitis n inflammation of a sacroiliac joint. Involvement of both joints characterizes such conditions as ankylosing spondylitis, Reiter's syndrome and psoriatic arthritis.

sacrolumbar adj pertaining to the sacrum and the lumbar area (loins).

sacroposterior adj describes a breech presentation in midwifery. The fetal sacrum is directed to one or other sacroiliac joint of the mother — **sacroposteriorly** adv.

sacrum n the triangular bone lying between the fifth lumbar vertebra and the coccyx. It consists of five vertebrae fused together, and it articulates on each side with the innominate bones of the pelvis, forming the sacroiliac joints — **sacral** adj.

SAD abbr seasonal affective disorder.

saddle nose one with a flattened bridge; often a sign of congenital syphilis.

sadism n the obtaining of pleasure from inflicting pain, violence or degradation on another person, or on the sexual partner. ⟶ masochism ant.

safe-handling or no-lifting policies npl policies that provide risk assessment, staff training with regular updates, and equipment that includes: hoists, slings, sliding devices, transfer boards, belts etc.

SaFFs abbr Service and Financial Frameworks.

sagittal adj resembling an arrow. In the anterior/posterior plane of the body. sagittal section section made by cutting through a specimen from top to bottom so there are equal right and left halves. sagittal sinuses venous channels draining blood from the brain. sagittal suture the immovable joint formed by the union of the two parietal bones.

SAH abbr subarachnoid haemorrhage.

Salem nasogastric tube a tube which has a double lumen to allow swallowed air to escape. It is used in whole gut irrigation.

salicylates npl a group of nonsteroidal anti-inflammatory drugs, e.g. aspirin which is an effective analgesic for minor painful disorders, such as headache, toothache or muscle strain. It may be used as an antipyretic. It also reduces inflammation in a variety of diseases affecting the musculoskeletal system. It also reduces platelet stickiness and inhibits platelet aggregation and prevents clotting; it is used in the prophylaxis of myocardial infarction and strokes. Aspirin should not be used for children under 12 years of age as it is associated with Reye's syndrome; it may, however, be specifically indicated for juvenile rheumatoid arthritis.

salicylic acid used topically, it is a keratolytic with fungicidal and bacteriostatic properties, and is used in a variety of hyperkeratotic (excess keratin) skin conditions, e.g. psoriasis. Used to remove corns and warts.

saline n a solution of salt and water. Normal or physiological saline is a 0.9% (0.9g/100ml) solution with the same osmotic pressure as that of blood. ⇒ hypertonic. ⟶ hypotonic ⇒ isotonic.

saliva n the secretion of the salivary glands. It contains water, mucus and salivary amylase — **salivary** adj.

salivary adj pertaining to saliva. salivary calculus a stone formed in the salivary ducts. salivary glands the exocrine glands which secrete saliva, i.e. the parotid, submandibular (submaxillary) and sublingual glands.

salivation n an increased secretion of saliva.

Salk vaccine a preparation of killed poliomyelitis virus used as an antigen to produce active artificial immunity to poliomyelitis. It is used for certain individuals, such as those who are immunocompromised. It is given by injection.

Salmonella n a genus of bacteria. Gram-negative bacilli. Parasitic in many animals and humans, in whom they are often pathogenic. Some species, such as Salmonella typhi and Salmonella paratyphi, are host-specific, infecting only humans, in whom they cause the enteric fevers (typhoid and paratyphoid respectively). Others, such as *Salmonella typhimurium*, may infect a wide range of host species, usually through contaminated foods. *Salmonella enteritidis* a motile Gram-negative rod, widely distributed in domestic animals, particularly poultry, and wild animals, e.g. rodents, and sporadic in humans as a cause of food poisoning.

salpingectomy *n* excision of a uterine tube.

salpingitis *n* acute or chronic inflammation of the uterine tubes. ⇒ hydrosalpinx. ⇒ pyosalpinx.

salpingogram *n* radiological examination of patency of the uterine tubes by retrograde introduction of contrast medium into the uterus and along the tubes — **salpingographically** *adv*.

salpingo-oophorectomy *n* excision of a uterine tube and ovary.

salpingostomy *n* the operation performed to restore tubal patency.

salpinx a tube, especially the uterine tube or the pharyngotympanic tube.

salt *n* a substance formed by the combination of an acid and alkali (base), such as sodium chloride.

salve *n* an ointment.

Samaritans *npl* a voluntary befriending service, available 24 hours to suicidal or despairing people who phone in, visit local branches or make contact via e-mail.

sample the subset selected from a population.

sandfly *n* an insect (*Phlebotomus*) responsible for transmitting viral diseases, such as sandfly fever. Likewise they transmit protozoa that causes leishmaniasis.

sanguineous *adj* pertaining to or containing blood.

SANS *abbr* Schedule for Assessment of Negative Symptoms.

saphenous *adj* apparent; manifest. The name given to two superficial veins in the leg, the long and short, and to the nerves accompanying them.

saprophyte *n* free-living micro-organisms obtaining food from dead and decaying animal or plant tissue — **saprophytic** *adj*.

sarcoid *adj* a term applied to a group of lesions in skin, lymph nodes, lungs or other organs, which resemble tuberculous foci in structure.

sarcoidosis *n* a granulomatous disease of unknown aetiology in which histological appearances resemble tuberculosis. May affect any organ of the body, but most commonly presents as a condition of the skin, lymph nodes, liver, spleen, lungs, eyes, parotid glands or the bones of the hand. The early stage disease usually requires no treatment but systemic corticosteroids may be required. ⇒ Kveim test.

sarcoma *n* malignant growth of mesodermal tissue (e.g. connective tissue, muscle, bone). ⇒ mesoderm — **sarcomatous** *adj*.

Sarcoptes *n* a genus of Acerina. *Sarcoptes scabiei* is the itch mite which causes scabies.

sartorius *n* the 'tailor's muscle' of the thigh, since it flexes one leg over the other.

satisfaction *n* a positive feeling. *job satisfaction* a term which is used when people, including nurses, experience positiveness in relation to their work: lack of it can lead to low morale. ⇒ burnout. *consumer satisfaction* ⇒ quality assurance.

saturated a solution into which no more solute can be dissolved. *saturated fatty acids* fatty acids that have no double bonds in their structure. Mainly derived from animal sources but some are found in plants. High dietary intake is associated with elevated serum cholesterol levels and an unfavourable HDL:LDL ratio, both of which are linked with atherosclerosis. ⇒ fatty acids. ⇒ lipoprotein. ⇒ monounsaturated fatty acids. ⇒ polyunsaturated fatty acids.

SBS *abbr* short bowel syndrome.

scab *n* a dried crust forming over an open wound.

scabies *n* a parasitic skin disease caused by the itch mite. Highly contagious. There is severe itching as the mite burrows into the skin, especially between the fingers, on the genitalia and buttocks. Secondary bacterial skin infection may occur. Treatment involves topical applications of benzyl benzoate.

scald *n* an injury caused by moist heat (hot liquids and vapours). ⇒ burn.

scalded skin syndrome ⇒ toxic epidermal necrolysis.

scale 1. the layers of dead epidermal cells that are shed from the skin. **2.** to remove tartar deposits from the teeth. **3.** a device or graded system used for measurement.

scalenus syndrome pain and tingling in arm and fingers, often with loss of power and muscle wasting, because of compression of the lower trunk of the brachial plexus behind scalenus anterior muscle at the thoracic outlet.

scalp *n* the hair-bearing and fairly movable skin which covers the cranium. *scalp cooling* the application of a cap made of coils through which flows cold water or malleable ice packs; research shows that cooling helps to prevent the hair loss associated with some types of chemotherapy used for the treatment of cancer.

scan *n* a diagnostic procedure where detailed images of organs or tissues, and sometimes their functions, are produced. ⇒ computed tomography. ⇒ imaging techniques. ⇒ magnetic resonance imaging. → positron emission tomography. ⇒ radionuclide imaging/scanning. ⇒ ultrasonography.

scanning speech staccato speech. A form of dysarthria characteristic of cerebellar disease. The speech is jumpy or slow with hesitation between syllables which are equally stressed.

scaphoid *n* boat shaped, as a bone of the tarsus and carpus. *scaphoid abdomen* concavity of the anterior abdominal wall, often associated with emaciation.

scapula *n* the shoulder-blade, a large, flat triangular bone that articulates with the humerus and clavicle — **scapular** *adj.*

scar *n* (*syn* cicatrix) the dense, avascular white fibrous tissue, formed as the end-result of healing, especially in the skin. ⇒ keloid.

scarification *n* the making of a series of small, superficial incisions or punctures in the skin to allow a vaccine to enter the body.

scarlet fever *n* scarlatina. Infectious disease with an incubation period of 2–4 days. Follows infection by a strain of Group A β-haemolytic streptococcus. Occurs mainly in children. Begins commonly with a throat infection, leading to fever and the outbreak of a punctate erythematous rash on the skin of the trunk which is followed by desquamation. Characteristically the area around the mouth escapes (circumoral pallor). Usually treated with penicillin.

SCAT *abbr* sheep cell agglutination test. A rheumatoid factor in the blood is detected by the sheep red cell agglutination titre.

SCBU *abbr* special care baby unit.

SCC *abbr* spinal cord compression.

Schedule for Assessment of Negative Symptoms (SANS) a scale used to assess twenty negative symptoms in schizophrenia, e.g. affective flattening, alogia, avolition/apathy, anhedonia and attention. Symptoms are rated on a 0–5 scale of increasing severity.

Scheuermann's disease osteochondritis of the spine affecting the ring epiphyses of the vertebral bodies. Occurs in adolescents and leads to kyphosis.

Schick test a skin test used to determine a person's susceptibility or immunity to diphtheria. It involves the intradermal injection of diphtheria toxin. A positive reaction is recognized by the appearance of a round red area within 24–48 hours and indicates a susceptibility to the disease. The presence of immunity is indicated by a negative reaction to the toxin, i.e. no redness or swelling.

Schilder's disease ⇒ adrenoleucodystrophy.

Schilling test used to confirm the diagnosis of pernicious anaemia. The absorption of ingested radioactive vitamin B_{12} is assessed by measuring urinary excretion of the labelled vitamin.

Schistosoma *n* (*syn* Bilharzia) a genus of trematodes (blood flukes) which require fresh water snails as an intermediate host before infesting humans. *Schistosoma haematobium* is found mainly in Africa and the Middle East. *Schistosoma japonicum* is found in Japan, the Philippines, China and the Far East. *Schistosoma mansoni* is indigenous to Africa, the Middle East, the Caribbean and South America. ⇒ schistosomiasis.

schistosomiasis *n* (*syn* bilharziasis) infestation of the human body by *Schistosoma* which enter via the skin or mucous membrane. (See Figure 56). A single fluke can live in one part of the body, depositing eggs frequently, for many years. Treatment is with the anthelmintic

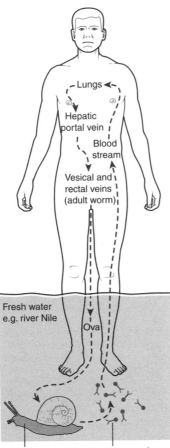

Lungs

Hepatic
portal vein

Blood
stream

Vesical and
rectal veins
(adult worm)

Fresh water
e.g. river Nile

Ova

Fresh-water snail   Immature form
(intermediate host)

Figure 56   Schistosoma (life cycle). (Adapted from Macleod et al 1987 with permission.)

praziquantel. Prevention is by chlorination of drinking water, proper disposal of human waste and eradication of fresh water snails. Schistosomiasis is a serious problem in the tropics and the Orient. There may be irritation at the entry site and after 3–5 weeks there are signs due to larval movement, e.g. eosinophilia, fever, hepatitis and pneumonitis. Later, the eggs are deposited and the effects are site and type dependent, e.g. hepatitis, hepatic portal hypertension, colitis, lesions in the CNS, skin lesions, cystitis and haematuria. Years later, there may be hepatic fibrosis and hepatic portal hypertension, urinary tract damage and pulmonary hypertension.

schistosomicide *n* any agent lethal to *Schistosoma* — **schistosomicidal** *adj*.

schizophrenia *n* a psychotic disorder, one of the commonest psychiatric illnesses. See Box – Schizophrenia. ⇒ Knowledge About Schizophrenia Interview. ⇒ Relatives Assessment Interview for Schizophrenia in a Secure Environment. ⇒ Schizophrenia Nursing Assessment Protocol. ⇒ Schneider's first rank. Symptoms may be subgrouped into: *catatonic schizophrenia* characterized by episodes of immobility with muscular rigidity or stupor, interspersed with periods of acute excitability; *hebephrenic schizophrenia* ⇒ hebephrenia; *simple schizophrenia* characterized by apathy and withdrawal – hallucinations and delusions are absent; and *paranoid schizophrenia* where hallucinations and paranoid delusions are present.

Schizophrenia Nursing Assessment Protocol (SNAP) used by mental health nurses to assess all family members, including the client. It covers four main areas in a semistructured interview format: clients' relationship with people with whom they live; clients' psychiatric and personal history; nature of present episode; and families' understanding/knowledge of the illness. Particularly useful for quick assessment of main problem areas.

schizophrenic *adj* pertaining to schizophrenia.

Schlatter's disease (*syn* Osgood-Schlatter's disease) osteochondritis of the tibial tubercle.

Schlemm's canal a canal in the inner part of the sclera, close to its junction with the cornea, which it encircles. It drains excess aqueous humor to maintain normal intraocular pressure. Failure of drainage results in raised intraocular pressure. ⇒ glaucoma.

Schneider's first rank symptoms list of 'first rank' symptoms used in the diagnosis and classification of schizophrenia. They include: certain types of delusions, hallucinatory voices and feelings of passivity.

Schönlein's disease ⇒ Henoch-Schönlein purpura.

school nurse a registered nurse with a specialist qualification in the specific health needs of school-age children. Their expanding role includes: health surveil-

Schizophrenia

Schizophrenia is one of the major diagnostic categories of mental illness. The diagnostic criteria (ICD-10) relies on identifying a number of key ('first rank') symptoms (Craig, 2000). These are: Any one of (a) to (d) or any two of (e) to (h) for one month or more on most days and not due to organic brain disease, alcohol or drug intoxication.

(a) thought echo, insertion, withdrawal, or broadcasting;

(b) delusions of control, influence or passivity, clearly referred to body or limb movements or specific thoughts, actions or sensations, delusional perception;

(c) third person auditory hallucinations, either running commentary on actions or discussing the client amongst themselves;

(d) persistent delusions that are culturally inappropriate and completely impossible;

(e) persistent hallucinations when accompanied by fleeting or half formed delusions without clear affective content, or by persistent overvalued ideas or when occurring every day for weeks or months on end;

(f) breaks or interpolations in the train of thought, incoherence, irrelevant speech or neologisms;

(g) catatonic behaviour;

(h) negative symptoms of apathy, paucity of speech and blunting or incongruity of affect, usually resulting in social withdrawal. Not due to depression or neuroleptic medication.

Symptoms can be grouped as positive and negative. Positive symptoms include hallucinations and delusions or hearing voices and/or having strange thoughts. Negative symptoms include social withdrawal and lack of energy or motivation. The negative symptoms are harder to recognize, they are often ascribed to reasons other than the illness such as personality or laziness or unwanted effects of medication.

The causes of schizophrenia are uncertain. There is a clear genetic link – if one parent has the illness there is a 10% chance that a child will have schizophrenia, but if both parents are affected there is a 50% chance. The theory that families can cause a member to develop schizophrenia have long been discredited, because concepts of dysfunctional parent-child relationships and interactions stigmatized families and made them believe that their behaviour induced or caused schizophrenia in their relatives (Harding and Zahniser 1994). Now, other causes are being investigated and these include viral infection during pregnancy and fetal abnormalities.

The incidence of schizophrenia is more than one in every one hundred persons. Schizophrenia frequently remains undetected by primary care services in its early stages. The sooner the illness is identified and treatment started the better the prognosis. One in four people will have only one illness episode. The remainder will always have some symptoms that can be more or less controlled depending: on how soon treatment begins, how able someone is to develop insight into their problems and how supportive and informed their carers or family are. Indeed, the work on expressed emotion (EE) has helped to provide evidence that certain living environments can either exacerbate or reduce the chance of someone with the illness relapsing.

Until very recently medication has been the first and generally only treatment of choice. Despite the introduction of new 'atypical neuroleptics', the drugs generally produce a range of unwanted and unpleasant side effects. Although drugs remove positive symptoms, they only do so entirely in a minority of cases. Most people continue to have a level of residual symptoms and the user movement has been actively campaigning for alternative treatments. New forms of treatment include social skills training, cognitive behavioural and psychosocial interventions. Helping clients and their carers understand the illness and its symptoms and enabling them to develop practical solutions to problems that the illness brings has proved very effective. The stress vulnerability model (Zubin and Spring 1977) is a useful model for considering the illness. This model suggests that we all have a different level of vulnerability to a mental health problem. If we become sufficiently stressed we can cross the vulnerability threshold and become mentally unwell. Therefore, educating people who have schizophrenia and their families to be alert to stress levels and learn strategies to moderate stress helps to reduce the impact of the illness.

References

Craig T K J 2000 Severe mental illness: symptoms, signs and diagnosis. In: Gamble C, Brennan G Working with Serious Mental Illness: A manual for clinical practice. Baillière Tindall, Edinburgh

Harding C M, Zahniser J H 1994 Empirical correction of seven myths about schizophrenia with implications for treatment. Acta Psychiatrica Scandinavica 90(suppl 384):140–146

Zubin J, Spring B 1977 Vulnerability: a new view of schizophrenia. Journal of Abnormal Psychology 86:260–266 lance and screening; monitoring growth and development; child protection; being accessible to pupils/students seeking advice; providing age-appropriate nurse-led clinics; advising and supporting the school management team on initiatives aimed at creating healthy schools, health and safety matters and the curriculum requirements of personal and social education and sex education. They are concerned with the provision for children with *special* educational needs, such as children with learning disability, behavioural problems and physical conditions that require extra care and support to enable them to benefit from inclusion in mainstream schools.

school refusal a situation where a child or young person will not attend school. Reasons include: an irrational fear of school with anxiety, boredom or bullying.

Schultz-Charlton test a blanching produced in the skin of a patient showing scarlatinal rash, around an injection of serum from a convalescent case, indicating neutralization of toxin by antitoxin.

Schwann cell *n* specialized neuroglial cells of the peripheral nervous system. They produce layers of neurilemma which form the myelin sheath enclosing some nerve fibres. ⇒ neuroglia.

sciatica *n* pain in the line of distribution of the sciatic nerve (buttock, back of thigh, calf and foot). Commonly caused by a prolapsed intervertebral disc. ⇒ backache.

scintillography *n* scintiscanning. Visual recording of radioactivity over selected areas after administration of suitable radioisotope, e.g. to diagnose cancer.

scirrhous *adj* hard; resembling a scirrhus. Describes malignant tumours that are hard.

scirrhus *n* a carcinoma containing connective tissue that makes it gritty and hard, such as in the breast.

scissor leg deformity the legs are crossed in walking, following double hip-joint disease, or as a manifestation of Little's disease (spastic cerebral diplegia).

scissors gait ⇒ gait.

sclera *n* the 'white' of the eye; the opaque bluish-white fibrous outer coat of the eyeball covering the posterior five-sixths; it merges into the cornea at the front — **scleral** *adj*.

scleritis *n* inflammation of the sclera.

sclerocorneal *adj* pertaining to the sclera and the cornea, as the circular junction of these two structures.

scleroderma *n* a group of connective tissues diseases that lead to fibrosis and degenerative changes in many organs and the skin. Localized disease causes oedema of the skin, hardening, atrophy, deformity and ulceration. Occasionally it becomes generalized, producing immobility of the face and contraction of the fingers. Diffuse fibrosis may occur in the myocardium, kidneys, digestive tract and lungs. When confined to the skin it is termed morphoea. ⇒ collagen. ⇒ dermatomyositis. ⇒ sclerosis.

scleromalacia softening and thinning of the sclera.

sclerosis *n* a word used in pathology to describe abnormal hardening or fibrosis of a tissue. ⇒ multiple sclerosis. ⇒ tuberous sclerosis.

sclerotherapy *n* injection of a sclerosing agent for the treatment of oesophageal varices, haemorrhoids and varicose veins. Sclerotherapy for oesophageal varices is performed via an endoscope — **sclerotherapeutically** *adv*.

sclerotic *adj* pertaining to or exhibiting the symptoms of sclerosis.

scolex *n* the head of the tapeworm by which it attaches itself to the intestinal wall, and from which the segments (proglottides) develop.

scoliosis *n* lateral curvature of the spine, which can be congenital or acquired, and is due to abnormality of the vertebrae, muscles and nerves.

scorbutic *adj* pertaining to scorbutus, the old name for scurvy.

scotoma *n* a blind spot in the field of vision. May be normal or abnormal — **scotomata** *pl*.

screening *n* 1. a preventive measure to identify potential or incipient disease at an early stage when it may be more easily treated. It is carried out in a variety of settings, including hospitals, and clinics for antenatal care, well babies, well men and well women. Screening checks include: breast screening with mammography, cervical cytology, blood pressure checks, faecal occult blood, triple blood test during pregnancy. The screening process may raise anxiety even when it yields a negative result (no disease or pathology found). ⇒ disease prevention. ⇒ sensitivity. ⇒ specificity. **2.** common name for fluoroscopy units.

scrofula *n* obsolete term for tuberculosis of bone or lymph node.

scrofuloderma *n* obsolete term for a skin condition resulting from tuberculous affecting the lymph nodes or other underlying structures.

scrotum *n* the bag of pigmented skin and fascia in the male which contains the testes — **scrotal** *adj*.

scrub typhus *n* → rickettsial fevers.

scurf *n* a popular term for dandruff.

scurvy *n* a deficiency disease caused by lack of vitamin C (ascorbic acid) in the diet. Clinical features in adults include: swollen and spongy gums that bleed, loose teeth, bleeding around hair follicles, petechial haemorrhages, spontaneous bruising with large ecchymoses, epistaxis, poor wound healing and anaemia. In infants there may be swelling of the costochondral junctions and painful subperiosteal haemorrhage. Affected infants may be lethargic with a poor appetite. Treatment is with oral vitamin C and correction of any other nutritional deficiencies.

scybala *npl* rounded, hard, faecal lumps — **scybalum** *sing*.

SD *abbr* standard deviation.

SDAT *abbr* senile dementia Alzheimer's type.

SE *abbr* standard error.

seasonal affective disorder (SAD) a disorder of mood where individuals experience depression and lethargy as the days shorten as winter approaches. It is linked to the amount of melatonin secreted by the pineal body (gland), which is light dependent. The treatment of choice is exposure to special lights during the autumn and winter, in addition to natural light, as spontaneous improvement occurs as the days lengthen in spring.

sebaceous *adj* literally, pertaining to fat; usually refers to sebum. *sebaceous cyst* (*syn* wen) a retention cyst in a sebaceous gland in the skin. Such cysts are most commonly found on the scalp, scrotum and vulva. *sebaceous glands* the cutaneous glands which secrete an oily substance called sebum. The ducts of these glands are short and straight and open into the hair follicles. ⇒ pilosebaceous.

seborrhoea *n* greasy condition of the scalp, face, sternal region and elsewhere due to overactivity of sebaceous glands. The seborrhoeic type of skin is especially liable to conditions such as alopecia, seborrhoeic eczema, acne, etc.

sebum *n* the normal secretion of the sebaceous glands; it contains fatty acids, cholesterol and dead cells.

seclusion *n* a nursing intervention for mentally ill patients: they are isolated in a special room to decrease stimuli which might be causing or exacerbating their emotional distress. The use of seclusion is strictly controlled, monitored and audited.

second intention ⇒ wound healing.

secondary *adj* second in order. *secondary care* care that requires admission to hospital, rather than provided in the community. ⇒ primary health care. → tertiary care. *secondary prevention* ⇒ disease prevention. *secondary tumour* or *cancer* refers to spread of the primary cancer; can occur via blood, lymph, tissue extension or through a body cavity. ⇒ metastasis. ⇒ neoplasm

secretin *n* a hormone produced in the duodenal mucosa, which stimulates pancreatic secretion. It is part of a group of regulatory peptides that inhibit gastric secretion and motility as partially digested food enters the duodenum. → enterogastric reflex.

secretion *n* a fluid or substance, formed or concentrated in a gland and passed into the alimentary canal/tract, the blood or to the exterior.

secretory *adj* involved in the process of secretion: describes a cell or gland which secretes. *secretory phase* the stage of the menstrual cycle that starts after ovulation and lasts until the next menstruation. It is characterized by the thickening of the endometrium and the development of glands and blood vessels. It corresponds to the luteal phase of the ovarian cycle.

secular beliefs not overtly or specifically religious. Words such as spirit, spiritual and spirituality are used in a nonreligious context; for instance, summing up a person who is undergoing a stressful period, one might say 'but he's in good spirits'; the term is concerned with hopefulness, optimism and positiveness. Those who use words in this way often have strong nonreligious beliefs/convictions which guide their concepts of right and wrong that affect everyday living. ⇒ spiritual beliefs.

sedation *n* the production of a state of lessened functional activity.

sedative *n* any agent which lessens functional activity by acting on the nervous system. Reduces tension, anxiety and excitement. Includes drugs such as the benzodiazepines which have sedating effects. ⇒ hypnotic. ⇒ narcotic.

segment *n* a small section; a part — **segmentation** *n*.

segregation *n* in genetics, the separation from one another of two alleles, each carried on one of a pair of chromosomes; this happens during meiosis when the haploid gametes (oocytes and spermatozoa) are produced. ⇒ Mendel's law.

seizure convulsion or fit.

Seldinger catheter a special catheter and guide wire for insertion into an artery, along which it is passed, e.g. to the heart.

selective (o)estrogen receptor modulators (SERMs) *npl* tissue selective drugs that modulate oestrogen receptors in some tissues and not others. They may have oestrogen-agonist or oestrogen-antagonist effects. SERMs are used in the management of postmenopausal problems: their oestrogen-agonist effects have a beneficial effect on the cardiovascular system, brain and on bone, helping to prevent osteoporosis. They are oestrogen-antagonist at the receptors in the uterus and breast, so avoid the oestrogenic effects on these structures associated with the use of HRT. Current examples, such as raloxifene, do not, however, alleviate the hot flushes or vaginal dryness associated with the climacteric. Research continues into the development of SERMs for the prevention and treatment of some breast cancers.

selective serotonin re-uptake inhibitors (SSRIs) *npl* a group of widely prescribed antidepressants that include: fluoxetine, paroxetine and sertraline. They take 2–4 weeks to become effective and act by blocking the re-uptake of 5-hydroxytryptamine (serotonin) by nerve cells. They have fewer side-effects than MAOIs and TCAs, but nausea, anorexia and insomnia are common.

Selectron *n* a proprietary device used to deliver brachytherapy by remote controlled afterloading. The radioactive sources are propelled along tubes connecting the Selectron to previously placed applicators in body cavities, such as cervix, vagina, bronchus.

selenium (Se) *n* a trace element required by the body for reactions that protect cells against oxidative damage. It is an antioxidant.

self-actualization according to Maslow, this is the highest human need. Being able to develop and use one's abilities to the full.

self-advocacy ⇒ advocacy.

self-catheterization both male and female patients can be taught to pass a nonretaining catheter into the urinary bladder to evacuate urine intermittently.

self-concept the view that the individual has of their total characteristics, ideas, feelings, qualities and negative features.

self-esteem the value or worth a person places on themselves.

self-fulfilling prophecy an event whereby our expectations of another person makes us behave in such a way as to cause the exact response that we expected.

self-harm deliberate self-inflicted injuries. ⇒ parasuicide.

self-image the total concept of what one believes oneself to be vis-à-vis one's role in society.

self-infection endogenous infection. The unwitting transfer of normal flora microorganisms from one part of the body to another in which they produce infection. For example, *Escherichia coli* from the bowel may cause urinary tract or wound infection.

self-injurious behaviour ⇒ parasuicide.

self-retaining catheter a catheter which, when inserted into the urinary bladder, can be secured in position by the inflation of a small balloon surrounding the tip.

sella turcica *n* pituitary fossa of the sphenoid bone.

semantic memory that part of memory that stores general information about the world, e.g. where polar bears are found.

semen *n* seminal fluid. The alkaline fluid produced at ejaculation. It contains spermatozoa from the testes and the secretions from the accessory glands: prostate, seminal vesicles and bulbourethral glands.

semicircular canals *npl* three fluid-filled canals contained within the bony labyrinth of the internal ear. Orientated in the three planes of space they are part of the vestibular apparatus concerned with dynamic equilibrium (responding to rotational movements of the head) and balance. ⇒ ear.

semicomatose *adj* a state of altered consciousness from which the person can be roused by suitable stimuli. ⇒ Glasgow coma scale.

semilunar *adj* 1. shaped like a crescent or half moon. *semilunar cartilages* the two crescentic cartilages of the knee joint (menisci) between the femur and tibia. Very commonly injured and torn, especially during certain sports and other activities. ⇒ meniscectomy. 2. heart valves at the entrance to the aorta and pulmonary artery that prevent the back flow of blood into the ventricles.

seminal *adj* pertaining to semen. *seminal vesicles* two tubular accessory glands situated posterior to the male bladder. They secrete a viscous alkaline fluid containing nutrients, enzymes and prostaglandins, which forms around 60% of the volume of semen.

seminiferous *adj* carrying or producing semen. *seminiferous tubules* coiled tubules within the testes; the site of spermatogenesis.

seminoma *n* a common malignant tumour of the testis. ⇒ testicular — **seminomatous** *adj*.

semipermeable *adj* describes a membrane which is selectively permeable to some substances in solutions, but not to others. It allows molecules of a certain size to pass through, but not larger molecules. ⇒ osmosis.

semipermeable films *n* an adhesive polyurethane membrane designed to retain wound exudate, thereby creating a moist wound environment. It permits the exchange of oxygen and carbon dioxide and has varying degrees of water vapour permeability, but it is impermeable to micro-organisms and water. It therefore fulfils the requirements for moist wound healing with its many advantages. It can be used for low exudate wounds (nonabsorbent); as a secondary dressing, e.g. to secure a hydrogel dressing; and in the prevention of pressure ulcers, when it is placed over intact skin. It must be removed with care (according to the manufacturer's instructions) to prevent skin trauma. Transparent, thus allowing wound inspection.

senescence *n* normal changes of mind and body in increasing age — **senescent** *adj*.

Sengstaken-Blakemore tube an oesophageal tube that incorporates a balloon which, after being positioned in the lower oesophagus, is inflated to apply pressure to bleeding oesophageal varices. (See Figure 57).

senile *adj* relating to the involutional changes occurring during old age or senescence. ⇒ dementia — **senility** *n*.

senna *n* leaves and pods of a purgative plant. ⇒ laxatives.

sensation *n* consciousness of perceiving a state or condition of one's body or any part of it; one's senses; one's mind or its emotions.

senses *npl* the special senses; hearing, vision, smell, proprioception and tactile feeling and tasting.

sensible *n* detectable by the senses.

sensitivity *n* the ability of a test to accurately identify affected individuals, such as a screening test.

sensitivity training group in a supportive atmosphere, members learn about what occurs during their interactions with others. They can test and refine new behavioural responses in the light of feedback about previously evoked reactions; they are encouraged to enact the positively modified behaviours in circumstances other than the group.

sensitization *n* rendering sensitive. Production of an immunological state in which there is a disproportionate response to certain antigenic substances, such as in allergies. One may become sensitive to a variety of substances, which

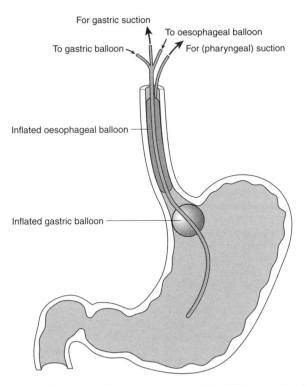

For gastric suction

To oesophageal balloon

To gastric balloon

For (pharyngeal) suction

Inflated oesophageal balloon

Inflated gastric balloon

Figure 57 Sengstaken-Blakemore tube. (Reproduced from Bruce & Finlay 1997 with permission.)

may be food (e.g. shellfish), bacteria, plants, chemical substances, drugs, sera, etc. Liability is much greater in some persons than others. ⇒ allergy. ⇒ anaphylaxis. ⇒ atopy. ⇒ hypersensitivity.

sensorineural *adj* pertaining to sensory neurons. *sensorineural deafness* or perceptive deafness; a discriminating term for nerve deafness.

sensory *adj* pertaining to sensation. *sensory cortex* the region of the cerebral cortex where sensory inputs are received. The main area is posterior to the central sulcus in the parietal lobes in both hemispheres. *sensory nerves* afferent nerves which convey impulses from the peripheral receptors to the brain and spinal cord.

sensory deprivation absence of usual sensory stimuli, e.g. for patients in intensive care units. Continued sensory deprivation may lead to mental changes, such as anxiety, depression and visual/auditory hallucinations.

sensory impairment/loss reduced function or total loss of any of the five special senses, i.e. sight, hearing, smell, taste and touch.

sensory overload a situation where patients are exposed to an excess of sensory stimuli, such as bright lights, constant noise of machines and people talking. It may occur in intensive care units.

separation anxiety a complication occurring in preschool children separated from their mothers for periods of time, such as due to hospital admission. It is characterized firstly by protest and then despair/depression, detachment and regression, such as loss of continence, clinging to parents or refusing to eat. The degree of distress is influenced by many factors, e.g. parental involvement/partnership in care, parenting styles, parent's response, the gender of the nurse etc. The features of regression and emotional instability may continue long after discharge home but gradually resolves.

sepsis *n* the state of being infected with pus-producing (pyogenic) micro-organisms — **septic** *adj*.

septic abortion ⇒ abortion.

septic arthritis joint inflammation caused by micro-organisms: bacteria, fungi and viruses. It may accompany septicaemia, follow joint trauma, injection or surgery, complicate immunosuppression and rheumatoid arthritis. Management includes treatment with appropriate antimicrobial drugs.

septic shock shock occurring as a result of infection and an overwhelming inflammatory response. ⇒ systemic inflammatory response syndrome.

septicaemia *n* the persistence and multiplication of bacteria in the bloodstream — **septicaemic** *adj*.

septoplasty *n* an operation to straighten the nasal septum, usually undertaken for septal dislocation. There is minimal removal of cartilage and repositioning of the septum in the normal midline position.

septostomy surgical procedure to form an opening in a septum, as in the heart. → Rhashkind's septostomy.

septum *n* a partition between two cavities, e.g. between the nasal cavities and between the left and right sides of the heart — **septate, septal** *adj. septal defect* congenital abnormality where an opening exists in the septum between the two atria or the two ventricles of the heart. ⇒ atrial septal defect. ⇒ ventricular septal defect. *septal haematoma* of nasal septum following surgery or trauma.

sequela *n* pathological consequences of a disease — **sequelae** *pl*.

sequestrectomy *n* excision of a sequestrum.

sequestrum *n* a piece of dead bone which separates from the healthy bone but remains within the tissues — **sequestra** *pl*.

serine *n* a nonessential (dispensable) amino acid.

SERMs *abbr* selective (o)estrogen receptor modulators.

serology *n* the branch of science dealing with the study of sera and blood — **serological** *adj*.

seropurulent *adj* containing serum and pus.

serosa *n* a serous membrane. Includes the pleura, pericardium and the peritoneum — **serosal** *adj*.

serosanguineous *adj* containing serum and blood.

serositis *n* inflammation of a serous membrane.

serotonin *n* Also known as 5-hydroxytryptamine (5-HT). A monoamine derived from the amino acid tryptophan. It is found in three main body situations: (a) the gastrointestinal tract wall, where it acts as a neurotransmitter affecting secretion and motility; (b) in platelets, which release 5-HT when tissue is damaged. This causes vasoconstriction and platelet aggregation and is part of haemostasis; (c) the central nervous system, where it acts as a central neurotransmitter. 5-HT is present in the pineal body (gland) and acts with melatonin to affect sleep–wake cycles. It is also involved in the transmission and perception of pain. Disturbances in release of 5-HT have been linked to conditions that include migraine and depression. ⇒ SSRIs.

serotyping classification of micro-organisms based on their antigenic features.

serous *adj* pertaining to serum. *serous membrane* → membrane.

serpiginous *adj* snake like, coiled, irregular; used to describe the margins of skin lesions, especially ulcers and ringworm.

Serratia *n* a genus of Gram-negative bacilli, such as *Serratia marcescens*, capable of causing infection in humans. It is an endemic hospital resident and is a cause of nosocomial pneumonia and urinary tract infection. Many strains have developed resistance to antibiotics. ⇒ infection.

serration *n* a saw-like notch — **serrated** *adj*.

serum *n* the clear fluid which remains after blood has clotted, i.e. plasma minus the coagulation factors and blood cells. *serum sickness* the allergic illness occurring 7–10 days after the injection of foreign serum for treatment or prophylaxis of infection. A rare event now that serum from other species has been replaced by the use of human immunoglobulins — **sera** *pl*.

Service and Financial Frameworks (SaFFs) the plans that quantify what will be required to achieve the health improvement targets identified for the local Health Improvement Programme (HImP).

Service Level Agreement (SLA) agreement between different departments or directorates within an organization which agree the level of service to be provided by one to another at an agreed price.

sesamoid bone *n* small foci of bone formation in the tendons of muscles. The patella is the largest example.

severe acute asthma (*syn* status asthmaticus) life-threatening attacks of asthma. It is characterized by respiratory distress, unproductive cough, central cyanosis, tachycardia, sweating, exhaustion and severe hypoxia. It is a medical emergency requiring immediate treatment with high concentration oxygen, intravenous access, systemic corticosteroids and inhaled β_2-adrenoceptor agonists, e.g. terbutaline. Where response is poor, the person may require respiratory support. ⇒ mechanical ventilation.

sex chromosomes *n* the pair of chromosomes that determine genetic sex; XY in males and XX in females.

sex education an essential part of any health education programme. It includes teaching about the male and female body so that the learner can understand expressing sexuality and recognize the onset of puberty: knowledge about personal relationships, knowledge about contraception, sexually transmitted infections, pregnancy, childbirth, bonding, parenting and family living.

sexism *n* a belief that members of one sex are superior to members of the other, and thereby have advantages over them. It leads to discrimination and can act as a limiting factor, e.g. in educational and professional development.

sex-linked *adj* refers to genes which are located on the sex chromosomes or, more especially, on the X-chromosome. To avoid confusion, it is now customary to refer to the latter genes (and the characteristics determined by them) as X-linked.

sexual abuse performing a sexual act with a child or with an adult against the person's wishes. The most common type of sexual abuse occurs between a father (or father figure) and daughter. See Box – Sexual abuse of children. ⇒ incest.

sexual counselling ⇒ counselling. ⇒ psychosexual counselling.

sexual dysfunction a lack of desire or the ability to achieve coitus in one or both partners. ⇒ dyspareunia. ⇒ erectile dysfunction. ⇒ frigidity. ⇒ impotence. ⇒ libido. ⇒ vaginismus.

sexual intercourse coitus.

sexual orientation denotes a person's sexual attraction towards people of the same sex (homosexuality), the opposite sex (heterosexuality) or both sexes (bisexuality). It may be transitory or life-long.

sexual problems ⇒ sexual dysfunction.

sexuality *n* the sum of the structural, functional and psychological attributes as they are expressed by one's gender-identity and sexual behaviour.

sexuality, expressing increasingly in a nursing context, the term is being accepted as an activity of living. It includes the many ways in which a person expresses gender to other people: by the clothes, perfume, jewellery and toilet articles used; make-up worn; behaviour; attitude to, and behaviour with, members of the opposite sex. ⇒ heterosexual. ⇒ homosexuality. ⇒ sexuality.

Sexual abuse of children

Sexual abuse involves adults seeking sexual gratification by using minors. This may be having sexual intercourse or anal intercourse, engaging the child in fondling, masturbation or oral sex, and includes encouraging them to watch sexually explicit behaviour or pornographic material. Kempe and Kempe (1984) provide the most common specific definition of sexual abuse in children: ... "*the involvement of dependent, developmentally immature children and adolescents in sexual activities they do not truly comprehend, to which they are unable to give informed consent, or that violate the taboos of family roles*".

Reference

Kempe R, Kempe C 1984 The Common Secret: Sexual abuse of children and adolescents. Freeman, New York

sexually transmitted disease (STD) ⇒ sexually transmitted infection.

sexually transmitted infection (STI) *n* the contagious conditions, including those defined legally as venereal, which are usually transmitted through sexual contact, but not exclusively so. They include: AIDS, candidiasis, chlamydial infection, genital herpes, genital warts, gonorrhoea, hepatitis, nonspecific urethritis, syphilis and trichomoniasis.

SFS *abbr* Social Functioning Scale.

shaken baby syndrome a syndrome characterized by unexplained long bone fractures and evidence of subdural haematoma. The injuries result from child abuse that involves violent shaking.

sharps *n* include used needles, razor blades, intravenous giving sets, central venous lines and cannulae. They should be put immediately into a rigid sharps' container of distinctive colour which is disposed of when three quarters full. It is sealed in such a way that used needles cannot be recovered for misuse. Arrangements have to be made for safe disposal of those used by people in their own homes, district nurses, at health centres and doctors' surgeries.

shaving *v* shaving may still be used preoperatively to remove hair from the operation site. However, scanning electron micrographs have shown that every skin shave causes epidermal damage, therefore where it is to be performed it should be done immediately prior to surgery to reduce bacterial colonization of damaged areas. It is preferable to use a disposable razor with foam rather than soap, or an electric razor with a removable head which can be disinfected. The use of depilatory creams is associated with a reduced incidence of infection

shearing force when any part of the supported body is on a gradient, the deeper tissues near the bone 'slide' towards the lower gradient while the skin remains at its point of contact with the supporting surface because of friction which is increased in the presence of moisture. The deep blood vessels are stretched and angulated, thus deeper tissues become ischaemic with consequent necrosis. ⇒ pressure ulcer.

Sheehan's syndrome *n* hypopituitarism that results from postpartum pituitary necrosis.

shelf operation an operation to deepen the acetabulum in developmental dysplasia of the hip (congenital dislocation), involving the use of a bone graft. May be performed where conservative treatment is unsuccessful.

shiatsu *n* an ancient form of Japanese health care similar in principle to acupuncture. Specific points along the surface of the body are pressed using the thumbs, fingers or palms to stimulate the body's own energy flow and to initiate the self-healing mechanisms. It is believed that an imbalance in an individual's energy may manifest in a range of physical symptoms. Shiatsu aims to restore the equilibrium in self-healing energy and so promote health and well-being.

Shigella *n* a genus of Gram-negative bacilli of the family Enterobacteriaceae. Several species cause dysentery. *Shigella boydii*, *Shigella dysenteriae* and *Shigella flexneri* cause dysentery epidemics in tropical and subtropical regions. *Shigella sonnei* causes dysentery in temperate regions and is the most common in the UK. It commonly affects young children in nurseries, and is spread by the faecal-oral route. The organism may be present in the faeces for a few weeks following an acute episode. ⇒ dysentery.

shin bone the tibia, the medial bone of the foreleg.

shingles *n* results from a reactivation of the varicella/zoster virus (VZV) that remains dormant in a sensory nerve ganglion following an earlier attack of chickenpox. It occurs in middle-aged and older people, or in individuals who are immunocompromised, such as those with cancer or AIDS. The person with shingles may infect another person with chickenpox. It is characterized by severe pain and the appearance of vesicles along the distribution of a sensory nerve (usually unilateral). Infection of the trigeminal nerve ganglion results in corneal vesicles which can lead to ulceration and corneal scarring. Early treatment with an antiviral drug, e.g. topical idoxuridine or acyclovir, can lessen the intensity of the infection. Post-herpetic neuralgia may be particularly resistant to treatment. ⇒ capsaicin. ⇒ herpes zoster. ⇒ Ramsay Hunt syndrome.

Shirodkar's operation placing of a purse-string suture around an incompetent cervix during pregnancy to prevent late miscarriage. It is usually removed around the 38th week, or before if labour commences.

shivering *n* an involuntary response occurring while the core body temperature is rising, either as a result of the release of pyrogens after injury, including surgery, or infection.

shock *n* acute circulatory disturbance leading to cell hypoxia through inappropriate or inadequate tissue perfusion. There is discrepancy between the circulating blood volume and the capacity of the vascular bed. Its features include a fall in blood pressure, rapid pulse, pallor, restlessness, thirst, oliguria and a cold clammy skin. ⇒ cardiogenic shock. ⇒ hypovolaemic shock. ⇒ neurogenic shock. ⇒ septic shock.

short bowel syndrome (SBS) *n* see Box – Short bowel syndrome.

short term memory (STM) the part of memory that deals with retention of information for a few seconds only. It can only be retained if it is rehearsed or moved to LTM. Also known as working memory. ⇒ chunking. ⇒ rehearsal in memory.

shortsightedness *n* ⇒ myopia.

shoulder joint formed by the humerus, scapula and clavicle. ⇒ frozen shoulder. *shoulder girdle* ⇒ pectoral girdle. *shoulder presentation* a variety of transverse lie which must be converted to vertex or breech presentation before vaginal delivery is possible.

'show' *n* a popular term for the slightly bloodstained mucoid vaginal discharge common at the commencement of labour. ⇒ operculum.

shunt *n* a term applied to the passage of blood through other than the usual channel. It may be congenital, due to acquired disease, or surgery, such as arteriovenous shunt.

SI *abbr* Système International d'Unités.

sialagogue *n* an agent which increases the flow of saliva.

sialogram *n* radiographic image of the salivary glands and ducts, after injection of a contrast medium — **sialographically** *adv*.

sialolith *n* a stone in a salivary gland or duct.

SIB *abbr* self-injurious behaviour.

sibling *n* one of a family of children having the same parents.

sick building syndrome a recognized condition affecting those who work in open-plan offices. The symptoms include lethargy, headache, dry itching skin and dry throat.

sick role a sociological term which signifies changes in a person's role because he or she is ill. In acute illness, the person is relieved of usual activities and responsibilities, and can accept assistance from, and perhaps dependence on, others. In exchange, the person complies with the treatment and relinquishes the sick role at an appropriate time. The concept is less useful when considering a person with chronic illness.

Short Bowel Syndrome

Short bowel syndrome (SBS)is a malabsorptive disorder which, in children, is commonly caused by congenital anomalies (jejunal and ileal atresia, gastroschisis), ischaemia (necrotizing enterocolitis) and trauma or vascular injury (volvulus).

Care centres around maintaining optimum nutrition by enteral feeding to ensure optimum growth and development while intestinal adaptation occurs. The initial phase of nutrition is via total parenteral nutrition (TPN) which helps to stimulate the adaptation response of the small intestine. In children, SBS results in a compensatory increase in the mucosal surface area, mostly by villus hyperplasia, and a small increase in the length and diameter of the small intestine. These changes enable a gradual increase in the absorption of nutrients.

Nursing care centres around the administration and maintenance of enteral feeding and the prevention of complications associated with long term TPN (infection and peritonitis, electrolyte/glucose disturbances, liver dysfunction as well as technical complications with the central venous catheter).

Further reading
Moules C, Ramsay J 1998 The textbook of children's nursing (p332–7). Stanley Thornes, London

sickle-cell disease an inherited haemoglobinopathy which is due to an abnormal haemoglobin (HbS). Seen in individuals from areas where falciparum malaria is endemic (equatorial Africa, part of India and part of the Eastern Mediterranean) and their descendants in Europe, West Indies and the USA. The red cells become sickle-shaped, in hypoxia, dehydration or infection, which leads to reduced oxygen-carrying capacity, blood vessel blockage with pain and infarction and a chronic haemolytic anaemia as the abnormal red cells are destroyed in the spleen. When a sickle-cell crisis occurs, the person requires urgent rehydration and pain relief. At risk populations should be screened for the abnormal HbS. ⇒ anaemia. ⇒ malaria.→ thalassaemia.

sickness certificate in the UK, when a person is ill and unable to go to work, a self-certification form is completed and forwarded to the employer. Absence from the 5th day onwards is notified by a doctor's signature on a sickness certificate, and, if necessary, thereafter at a time interval as determined by the doctor on the certificate.

side-effect any physiological change other than the desired one from drug administration, e.g. the antispasmodic drug propantheline causes the side-effect of dry mouth in some patients. The term also covers undesirable drug reactions. Some are predictable, being the result of a known metabolic action of the drug, e.g. hyperglycaemia with corticosteroids, loss of hair with cyclophosphamide. Unpredictable reactions can be: (a) immediate: anaphylactic shock, angio-oedema (angioneurotic oedema); (b) erythematous: all forms of erythema, including nodosum and multiforme and purpuric rashes; (c) cellular eczematous rashes and contact dermatitis; (d) specific, e.g. light-sensitive eruptions with ledermycin and griseofulvin. ⇒ adverse drug reactions. ⇒ yellow card reporting.

sideroblastic anaemias npl rare anaemias caused by an inherited or acquired abnormality of iron metabolism.

sideropenic dysphagia ⇒ Plummer-Vinson syndrome.

siderosis n excess of iron in the blood or tissues. Inhalation of iron oxide into the lungs can cause one form of pneumoconiosis.

SIDS abbr sudden infant death syndrome.

sievert (Sv) the SI unit (International System of Units) for radiation dose equivalent, it replaces the rem.

sigmoid adj shaped like the letter S, such as the sigmoid colon. *sigmoid sinus* venous channel draining blood from the brain. ⇒ flexure.

sigmoidoscope n an endoscope for visualizing the rectum and sigmoid colon. Both flexible fibreoptic types and rigid metal types are in use. ⇒ endoscope — **sigmoidoscopy** n.

sigmoidostomy n opening in the sigmoid colon.

sign n any objective evidence of disease that can be seen or elicited. ⇒ vital signs.

sign language a form of nonverbal language using the hands and upper body to make signs, whereby deaf people can communicate with each other and with family members and friends. When a profoundly deaf person who uses sign language is admitted to hospital, special arrangements need to be made so that a person skilled in using sign language is present most of the time. ⇒ British sign language. ⇒ finger spelling. ⇒ Makaton.

significant other a term used to designate the person that the patient or client wants the nursing staff to consult when relevant, for instance when making arrangements for transfer or discharge, or to be notified in the case of emergency.

silicone n an organic compound which is water-repellant. Used as sheets (gels or contact layer) in dressings that fit exactly the contours of a granulating wound in which it encourages healing, on newly healed wounds to minimize scarring, and on fragile wounds or those with large amounts of exudate (with an absorbent dressing). Silicone implants may be used in breast reconstruction following mastectomy or in breast augmentation.

silicosis n a form of pneumoconiosis or 'industrial dust disease' found in metal grinders, stone-workers, etc. Results in fibrotic lung disease.

silver nitrate in the form of small sticks, is used as a caustic for warts.

silver sulfadiazine (sulphadiazine) silver derivative of sulfadiazine (sulphadiazine). Topical bacteriostatic agent, used to control bacterial infection in burns patients.

Sim's position an exaggerated left lateral position with the right knee well flexed and the left arm drawn back over the edge of the bed. Used for demonstration of vaginal prolapse and stress incontinence. ⇒ speculum.

Sim's speculum *n* ⇒ speculum.

SIMV *abbr* synchronized intermittent mandatory ventilation.

sinew *n* a ligament or tendon.

sinoatrial node the pacemaker of the heart. An area of specialized autorhythmic cells situated at the opening of the superior vena cava into the right atrium. They regulate the cardiac impulse and the muscular contraction which then spreads over the heart. ⇒ atrioventricular bundle. ⇒ atrioventricular node.

sinus *n* **1.** a hollow or cavity. Especially the paranasal (air) sinuses, the air-filled cavities, frontal, maxillary, ethmoidal and sphenoidal, that give the voice resonance and lighten the skull. **2.** a channel containing blood, especially venous blood, such as those in the brain (cavernous, straight, sigmoid, transverse and sagittal sinuses), or the heart. ⇒ cavernous sinuses. ⇒ coronary sinus. **3.** a recess or cavity within a bone. **4.** any suppurating tract or channel leading from an abscess or internal structure to an external opening. ⇒ pilonidal sinus. *sinus arrhythmia* an increase of the pulse rate on inspiration, decrease on expiration. *sinus rhythm* the normal heart rhythm. ⇒ carotid sinus. ⇒ electrocardiogram. ⇒ PQRST complex.

sinusitis *n* inflammation of a sinus, especially infection affecting the mucosal lining of the paranasal sinuses. It may be acute or chronic and may follow an upper respiratory tract infection or a dental infection. There is rhinorrhoea or postnasal drip with localized headache and facial pain, nasal obstruction, hyposmia and pyrexia. It may be complicated by orbital cellulitis or intracerebral abscess and venous sinus thrombosis. Management includes: analgesia, antibiotics, steam inhalations and decongestants. Where these measures fail, it may be necessary to wash out the maxillary sinus or undertake surgery to improve the drainage. ⇒ antrostomy. ⇒ functional endoscopic sinus surgery.

sinusoid *n* a dilated channel into which arterioles or veins open in some organs and which take the place of the usual capillaries, such as in the spleen and liver.

SIRS *n* systemic inflammatory response syndrome.

sitz-bath *n* a hip bath.

Sjögren syndrome an autoimmune condition of unknown cause. It is characterized by keratoconjunctivitis and xerostomia with reduced secretions from lacrimal and salivary glands associated with connective tissue disease such as rheumatoid arthritis. Usually affects older women.

Sjögren-Larsson syndrome a genetic condition inherited as an autosomal recessive trait. It is characterized by congenital ectodermosis, learning disability and spasticity.

skeletomuscular *adj* pertaining to the skeletal and muscular systems. ⇒ musculoskeletal.

skeleton *n* the bony framework of the body, supporting and protecting the soft tissues and organs and providing an attachment for muscles. Adults have 206 bones. *appendicular skeleton* pectoral girdle, upper limbs, pelvic girdle and lower limbs. *axial skeleton* skull, spine, sternum, ribs and hyoid bone — **skeletal** *adj* pertaining to the skeleton. ⇒ traction

Skene's glands two small glands situated in the vestibule; they open into the female urethral meatus. Also known as the lesser vestibular glands. ⇒ Bartholin's glands. ⇒ vestibule.

skewed distribution *n* in statistics. Any distribution of scores where there are more values on one side of the mean than the other, i.e. not symmetrical. ⇒ normal distribution curve.

skill *n* a specific or a complex of abilities required to carry out a particular task, which may be of a cognitive, affective or psychomotor nature, or a mix of these. *skill analysis* identification of the components needed for its execution.

skill mix the level, range and variety of skills of the staff in a department, unit, team or ward which is required to meet the outcomes of the organization. Agreement is reached as to the skill mix required in each clinical area.

skin *n* the outer covering of the body consisting of the epidermis (outer), dermis and the appendages: nail, hairs and glands. Its functions include: sensory, protective, storage, excretory, temperature regulation, absorption and synthesis. *skin fold thickness* an anthropometric measurement used, with others, to assess nutritional status. *skin patch* the topical application of a drug-impregnated adhesive patch. The drug, e.g. oestrogen, is absorbed gradually so that its blood level is maintained throughout each 24 h. A method of drug administration that avoids the 'first pass' metabolism in the liver associated with oral drugs. *skin shedding* skin is continually shedding its outer keratinized cells as scales. As the skin has a natural bacterial flora, the scales are a potential source of infection for susceptible patients. *skin traction* ⇒ traction. ⇒ psoriasis.

skull *n* the bony framework of the head; the bones of the cranium and face.

SLA *abbr* Service Level Agreement.

SLE *abbr* systemic lupus erythematosus.

sleep *n* periods where the body and mind are at rest. There is an alteration in consciousness (which is easily reversed), suspension of volition and reduced activity. Typically, sleep consists of alternating cycles of non-rapid eye movement sleep (NREM) or orthodox sleep, which has four stages, and rapid eye movement sleep (REM) or paradoxical sleep, *sleep apnoea* ⇒ apnoea. *sleep deprivation* a cumulative condition arising when there is interference with a person's established rhythm of REM sleep. It leads to sleep deficit. It can result in slurred rambling speech, irritability, disorientation, poor concentration, slowed reaction time, malaise, progressing to illusions, delusions, paranoia and hyperactivity. *sleep terrors* sudden wakening in a state of extreme fear, disorientation and agitation. *sleep walking* ⇒ somnambulism. (See Figure 58).

sleeping pills a general term which includes sedatives, hypnotics, narcotics.

sleeping sickness a disease endemic in Africa, characterized by increasing sleepiness (somnolence) caused by infection of the brain by trypanosomes. ⇒ trypanosomiasis.

sleeplessness *n* some people take a long time, 30–90 minutes, to get off to sleep; others have one or more wakeful periods

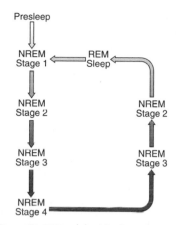

Figure 50 Sleep cycle in adults. (Reproduced from Heath 1995 with permission.)

during the night, and yet others experience early morning wakening. Detailed assessment data will reveal a patient's or client's individual sleeping habits.

sleepwalking ⇒ somnambulism.

sliding board *n* a device used to move patients as part of safe-handling or no lifting policies.

sliding filament hypothesis *n* an explanation of muscle contraction that proposes that the filaments slide against each other to produce shortening.

slipped disc *n* prolapsed intervertebral disc. ⇒ prolapse.

slipped epiphysis displacement of an epiphysis, especially the upper femoral one.

slough *n* tissue which becomes necrosed and eventually separates from the healthy tissue.

slow release (SR) drugs sustained release. Drug formulations which do not dissolve in the stomach but in the small intestine where the drug is slowly released and absorbed. Many drugs, e.g. hormones, are now incorporated into a skin patch, which, after application, permits slow release.

slow virus *n* an infective agent known as a prion which only produces infection after a long latent period, and many cases may never develop overt symptoms but may still be a link in the chain of infectivity. ⇒ bovine spongiform encephalopathy. ⇒ Creutzfeldt-Jakob disease.

SLT *abbr* speech and language therapy.

small-for-dates ⇒ low birthweight.

smallpox *n* (*syn* variola) serious viral disease; eradicated following a world-wide programme of disease control by the World Health Organization (WHO). Prophylaxis against the disease is by vaccination. ⇒ vaccinia.

small stomach syndrome a complication of gastric surgery. Feelings of fullness and discomfort after meals restricts intake and may contribute to malnutrition.

SMBR *n* standardized morbidity ratio.

smear *n* a film of material spread out on a glass slide for microscopic examination. *cervical smear* microscopic examination of cells scraped from the cervix to detect carcinoma-in-situ. ⇒ cervical intraepithelial neoplasia (CIN). ⇒ colposcope. ⇒ exfoliative cytology. ⇒ Papanicolaou test.

smegma *n* the sebaceous secretion which accumulates beneath the prepuce of the glans penis and clitoris. It should be removed by uncircumcized males retracting the prepuce before washing the penis.

Smith-Petersen nail a trifid, cannulated metal nail used to provide internal fixation for intracapsular fractures of the femoral neck.

smokers' blindness (*syn* tobacco amblyopia) ⇒ amblyopia.

smoking, passive *v* involuntary inhalation of smoke from tobacco products by non-smokers. Associated with an increased incidence of smoking-related diseases, such as lung cancer, coronary heart disease, hypertension, chronic obstructive pulmonary disease (bronchitis and emphysema); may also trigger an asthma attack. Environmental tobacco smoke is a hazard at work and considerable health promotion effort is used to reduce occupational risk by encouraging employers to support smoking cessation programmes and to have no smoking policies. Certain occupations are a particular health hazard where employees are exposed to persistently high levels of smoke, e.g. bar, club and restaurant staff. Children are particularly vulnerable and have little choice over their exposure to tobacco smoke. ⇒ sudden infant death syndrome.

SMR *n* standardized mortality ratio.

SNAP *acr* Schizophrenia Nursing Assessment Protocol.

snare *n* a surgical instrument with a wire loop at the end; used for removal of polypi.

Snellen's test types a chart of different sized letters used for testing visual acuity. The letters are arranged in lines that can be read by a normal (emmetropic) eye at 60, 36, 24, 18, 12, 9, 6 and 5 metres. Acuity is checked in each eye separately and expressed as 6 over the smallest line of letters that can be read, e.g. a person able to read the 6 metre line at 6 metres is said to have a visual acuity of 6/6. Special E test-type charts (different orientations of the letter E) are used to test children and others unable to read the letters.

snoring *n* flaccid muscles in the upper respiratory tract are thought to be responsible for turbulent airflow and hence snoring. Loud snoring may be associated with upper airway closure (sleep apnoea), resulting in repetitive awakenings and severe sleep disturbance.

snow *n* solid carbon dioxide. Used for local freezing of the tissues in minor surgery. ⇒ cryosurgery.

snuffles *n* a snorting inspiration due to congestion of nasal mucous membrane. It is a sign of early congenital (prenatal) syphilis when the nasal discharge may be purulent or blood-stained.

social class the classification of people into social groups. Currently in the UK, the Office of Population Censuses and Surveys uses a five category socioeconomic classification based on the occupation of the householder: I – professional, e.g. lawyer; II – intermediate, e.g. nurse; III – skilled, (nonmanual), e.g. secretary and (manual), e.g. carpenter; IV – semi-skilled, e.g. agricultual worker; V – unskilled, e.g. cleaner. Other classifications are also in use.

social cognition mental processes involved in the manner that individuals perceive and react to social situations.

social construction describes the influence of social processes on instinctive behaviours.

social deprivation measurement a way of measuring deprivation by the use of a scale or index. National census data regarding occupation can be used to link morbidity and mortality to social class, but much more sensitive scales are needed to assess levels of deprivation in an area. Various indices exist, Jarman index, Townsend index etc, but these have limitations such as excluding people aged 65 years and over, and some may be more appropriate for use in urban areas rather than sparsely populated rural locations.

social exclusion refers to the multiple deprivation experienced by certain population groups who can become socially isolated in their neighbourhood and unable to participate in mainstream activities such as work or education. Refugees, rough sleepers, teenage mothers and many young people can be socially excluded.

social exclusion unit government unit set up to study and report on social exclusion and measures aimed at reducing the problem, such as new ways of decreasing the number of teenage pregnancies.

social functioning describes the everyday activities and abilities that enable social interaction, interpersonal relationships and independent living. Social functioning ability may be severely affected by mental health problems, such as depression and schizophrenia. ⇒ Social Functioning Scale.

Social Functioning Scale (SFS) used to assess aspects of day-to-day social functioning which are adversely affected by clients' mental health difficulties. It covers seven main areas of social functioning, e.g. social engagement, interpersonal behaviour, independence in living skills (competence and performance). The scale can provide a guide to goals and interventions, as well as measure progress and outcome.

social groups groupings of individuals who engage in interaction at various levels, e.g. tribes, clans, nations etc.

social isolation a term which can be applied to one person, a family or a group of people. Those 'isolated' do not interact with other human beings in the usual pattern for any one of a number of reasons, that may include poor health, poverty, rural isolation etc.

social justice ⇒ justice. ⇒ social exclusion.

social mobility describes the movement of individuals between social classes.

social norms *npl* socially acceptable forms of behaviour. Norms may forbid certain types of behaviour and prescribe others. ⇒ anomie.

social stratification describes the process of dividing populations into unequal strata using various characteristics that include: age, influence, religion, status, income, wealth, ethnicity, gender etc.

socialization in sociology, it describes the processes by which people learn the social norms and the value of adhering to them. Socialization occurs informally in the family and with friends, and more formally at school and in the workplace.

socially clean a term used when articles require to be scrupulously clean, a condition achieved without using disinfectants. To prevent nosocomial infection, it must characterize all articles which patients use, including baths, bath mats, showers, sieved water outlets, sinks and washbowls. ⇒ asepsis. ⇒ disinfection. ⇒ sterilization.

sociocultural *adj* pertaining to culture in its sociological setting.

sociology *n* the scientific study of interpersonal and intergroup social relationships within society or the social system — **sociological** *adj*.

sociomedical *adj* pertaining to sociology and medicine. Social factors that can precipitate or predispose to medical conditions, for example homelessness and poor housing may cause bronchitis, tuberculosis, hypothermia, etc.

sodium (Na) *n* a metallic element. It is a major extracellular cation concerned with the integrity of fluid compartments and neuromuscular function. *sodium bicarbonate (hydrogen carbonate)* important buffer in the blood. Used intravenously to correct metabolic acidosis, *sodium chloride* used extensively in intravenous fluids to replace fluids and correct electrolytes. *sodium citrate* used as an in vitro anticoagulant, such as for stored blood. *sodium hypochlorite* a powerful disinfectant used, in suitable dilutions, in many situations, e.g. dealing with environmental contamination with blood or body fluids. *sodium pump* an active transport mechanism, requiring ATP, whereby sodium ions are pumped through selectively permeable membranes.

soft sore the primary ulcer of the genitalia occurring in the venereal disease chancroid.

soft tissue mobilization (mobilisation) See Box – Soft tissue mobilization (mobilisation).

soft tissue rheumatism ⇒ fibromyalgia. ⇒ fibrositis. ⇒ rheumatism.

software a general term describing computer data and programs. ⇒ program.

solar plexus a large network of sympathetic (autonomic) nerves and ganglia in the upper abdomen that supplies the abdominal organs.

soleus muscle in the calf.

solute *n* that which is dissolved in a solvent.

solution *n* a fluid (solvent) which contains a dissolved substance or substances (solute). *saturated solution* one in which the maximum possible quantity of a particular substance is dissolved, and further additions of the substance remain undissolved.

solvent *n* an agent which is capable of dissolving other substances (solutes). The component of a solution which is present in excess. *solvent abuse* previously called glue sniffing. Popular practice amongst some groups of adolescents. The practice of inhaling volatile substances, such as those present in some adhesives, solvents and fuels, to produce euphoria and intoxication. Signs include lingering smell on clothes and hair, changed behaviour, and redness and blistering around the nose and mouth. It results in addiction, damage to the nasal mucosa and organ damage, e.g. the brain. Death may occur from asphyxia or toxicity. ⇒ drug misuse.

somatic *adj* pertaining to the body. *somatic cells* body cells, as distinct from the gametes or germ cells. *somatic nerves* nerves controlling the activity of striated, skeletal muscle.

somatoagnosia ⇒ agnosia.

somatostatin *n* also known as growth hormone inhibiting hormone (GHIH). A hormone released by the hypothalamus, pancreas and the intestinal cells. Apart from inhibiting the release of growth hormone, it also inhibits the release of insulin, glucagon, pancreatic digestive enzymes and influences gastric secretion, motility and emptying.

somatotropin *n* ⇒ growth hormone.

somnambulism *n* (*syn* sleepwalking) a state of dissociated consciousness in which sleeping and waking states are combined. Considered normal in children but as an illness in adults.

somnolence *n* sleepiness, drowsiness.

Somogyi phenomenon rebound hyperglycaemia followng hypoglycaemia; seen in people with insulin dependent diabetes mellitus. ⇒ dawn phenomenon.

Sonicaid *n* proprietary name for diagnostic ultrasound machine used to detect movement inside the body.

Sonne dysentery bacillary dysentery caused by infection with *Shigella sonnei* (Sonne bacillus), the commonest form of dysentery in the United Kingdom. The organism is excreted by cases and carriers (not long-term) in their faeces, and contaminates hands, food and water, from which new hosts are infected. It causes mild diarrhoea. Outbreaks have occurred in nursery schools and other situations where there is poor hand hygiene after defaecation. ⇒ dysentery.

sonograph *n* graphic record of sound waves. ⇒ ultrasonography.

sonography *n* the process by which a sonograph is recorded and interpreted; considered safer than X-rays for use during pregnancy.

Soft tissue mobilization (mobilisation)
Massage is an art that has been practised since someone first rubbed something better. Slow, gentle stroking is a soothing form that is almost instinctive. Other techniques are used for specific purposes and, although it was referred to as 'medical rubbing' at the beginning of the 20th century, skillful therapeutic massage requires many hours of practice under the guidance of a competent teacher. Physiotherapists and sports therapists use pétrissage or kneading techniques with the whole hand or the finger pads to stretch retracted muscles and tendons, relieve spasm and assist removal of waste products from muscles. Kneading with the finger pads is also used in some natural childbirth methods. Physiotherapists employ percussive manipulations, collectively called tapôtement, to dislodge viscid fluids in the lungs and assist expectoration. Masseurs may also learn the techniques of special methods such as connective tissue manipulation and Chinese massage.

Further reading
Holey E A, Cook E M (1997) Therapeutic massage.
    W B Saunders, London

soporific *adj, n* (describes) an agent which induces profound sleep.

sorbitol a sweet-tasting substance made from sugars. Used as a food sweetener.

sordes *npl* dried, brown crusts which form in the mouth, especially on the lips and teeth, in situations where normal oral hygiene mechanisms are impaired, such as with dehydration and pyrexia. ⇒ mouth care.

souffle *n* puffing or soft blowing sound. *funic souffle* auscultatory murmur of pregnancy. Synchronizes with the fetal heartbeat and is caused by pressure on the umbilical cord. *uterine souffle* soft, blowing murmur which can be auscultated over the uterus after the fourth month of pregnancy.

sound *n* an instrument to be introduced into a hollow organ or duct to detect a stone or to dilate a stricture.

source isolation is for patients who are sources of micro-organisms which may spread from them to infect others. *strict source isolation* is for highly transmissible and dangerous diseases. *standard source isolation* is for other communicable disease.

soya bean a legume containing high levels of protein and nonstarch polysaccharides. Soya products include flour which is used extensively in processed foods. Soya protein is used to produce a milk substitute for individuals who have a food sensitivity to cow's milk or for people who exclude milk from their diet, e.g. vegans and some vegetarians. ⇒ genetically modified food.

spansules *n* a chemically prepared formulation for drugs designed to obtain controlled release via oral route.

spasm *n* 1. sudden convulsive, involuntary movement. 2. sudden muscle contraction, the effects of which depend upon the structures involved. ⇒ bronchospasm. ⇒ carpopedal spasm. ⇒ coronary arteries.

spasmodic dysmenorrhoea ⇒ dysmenorrhoea.

spasmolytic *adj, n* current term for antispasmodic drugs — **spasmolysis** *n*.

spastic *adj* 1. pertaining to spasm. 2. in a state of muscular rigidity or spasm, e.g. spastic diplegia (Little's disease). *spastic colon* old term for irritable bowel syndrome. *spastic dystonic syndrome* abnormality of gait and foot posture, usually due to brain damage at birth. Difficult to treat because imbalance in various opposing muscles has developed over a long period. *spastic gait* ⇒ gait. *spastic paralysis* results mainly from upper motor neuron lesions. There are exaggerated tendon reflexes.

spasticity *n* condition of rigidity or spasm of muscle.

spatial appreciation the ability to perceive the space relationships of things in the environment, one to the other, and to one's body. Defects can cause a person to, for instance, put a glass down before it is safely over the table, consequently it lands on the floor.

spatula *n* a flat, flexible knife with blunt edges for spreading ointment. *tongue spatula* a rigid, blade-shaped instrument for depressing the tongue.

special care baby unit (SCBU) a unit that provides specialist care for preterm, sick and small-for-dates babies. It is staffed by health professionals with the necessary qualifications, skills and experience. It does not offer facilities for neonates requiring very specialized intensive care. ⇒ neonatal intensive care unit.

special needs a phrase usually applied to the particular (educational) needs of a child or adult with a learning disability. It can also apply to individuals who do not have a learning disability, e.g. the special educational needs of a child who is particularly gifted. ⇒ statement of special educational needs.

specialist community practitioner a nurse with a specialist qualification (advanced diploma or degree) in primary or community health care. They include: community children's nurse, community learning disability nurse, community psychiatric (mental health) nurse, district nurse, health visitor (public health nurse), practice nurse and school nurse.

specialist nursing practice a new level of nursing practice agreed by the UKCC as part of its framework for postregistration education and practice (PREP). The specialist practitioner is a nurse who demonstrates higher levels of clinical decision-making and who is involved in monitoring and developing nursing practice programmes of study leading to a specialist practice. Qualifications are at degree level. ⇒ higher level practice (advanced). ⇒ clinical nurse specialist.

species *n* a systematic category, subdivision of genus. Natural groups of organisms actually or potentially interbreeding but biologically different so that they are reproductively isolated from one another. The individuals within a species group have common characteristics and generally differ fairly clearly from those of a related species.

specific *adj* special; characteristic; peculiar to. *specific disease* one that is always caused by a specified organism. *specific gravity* the density of a fluid compared with that of an equal volume of pure water, the latter being represented by 1000. It depends on the quantity of solids dissolved in the fluid.

specificity the ability of a test to accurately identify nonaffected individuals, such as a screening test.

specimens *npl* substances which are sent to the laboratory for analysis of contents or for culture to discover the infecting micro-organisms. They include blood, cerebrospinal fluid, faeces, pus, urine, sputum, swabs from nose, mouth, throat, eye, wound and vagina. ⇒ biopsy.

SPECT *abbr* single photon emission computed tomography.

spectrin *n* a protein in the red blood cell membrane that controls and stabilizes cell shape. This allows the red cell to disort to negotiate capillaries.

spectrometer *n* an instrument used to measure wavelengths of light and other electromagnetic waves. ⇒ spectrophotometer. ⇒ spectroscope — **spectrometry** *n* measuring the wavelengths of light and other electromagnetic waves using a spectrometer. ⇒ spectrophotometry.

spectrophotometer *n* a spectroscope combined with a photometer for quantitatively measuring the relative intensity of different parts of a light spectrum.

spectrophotometry analytical technique that uses a spectrophotometer to determine the amount of a substance present by measuring the light absorbed by its molecules.

spectroscope *n* an instrument for observing spectra of light.

spectroscopy analytical technique that detects and measures substances by examination of their individual absorption spectra.

spectrum *n* **1.** a range of increasing or decreasing features or activity such as the types of electromagnetic waves arranged by wavelength or frequency. **2.** the activity range of an antimicrobial agent, e.g. broad spectrum drugs are effective against several micro-organisms.

speculum *n* an instrument used to hold the walls of a cavity apart, so that the interior of the cavity can be examined. Also used to facilitate treatments. *nasal speculum* used for examination of the nose. Also allows visualization for treatments, such as nasal cautery and packing. *vaginal speculum* used to examine the vagina and cervix, for taking swabs and smears and for some treatments. Commonly used types include: Cuscoe's bivalve and Sim's (used in Sim's position) — **specula** *pl.*

speech and language therapist the professionals responsible for the assessment, diagnosis and treatment of speech and language disorders in children and adults. Known as speech pathologists in the USA and Australia.

speech and language therapy (SLT) one of the professions allied to medicine. The therapy provided by a speech and language therapist to clients with communication impairment, such as stammering, aphasia, dysarthria, and also disorders of swallowing (dysphagia). See Box – Speech and Language Therapy.

speech mechanism involves the processes of breathing, phonation, articulation, resonance and rhythm. It is disturbed in various combinations in dysarthria and aphasia.

speech pathology includes such conditions as stammering, stuttering, slurring, explosive and staccato speech. Aphasia, dysarthria and dysphasia may be part of the disorder, such as stroke or head injury, for which the affected person is in the care of the health service.

sperm *n* an abbreviated form of the word spermatozoon or spermatozoa. *sperm bank* storage of semen at very low temperatures prior to its use in artificial insemination. Semen can be stored in this way before treatments, such as chemotherapy, which damage spermatogenesis. *sperm count* a test for male infertility. Where semen is examined for volume, chemical composition and sperm numbers, morphology and motility.

Usually the volume of semen produced at each ejaculation is 2–6 millilitres containing 50–150 million sperm per millilitre.

spermatic *adj* pertaining to or conveying semen. *spermatic cord* suspends the testis in the scrotum and contains the spermatic artery and vein and the vas deferens.

spermatocele *n* cystic swelling of the epididymis or rete testis containing spermatozoa.

spermatogenesis *n* the formation and development of spermatozoa within the testes — **spermatogenetic** *adj*.

spermatorrhoea *n* involuntary discharge of semen without orgasm.

spermatozoon *n* a mature, male germ cell or gamete. It consists of a head containing the genetic material, a midpiece containing many mitochondria and a tail for motility. ⇒ acrosome. ⇒ flagellum. ⇒ spermatogenesis — **spermatozoa** *pl*.

spermicide, spermatocide *n* an agent that kills spermatozoa, e.g. nonoxinol in foams, creams and pessaries, used in conjunction with other contraceptive methods — **spermicidal** *adj*.

sphenoid *n* a wedge-shaped bone at the base of the skull containing a cavity, the sphenoidal sinus — **sphenoidal** *adj*.

spherocyte *n* an abnormal red blood cell that is spherical rather than the normal biconcave disc — **spherocytic** *adj*.

spherocytosis *n* the presence in the blood of spherocytes. It may be hereditary, inherited as an autosomal dominant disorder, or a feature of some haemolytic anaemias. The inherited type is caused by a deficiency of spectrin, a red cell membrane protein. There is increased haemolysis of the abnormal red cells by the spleen, resulting in anaemia, jaundice and splenomegaly.

sphincter *n* a circular muscle, contraction of which serves to close an orifice; may be under voluntary or involuntary control, such as the anal sphincter. *sphincter of Oddi* muscular sphincter around the opening of the common bile duct into the duodenum.

sphincterotomy *n* surgical division of a muscular sphincter.

sphingolipid *n* sphingosine and a lipid. A component of biological membranes, especially in the brain and other nervous tissue.

sphingomyelin *n* a phospholipid formed from sphingosine found as a component of biological membranes. It is primarily found in the nervous system and in blood lipids.

sphingomyelinase *n* an essential enzyme in lipid metabolism and storage.

sphingosine *n* an amino alcohol with an unsaturated hydrocarbon chain. A constituent of sphingolipids and sphingomyelin.

Speech and language therapy

Speech and language therapy (SLT) aims to assist the millions of individuals with difficulties in communication (one per cent of the normal population). Both children and adults may have difficulties with communication. They may be dysfluent (stammer), have a hearing impairment, have language difficulties including problems with vocabulary and grammar and the social use of language, they may have problems producing the correct sounds for speech so that they are difficult to understand, or have difficulties with their voice. Speech and language therapists (SLTs) also work with people who have dysphagia (difficulties swallowing).

SLT includes assessment and treatment of these difficulties. Therapy with adults is usually carried out within an NHS setting, including hospitals and nursing homes, and although children may be seen in health centres there is an increase in the number of SLT services being offered in educational settings, including mainstream schools. SLT aims to achieve the best level of communication possible for the individual concerned. As well as working with individual patients, SLTs may work with small groups of patients, or may set up programmes for other staff such as nurses to carry out. SLTs can provide other members of the multidisciplinary team with advice on how to achieve optimum communication with a person who has difficulty in communicating. SLTs also provide alternative and augmentative communication systems for individuals who require these systems.

Further reading
Wright JA, Kersner M 1998 Supporting children with communication problems: Sharing the workload. David Fulton Publishers, London

sphygmocardiograph *n* an apparatus for simultaneous graphic recording of the radial pulse and heartbeats — **sphygmocardiographically** *adv.*

sphygmograph *n* an apparatus attached to the wrist, over the radial artery, which records the movements of the pulse beat — **sphygmographic** *adj.*

sphygmomanometer *n* an instrument used for the noninvasive measurement of arterial blood pressure.

spica *n* 1. a bandage applied in a figure-of-eight pattern. 2. the application of a plaster cast to hold a joint at the required angle and position, e.g. hip, shoulder or thumb. *double hip spica* enclosure of both lower limbs and lower trunk in a plaster cast. The toes are exposed for observation of complications such as swelling, blanching, cyanosis, inability to move them, lack of sensation in them. *shoulder spica* enclosure of an upper limb and upper trunk in a plaster cast. Digits observed as for double hip spica. *single spica* enclosure of one lower limb and the lower trunk in a plaster cast. See *double hip spica* re observation of digits.

spicule *n* a small, spike-like fragment, especially of bone.

spider telangiectasia a branched pattern of dilated capillaries arising from a central arteriole, resembling a spider's web. A feature of liver cirrhosis.

spigot *n* a peg (usually plastic), used to close a tube.

spina bifida a congenital neural tube defect in which there is incomplete closure of the neural canal, usually in the lumbosacral region. It is associated with a deficiency of folates in the diet and all women of child bearing age are encouraged to have sufficient amounts; this is especially important around the time of conception and during early pregnancy, when they should supplement their intake. The condition can be detected during pregnancy by testing for increased concentration of alpha-fetoprotein in the amniotic fluid or maternal blood, or by ultrasonography. Spina bifida varies in severity and may be associated with meningocele or meningomyelocele. *spina bifida occulta* the defect does not affect the spinal cord or meninges. It is often marked externally by pigmentation, a haemangioma, a tuft of hair or a lipoma which may extend into the spinal canal.

spinal *adj* pertaining to the spine. *spinal anaesthetic* ⇒ anaesthetic. *spinal canal* canal formed by the vertebrae, contains the spinal cord. Also known as the vertebral canal. *spinal caries* disease of the vertebral bones. *spinal column* ⇒ vertebral column. *spinal cord* that part of the central nervous system within the spinal canal. It extends from the medulla oblongata down the spinal canal to the level of the first or second lumbar vertebra in adults. In young children the cord may extend to the third lumbar vertebra. *spinal curves* the normal curves are two primary, thoracic and sacral, and two secondary curves, the cervical and lumbar. ⇒ kyphosis. ⇒ lordosis. ⇒ scoliosis. *spinal nerves* 31 pairs of mixed nerves that leave the spinal cord and pass out of the spinal canal to form the peripheral nerves of the neck, trunk and limbs.

spinal cord compression (SCC) pressure on the spinal cord caused by tumour which, in most cases, is metastatic tumour from breast, lung or gastrointestinal cancers. Most cases present with pain, and prompt diagnosis is vital to prevent permanent paralysis. Treatment is with corticosteroids and radiotherapy.

spindle structure formed during mitosis and meiosis. ⇒ centriole. ⇒ centromeres.

spine *n* 1. a popular term for the bony spinal or vertebral column. 2. a sharp process of bone — **spinous, spinal** *adj.*

spinhaler *n* a sophisticated nebulizer (atomizer) which delivers a preset dose of the contained drug.

spinnbarkeit the slippery, elastic cervical mucus which can be drawn out on a glass slide. It is associated with ovulation and can be used to determine peak fertility. ⇒ natural family planning.

spinocerebellar pertaining to the spinal cord and cerebellum such as the sensory tracts that carry proprioceptor and touch impulses to the cerebellum.

Spirillum *n* a genus of small spiral bacteria. Common in water and organic matter. *Spirillum minus* is found in rodents and may infect humans, in whom it causes one form of rat bite fever — **spirillary** *adj.*

spiritual beliefs a person may choose a system of beliefs ascribed by a particular religion; may be a modified version of these, arrived at after questioning, thinking and reasoning. Some people, after going through this process, develop strong nonreligious beliefs to guide their concept of right and wrong, and to find meaning in human life on earth. ⇒ secular beliefs.

spiritual distress when a person's spiritual beliefs are derived from a particular religion, which transmits relevant practices in some of the everyday living activities, e.g. the way in which food is prepared, the type of food eaten, periods of fasting, attending public worship, praying, handwashing, perineal toilet and the type of clothes, it is natural that they will be distressed when these religion based activities are not carried out, e.g. in hospital. These are points to have in mind when assessing patients' religious/spiritual concepts.

spirochaetaemia *n* spirochaetes in the bloodstream. This kind of bacteraemia occurs in the secondary stage of syphilis — **spirochaetaemic** *adj*.

spirochaete *n* an order of tiny spiral bacteria that includes the genera Borrelia, Leptospira and Treponema. *Treponema pallidum*, which causes syphilis, is an example — **spirochaetal** *adj*.

spirograph *n* an apparatus that records respiratory movements — **spirographically** *adv*.

spirometer *n* instrument for measuring the amount of air moved in and out of the lungs, from which various lung capacities and changes in volumes can be calculated. Used as part of respiratory (pulmonary) function assessment. ⇒ respiratory function tests — **spirometry** *n*.

Spitz-Holter valve a regulatory valve used as part of a drainage system designed to treat hydrocephalus by draining cerebrospinal fluid from a lateral ventricle of the brain into the venous circulation; the right atrium of the heart or the superior vena cava.

splanchnic *adj* pertaining to or supplying the viscera. *splanchnic nerves* group of sympathetic nerve fibres that supply the viscera.

splanchnicectomy *n* surgical removal of the splanchnic nerves, whereby the viscera are deprived of sympathetic impulses. Performed rarely for the relief of certain kinds of visceral pain.

splanchnology *n* the study of the structure and function of the viscera.

spleen *n* a lymphoid, vascular organ immediately below the diaphragm, at the tail of the pancreas, behind the stomach. It forms part of the monocyte-macrophage system (reticuloendothelial). Its functions include: destruction, by macrophages, of old red cells and platelets; filtering blood and destroying any micro-organisms, toxins and debris; site of lymphocyte proliferation and immunoglobulin (antibody) production; storage of platelets and red cell breakdown products; fetal red cell production and acting as a reservoir for blood — **splenic** *adj* pertaining to the spleen. Applied to the artery and vein.

splenectomy *n* surgical removal of the spleen.

splenitis *n* inflammation of the spleen.

splenocaval *adj* pertaining to the spleen and inferior vena cava, usually referring to anastomosis of the splenic vein to the latter. A surgical procedure used to relieve hepatic portal hypertension.

splenomegaly *n* enlargement of the spleen.

splenoportal *adj* pertaining to the spleen and hepatic portal vein.

splenoportogram *n* radiographic demonstration of the spleen and hepatic portal vein after injection of contrast medium — **splenoportographically** *adv*.

splenorenal *adj* pertaining to the spleen and kidney, as anastomosis of the splenic vein to the renal vein; a surgical procedure used to relieve hepatic portal hypertension.

SPOD *abbr* sexual problems of the disabled. A department which offers help to disabled people: it is part of the Royal Association of Disability and Rehabilitation.

spondyl(e) *n* a vertebra.

spondylitis *n* inflammation of one or more vertebrae. *ankylosing spondylitis* a chronic rheumatic condition characterized by abnormal ossification and ankylosis affecting the spine and sacroiliac joints. Loss of joint space leads to fusion with immobility. It occurs chiefly in young men — **spondylitic** *adj*.

spondylography *n* a method of measuring and studying the degree of kyphosis by directly tracing the line of the back.

spondylolisthesis *n* forward displacement of lumbar vertebral bodies, causing pressure on the nerve roots — **spondylolisthetic** *adj*.

spondylosis ankylosis of the vertebral joints. The intervertebral disc is affected by degenerative diseases that include osteoarthritis.

spongioblastoma multiforme a highly malignant rapidly growing brain tumour. A type of glioma. ⇒ astrocytoma.

sporadic *adj* scattered; occurring in isolated cases; not epidemic — **sporadically** *adv*.

spore *n* **1.** a phase in the life cycle of a limited number of bacterial genera (Clostridium and Bacillus) where the vegetative cell becomes encapsulated and metabolism almost ceases. These spores are highly resistant to environmental conditions such as heat and desiccation. ⇒ endospore. **2.** reproductive body produced by certain plants, particularly fungi, and by protozoa.

sporicidal *adj* lethal to spores — **sporicide** *n*.

sporotrichosis *n* a chronic, subcutaneous infection caused by the fungus *Sporothrix schenkii*, a species found in soil and decaying vegetation. Usually an abscess or ulcer develops, then lymphatic spread occurs. Enters the skin by traumatic injury (particularly amongst agricultural workers).

sporulation *n* the formation of spores by bacteria.

spotted fever an acute febrile disease caused by *Rickettsia rickettsii* and transmitted by ticks. Also known as Rocky Mountain spotted fever, as this was where it was initially recognized. ⇒ rickettsial fevers.

sprain *n* injury to the soft tissues surrounding a joint, resulting in discolouration, swelling and pain. It is caused by sudden overstretching of the surrounding ligaments and tendons without fracture or dislocation.

spreadsheet a computer program that manipulates data in cells arranged in rows and columns.

Sprengel's shoulder deformity congenital high scapula, a permanent elevation of one or both shoulders, often associated with other congenital deformities, e.g. the presence of a cervical rib or the absence of vertebrae.

sprue *n* a chronic malabsorption disorder associated with various conditions and occurring in a nontropical and tropical form. It is characterized by glossitis, abdominal pain, diarrhoea, weight loss, steatorrhoea, weakness and anaemia.

SPSS *abbr* Statistical Package for the Social Sciences.

spurious not what it appears to be. *spurious diarrhoea* the leakage of fluid faeces past a solid impacted mass of faeces. More likely to occur in children and older people. It is vital that a thorough nursing assessment is used to differentiate this condition from true diarrhoea.

sputum *n* mucus/matter expectorated from the lower respiratory tract by the force of coughing. Sputum may be mucoid, mucopurulent in infection, rusty in appearance (altered blood), frothy in pulmonary oedema or bloodstained. ⇒ cough. ⇒ expectorate. ⇒ postural drainage.

squamous *adj* scaly. *squamous cell carcinoma (SCC)* carcinoma arising in squamous epithelium; epithelioma. Accounts for around 50% of bronchial cancers. Also applied specifically to a form of skin cancer affecting keratinocytes. It is associated with skin damage from longterm exposure to sunlight and other forms of radiation. The lesions are common on the lip and the oral cavity, and some types may metastasize to distant sites. ⇒ leukoplakia. *squamous epithelium* the nonglandular epithelial covering of the body surfaces.

squint *n* ⇒ strabismus.

SSPE *abbr* subacute sclerosing panencephalitis.

SSRI *abbr* selective serotonin re-uptake inhibitors.

stable factor (proconvertin) *n* factor VII in coagulation.

staff development all registered nurses should have access to staff development or continuing professional development to maintain and enhance their knowledge, experience and skills. ⇒ Postregistration Education and Practice.

staff nurse the title accorded registered nurses.

staging a way of classifying malignant tumours according to type and extent. Each cancer has specific classification criteria, but the TNM classification system enables clinicians to assess, either by clinical (TMN) or pathological investigation (pTMN), the size of the tumour (T), the absence or presence and extent of regional lymph node metastases (N) and the absence or presence of distant metastasis (M). TNM staging may be supported with histopathological grading. Patients with localized disease usually have a better prognosis than those with widespread disease. Information about the stage of the disease allows the clinician to assess the likely prognosis and choose the most effective and appropriate treatment modality.

stagnant loop syndrome ⇒ blind loop syndrome.

stakeholders individuals and groups of people or organizations that have a legitimate interest in an activity, e.g. developing the HImP.

stammering *n* a disorder characterized by dysfluency of speech with sound, syllable and/or word repetitions. The term is used synonymously with stuttering. May occur developmentally or following brain injury.

standard a level or measure against which the performance of an activity can be monitored.

standard deviation (SD) in statistics, a measure of dispersion of scores around the mean value. ⇒ variance.

standard error (SE) a measure of variability of many mean values of different samples from a population. Used to calculate the chance of a sample mean being smaller or bigger than the mean for the population. Often used inappropriately in place of standard deviation (SD). SD should be used to measure variability of individuals within a sample, SE is used for variability of samples within a population.

St Anthony's fire historical term for the mental disturbances and painful vasoconstriction leading to gangrene of the extremities caused by ergot poisoning (ergot alkaloids present in a fungus that infests rye).

stapedectomy *n* removal of the stapes. The surgical treatment of choice for patients with otosclerosis.

stapes *n* the stirrup-shaped bone. One of the three middle ear ossicles. ⇒ incus. ⇒ malleus — **stapedial** *adj*.

Staphylococcus *n* a genus of bacteria. Gram-positive cocci occurring in clusters. Some staphylococci are commensal on the skin and may be found in the nasopharynx, axillae and perineum of some individuals. Staphylococcal infections include: boils, impetigo, wound infection, endocarditis, pneumonia, osteomyelitis, toxic shock syndrome and septicaemia. Staphylococci are an important cause of nosocomial infection. The genus includes the major pathogen *Staphylococcus aureus* which produces the enzyme coagulase, some strains produce a powerful exotoxin, and others are methicillin resistant. ⇒ Methicillin resistant *Staphylococcus aureus*. *Staphylococcus epidermidis* is a skin commensal that does not produce coagulase. It causes wound infection and is increasingly responsible for infection involving prosthetic valves, intravascular devices and peritoneal dialysis catheters. Treatment is difficult because the organism possesses a natural resistance to many antibiotics — **staphylococcal** *adj*.

staphyloma *n* a protrusion of the cornea or sclera of the eye — **staphylomata** *pl*.

starch *n* carbohydrate. A storage polysaccharide of plants consisting of many monosaccharide (glucose) units, e.g. amylose and amylopectin. It is present in cereals, e.g. wheat, rice, oats and maize and in their products, such as bread, pasta, breakfast cereals and chapatis, and vegetables that include potatoes and yams. They provide energy and some indigestible fibre.

Starling's law of the heart the force of myocardial contraction is proportional to the length (stretching) of the ventricular muscle fibres. As the heart fills during diastole the fibres stretch and the next contraction is more powerful. This relationship between length and tension is known as Starling's law.

start up costs the costs, such as the purchase of a building, purchasing of equipment that occur when a project commences.

stasis *n* stagnation, such as blood flow; cessation of motion. It may be gravitational. *intestinal stasis* sluggish bowel contractions resulting in constipation.

statement of special educational needs used in relation to educational provision for children with a learning disability. A statement of the special educational needs of a particular child may be drawn up, following formal assessment, in order to determine whether the child's needs can be met in mainstream schooling, perhaps with additional staff provision, or in special schools.

statins ⇒ HMG-CoA reductase inhibitors.

Statistical Package for the Social Sciences. *n* software package commonly used to analyse quantitative data.

statistical significance in research, an expression of how likely it is that the results occurred by chance, e.g. 0.05, 0.01 and 0.001 levels. ⇒ *P* value.

statistics science of numerical data collection, analysis and evaluation — **statistic** a specific statistical test, such as chi-square statistic.

status *n* state; condition. *status asthmaticus* ⇒ severe acute asthma. *status epilepticus* describes epileptic seizures following each other almost continuously. It is a medical emergency and requires immediate treatment to protect the airway, control seizures with intravenous diazepam or phenytoin, and monitor condition in HDU.

statute law statutory. Law made by Acts of Parliament.

STD *abbr* sexually transmitted disease.

steatorrhoea *n* excessive fat in the faeces due to defective fat digestion or malabsorption from the gut, characterized by the passage of pale, bulky, greasy, foul-smelling stools.

steatosis *n* fatty degeneration. Fat droplets appear in the parenchymal cells of the liver, heart and kidney. A particular feature of alcohol induced liver disease.

stegomyia *n* a genus of mosquitoes, some of which transmit the malaria parasite. Found in most tropical and subtropical regions.

Stein-Leventhal syndrome polycystic ovary syndrome. An increase in ovarian and adrenal androgen secretion leads to menstrual irregularities, secondary amenorrhoea, infertility, obesity, hirsutism and multiple follicular ovarian cysts.

Steinmann's pin wide diameter pin inserted through a bone in order to apply extension in the case of fractures. Used for heavy skeletal traction. An alternative to the use of a Kirschner wire.

stellate *adj* star-shaped. *stellate ganglion* a large collection of nerve cells (ganglion) on the sympathetic chain in the root of the neck. *stellate ganglionectomy* surgical removal of the stellate ganglion.

Stellwag's sign occurs in exophthalmic goitre (hyperthyroidism). The affected person does not blink as often as usual, and the eyelids close only imperfectly when he or she does so.

stem cell *n* ⇒ pluripotent stem cell.

stenosis *n* narrowing of a channel or opening, such as heart valves. ⇒ pyloric stenosis. ⇒ pyloromyotomy — **stenotic** *adj*.

stent *n* device used in a variety of situations to provide a shunt or keep a tube or vessel open. Examples include: stent insertion into the bile duct to relieve obstructive jaundice associated with cancer of the pancreas, stenting the ureters to overcome urinary obstruction, and stenting the oesophagus for palliation of dysphagia caused by tumour. *transjugular intrahepatic portasystemic stent shunting (TIPSS)* a stent placed between the hepatic portal vein and the hepatic vein in the liver to reduce hepatic portal pressure by providing a shunt between the hepatic portal and systemic circulations. Used to prevent further bleeding from oesophageal varices.

stercobilin *n* the brown pigment of normal faeces. It is formed from the action of intestinal bacteria on stercobilinogen which is derived from the bile pigments.

stercobilinogen *n* faecal urobilinogen. A substance formed from the action of the intestinal bacteria on bilirubin. It is subsequently oxidized to form stercobilin.

stercoraceous *adj* pertaining to or resembling faeces — **stercoral** *adj*.

stereoscopic vision ability to perceive and assess distance, depth and speed resulting from the two eyes transmitting different images from different, but overlapping, visual fields (binocular vision).

stereotactic surgery a method of operating on the brain after the exact position has been determined by the use of three-dimensional measurements. ⇒ pallidectomy. ⇒ thalamotomy — **stereotaxy** *n*.

stereotype *n* a generalization about a behaviour, individual or a group; can be the basis for prejudice.

sterile *adj* 1. free from micro-organisms. 2. barren, unable to reproduce — **sterility** *n*.

sterilization *n* 1. the destruction of micro-organisms and spores, through the use of heat, radiation, chemicals or filtration. ⇒ autoclave. 2. rendering incapable of reproduction, such as by division/occlusion of the uterine tubes, or vasectomy. ⇒ tubal ligation.

sternoclavicular *adj* pertaining to the sternum and the clavicle.

sternocleidomastoid muscle a strap-like neck muscle arising from the sternum and clavicle, and inserting into the mastoid process of temporal bone. ⇒ torticollis.

sternocostal *adj* pertaining to the sternum and ribs.

sternotomy *n* surgical division of the sternum.

sternum *n* the breast bone — **sternal** *adj* pertaining to the sternum. *sternal puncture* ⇒ bone marrow puncture.

steroids *npl* a large group of organic compounds (lipids) having a common basic chemical configuration: three 6-carbon rings and a 5-carbon ring. They include: cholesterol (precursor of many steroids and a component of cell membranes), bile salts, vitamin D precursors, sex hormones and adrenal cortical hormones. ⇒ corticosteroids.

sterol *n* a subgroup of steroids that combine the basic steroid structure with an alcohol group. Examples include cholesterol and ergosterol.

stertor *n* loud snoring; sonorous breathing — **stertorous** *adj*.

stethoscope *n* an instrument used for listening to the various body sounds, especially those of the heart and chest — **stethoscopically** *adv*.

Stevens-Johnson syndrome severe bullous form of erythema multiforme with ulceration of the mucous membranes and fever. It is an acute hypersensitivity state and can follow a viral or bacterial infection or drugs such as long-acting sulphonamides, some anticonvulsants and some antibiotics. In some cases no cause can be found. Management involves treating the primary cause and systemic corticosteroids.

STI *abbr* sexually transmitted infection.

stigma *n* a defining characteristic of a person or an action usually perceived negatively by others — **stigmata, stigmas** *pl*.

stilette *n* a wire or metal rod for maintaining patency of hollow instruments.

stillbirth *n* birth of a baby, after 24 weeks gestation, that shows no sign of life. Parents, and other siblings if relevant, need opportunity to grieve for this occurrence.

stillborn *n* born dead. ⇒ stillbirth.

Still's disease systemic onset juvenile chronic arthritis. It is characterized by swollen joints, arthralgia, myalgia, fever, rashes with hepatosplenomegaly and lymphadenopathy. Occurs in infants and young children. There may also be pleurisy and pericarditis. ⇒ juvenile chronic arthritis.

stimulant *n* an agent, usually artificial, which excites or increases function.

stimulus *n* anything which excites functional activity in an organ or part.

STM *abbr* short term memory.

Stokes-Adams syndrome also called Adams-Stokes attacks. Recurrent fainting (syncope) attacks, commonly transient, resulting from second degree or complete heart block causing ventricular asystole. It can occur in patients with sinoatrial disease. If severe, may take the form of a convulsion, or patient may become unconscious. Patients may require an artificial pacemaker.

stoma *n* the mouth; any opening, e.g. opening of the bowel or ureters on to the abdominal surface. ⇒ colostomy. ⇒ ileostomy. ⇒ urostomy. *stoma bag* an appliance worn over a stoma to collect faeces or urine. (See Figure 59). *stoma nurse specialist* a nurse specialist qualified in the support and management of individuals with stomas. They may have other titles, such as stoma care nurse — **stomal** *adj*.

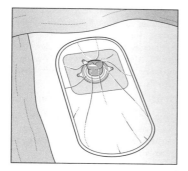

Figure 59 Stoma bag. (Reproduced from Nicol et al 2000 with permission.)

stomach *n* the most dilated part of the digestive tract, situated between the oesophagus and the beginning of the small intestine (duodenum); it lies in the epigastric, umbilical and left hypochondriac regions of the abdomen (see Figure 1). The wall is composed of four coats: serous, muscular, submucous and mucous. It produces gastric juice containing hydrochloric acid, enzymes and mucus. Gastric functions include: commencing protein digestion, mechanical churning of food to produce chyme, destruction of some micro-organisms and some absorption. ⇒ gastro-oesophageal sphincter. ⇒ pylorus.

stomatitis *n* inflammation of the mouth. *angular stomatitis* fissuring in the corners of the mouth consequent upon riboflavin deficiency. Sometimes misapplied to: (a) the superficial maceration and fissuring at the labial commissures in perléche and (b) the chronic fissuring at the site in older persons with sagging lower lip or malapposition of artificial dentures. *aphthous stomatitis* recurring crops of small ulcers in the mouth. May be a problem for patients with AIDS, where it is particularly important to maintain good oral hygiene. ⇒ aphthae. *gangrenous stomatitis* ⇒ cancrum oris. *ulcerative stomatitis* ⇒ Vincent's angina.

stone *n* calculus; a hardened mass of mineral matter.

stool *n* faeces or motion. An evacuation of the bowels.

stove-in chest an injury which may involve multiple anterior or posterior fractures of the ribs (causing paradoxical respiration) and fractures of sternum, or a mixture of such fractures. ⇒ flail chest.

strabismus *n* (*syn* squint) may be paralytic, which is due to a weakness in the muscles of the eyeball or neurological disorder, or concomitant, where there is a failure to maintain the correct position of an eye that has defective vision. The visual axes of the two eyes fail to meet at the objective point. The most common are *convergent squint* when the eyes turn towards the medial line, and *divergent squint* when the eyes turn outwards.

straight sinus venous channel draining blood from the brain.

strain 1. a group of micro-organisms within the same species, but having different characteristics. **2.** condition due to stretching or unsuitable use of a body part. **3.** to filter.

strangulated hernia ⇒ hernia.

strangulation *n* constriction which impedes the circulation — **strangulated** *adj*.

strangury *n* frequent painful desire to void small amounts of urine, due to muscle spasm associated with inflammation or irritation.

Strassman operation a plastic operation to make a bicornuate uterus a near normal shape.

strategic management the management function concerned with longer term future strategy. Financial and resource planning. ⇒ operational management.

stratified *adj* arranged in layers.

stratum *n* a layer or lamina, e.g. the various layers of the epithelium of the skin, i.e. stratum corneum, stratum lucidum, stratum granulosum, stratum spinosum and stratum basale.

strawberry tongue a characteristic of scarlet fever. The tongue is thickly furred with projecting red papillae. As the fur disappears the tongue is vividly red like an over-ripe strawberry.

Streptobacillus moniliformis *n* a bacterium that causes a type of rat bite fever.

Streptococcus *n* a genus of bacteria. Gram-positive cocci, often occurring in chains of varying length. Require enriched media for growth, and the colonies are small. Saprophytic and parasitic species. They have varying haemolytic ability (α, β and nonhaemolytic) and some types produce powerful toxin. Some streptococci are commensal in the alimentary canal/tract (*Streptococcus faecalis*) and respiratory tract (*Streptococcus viridans*). The commensal streptococci, along with the pathogens *Streptococcus pyogenes* and *Streptococcus pneumoniae*, cause serious infections that include: scarlet fever, tonsillitis, otitis media, erysipelas, endocarditis, wound infections, pneumonia , meningitis, urinary tract infection. Rheumatic fever and glomerulonephritis may be sequelae of some streptococcal infections. Group B streptococcus, a commensal of the gut and vagina, may cause meningitis, pneumonia and septicaemia in neonates infected by organisms present in the maternal genital tract. ⇒ Griffith's typing. ⇒ Lancefield's groups. ⇒ necrotizing fasciitis — **streptococcal** *adj*.

streptodornase *n* a streptococcal enzyme used with streptokinase in liquefying pus and blood clots. ⇒ proteolytic enzymes.

streptokinase *n* a streptococcal enzyme. Plasminogen activator. Its fibrinolytic effect is used to treat various thromboembolic conditions. → fibrinolytic therapy. Used with streptodornase in wound management.

streptolysins *npl* exotoxins produced by streptococci. Antibody produced in the tissues against streptolysin may be measured and taken as an indicator of recent streptococcal infection.

stress *n* the response of an organism to any demand made upon it by agents threatening physical or emotional well-being. Selye called such agents stressors, and said that they could be physical, physiological, psychological or sociocultural. Stress can be described as being either: *distress* which is viewed as a negative event, with long term effects on health when it becomes chronic, or *eustress* which accompanies pleasurable excitement and euphoria and is viewed more positively. *stress incontinence* ⇒ incontinence. *stress management* measures that reduce the negative effects of stress, such as relaxation techniques, biofeedback, autogenic therapy etc, or reducing stress, e.g. reducing workload through delegation. ⇒ burnout. ⇒ general adaptation syndrome.

stressors *npl* factors which initiate stress responses. They may be structural/physical, physiological, psychological and sociocultural, and include: pain, hunger, cold, blood loss, overwork, a life crisis such as divorce, poor housing or low income. ⇒ burnout.

striae *npl* streaks; stripes; narrow bands. Scars on the thighs and abdomen caused by stretching of the dermis and rupture of elastic fibres when the abdomen enlarges, such as with tumours, ascites, obesity and pregnancy, when the marks are known as *striae gravidarum* or stretch marks, which are red at first, becoming white. Striae may be associated with Cushing's disease or as a side-effect of glucocorticoid therapy — **striated** *adj* *striated muscle* striped voluntary muscle. ⇒ muscle.

stricture *n* a narrowing, especially of a tube or canal, due to inflammation, scar tissue, external pressure, spasm or tumour, such as urethral stricture.

stridor *n* a harsh sound in breathing, caused by air passing through constricted air passages — **stridulous** *adj*.

stroke *n* ⇒ cerebrovascular accident.

stroke volume (SV) *n* the difference between ventricular end diastolic volume (EDV) and end systolic volume (ESV), i.e. the amount of blood pumped out of the heart by each ventricular contraction. ⇒ cardiac output. ⇒ pulse.

stroma *n* the interstitial or foundation substance of a structure.

Strongyloides *n* a genus of small intestinal nematode worms, e.g. *Strongyloides stercoralis*. It infects humans, who are the natural host, but it can infect dogs. → strongyloidiasis.

strongyloidiasis *n* infestation with *Strongyloides stercoralis*. Common in the tropics and subtropics, but it also occurs in immunocompromised individuals, such as patients with AIDS. Systemic strongyloidiasis is an AIDS defining condition according to CDC/WHO. Infection is usually acquired through the skin from contaminated soil, but can be through mucous membrane. At the site of larval penetration there may be an itchy rash. The larvae migrate through the lungs and there may be pulmonary symptoms as the larvae are coughed up in sputum. The larvae reaching the pharynx are swallowed and they reach the intestine. There may be varying abdominal symptoms produced as the female worm burrows into the intestinal mucosa and submucosa. There is abdominal pain, diarrhoea with malabsorption and weight loss. Some patients may exhibit allergic features, e.g. urticaria and wheezing. Treatment is with anthelmintics: tiabendazole (thiabendazole), albendazole.

strontium (Sr) *n* a metallic element chemically similar to calcium and present in bone. Isotopes of strontium are used in radionuclide scanning of bone to detect abnormalities. *strontium*^{90} a radioactive isotope with a relatively long half-life (28 years) produced by atomic explosions. It becomes hazardous when it is incorporated into bone tissue where turnover is slow.

structuralism a sociological perspective based on the idea of organized social structures and institutions that influence people's lives.

Stryker bed a proprietary, turning bed, constructed so that a patient can be rotated as required to the prone or supine position. Used mainly for spinal conditions and burns.

Stuart-Prower factor *n* factor X in coagulation.

student's elbow olecranon bursitis.

Student's paired test *n* a parametric test for statistical significance. Used to test differences in mean values for two related measurements, for example on the same person. ⇒ Wilcoxon test.

Student's t test for independent groups *n* a parametric test for statistical significance. Used to test differences in mean values of two groups. ⇒ Mann Whitney test.

stupor *n* a state of marked impairment, but not complete loss, of consciousness. The victim shows gross lack of responsiveness, usually reacting only to noxious stimuli — **stuporous** *adj*.

Sturge-Weber syndrome (*syn* naevoid amentia) a genetically determined congenital ectodermosis, i.e. a capillary haemangioma above the eye may be accompanied by similar changes in vessels inside the skull, giving rise to epilepsy and other cerebral manifestations.

St Vitus' dance ⇒ chorea.

stye *n* (*syn* hordeolum) an abscess in the follicle of an eyelash.

styloid *adj* long and pointed; resembling a pen or stylus. A process of the temporal bone, radius and ulna.

styptic *n* an astringent applied to stop bleeding. A haemostatic.

subacute *adj* the stage between the acute and chronic phases of disease. *subacute bacterial endocarditis* septicaemia due to bacterial infection of a heart valve. Petechiae of the skin and embolic phenomena are characteristic. The term infective endocarditis is now preferred, since other micro-organisms may be involved. *subacute combined degeneration of the spinal cord* demyelination of the posterior and corticospinal tracts of the spinal cord due to a deficiency of vitamin B_{12}. Associated with pernicious anaemia. *subacute sclerosing panencephalitis (SSPE)* a slow virus infection caused by the measles virus; characterized by diffuse inflammation of brain tissue.

subarachnoid *n* below the arachnoid mater. *subarachnoid space* the space between the arachnoid and the pia mater which contains cerebrospinal fluid. ⇒ subarachnoid haemorrhage.

subarachnoid haemorrhage (SAH) bleeding into the subarachnoid space, usually due to rupture of an intracranial aneurysm, but may be caused by trauma or the extension of an intracerebral bleed. It is accompanied by sudden, severe headache and often by vomiting and a stiff neck. Blood is present in the CSF. CT scanning is used for diagnosis, and cerebral angiography reveals the site of bleeding which may be resolved by surgical clipping of the aneurysm.

subcarinal *adj* below a carina, usually referring to the carina at the bifurcation of the trachea.

subclavian *adj* beneath the clavicle, such as the artery and vein.

subclinical *adj* without obvious signs and symptoms of the disease.

subconjunctival *adj* below the conjunctiva — **subconjunctivally** *adj*.

subconscious *adj, n* that portion of the mind outside the range of clear consciousness, but capable of affecting conscious mental or physical reactions.

subcostal *adj* beneath the rib.

subculture the customs and values of a subgroup that is different from, but is related to, the dominant cultural group in that society.

subcutaneous *adj* beneath the skin. ⇒ injection — **subcutaneously** *adv* subcutaneous oedema is demonstrable by the 'pitting' produced by pressure of the finger.

subcuticular *adj* beneath the cuticle, as a subcuticular abscess.

subdural *adj* beneath the dura mater; between the dura and arachnoid maters. *subdural haematoma* the bleeding comes from a small vein or veins lying between the dura and brain. Usually caused by trauma, it may develop slowly and may present as a space-occupying lesion with vomiting, papilloedema, fluctuating level of consciousness, weakness and usually a hemiplegia on the opposite side to the clot. Finally there is a rise in blood pressure and a fall in pulse rate.

subendocardial *adj* immediately beneath the endocardium.

subhepatic *adj* beneath the liver.

subinvolution *adj* failure of the gravid uterus to return to its normal size, shape and position within a normal time after childbirth. ⇒ involution.

subjective *adj* internal, personal; arising from the senses and not perceptible to others. → objective *ant*.

sublimate *n* a solid deposit resulting from the condensation of a vapour.

sublimation *n* a mental defence mechanism whereby unacceptable instinctive drives are unconsciously diverted to, and expressed through, personally approved and socially accepted behaviour, such as aggression diverted to physical exercise and sport.

subliminal *adj* inadequate for perceptible response. Below the threshold of consciousness. ⇒ liminal.

sublingual *adj* beneath the tongue. *sublingual glands* ⇒ salivary glands.

subluxation *n* incomplete dislocation of a joint. ⇒ luxation.

submandibular *adj* below the mandible. *submandibular glands* ⇒ salivary glands.

submaxillary *adj* beneath the maxilla.

submucosa *n* the layer of connective tissue beneath a mucous membrane — **submucous, submucosal** *adj*.

submucous *adj* beneath a mucous membrane. *submucous resection (SMR)* surgical procedure to correct a deviated nasal septum.

suboccipital *adj* beneath the occiput; in the nape of the neck.

subperiosteal *adj* beneath the periosteum of bone.

subphrenic *adj* beneath the diaphragm. *subphrenic abscess* collection of pus under the diaphragm.

subpoena an order of the court requiring a person to appear as a witness (subpoena ad testificandum) or to bring records/documents (subpoena duces tecum).

substance misuse 1. a general term which includes drug and solvent abuse. 2. an all-inclusive term which describes misuse of alcohol, drugs and tobacco to the point where health and/or social functioning is adversely affected. Drugs involved may be over the counter, prescribed or those obtained illegally. Groups of drugs involved include: amfetamines (amphetamines), barbiturates, benzodiazepines, cannabis, cocaine, heroin, morphine and hallucinogens. ⇒ Misuse of Drugs Act.

substernal *adj* beneath the sternum. *substernal goitre* one where part of the enlarged thyroid gland is under the sternum.

substrate *n* the chemical which a specific enzyme works on.

subungual *adj* beneath a nail. *subungual haematoma* a collection of blood under a nail usually resulting from trauma. Extremely painful until the blood is released.

succussion *n* 1. splashing sound produced by fluid in a hollow cavity when the patient moves, e.g. liquid content of dilated stomach in pyloric stenosis. 2. in homeopathy, the process whereby natural diluted substances are shaken vigorously.

sucrase *n* an intestinal enzyme which splits sucrose into glucose and fructose.

sucrose *n* a disaccharide present in cane and beet sugar and maple syrup. It consists of a glucose and fructose molecule.

sudamina *n* sweat rash.

Sudan blindness a form of onchocerciasis.

sudden infant death syndrome (SIDS) (*syn* cot death) the unexpected sudden death of an infant, usually occurring overnight while sleeping in a cot, but may occur under other circumstances.

The commonest mode of death in infants between the ages of 1 month and 1 year, neither clinical nor postmortem findings being adequate to account for death. Overheating, sleeping in the prone position, respiratory illness and infection, and being in an environment where people smoke have all been implicated as risk factors. Parents/carers are now recommended to put babies to sleep on their backs, at the foot of the cot to prevent them wriggling under bedclothes, not to overheat the room, not to smoke in the same room and seek advice from a health professional if the baby seems unwell.

sudor *n* sweat — **sudoriferous** *adj.*

sudorific *n* any agent that stimulates or promotes sweating. ⇒ sweat test.

suggestibility *n* abnormal susceptibility to suggestion. May be heightened in hospital patients due to the dependence on others that illness brings, in children and in people with learning disabilities.

suicide *n* intentional taking of one's own life. Usually related to depression and hopelessness. Attitudes to suicide are culturally determined, and stigma may exist in some groups. ⇒ Beck Hopelessness Scale. ⇒ Beck Scale for Suicide Ideation. ⇒ parasuicide.

sulcus *n* a furrow or groove, particularly those separating the gyri or convolutions of the cortex of the brain. Deep sulci divide the lobes of the cerebral hemispheres — **sulci** *pl.*

sulphaemoglobin *n* abnormal haemoglobin pigment. ⇒ sulphmethaemoglobin.

sulphaemoglobinaemia *n* a condition of circulating sulphmethaemoglobin in the blood.

sulphate *n* salt of sulphuric acid, such as magnesium sulphate.

sulphmethaemoglobin *n* (*syn* sulphaemoglobin) a sulphide oxidation product of haemoglobin, produced in vivo by certain drugs. This compound cannot transport oxygen or carbon dioxide and, not being reversible in the body, is an indirect poison.

sulphonamides *npl* a group of antibacterial agents, e.g sulfadimidine (sulphadimidine), sulfasalazine (sulphasalazine) etc. They act as antimetabolites by inhibiting the conversion of para-aminobenzoic acid to folic acid, which is required for bacterial metabolism.

sulphones *npl* a group of synthetic drugs related to the sulphonamides, e.g. dapsone, used for treating leprosy and malaria.

sulphonylureas *npl* ⇒ hypoglycaemic drugs.

sulphur *n* an insoluble yellow powder. Used in lotions, ointments and baths for acne and other skin disorders.

sulphuric acid *n* corrosive inorganic acid.

summation the accumulation of effects such as those concerned with sensory stimuli, transmission of nerve impulses or muscle contraction. It may be spatial or temporal.

sunstroke *n* ⇒ heatstroke.

superego according to Freud, one of the three main aspects of the personality (the other two are id and ego); the part of the mind concerned with morality and self-criticism, it operates at a partly conscious, but mostly unconscious, level and corresponds roughly to what is called 'conscience'.

superficial *adj* near the surface, such as the superficial veins of the leg.

superinfection *n* an infection that follows destruction of the normal flora with broad spectrum antibiotics. This allows other micro-organisms, such as *Clostridium difficle*, to flourish in the bowel without competition from micro-organisms of the normal flora. ⇒ pseudomembranous colitis. ⇒ pseudomonas.

superior *adj* in anatomy, the upper of two parts — **superiorly** *adj.*

supernumerary *n* in excess of the normal number; additional. Such as with students of nursing undertaking clinical placements.

superovulation *n* process used in various assisted conception techniques. Ovarian activity is controlled, follicular growth encouraged and ovulation stimulated at a specified time using a complex programme of hormone injections. It may be preceded by a period of down-regulation. Progress is monitored by ultrasound scan.

superoxide ⇒ free radical.

supinate *vt* turn or lay face or palm upward. ⇒ pronate *ant.*

supinator *n* that which supinates, usually applied to a muscle, such as the biceps brachii muscle of the arm. ⇒ pronator *ant.*

supine *adj* **1.** lying on the back with face upwards. **2.** of the hand, with the palm upwards. ⇒ prone *ant.*

support *n* can be of a physical nature as when the hands are placed over an abdominal wound during coughing. It can be of a psychological nature as when a nurse listens actively to a patient, or holds the hand of someone who is dying. It can be of a social nature as when a district nurse arranges for a voluntary visitor to spend time with a lonely housebound patient.

support worker ⇒ healthcare assistant.

suppository *n* medicament in a base that melts at body temperature. Inserted into the rectum (blunt end first to aid retention). (See Figure 60)

suppression *n* in psychology, a mental defence mechanism, whereby individuals voluntarily force painful thoughts out of the mind; it can precipitate a neurosis.

suppuration *n* the formation of pus — **suppurate** *vi.*

supraclavicular *adj* above the clavicle.

supracondylar *adj* above a condyle. *supracondylar fracture* a fracture involving the area between the condyles at the lower end of the femur or the humerus. Those affecting the humerus may interfere with the blood supply to the forearm. Nursing observation should include radial pulse on the affected side, skin colour and temperature and complaints of pain or abnormal sensation ⇒ Volkmann's ischaemic contracture.

supraoptic nucleus a hypothalamic nucleus with nerve fibres extending to the posterior pituitary gland. Together with the paraventricular nucleus it produces antidiuretic hormone and oxytocin.

supraorbital *adj* above the orbits. *supraorbital ridge* the ridge of the frontal bone covered by the eyebrows.

suprapubic *adj* above the pubis. *suprapubic catheter* a catheter inserted into the urinary bladder via the abdominal wall. ⇒ catheterization.

suprarenal *adj* above the kidney. *suprarenal gland* ⇒ adrenal gland.

suprasternal *adj* above the sternum.

supraventricular *adj* above the ventricles, such as abnormal heart rhythms arising in the atria.

supraventricular tachycardia *n* cardiac rhythm with a rate >100 beats per minute that arises from a focus above the ventricles, such as in the SA node, atria or A-V node. It is termed junctional tachycardia where the abnormal focus is situated in the junctional tissue present in the A-V node.

Sure Start a Government initiative that aims to provide innovative services for families with children aged 0–4 years to ensure the best start in life. It depends on collaborate multidisciplinary and multiagency working with socially and economically disadvantaged families.

surfactant *n* a phospholipid fluid secreted by type II pneumocytes reduces surface tension in the alveoli and allows lung inflation. Surfactants prevent alveolar collapse between breaths and reduce the effort required to reinflate the alveoli on inspiration. A deficiency in pre-term babies can lead to respiratory distress syndrome. Intratracheal administration of surfactants may form part of the management of affected babies

surgeon *n* a person qualified to carry out surgical operations.

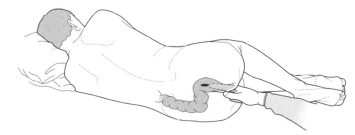

Figure 60 Administration of suppositories. (Reproduced from Nicol et al 2000 with permission.)

surgery *n* that branch of medicine which treats diseases, deformities and injuries, wholly or in part, by manual or operative procedures.

surgical *adj* relating to surgery. *surgical emphysema* air in the subcutaneous tissue planes following the trauma of surgery or injury. *surgical neck* narrow part of the humerus, below the tuberosities. ⇒ tuberosity.

surrogate a substitute for a person or an object. *surrogate motherhood* where one woman agrees to have a child for an infertile couple. Surrogacy is allowed in the UK, where women can only receive reasonable financial expenses. There are, however, many informal arrangements for surrogacy. It remains controversial and is fraught with emotional, ethical and legal problems.

surveillance the process that monitors, analyses and reports on the occurrence of disease, such as wound infections with a particular micro-organism or the number of cases of a notifiable infection in a population.

survey a data collection method. It may be postal, telephone, interview or via the internet.

susceptibility *n* the opposite of resistance. Includes a state of reduced capacity to deal with infection.

suspensory supporting. *suspensory bandage* applied so that it supports and suspends, such as the lower jaw or scrotum. *suspensory ligament* suspends or supports a body part, such as that supporting the lens of the eye.

suture *n* **1.** the junction of cranial bones. **2.** in surgery, a suture is a stitch used to close a wound, either deep, of the layers, or superficial. They are made of various materials and may be absorbable or non-absorbable.

SVGA *abbr* super video graphics array. A type of screen display supporting high resolution colour images.

SVQs *abbr* Scottish Vocational Qualifications.

SVR *abbr* systemic vascular resistance.

SVT *abbr* supraventricular tachycardia.

swab *n* **1.** a small piece of cotton wool or gauze. **2.** a small piece of sterile cotton wool, or similar material, on the end of a shaft of wire, plastic or wood, enclosed in a protecting tube. It is used to collect material for microbiological examination.

swallowing *n* deglutition. A complex activity with three stages: oral (buccal), pharyngeal and oesophageal. It is part voluntary and part involuntary. It involves chewed food in the form of a bolus being enclosed by the muscles of the pharynx and moved into the oesophagus. Peristalsis moves the bolus to the stomach. ⇒ dysphagia.

sweat *n* the secretion from the sweat (sudoriferous) glands. Contains water, electrolytes (mainly sodium and chloride) and waste (nitrogenous, drug and food residues). Sweat production is determined by skin temperature and emotional state. Sweat production is concerned with temperature regulation and also has a minor excretory role. *sweat glands* ⇒ apocrine. ⇒ eccrine.

sweat test a test to measure the amount of sodium and chloride in sweat, used to confirm a diagnosis of cystic fibrosis. The drug pilocarpine is introduced into the skin by iontophoresis to stimulate the sweat glands and induce sweating. The sweat is collected and tested.

sycosis barbae (*syn* barber's itch) a pustular folliculitis of the beard area in men.

sycosis nuchae a folliculitis at the nape of the neck.

symbiosis *n* a relationship between two or more organisms in which the participants are of mutual aid and benefit to one another. ⇒ antibiosis *ant* — **symbiotic** *adj*.

symblepharon *n* adhesion of the lid to the eyeball.

Syme's amputation amputation just above the ankle joint. Provides an endbearing stump.

symmetrical family a family where household tasks are evenly divided between women and men. ⇒ family.

sympathectomy *n* surgical excision or chemical blockade of part of the sympathetic nervous system.

sympathetic chain a paired chain of ganglia joined by nerve fibres. Running either side of the vertebral column it extends from the cervical to the lumbar region. This arrangement enables sympathetic nerves (which only have thoracolumbar outflow) to supply a larger area of the body. Also known as the paravertebral ganglia.

sympathetic nervous system *n* part of the peripheral nervous system (PNS), it describes the division of the autonomic nervous system (ANS) consisting of a chain of ganglia (joined by nerve fibres) on either side of the vertebral column and nerve fibres having thoracolumbar outflow. Opposing the parasympathetic nervous system its actions are usually concerned with stimulation, the flight or fight response which includes dilation of pupil and bronchi, increased heart rate and cessation of digestion. Catecholamine hormones, adrenaline (epinephrine) and noradrenaline (norepinephrine), from the adrenal medulla, augment the effects of the sympathetic system. ⇒ parasympathetic nervous system. → sympathetic chain.

sympatholytic *n* an antagonist. A drug which opposes or blocks the effects of the sympathetic nervous system, e.g. propranolol, a nonselective beta (β)-adrenoceptor antagonist. ⇒ alpha (α)-adrenoceptor antagonist. ⇒ beta (β)-adrenoceptor antagonist.

sympathomimetic *adj* an agonist. Capable of producing changes similar to those produced by stimulation of the sympathetic nerves, e.g. the beta (β)-adrenoceptor agonist salbutamol, ⇒ alpha (α)-adrenoceptor agonist. ⇒ beta (β)-adrenoceptor agonist.

symphisiotomy *n* pubiotomy. Cutting of the connective tissue of the symphysis pubis to facilitate delivery of a baby when caesarian section is impractical or dangerous.

symphysis *n* a type of slightly movable cartilaginous joint where a pad of fibrocartilage separates the two bones. *symphysis pubis* the joint formed by the two pubic bones — **symphyseal** *adj*.

symptom *n* a subjective phenomenon or manifestation of disease. *symptom complex* a group of symptoms which, occurring together, typify a particular disease or syndrome — **symptomatic** *adj*.

symptomatology *n* 1. the branch of medicine concerned with symptoms. 2. the combined symptoms typical of a particular disease.

synapse *n* the gap between the axon of one neuron and the dendrites of another, or the gap between an axon and an effector cell, such as a gland or muscle. Synapses allow nerve impulses to continue across the gap by electrical or more commonly chemical means. Transmission of the nerve impulse across the gap/cleft in a chemical synapse depends upon the release of calcium and a chemical neurotransmitter such as acetylcholine (see Figure 61) — **synaptic** *adj*.

synapsis *n* pairing of homologous chromosomes to form a bivalent during meiosis.

synarthrosis *n* fibrous, immovable joint.

synchondrosis *n* cartilaginous, slightly movable joint formed from the epiphyseal plates of long bones during growth.

synchronized intermittent mandatory ventilation (SIMV) ⇒ mechanical ventilation.

syncope *n* (*syn* faint) literally, sudden loss of strength. Caused by reduced cerebral circulation often following a fright, when vasodilation is responsible. May be symptomatic of cardiac arrhythmia, e.g. heart block.

syncytium *n* a mass of tissue with many nuclei. A tissue where boundaries between individual cells are absent or poorly defined (pseudosyncytium). This arrangement allows the rapid transmission of impulses, contraction waves, etc. across the tissue, such as in myocardial contraction.

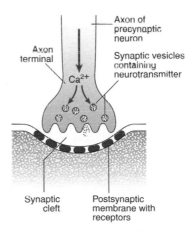

Figure 61 A synapse. (Reproduced from Brooker 1998 with permission.)

syndactyly, syndactylism, syndactylia *n* webbed fingers or toes — **syndactylous** *adj.*

syndrome *n* a group of symptoms and/or signs which, occurring together, produce a pattern or symptom complex, typical of a particular disease. *syndrome X* insulin resistance, hypertension, obesity and hyperlipidaemia associated with NIDDM.

synechia *n* abnormal union of parts, especially adhesion of the iris to the cornea in front, or the lens capsule behind — **synechiae** *pl.*

synergist *n* an agent cooperating with another. One partner in a synergic action, such as a drug or muscle.

synergistic action ⇒ action.

synergy, synergism *n* the harmonious working together of two agents, such as drugs, micro-organisms, muscles etc — **synergic** *adj.*

synkinesis *n* the ability to carry out precision movements.

synovectomy *n* excision of synovial membrane. Frequently used for rheumatoid arthritis.

synovial pertaining to the special membrane, fluid and the joints that contain them. *synovial fluid* viscous lubricating fluid secreted by the synovial membrane lining the cavity of freely movable joints. *synovial joint* diarthrosis. A freely movable joint whose cavity is lined with synovial membrane except for the articulating surfaces. *synovial membrane* ⇒ membrane.

synovioma *n* a tumour of synovial membrane, benign or malignant.

synovitis *n* inflammation of a synovial membrane.

synthesis *n* the process of building complex substances from simpler substances by chemical reactions — **synthetic** *adj.*

syphilide *n* a syphilitic skin lesion.

syphilis *n* a sexually transmitted infection caused by the spirochaete *Treponema pallidum*. It may be congenital or acquired. *acquired syphilis* contracted during sexual contact with an infected person. There are four stages: (a) primary with chancre development and lymphadenopathy; (b) secondary with rash, fever, condylomata lata, mucosal ulcers (snail track) and lymphadenopathy; (c) tertiary may occur after many years with skin lesions such as gumma; (d) quaternary with cardiovascular and nervous system involvement. ⇒ neurosyphilis. *congenital syphilis* transmitted from mother to fetus via the placenta. The affected infant may exhibit certain characteristic features which include: rash, abnormal teeth and keratitis — **syphilitic** *adj.*

syringe *n* a device for injecting, instilling or withdrawing fluids.

syringomyelia *n* an uncommon, progressive disease of the nervous system, beginning mainly in early adult life. Cavitation and surrounding fibrous tissue reaction, in the upper spinal cord and brainstem, interfere with sensation of pain and temperature, and sometimes with the motor pathways. The characteristic symptom is painless injury, particularly of the exposed hands. Touch sensation is intact. ⇒ Charcot's joint.

syringomyelocele *n* a severe form of spina bifida. The central canal is dilated and the thinned out posterior part of the spinal cord is in the hernia.

systematic desensitization a technique that utilizes classical conditioning to treat phobias and anxiety. ⇒ conditioning. ⇒ desensitization.

systematic review *n* a systematic approach to literature reviews (published and unpublished material) that reduces random errors and bias.

Système International d'Unités (International System of units) system of measurement used for scientific, technical and medical purposes in most countries. It consists of seven base units: metre, kilogram, kelvin, second, mole, ampere and candela, and various derived units, e.g. pascal, becquerel etc.

systemic *adj* relating to the body as a whole. ⇒ circulation.

systemic inflammatory response syndrome (SIRS) *n* see Box – Systemic inflammatory response syndrome/multiple organ dysfunction syndrome. ⇒ multiple organ dysfunction syndrome.

systemic lupus erythematosus (SLE) *n* a connective tissue disease with auto-antibodies and immune complexes affecting many body systems. The aetiology is multifactorial with genetic, immunological, environmental (sunlight,

Systemic inflammatory response syndrome/multiple organ dysfunction syndrome

Systemic inflammatory response syndrome (SIRS) and multiple organ dysfunction syndrome (MODS) frequently coexist in critically ill patients and are commonly seen conditions in intensive care units. Previously, septic shock, sepsis or septicaemia were terms used to describe the clinical scenario of pyrexia, tachycardia, tachypnoea and deranged white cell count. It was then discovered that a number of other factors, i.e. in the complete absence of infection, could also precipitate the same clinical features, including trauma, reduced perfusion, major burns and pancreatitis. This resulted in the adoption of the term SIRS. Regardless of the cause, SIRS results in a response of the inflammatory system which is unnatural, in that it is exaggerated and not localized, causing widespread physiological derangement and damage.

MODS describes alteration of organ function that is significant enough to require intervention to maintain body function and stability. MODS may be as a result of SIRS or following a direct insult. MODS was previously known as multiple

organ failure or multisystem organ failure. The physiological damage is an accumulative result of: the inflammatory response; mediator, toxin and enzyme production; reduced perfusion and reduced oxygen delivery to the cells.

Organ systems commonly affected are: the lungs – acute respiratory distress syndrome (ARDS) where mechanical ventilation is usually required; the kidneys – acute tubular necrosis where haemofiltration is required; and the cardiovascular system where fluids and inotrope drugs are needed.

Other organ systems can also be affected. The central nervous system with confusion, encephalopathy and neuropathy; the coagulation system as shown by disseminated intravascular coagulation (DIC); the gastrointestinal system with pancreatitis, reduced motility and ulceration; and the hepatobiliary system with liver dysfunction and acalculous cholecystitis.

Further reading
American College of Chest Physician/Society of Critical Care Medicine. 1992 Consensus Conference: definitions for sepsis and organ failure and guidelines for the use of innovative therapies in sepsis. Critical Care Medicine, 20: 864–74

drugs) and a possible infective element. It affects the skin, joints, kidneys, lungs, heart and blood vessels. The presentation depends on areas affected, but may include: pyrexia, alopecia, skin changes, rash (typically butterfly-shaped on the face) pleurisy, thickening pericarditis, arthritis and renal damage. Occurs most commonly in younger women. Management may include: corticosteroids, immunosuppressive drugs, plasma exchange and system specific treatment as required.

systemic vascular resistance *n* the resistance against which the left ventricle must eject blood into the systemic circulation. SVR is predominantly influenced by the degree of vasoconstriction in the peripheral arterioles. ⇒ peripheral resistance.

systole *n* the contraction phase of the cardiac cycle when the heart contracts. ⇒ diastole — **systolic** *adj* pertaining to systole. ⇒ blood pressure.

systolic murmur a cardiac murmur occurring between the first and second heart sounds due to valvular disease, e.g. mitral systolic murmur.

T

T_3 *abbr* triiodothyronine.

T_4 *abbr* thyroxine.

tabes *n* wasting away. *tabes dorsalis* is a variety of neurosyphilis in which the posterior (sensory) roots of the spinal cord are infected with *Treponema pallidum*. Results in 'lightening pains', loss of proprioception, staggering gait and Charcot's joint. ⇒ locomotor ataxia — **tabetic** *adj*.

taboo behaviours banned by individual societies, such as incest.

taboparesis *n* paralysis arising from neurosyphilis.

tachycardia *n* rapid heart rate (in excess of 100 beats per minute in adults). ⇒ arrhythmia. ⇒ paroxysmal atrial tachycardia. ⇒ supraventricular tachycardia.

tachyphasia *n* extreme rapidity of flow of speech, occurring in some mental disorders.

tachypnoea *n* abnormally rapid respiratory rate — **tachypnoeic** *adj*.

tactile *adj* pertaining to the sense of touch.

taenia *n* a flat band. *taenia coli* three flat bands of longitudinal muscle fibres running the length of the large intestine. They are shorter than the large intestine and produce puckering or haustrations.

Taenia *n* a genus of flat, parasitic worms; cestodes or tapeworms. *Taenia saginata* larvae present in infested, undercooked beef; the commonest species in Britain. In humans (the definitive host) the worm matures in the intestinal lumen and the adult tapeworm, which has four suckers on the scolex, is able to attach itself to the gut wall. *Taenia solium* resembles *Taenia saginata* but has hooklets as well as suckers. Commonest species in Eastern Europe. The larvae are ingested in infested, undercooked pork; humans can also be the intermediate host for this worm by ingesting eggs which, developing into larvae in the stomach, pass via the bowel wall to reach organs, and there develop into cysts. In the brain these may give rise to epilepsy. ⇒ cysticercosis. ⇒ Echinococcus. ⇒ tapeworm.

taeniacide *n* an agent that destroys tapeworms — **taeniacidal** *adj*.

taeniafuge *n* an agent that expels tapeworms.

Takayasu's disease ⇒ 'pulseless' disease.

talc a naturally occurring soft white powder, consisting of magnesium silicate.

talipes *n* clubfoot. Any of a number of deformities of the foot and ankle, often congenital. *talipes calcaneus* heel projected downwards. *talipes equinus* heel lifted from the ground. *talipes valgus* eversion, the foot turned outwards. *talipes varus* inversion, the foot turned inwards. Combinations of these four basic types also exist, e.g. *talipes equinovarus*.

talus *n* the second largest bone of the ankle, situated between the tibia proximally and the calcaneus distally, thus directly bearing the weight of the body.

tampon a plug used in the nose, vagina or other orifice to absorb blood or secretions. *tampon shock syndrome* ⇒ toxic shock syndrome.

tamponade *n* the surgical use of tampons to control haemorrhage or absorb secretions. ⇒ cardiac tamponade.

tapeworm *n* cestodes. Humans are infected by eating contaminated undercooked meat (beef or pork). ⇒ Taenia. Or from undercooked fish contaminated with *Diphyllobothrium latum* (the tapeworm found in fish). Treatment is with the anthelmintic praziquantel. Cats and dogs are the definitive host for the tapeworm *Dipylidium caninum* which occasionally infects humans. ⇒ proglottis.

tapôtement *n* (*syn* tapping) massage manipulations in which the hands strike, or percuss, the body alternately and rhythmically; used to eliminate secretions, as in postural drainage, and in an invigorating massage; *beating* with loosely clenched fists, *clapping* with clapped hands producing a deep-toned sound, *hacking* with the ulnar (little finger side) borders of the hands and fingers, and *pounding* with the ulnar sides of loosely clenched fists.

tapping *n* 1. ⇒ aspiration. 2. ⇒ tapôtement.

tardive dyskinesia a disorder characterized by repeated involuntary movements of limbs, trunk and face. May be seen as a side effect of treatment with the typical neuroleptics, especially the phenothiazines. ⇒ parkinsonism.

target cells *npl* abnormal red cells that are flat with a pale ring around a central mass of haemoglobin and an outer ring of haemoglobin. They are seen in haemoglobinopathies, liver and spleen disease.

tarsalgia *n* pain in the foot.

tarsometatarsal *adj* pertaining to the tarsal and metatarsal region.

tarsoplasty *n* any plastic operation to the eyelid.

tarsorrhaphy *n* suturing of the lids together in order to protect the cornea, or to allow healing of an abrasion.

tarsus *n* 1. the seven small bones of the ankle. 2. the thin elongated plates of dense connective tissue found in each eyelid, contributing to its form and support — **tarsal** *adj*.

tartar *n* the deposit, calculus, which forms on the teeth.

task *n* a part or stage of an activity.

taste *n* the chemical sense of gustation. It is closely linked with smell. *taste buds* specialized sensory receptors found on the tongue, epiglottis and pharynx. They are sensitive to four basic tastes: sweet, bitter, sour and salty. Taste changes with normal aging and can be distorted, particularly after cancer treatment.

taxonomy *n* biological classification.

Tay-Sachs' disease an inherited lipid storage disease with accumulation of the GM$_2$ganglioside (carbohydrate-rich sphingolipid) within the nervous system, caused by a deficiency of the enzyme βN-acetylhexosaminidase. It results in mental deterioration, blindness and death. The autosomal recessive gene is most commonly carried by people of Ashkenazic Jewish origins. The alternative name is gangliosidosis.

Tay's choroiditis ⇒ choroiditis.

T-bandage used to hold a dressing on the perineum in position.

TBI *abbr* ⇒ total body irradiation.

TCA *abbr* tricyclic antidepressants.

T-cell *n* a lymphocyte (thymus dependent) responsible for cell-mediated immunity. ⇒ lymphocyte.

T-cytotoxic or killer cells *n* T cells that are activated by T-helper cells and which circulate in the blood and lymphatic systems, searching for the body cells displaying antigens to which they have been sensitized (also called T8 or CD8 cells). Main target are virus infected cells but also attack cells infected by intracellular bacteria.

T-delayed hypersensitivity cell *n* T-cells involved with macrophages and other T-cells in chronic inflammation and cell-mediated delayed hypersensitivity (also known as T4 or CD4 cells).

team nursing a method of care delivery designed to provide maximum continuity of patient-centred care. A small team of nurses, working together but led by one registered nurse, is responsible and accountable for the assessment, planning and implementation of the care of a particular group of patients for the length of time they require care in a particular setting. It differs from patient allocation or primary nursing in that it is based on the belief that a small group of nurses working together can give better care than if working individually, using the skills of all the team members to the benefit of each patient, but retaining continuity of care. Effective verbal and written communication between the team members is vital. ⇒ named nurse. ⇒ primary nursing.

tears *npl* the secretion formed by the lacrimal gland. They contain the bactericidal enzyme lysozyme.

technetium (Tc) *n* a radioactive element. The isotope ^{99m}Tc produced from molybdenum is used in radionuclide scanning (imaging).

TEDs *acr* ThromboEmbolic Deterrents. ⇒ antiembolic.

teeth *npl* the structures used for mastication. In humans, the first teeth (milk or deciduous teeth) are called *first or primary dentition* and are normally 20 in number. They erupt between five to six months and two and a half years (see Figure 62A). The adult, permanent teeth are known as the *second or secondary dentition* and are normally 32 in number. They start to replace the deciduous teeth at about six years, and the process is nearly complete by twelve years of age with only the third molars (wisdom teeth), if they erupt, appearing between eighteen and twenty five (see Figure 62B). *bicuspid teeth* ⇒ bicuspid. *canine* or *eye teeth* have a sharp fang-like edge for tearing food. ⇒ canine. *incisor teeth* have a knife-like edge

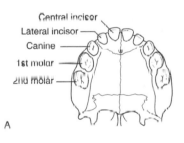

Central incisor
Lateral incisor
Canine
1st molar
2nd molar

A

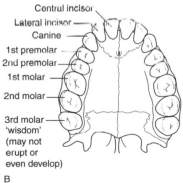

Central incisor
Lateral incisor
Canine
1st premolar
2nd premolar
1st molar
2nd molar
3rd molar 'wisdom' (may not erupt or even develop)

B

Figure 62 A First dentition. B Second dentition. (Reproduced from Brooker 1996 with permission.)

for biting food. ⇒ incisors. *molar* and *premolar teeth* have a squarish termination for chewing and grinding food. ⇒ molar teeth. ⇒ premolar teeth. *wisdom teeth* are the last four molar teeth, one at either side of each jaw. ⇒ Hutchinson's teeth. ⇒ tooth.

teething discomfort, often associated with the signs of inflammation, during the eruption of teeth in infants.

tegument *n* the skin or covering of the animal body.

telangiectasis *n* dilatation of the capillaries on a body surface. *hereditary haemorrhagic telangiectasis* inherited as an autosomal dominant condition, it gives rise to telangiectasia and aneurysms on the fingertips, the face, nasal passages and gastroinestinal tract.

telencephalon part of the developing brain above the diencephalon, it forms the cerebrum.

teletherapy *n* treatment using a source of radiation that is remote from the patient, e.g. X-rays, cobalt-60 (^{60}Co). ⇒ linear accelerator — **teletherapeutically** *adv.*

telomeres *npl* protective covering present on the ends of chromosomes. They normally prevent chromosomal damage during cell division, but after 50 or so divisions the telomeres no longer function properly. This eventually leads to genetic disruption and cell death. ⇒ apoptosis.

telophase the last stage of mitosis and meiosis.

temperament *n* the habitual mental attitude of the individual.

temperature *n* ⇒ body temperature. ⇒ clinical thermometer. ⇒ clinical thermometry.

temple *n* that part of the head lying between the outer angle of the eye and the top of the earflap.

temporal *adj* relating to the temple. *temporal bones* one on each side of the head below the parietal bone, containing the middle ear. *temporal lobe* cerebral lobe containing the auditory and olfactory cortex. *temporal lobe epilepsy* ⇒ epilepsy.

temporomandibular *adj* pertaining to the temporal region or bone, and the mandible. *temporomandibular joint* the synovial joint between the mandible and the temporal bone.

temporomandibular joint syndrome (TMJ) pain in the region of the temporomandibular joint, frequently caused by malocclusion of the teeth, resulting in malposition of the condylar heads in the joint and abnormal muscle activity, and by bruxism. There may be clicking and impaired jaw movement.

TEN *abbr* toxic epidermal necrolysis. ⇒ toxic.

Tenckhoff catheter a silicone-coated tube with spaced perforations in the last 7 cm of the tube, suitable for continuous ambulatory peritoneal dialysis.

tendon *n* a firm, white, fibrous inelastic cord which attaches muscle to bone — **tendinous** *adj.*

tendonitis *n* inflammation of a tendon.

tenesmus *n* painful, ineffectual straining to empty the bowel or bladder.

tenoplasty a reconstructive operation on a tendon — **tenoplastic** *adj.*

tenorrhaphy *n* the suturing of a tendon.

tenosynovitis *n* inflammation of the tendon sheath. The causes include: mechanical irritation, metabolic abnormalities and rheumatoid arthritis.

tenotomy *n* division of a tendon.

TENS *acr* transcutaneous electrical nerve stimulation.

tentorial *adj* pertaining to the tentorium. *tentorial herniation* a bulging of brain tissue into the tentorium resulting from raised intracranial pressure.

tentorium cerebelli *n* a fold of dura mater between the cerebrum and cerebellum. Damage during birth may result in haemorrhage.

teratogen *n* any agent capable of disrupting embryonic or fetal development and growth, and producing malformation. Classified as drugs, e.g. thalidomide, cytotoxic drugs, anticonvulsants, antithyroid drugs, tetracyclines etc; poisons, e.g. alcohol; radiation; micro-organisms, e.g. rubella, syphilis, toxoplasmosis etc; environmental pollutants and rhesus and thyroid antibodies. Also dysmorphogenic — **teratogenic** *adj* — **teratogenicity, teratogenesis** *n.*

teratology *n* the scientific study of teratogens and their mode of action — **teratologically** *adv.*

teratoma *n* a tumour of embryonic origin, most commonly found in the ovaries and testes, the majority being malignant. It is a common cancer in young men aged 20–40 years, but responds well to treatment if detected early. → testicular — **teratomatous** *adj.*

terminal hair *n* coarse, pigmented hair of the scalp and eyebrows.

termination of pregnancy (TOP) *n* an induced therapeutic abortion which fulfils the criteria of the relevant legislation, e.g. Abortion Act 1967 (amended 1990). The methods employed depend upon the stage of gestation and include: an oral progesterone agonist (mifepristone) with vaginal prostaglandin used as an alternative to surgical termination (within 49 days of the LMP), suction evacuation, dilatation and curretage and prostaglandins or other substances administered transcervically, abdominally in the amniotic sac or intravenously.

tertian recurring every 48 hours. ⇒ malaria

tertiary *adj* third in order. *tertiary care* hospital care in a specialized, regional centre, e.g. specializing in cardiac surgery or cancer treatment. → primary health care. ⇒ secondary care. *tertiary prevention* ⇒ disease prevention.

testicle *n* ⇒ testis

testicular *adj.* pertaining to the testicle. *testicular cancer* is a major contributor to young male mortality but, if detected early, the cancer is eminently curable. A risk factor is undescended testes, therefore surgery is usually recommended to reduce the risk of malignancy. The cancer is characterized by a firm, but painless mass in the scrotum. Treatment is usually surgical removal of the testis and spermatic cord (radical orchidectomy) followed by radiation or cisplatin based chemotherapy. ⇒ seminoma. ⇒ teratoma. *testicular self examination* currently advocated to check for the appearance of lumps or irregularities which may be signs of testicular tumour. After a bath or shower to relax the scrotal skin, roll each testicle with the hand from the same side of the body gently between the thumb and fingers to feel any deviation from normal.

testis *n* a male gonad. One of two glandular bodies contained in the scrotum of the male; they form spermatozoa and also the

male sex hormones. ⇒ spermatogenesis. ⇒ testosterone. *undescended testis* the organ remains within the bony pelvis or inguinal canal and fails to migrate to scrotum. ⇒ cryptorchism — **testes** *pl.*

testosterone *n* the major androgen, a steroid hormone derived from cholesterol. It is produced by the testes and is responsible for the development of the male secondary sexual characteristics and reproductive functioning. Used therapeutically to treat male sexual underdevelopment, some menstrual problems and breast tumours in the female.

test-tube baby one produced by in vitro fertilization. First achieved in 1978.

tetanus *n* 1. (*syn* lockjaw) disease caused by the bacterium *Clostridium tetani*, an anaerobic spore-forming bacteria which is commensal in the gut of humans and domestic animals, found in manure, soil and dust. The organism enters through penetrating wounds contaminated with soil. In neonates the organism may gain entry via the umbilical cord stump. Its powerful exotoxin affects motor nerves causing muscle spasm, convulsions and rigidity. Active immunization with tetanus toxoid is available as part of the routine programme: in conjunction with diphtheria and pertussis, as regular booster doses and at times of increased risk. Passive immunization with tetanus immunoglobulin is also available — opisthotonos. ⇒ risus sardonicus. ⇒ trismus. 2. In muscle contraction, the summation which increases force by increasing the frequency of stimulation to the maximum to produce a sustained contraction — **tetanic** *adj*

tetany *n* condition of muscular hyperexcitability in which mild stimuli produce cramps and spasms in the hands and feet (carpopedal spasm). It is due to hypocalcaemia or in alkalosis where the amount of available calcium is reduced. Causes include hypoparathyroidism, rickets, hyperventilation and excessive ingestion of alkalis. ⇒ Chvostek's sign. ⇒ Trousseau's sign.

tetracoccus *n* coccal bacteria arranged in cubical packets of four.

tetracyclines *npl* a group of broad spectrum antibiotics, e.g. doxycycline, minocycline, oxytetracycline etc. They are effective against bacteria, rickettsiae, chlamydiae, some amoeba and mycoplasma, and are used to treat respiratory, skin and genital infections. There are problems with super-infection causing gastrointestinal disturbances and vitamin B deficiency, and bacterial resistance. The tetracyclines are deposited in bone and teeth and should not be prescribed during pregnancy, lactation or childhood because they can cause discolouration of the permanent teeth and bone deformities.

tetradactylous *adj* having four digits on each limb.

tetralogy *n* a series of four. *tetralogy of Fallot* ⇒ Fallot's tetralogy.

tetraplegia *n* (*syn* quadriplegia) paralysis of all four limbs — **tetraplegic** *adj*.

tetravalent having a valence of four, such as carbon.

thalamotomy *n* usually operative (stereotactic) destruction of a portion of thalamus. Can be done for intractable pain.

thalamus *n* a paired collection of grey matter at the base of the cerebrum. Sensory impulses from the whole body pass through on their way to the cerebral cortex — **thalamic** *adj*.

thalassaemias *npl* a group of inherited haemoglobinopathies resulting from reduced or absent synthesis of globin chains producing haemolytic anaemia. They are inherited in an autosomal recessive pattern. They are seen most commonly in populations around the Mediterranean and in South East Asia. There are three main types: (a) *β thalassaemia major* Cooley's anaemia. A severe form where individuals are unable to synthesize β chains of adult haemoglobin (HbA). It is caused by inheriting two abnormal genes (homozygous). There is severe anaemia, jaundice and hepatomegaly and splenomegaly. Treatment includes bone marrow transplant, blood transfusion, folic acid and chelating agents, such as desferrioxamine for iron overload; (b) *β thalassaemia minor* denotes the carrier state where the individual has only one abnormal gene (heterozygous). They may be asymptomatic or have mild microcytic, hypochromic anaemia with target cells and punctate basophilia; (c) *α thalassaemia* a form where individuals are unable to synthesize α chains because the genes (4) have been deleted. The effects

depend on the number of genes deleted; i.e. one gene has no effects, two genes deleted cause mild anaemia, if three genes are deleted the person has haemoglobin H disease requiring treatment with folic acid, and stillbirth occurs where all four are deleted. ⇒ anaemia.

thallium (Tl) *n* a metallic element. Many of its compounds are highly toxic. A radioactive isotope is used in radionuclide scanning.

thanatology *n* the scientific study of death, including its aetiology and diagnosis.

The Health Act (1999) in the UK an act of Parliament passed in June 1999 that implements the measures within the white paper *The New NHS* and the variations in Scotland, Wales and Northern Ireland.

theca *n* an enveloping sheath, especially of a tendon or the dura mater of the spinal cord. *theca folliculi* the hormone secreting covering of a developing ovarian follicle — **thecal** *adj*.

T-helper cell *n* a T-cell that activates B cells to release antibodies and killer T-cells to destroy cells having a specific antigenic makeup (also called T4 or CD4 cells).

thenar *adj* pertaining to the palm of the hand and the sole of the foot. *thenar eminence* the palmar eminence below the thumb.

therapeutic index *n* an indicator of the difference between the drug dose that produces a therapeutic effect and the dose which causes toxic effects. It alerts the prescriber to the safety margin for a particular drug, but the therapeutic index will vary between people who all process drugs in an individual way.

therapeutic touch 1. a non-touch therapy directed towards initiating the body's self-healing mechanisms. It is based upon the idea that healing occurs through an energy field interaction between therapist and client. The aim is to rebalance or repattern an individual's energy towards health or well-being. **2.** the use of touch as a therapeutic intervention in its own right, rather than as a necessary function of nursing activity. It may involve therapeutic massage or simply appropriate bodily contact, indicating empathy and support.

therapeutics *n* the branch of medical science dealing with the treatment of disease — **therapeutically** *adv*.

therapy *n* treatment of a physical or psychological condition. ⇒ occupational therapy. ⇒ physiotherapy. ⇒ speech and language therapy.

thermal *adj* pertaining to heat. *thermal dilution* a method of measuring cardiac ouput.

thermistor *n* a device able to detect minute temperature changes.

thermogenesis *n* the production of heat — **thermogenetic** *adj*.

thermography *n* the detection of minute differences in temperature over regions of the body using an infrared device (thermograph) sensitive to radiant heat. It is a technique that can be used to study blood flow disorders, the viability of skin grafts and the detection of malignancies, such as breast cancer, that show up as a 'hot spot'.

thermolabile *adj* capable of being easily altered or discomposed by heat.

thermolysis *n* heat-induced chemical dissociation. Dissipation of body heat — **thermolytic** *adj*.

thermometer *n* device for measuring and recording temperature. ⇒ clinical thermometer — **thermometric** *adj*.

thermophile *n* a bacterium accustomed to growing at a high temperature between 55–90°C. They are not human pathogens — **thermophilic** *adj*.

thermoregulation the maintenance of body temperature within a normal range, through homeostaic processes.

thermostable *adj* unaffected by heat. Remaining unaltered at a high temperature, which is usually specified **thermostability** *n*.

thermotherapy *n* heat treatment, such as warm compresses. ⇒ hyperthermia.

thiamine *n* vitamin B_1. Also known as thiamin. Coenzyme concerned in the metabolism of carbohydrates, fat and alcohol. It is present in many foods, e.g. milk, offal, wholegrain cereals, and their products, fortified breakfast cereals, eggs, fruit and vegetables. Deficiency results in beri-beri. ⇒ Korsakoff's psychosis, syndrome. ⇒ Wernicke's encephalopathy.

thiazide diuretics *npl* diuretics that act upon the first part of the distal tubule of the nephron, e.g. bendroflumethiazide (bendrofluazide). They reduce sodium and chloride reabsorption, this increases the excretion of water, sodium and chloride, and, in addition, potassium is lost and calcium conserved. They are used in hypertension, mild heart failure, oedema and in nephrogenic diabetes insipidus.

Thiersch skin graft a very thin skin graft.

thioxanthines a group of neuroleptic drugs, e.g. flupentixol (flupenthixol).

third intention → wound healing.

thirst *n* awareness of a dry mouth; part of the symptomatology of dehydration. ⇒ mouth care.

Thomas' splint also called Thomas' ring splint. A metal splint shaped like a hair pin, with a padded ring at the opened end. Used to immobilize fractures of the lower limb during transportation and to facilitate skeletal traction.

thoracentesis *n* aspiration of the pleural cavity.

thoracolumbar pertaining to the thoracic and lumbar regions.

thoracoplasty *n* an operation on the thorax in which the ribs are resected to allow the chest wall to collapse; previously used in the treatment of tuberculosis prior to the development of antitubercular drugs.

thoracoscope *n* an instrument which can be inserted into the pleural cavity through a small incision in the chest wall, to permit inspection of the pleural surfaces and division of adhesions by electric diathermy. *thoracoscopic sympathectomy* destruction of the sympathetic ganglia with low power unipolar diathermy through laparoscopic incisions. Performed for hyperhidrosis of the hands, axillae and feet, and for advanced Raynaud's phenomenon — **thoracoscopy** *n*.

thoracostomy *n* opening into the chest wall for the drainage of the fluid.

thoracotomy *n* surgical opening of the chest.

thorax *n* the chest cavity. Contains the heart, lungs and great vessels — **thoracic** *adj* pertaining to the thorax. *thoracic cage* bony framework which protects the thoracic organs and provides attachment for muscles. *thoracic cavity* the chest or thorax. *thoracic duct* large lymphatic vessel commencing in the abdomen as the cisterna chyli which collects lymph draining from the legs, abdomen, left side of chest and head and left arm. It returns fluid to the left subclavian vein. *thoracic inlet syndrome* ⇒ cervical rib.

Thorn initiative training programme see Box – Thorn initiative training programme.

threadworm *n Enterobius vermicularis.* Tiny threadlike worms that infest the intestine. ⇒ enterobiasis.

threonine *n* an essential (indispensable) amino acid.

thrill *n* vibration as perceived by the sense of touch.

thrombectomy *n* surgical removal of a thrombus from within a blood vessel.

thrombin *n* active enzyme generated from prothrombin (factor II). The extrinsic and intrinsic coagulation pathways lead to production of thrombin which converts soluble fibrinogen into insoluble fibrin. ⇒ coagulation.

thromboangiitis *n* clot formation within an inflamed vessel. *thromboangiitis obliterans* ⇒ Buerger's disease.

thromboarteritis *n* inflammation of an artery with clot formation.

thrombocyte *n* (*syn* platelet) small, disc-shaped cellular fragment present in the blood. Plays a vital part in the clotting of blood. ⇒ coagulation.

thrombocythaemia *n* a condition in which there is an increase in circulating blood platelets. Some of these may function abnormally. There may be bruising, bleeding and venous and arterial thrombosis. ⇒ myeloproliferative disorders. ⇒ thrombocytosis.

thrombocytopenia *n* a reduction in the number of platelets in the blood which can result in spontaneous bruising and prolonged bleeding after injury. Causes include: idiopathic, drugs, infections, malignancy affecting the marrow and radiation — **thrombocytopenic** *adj.*

thrombocytosis *n* an increase in the number of platelets in the blood. It can arise as a reaction to malignancy, chronic inflammatory conditions and with chronic blood loss, or as part of thrombocythaemia and other myeloproliferative disorders.

thromboembolic deterrents (TEDs) ⇒ antiembolic hose.

thromboembolism *n* embolism or clot which detaches from a blood clot and is carried to another part of the body in the bloodstream to block a blood vessel, such as pulmonary embolism arising from a deep vein thrombosis in the leg — **thromboembolic** *adj* pertaining to thromboembolism. ⇒ antiembolic

thromboendarterectomy *n* removal of a thrombus and atheromatous plaques from an artery. ⇒ endarterectomy.

thromboendarteritis *n* inflammation of the inner lining of an artery with clot formation.

thrombogenic *adj* capable of clotting blood — **thrombogenesis, thrombogenicity** *n.*

Thorn initiative training programme
Supported by funding from the Sir Jules Thorn Charitable Trust, the Thorn initiative training programme was established in 1991, in London, at the Institute of Psychiatry and at Manchester University. The programme provided mental health practitioners with the opportunity to develop skills in psychosocial interventions and management strategies to help reduce relapse rates. Initial evidence from the original programmes confirmed that training can enhance practitioners' knowledge and attitudes towards clients and their relatives who in turn derive significant benefits from the psychological interventions they receive.

In the light of the aforementioned outcomes and other recommendations made, more Thorn training initiatives have been developed, for example, South Bank, Greenwich, City, Nottingham, Bournemouth, Cheltenham, York University.

Further reading
Department of Health. 1994 Working in partnership: Report of the review of mental health nursing. HMSO, London
Department of Health. 1995 Report of a clinical standards advisory group on schizophrenia. Vol. I. HMSO, London
Gamble C 1997 The Thorn nursing programme: its past, present and future. Mental Health Care. I (3): 95–97
Sainsbury Centre for Mental Health. 1997 Pulling together: The future roles and training of mental health staff. The Sainsbury Centre for Mental Health, London

thrombokinase *n* ⇒ thromboplastin.

thrombolytic *adj* pertaining to disintegration of a blood clot. *thrombolytic therapy* ⇒ fibrinolytic — **thrombolysis** *n* ⇒ fibrinolysis.

thrombophlebitis *n* inflammation of a vein associated with the formation of a thrombus. *thrombophlebitis migrans* recurrent episodes of thrombophlebitis in various sites — **thrombophlebitic** *adj*.

thromboplastin *n* (*syn* thrombokinase) a lipoprotein released from damaged tissue which initiates the extrinsic coagulation pathway. *activated partial thromboplastin time (APTT)* a test of blood coagulation function. *intrinsic thromboplastin* produced by the interaction of several factors during the clotting of blood. Much more active than tissue thromboplastin. *tissue thromboplastin* factor III of blood coagulation, it joins with other factors to activate factor X needed for the formation of a fibrin clot.

thrombosis *n* intravascular clotting. Thrombus formation in the heart or blood vessels. ⇒ cavernous sinuses. ⇒ cerebral thrombosis. ⇒ coronary thrombosis. ⇒ deep vein thrombosis — **thrombotic** *adj*.

thrombosthenin *n* contractile protein in blood platelets that causes clot retraction.

thromboxanes *npl* part of a group of regulatory lipids derived from arachidonic acid (fatty acid). Released from platelets they cause vasospasm and platelet aggregation during platelet plug formation (a process of haemostasis). ⇒ leukotrienes. ⇒ prostaglandins.

thrombus *n* an intravascular blood clot at its site of formation — **thrombi** *pl*.

thrush *n* fungal infection. ⇒ candidiasis.

Thudichum's speculae a range of nasal speculae for examination of the anterior part of the nose.

thymectomy *n* surgical excision of the thymus gland.

thymine *n* nitrogenous base derived from pyrimidine. A component of deoxyribonucleic acid (DNA).

thymocytes *n* cells found in the dense lymphoid tissue in the lobular cortex of the thymus gland — **thymocytic** *adj*.

thymoma *n* a tumour arising in the thymus gland — **thymomata** *pl*.

thymopoietin *n* thymic peptide hormone. ⇒ thymus.

thymosins *n* thymic peptide hormone. ⇒ thymus.

thymus *n* a two-lobed lymphoid gland situated in the mediastinum, lying behind the breast bone and extending upward as far as the thyroid gland. It is well developed in infancy and attains its greatest size towards puberty; the lymphoid tissue is then replaced by fatty tissue. It consists of lymphoid tissue containing many lymphocytes. The thymic hormones, thymosin and thymopoietin, stimulate the proper development of T-lymphocytes which are concerned with cell mediated immunity. Various autoimmune conditions, such as myasthenia gravis, result from pathological activity of this gland — **thymic** *adj*.

thyrocalcitonin *n* ⇒ calcitonin.

thyroglobulin *n* a colloidal substance produced and stored in the thyroid follicles. With iodine molecules it forms thyroxine.

thyroglossal *adj* pertaining to the thyroid gland and the tongue. *thyroglossal cyst* a retention cyst around the hyoid bone associated with the persistence of an embryonic structure, the thyroglossal duct. *thyroglossal duct* the embryonic passage from the thyroid gland to the back of the tongue where its vestigial end remains. In this area thyroglossal cyst or fistula can occur.

thyroid *n* pertaining to the thyroid. *thyroid antibody test* the presence and severity of autoimmune thyroid disease is diagnosed by the levels of thyroid antibody in the blood. *thyroid cartilage* largest cartilage of the larynx (Adam's apple). *thyroid or thyrotoxic crisis* a sudden increase in metabolic rate characterized by tachycardia, pyrexia and dehydration. A very uncommon event seen after thyroidectomy in a person inadequately prepared with antithyroid drugs or infection in a person with hyperthyroidism. *thyroid gland* an endocrine gland consisting of two lobes, one either side of the trachea. It secretes three hormones: triiodothyronine (T_3) and thyroxine (T_4) under pituitary control which stimulate metabolism, and calcitonin from the follicular cells which regulates calcium and phosphate homeostasis. ⇒ hyperthyroidism. ⇒ hypothyroidism. *thyroid hormones* ⇒

calcitonin. ⇒ iodine. ⇒ thyroxine. ⇒ triiodothyronine. *thyroid-stimulating hormone (TSH)* pituitary hormone that stimulates the secretion of the thyroid hormones: thyroxine and triiodothyronine. *thyroid-stimulating hormone assay* radioimmunoassay of the level of thyroid-stimulating hormone in the serum. Useful in diagnosing mild hypothyroidism.

thyroidectomy *n* operation to remove part or all of the thyroid gland.

thyroiditis *n* inflammation of the thyroid gland. Autoimmune thyroiditis (Hashimoto's disease). ⇒ Riedel's thyroiditis.

thyrotoxicosis *n* ⇒ hyperthyroidism — **thyrotoxic** *adj.*

thyrotrophic *adj* describes a substance which stimulates the thyroid gland, e.g. thyrotrophin (thyroid stimulating hormone, TSH) secreted by the anterior pituitary gland.

thyroxine (T₄) *n* the principal hormone of the thyroid gland. It is essential for metabolism and development. It has four atoms of iodine and is formed from the amino acid tyrosine. Thyroxine is used in the treatment of hypothyroidism. ⇒ triiodothyronine.

TIA *abbr* transient ischaemic attacks.

tibia *n* the shin-bone; the larger of the two bones in the lower part of the leg; it articulates with the femur, fibula and talus — **tibial** *adj.*

tibiofibular *adj* pertaining to the tibia and the fibula.

tic *n* purposeless, involuntary, spasmodic muscular movements and twitchings. Usually affecting the face and neck.

tic douloureux (trigeminal neuralgia) ⇒ trigeminal.

tick *n* a blood-sucking parasitic arthropod. Some of them are involved in the transmission of relapsing fever, Rocky Mountain spotted fever and typhus, etc.

tidal volume the volume of air which passes in and out of the lungs in normal quiet breathing.

Tietze syndrome costochondritis which is self-limiting and of unknown aetiology. It is characterized by pain that may mimic that of myocardial ischaemia. Treatment is symptomatic, e.g. pain relief.

tight junction *n* a type of junction between cells, formed from an adaptation of the plasma membrane. It is so designed to prevent leakage from cells and the movement of molecules between cells. Tight junctions are important in the structure of the blood-brain barrier.

tincture *n* the solution of a drug in alcohol.

tine test skin test for tuberculosis. A multiple puncture device with several tines is used to inject tuberculin into the skin. The reaction is read in 48–72 h using a grading system. ⇒ Heaf test.

tinea *n* ringworm. A group of skin infections caused by a variety of dermatophyte fungi, e.g. *Trichophyton, Epidermophyton* and *Microspoum*. Each is named after the area of the body affected, i.e. *tinea barbae* sycosis barbae, ringworm of the beard area. *tinea capitis* ringworm of the head. *tinea corporis (syn* circinata) ringworm of the body. *tinea cruris (syn* dhobie itch) ringworm of the groin. *tinea pedis* ringworm of the foot (athlete's foot). *tinea unguium* ringworm affecting the nails.

tinnitus *n* a buzzing, thumping, roaring or ringing sound in the ears. A feature of conditions that include Menière's disease and otosclerosis.

TIPSS *abbr* transjugular intrahepatic portasystemic stent shunting.

tissue *n* a collection of specialized cells or fibres of similar function, e.g. muscle, connective, nervous and epithelium. *tissue culture* cells and tissues grown under artificial conditions. *tissue repair* ⇒ healing. ⇒ wound dressings. *tissue respiration* ⇒ respiration.

tissue plasminogen activator (t-PA) *n* chemical required to activate plasminogen. It is produced by endothelium lining the blood vessels.

titration *n* volumetric analysis by aid of standard solutions to determine the concentration of a substance in solution.

titre *n* a standard of concentration per volume, as determined by titration. Unit of measure used to assess antibody concentration in serum.

TLC *abbr* total lung capacity.

TLS *abbr* tumour lysis syndrome.

TMJ *abbr* temporomandibular joint syndrome.

TNF *abbr* tumour necrosis factor.

TNM classification *abbr* tumour, node and metastasis. ⇒ staging.

tobacco amblyopia ⇒ amblyopia.

tocography *n* process of recording uterine contractions (pressure changes) during labour, using a tocograph. ⇒ cardiotocography.

tocolytics *npl* agents that relax uterine muscle, e.g. the selective beta (β)-adrenoceptor agonists: terbutaline, ritodrine. They have limited use in the inhibition of preterm labour.

tocopherols *npl* group of compounds with vitamin E activity which includes the important α-tocopherols. They are widely distributed in many foods, e.g. cereals, egg yolk, vegetable oils and nuts. They are important as antioxidants in biological membranes.

tocotrienols *npl* group of compounds with vitamin E activity. They act as antitoxidants in biological membranes but less potent than tocopherols.

togaviruses *n* a family of RNA viruses that include the rubella virus and several spread by insects, e.g. yellow fever. ⇒ arboviruses.

tolerance *n* ability to resist the application or administration of a substance, usually a drug. ⇒ drug tolerance. *exercise tolerance* exercise accomplished without pain or marked breathlessness. American Heart Association's classification of functional capacity: Class I no symptoms on ordinary effort; Class II slight disability on ordinary effort (in Britain it is usual to subdivide this class into Class IIa, able to carry on with normal housework under difficulty, and Class IIb, cannot manage shopping or bedmaking except very slowly); Class III marked disability on ordinary effort which prevents any attempt at housework; Class IV symptoms at rest or heart failure.

tomography *n* a technique of using X-rays to create an image of a specific, thin layer through the body (rather than the whole body) — **tomographically** *adv*.

tone *n* the normal, healthy state of tension. Also describes a quality of sound.

tongue *n* the mobile muscular organ contained in the mouth and attached to the hyoid bone; it is concerned with speech,

mastication, swallowing and taste. ⇒ strawberry tongue.

tonic *adj* 1. used to describe a state of sustained or continuous muscular contraction. ⇒ clonic. ⇒ epilepsy. 2. popular term for a medicine that increases general well-being.

tonography *n* recording pressure of blood or intraocular pressure. ⇒ glaucoma. *carotid compression tonography* normally occlusion of one common carotid artery causes an ipsilateral fall of intraocular pressure. Used as a screening test for carotid insufficiency.

tonometer *n* an instrument for measuring intraocular pressure.

tonsillectomy *n* removal of the palatine tonsils. *tonsillectomy position* the three-quarters prone position to prevent inhalation (aspiration) pneumonia and asphyxiation.

tonsillitis *n* inflammation of the tonsils.

tonsilloliths *npl* concretions arising in the body of the tonsil.

tonsillopharyngeal *adj* pertaining to the tonsils and pharynx.

tonsils *npl* small patches of lymphoid tissue located around the pharynx. Forming part of body defences they contain macrophages and are a site for lymphocyte proliferation. *lingual tonsils* located under the tongue. *nasopharyngeal tonsils* found on the posterior wall of the nasopharynx. When enlarged they are known as adenoids. *palatine tonsils* located in the oropharynx, one on each side embedded in the fauces between the palatine arch. ⇒ Waldeyer's ring — **tonsillar** *adj*.

tooth *n* one of the structures in the mouth used to cut, tear and chew food. Each tooth consists of a root embedded in the jaw and an exposed crown; the bulk of the tooth is made of dentine surrounding a pulp chamber/cavity; the exposed portion is covered with enamel. ⇒ teeth.

TOP *acr* termination of pregnancy.

tophus *n* a small, hard concretion forming on the ear lobe, on the joints of the phalanges, etc in gout — **tophi** *pl*.

topical *adj* describes the local application of such things as anaesthetics, drugs, powders and ointments to skin and mucous membrane.

topography *n* a description of the regions of the body — **topographically** *adv*.

torsion *n* twisting.

tort a civil wrong, excluding breach of contract. It includes: negligence, trespass (to person, goods or land), nuisance, breach of statutory duty and defamation.

torticollis *n* (*syn* wryneck) contraction of one sternocleidomastoid muscle. The head is flexed and drawn towards the contracted side, with the face rotated over the other shoulder. It may result from damage during birth. After birth, it can occur acutely as a result of pain and muscle spasm associated with neck injuries. People with certain neurological problems can also develop painful spasmodic torticollis and other abnormal postures.

total body irradiation (TBI) used in the treatment of some cancers, e.g. diseases of the haemopoietic tissue. Usually carried out prior to bone marrow transplantation.

total lung capacity (TLC) *n* volume of air in the lungs following greatest inspiratory effort.

total parenteral nutrition (TPN) provision of the entire nutritional requirements using solutions containing all essential nutrients, administered by the intravenous route using a central vein catheter. ⇒ enteral feeding. ⇒ parenteral feeding.

total patient care 1. a therapeutic programme for a patient to which members of several professional groups contribute. **2.** a term used to signify inclusion of the physical, psychological and social dimensions of the person who requires nursing. ⇒ holistic.

Total Quality Management a whole organization approach to quality. It aims to ensure quality at every interface and improve effectiveness and flexibility throughout the organization. Everyone working in the organization is expected to take responsibility for quality.

touch *n* one of the special senses. There is increasing awareness of the value of therapeutic touch in nursing. ⇒ therapeutic touch.

Tourette's syndrome *n* Gilles de la Tourette syndrome. It is characterized by rude gestures and obscene speech. ⇒ coprolalia. ⇒ copropraxia.

tourniquet *n* an apparatus for the compression of the blood vessels of a limb. Designed for compression of a main artery to control bleeding. It is also often used to obstruct the venous return from a limb and so facilitate the withdrawal of blood from a vein. Tourniquets vary from a simple rubber band to a pneumatic cuff.

Townsend index an index that uses indirect measures of social deprivation, such as car ownership. These sort of factors are not always applicable to certain areas; for example, not owning a car in a remote rural area is more likely to indicate social deprivation than lack of a car in a city with good public transport.

toxaemia *n* a generalized poisoning of the body by the products of bacteria or damaged tissue — **toxaemic** *adj*.

toxic *adj* poisonous, caused by a poison. *toxic epidermal necrolysis* a serious condition characterized by severe skin rash, hyperpigmentation and extensive skin shedding. It can occur in response to serious drug reactions, staphylococcal infection, systemic illness, and it can be idiopathic. *toxic shock syndrome (TSS)* a potential complication of tampon use, but it does occur in men and nonmenstruating women. It is a rare occurrence caused by the toxins produced by the bacterium *Staphylococcus aureus* found at various sites including the perineal area in healthy people. Bacterial contamination of the tampon occurs and the bacteria multiply within the vagina. The toxins enter the blood to cause pyrexia, vomiting and diarrhoea, a rash, and sometimes life-threatening hypovolaemic shock. Prevention involves: hand hygiene, use of lowest absorbency tampons appropriate for the loss, changing tampons every four hours, using a sanitary pad at night, remembering to remove the tampon at the end of menstruation and reporting illness occurring during menstruation. Women with a history of TSS are advised to use sanitary pads rather than tampons.

toxicity *n* the quality or degree of being poisonous or toxic. See Box – Toxicity and cancer treatment.

toxicology *n* the science dealing with poisons, their mechanisms of action and antidotes to them — **toxicologically** *adv*.

Toxicity and cancer treatment

Toxicity refers to the degree that a substance is poisonous or to the resulting physical condition that follows exposure to a toxin. In cancer care it refers to the side-effects of chemotherapy and radiotherapy treatment. In most cases the higher the treatment dose the greater number of cancer cells that will be killed (Peterson and Goodman 1997), however cancer treatments cannot differentiate between healthy and cancer cells so patients inevitably suffer a degree of treatment-related toxicity. Cancer treatments predominantly affect rapidly dividing tissue therefore the most common toxicity is bone marrow depression, manifesting as anaemia, neutropenia and thrombocytopenia. Gastrointestinal toxicities include nausea and vomiting, anorexia, mucositis, stomatitis and diarrhoea, whilst the skin can be affected by rashes and blistering. Hair loss is common with some chemotherapy agents and head irradiation. Overall the patient who has received cancer therapies may suffer with extreme fatigue that persists for long periods of time. The nature and degree of toxicity depends on the drug administered, the treatment schedule, dose, route of administration and the individual response of the patient, and may be short or long term. The nursing role focuses on informing the patient, proactive care, monitoring for toxicity and providing support.

Reference
Peterson J, Goodman M 1997 Principles of chemotherapy. In: Gates R A, Fink R M (eds) *Oncology Nursing Secrets*. Hanley and Belfus, Philadelphia, pp 39–55

toxicomania *n* WHO definition: Periodic or chronic state of intoxication produced by repeated consumption of a drug harmful to the individual or society. Characteristics are: (a) uncontrollable desire or necessity to continue consuming the drug and to try to get it by all means; (b) tendency to increase the dose; (c) psychological and physical dependency as a result.

toxin *n* a poison, usually of bacterial origin that damages or kills cells. ⇒ endotoxin. ⇒ exotoxin.

Toxocara *n* genus of nematode roundworm of the cat and dog, particularly *Toxocara canis* which can infest humans. ⇒ toxocariasis.

toxocariasis infestation with *Toxocara*. Infestation occurs by eating with hands soiled from contact with affected animals, especially puppies. The ova can exist for several months in soil contaminated by infected faeces from dogs or cats. The worms cannot become adult in humans (incorrect host) so the larval worms wander through the body before dying. The migrating larvae cause problems in the liver and the eye, which are characterized by: fever, hepatomegaly and the possibility of blindness. Treatment is with the anthelmintic albendazole.

toxoid *adj* bacterial toxin treated to remove its pathogenicity while retaining its antigenicity. Used to produce active immunity to diseases such as diphtheria and tetanus.

Toxoplasma *n* a genus of protozoon, e.g. *Toxoplasma gondii*. The definitive host is the domestic cat and other felines and rodents are the intermediate host. It can cause serious infections in humans and other mammals, e.g. cattle, pigs and sheep can be infected. → toxoplasmosis.

toxoplasmosis *n* infection with *Toxoplasma gondii*. Infected animals contaminate the environment with faeces containing cysts. Humans are usually infected by handling infected animals, by environmental contact, such as during gardening, playing in contaminated sand and cleaning cat litter trays, or by eating undercooked meat. Most people are asymptomatic or may have a mild illness with fatigue and aching muscles. It causes serious disease in immunocompromised individuals, e.g. AIDS patients, who develop encephalitis and eye involvement. Patients having organ transplants may acquire toxoplasmosis from the donated organ, which is reactivated because of their immunosuppressed state. Women who have primary toxoplasmosis during pregnancy can pass the disease to the fetus via the placenta (vertical transmission). This is extremely serious and can result in stillbirth or the birth of an infant with central nervous system problems, e.g. microcephaly or hydrocephaly, convulsions or paralysis, or liver damage with jaundice, thrombocytopenia and purpura or eye involvement, e.g. choroidoretinitis. Infants who survive may have learning disability and develop liver cirrhosis, encephalitis and blindness.

TPHA *abbr Treponema pallidum* haemagglutination assay.

TPN *abbr* total parenteral nutrition.

TPR *abbr* temperature, pulse and respiration.

TQM *abbr* Total Quality Management.

trabeculae *npl* the fibrous bands or septa projecting into the interior of an organ, e.g. the spleen; they are extensions from the capsule surrounding the organ — **trabecular** *adj*.

trabeculotomy *n* operation for glaucoma. It aims to create a channel through the trabecular meshwork from the canal of Schlemm to the angle of the anterior chamber. ⇒ trabeculae.

trace elements elements required by the body in minute amounts for metabolic processes and homeostasis, e.g. copper, cobalt, manganese, fluorine, etc. ⇒ minerals.

tracer *n* a substance or instrument used to gain information about metabolic processes. Radioactive tracers can be used to investigate thyroid disease or possible brain tumours.

trachea *n* (*syn* windpipe) the air passage from the larynx to the bronchi. It is about 115 mm long and about 25 mm wide. It is fibrocartilaginous, consisting of incomplete C-shaped rings of cartilage, and is lined with ciliated mucous membrane — **tracheal** *adj* pertaining to the trachea. *tracheal intubation* insertion of an endotracheal tube into the trachea to secure a patent airway.

tracheitis *n* inflammation of the trachea; most commonly the result of a viral infection such as the common cold. ⇒ acute bronchitis.

trachelorrhaphy *n* operative repair of a uterine cervical laceration.

tracheobronchial *adj* pertaining to the trachea and the bronchi.

tracheobronchitis *n* inflammation of the trachea and bronchi. ⇒ acute bronchitis.

tracheo-oesophageal *adj* pertaining to the trachea and the oesophagus. *tracheo-oesophageal fistula* a congenital abnormality that usually occurs in conjunction with oesophageal atresia. The fistula usually connects the distal oesophagus to the trachea.

tracheostomy *n* an opening in the trachea, for establishment of a safe airway with the insertion of a plastic or metal tube. The tube may be inserted directly through an incision made between the tracheal cartilages, percutaneously or as a minitracheostomy. It may be performed to facilitate mechanical ventilation, where there is a respiratory obstruction, for the removal of secretions and following laryngectomy. May be temporary or permanent. (See Figure 63) — **tracheostome** *n*.

tracheotomy vertical slit in the anterior wall of the trachea at the level of the third and fourth cartilaginous rings. ⇒ tracheostomy.

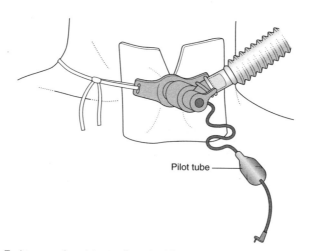

Pilot tube

Figure 63 Tracheostomy tube and dressing. (Reproduced from Nicol et al 2000 with permission.)

trachoma *n* contagious chlamydial kerato-conjunctivitis caused by *Chlamydia trachomatis*, a common cause of blindness in hot dry regions of the world. Infection may occur by contact, during birth an infant may become infected fom vaginal discharge, or from unhygienic use of fomites. Also called trachoma inclusion conjunctivitis (TRIC) — **trachomatous** *adj*.

trachoma inclusion conjunctivitis (TRIC) *n* serious keratoconjunctivitis caused by *Chlamydia trachomatis*, which also causes urethritis and genital tract disease. ⇒ conjunctivitis. ⇒ trachoma.

traction *n* a drawing or pulling. A steady pulling exerted on some part of the body, such as the skeleton or skin, by means of a series of weights, cords and pulleys in conjunction with frames and splints. *skeletal traction* applied on a bone by means of a pin or wire passed through a lower fragment. This keeps the fractured bone in the correct position and overcomes muscle contraction. Tongs are used to apply skull traction in cervical spine injuries. *skin traction or extension* achieved by applying weights to foam or extension plaster attached to the skin. This type of straight pull traction can be used prior to internal fixation of fractures of the femoral neck. ⇒ Balkan beam. ⇒ Braun's frame. ⇒ Bryant's traction. ⇒ halopelvic traction. ⇒ Hamilton-Russell traction. ⇒ Milwaukee brace. ⇒ Thomas' splint.

tractotomy *n* incision of a nerve tract for relief of intractable pain.

tragus *n* the projection in front of the external auditory meatus — **tragi** *pl*.

trait *n* an inherited or developed mental or physical individual characteristic.

trance *n* a term used for hypnotic sleep and for certain self-induced stuporous states.

tranquillizers *npl* drugs used to relieve anxiety or combat psychotic symptoms without significant sedation. ⇒ anxiolytics. ⇒ neuroleptics.

transabdominal *adj* through the abdomen, as the transabdominal approach for nephrectomy — **transabdominally** *adv*.

transactional analysis a form of psychotherapy predicated on the theory that inter-relationships between people can be analysed in terms of transactions with each other as representing 'child', 'adult' and 'parent'. The goal is to give the adult ego decision-making power over the child and parent egos.

transaminases ⇒ aminotransferases.

transamniotic *adj* through the amniotic membrane and fluid, as a transamniotic transfusion of the fetus for haemolytic disease.

transcription *n* the first stage in protein synthesis. Involves the transfer of genetic information (the base sequence) from DNA to mRNA. ⇒ translation.

transcultural nursing in multicultural societies, a nurse's knowledge of such factors as the customs and perceptions of health, ill health, diet, birth, circumcision, contraception, marriage, religion and death, can alert him or her to actual or potential health needs or problems.

transcutaneous *adj* through the skin, e.g. absorption of applied drugs or the monitoring by pulse oximetry. *transcutaneous electrical nerve stimulation (TENS)* a noninvasive method of pain relief; four electrodes are placed on either side of the spine to apply a mild electric current from a battery-operated apparatus which can be controlled by the patient.

transdermal through the skin. A method of drug administration using skin patches, gels and creams. Drugs administered in this way, e.g. nitrates and hormone replacement therapy, avoid first pass metabolism in the liver.

transducer *n* a device that transforms one form of energy into another to facilitate its electrical transmission.

transduction the term used to describe the sexual reproductive process whereby genetic material is transferred between bacteria by a bacteriophage. Allows genes for drug resistance to pass between bacterial strains. ⇒ conjugation. ⇒ transformation.

transection *n* the cutting across or mechanical severance of a structure.

transfer RNA (tRNA) *n* ⇒ ribonucleic acid.

transference in psychotherapy or psychoanalysis, the unconscious transfer of a client's emotions regarding a significant person in their life to the therapist. *countertransference* the conscious or unconscious emotional reaction of therapist to client.

transferrin *n* a protein to which iron is bound for safe transport around the body.

transformation the term used to describe the sexual reproductive process whereby genetic material is transferred between bacteria by being absorbed through the cell wall. Allows genes for drug resistance to pass between bacterial strains. ⇒ conjugation. ⇒ transduction.

transfrontal *adj* through the frontal bone; an approach used for hypophysectomy.

transfusion *n* the introduction of fluid into the tissue or into a blood vessel. *blood transfusion* the intravenous replacement of lost or destroyed blood by compatible human blood. Also used for severe anaemia with deficient blood production. Fresh blood from a donor may be used, but usually stored blood donated by healthy volunteers is used. It can be given as whole blood, or as plasma-reduced blood ('packed-cell' transfusion). Various components of blood can be transfused as required by the situation, such as platelet transfusion for thrombocytopenia. Before transfusion, the donor red cells are crossmatched against the patient's serum to ensure compatibility and prevent mismatched blood transfusions that result in severe reactions and may be fatal. ⇒ autologous blood transfusion. ⇒ blood groups. *intrauterine transfusion* may occasionally be used for a fetus endangered by Rhesus incompatibility. Rh-negative blood is transfused directly into the abdominal cavity of the fetus, on one or more occasions. This enables the induction of labour to be postponed until a time more favourable to fetal welfare.

transient ischaemic attacks (TIA) sudden attacks of cerebral ischaemia caused by emboli or platelet masses, where symptoms last less than 24 hours. They may be followed by complete recovery, but minor infarction does occur. May precede a more severe stroke. Management involves identifying and reducing risk factors, and long-term aspirin. Carotid endarterectomy can reduce the risk of TIA and stroke in patients with carotid artery disease. ⇒ drop attacks. ⇒ endarterectomy. ⇒ vertebrobasilar insufficiency.

translation *n* the second stage of protein synthesis. It involves tRNA and rRNA translating the base sequence required to make a new protein from amino acids within the ribosomes. ⇒ transcription.

translocation *n* transfer of a segment of a chromosome to a different site on the same chromosome (shift) or to a different one. Can be a direct or indirect cause of congenital abnormality.

translucent *adj* intermediate between opaque and transparent.

translumbar *adj* through the lumbar region. Route used for injecting aorta prior to aortography.

transmethylation *n* a process in the metabolism of amino acids in which a methyl group is transferred from one compound to another.

transmural *adj* through the wall, e.g. of a cyst, organ or vessel.

transonic *adj* allowing the passage of ultrasound.

transperitoneal *adj* across or through the peritoneal cavity. ⇒ dialysis. ⇒ laparoscopy.

transplacental *adj* through the placenta — **transplacentally** *adv*.

transplant *n* customarily refers to the surgical operation of grafting an organ, which has been removed from a person who has been declared brain-dead, or from a living relative. If the recipient's malfunctioning organ is removed and the transplant is placed in its bed, it is referred to as an *orthotopic transplant* (e.g. liver and heart). If the transplanted organ is not placed in its normal anatomical site, the term *heterotopic transplant* is used — **transplantation** *n* ⇒ graft.

transposition *n* 1. displacement of any internal organ to the other side of the body. *transposition of the great vessels* a congenital abnormality of the heart in which the aorta and the pulmonary artery are transposed, with the aorta arising from the right ventricle and the pulmonary artery from the left ventricle. 2. the operation which attaches a piece of tissue to one part of the body from another, delaying complete separation until it has become established in its new location. 3. in genetics, the movement of genetic material between chromosomes.

transrectal *adj* through the rectum — **transrectally** *adv*.

trans-sexualism situation where a person feels that they are of the opposite gender to their biological gender. This may lead to considerable conflict, with severe psychological, emotional and social problems. Hormonal and surgical modification, following counselling, may eventually be undertaken to change the individual's ender to conform with his or her wishes.

trans-sphenoidal *adj* through the sphenoid bone; an approach used for hypophysectomy.

transthoracic *adj* across or through the chest, as in transthoracic needle biopsy of a lung mass, transthoracic echocardiography.

transudate *n* a fluid that has passed out through a membrane or from a tissue. An example is ascitic fluid in the peritoneal cavity.

transurethral *adj* by way of the urethra. ⇒ prostatectomy.

transvaginal *adj* through the vagina, as an incision to drain the rectouterine pouch, transvaginal injection into a tumour, pudendal block or culdoscopy — **transvaginally** *adv*.

transventricular *adj* through a ventricle. Term used mainly in cardiac surgery — **transventricularly** *adv*.

transverse across. *transverse colon* ⇒ colon. *transverse sinuses* venous channels draining blood from the brain.

transvesical *adj* through the bladder, by custom referring to the urinary bladder. ⇒ prostatectomy — **transvesically** *adv*.

trapezium *n* one of the carpals or wrist bones.

trapezius *n* large triangular muscle of the neck and thorax.

trapezoid *n* one of the carpals or wrist bones.

trauma *n* 1. bodily injury. 2. emotional shock — **traumatic** *adj*.

traumatologist *n* a surgeon who specializes in traumatology.

traumatology *n* the branch of surgery dealing with injury caused by accident — **traumatologically** *adv*.

trematodes *n* a class of parasitic flukes which include many human pathogens such as *Schistosoma* a blood fluke causing schistosomiasis.

tremor *n* involuntary trembling. *intention tremor* an involuntary tremor which only occurs on attempting voluntary movement; a characteristic of multiple sclerosis.

trench foot (*syn* immersion foot) occurs in frostbite or other conditions of exposure where there is deprivation of local blood supply and secondary bacterial infection.

Trendelenburg's operation ligation of the long saphenous vein in the groin at its junction with the femoral vein. Used in cases of varicose veins.

Trendelenburg's position lying on an operating or examination table, with the head lowermost and the legs raised.

Trendelenburg's sign a test of the stability of the hip, and particularly of the ability of the hip abductors (gluteus medius and minimus) to steady the pelvis upon the femur. Normally, when one leg is raised from the ground, the pelvis tilts upwards on that side, through the hip abductors of the standing limb. If the abductors are inefficient (e.g. in poliomyelitis, severe coxa vara and developmental dysplasia of the hip), they are unable to sustain the pelvis against the body weight and it tilts downwards instead of rising.

trephine *n* an instrument with sawlike edges for removing a circular piece of tissue, such as the cornea or skull.

Treponema *n* a genus of slender spirochaete (spiral-shaped) bacteria which are actively motile. Best visualized with dark-ground illumination. Cultivated in the laboratory with great difficulty. *Treponema pallidum* is the causative organism of syphilis; *Treponema pertenue* the spirochaete that causes yaws; *Treponema carateum* the spirochaete that causes pinta — **treponemal** *adj*.

Treponema pallidum haemagglutination assay (TPHA) *n* a specific serological test for syphilis.

treponemal enzyme-linked immunosorbent assay *n* a specific serological test for syphilis. ⇒ ELISA.

treponematosis *n* the term applied to the treponemal diseases.

treponemicide *n* lethal to *Treponema* — **treponemicidal** *adj*.

trespass against the person a wrongful direct interference with another person. Harm does not have to be proved; it includes both assault and battery.

Trexler isolator a flexible film, negative pressure, bed isolator for dangerous infections such as viral haemorrhagic fevers or immunocompromised patients. They are so designed as to allow healthcare staff to provide care without having any contact with the patient.

triacylglycerol *n* ⇒ triglyceride.

triage *n* a system of priority classification of patients in any emergency situation. *triage nurse* the nurse given this specific responsibility in an accident and emergency department.

triangular bandage useful for arm slings, for securing splints, in first aid work and for inclusive dressings of a part, as a whole hand or foot.

TRIC *abbr* trachoma inclusion conjunctivitis.

tricarboxylic acid cycle (TCA) *n* ⇒ Krebs' cycle.

triceps *n* muscles with three heads. *triceps brachii* muscle on the back of the upper arm that extends the elbow. *triceps skin fold* a measurement of the mid-arm fat layer. Used as part of nutritional assessment.

trichiasis *n* abnormal ingrowing eyelashes causing irritation from friction on the cornea.

Trichinella *n* a genus of parasitic nematode worms. *Trichinella spiralis* is a parasite of pigs and rats, and causes human disease. ⇒ trichinosis.

trichinosis *n* also called trichiniasis. Infestation with the roundworm *Trichinella spiralis*, a parasite of pigs and rats. The infestation is caused by eating undercooked pig meat. The female worms living in the small bowel produce larvae which invade the body and, in particular, form cysts in skeletal muscles. It is characterized by diarrhoea, nausea, colic, fever, facial oedema, muscular pains and stiffness. Migration of larvae can cause encephalitis or myocarditis. Treatment is with anthelmintics, such as tiabendazole (thiabendazole).

Trichomonas *n* a genus of motile protozoan parasites that infect humans. *Trichomonas vaginalis* produces vaginitis in females and genitourinary infection in males. The organism is easily recognized by wet microscope preparations of the vaginal discharge. ⇒ protozoa. ⇒ trichomoniasis.

trichomoniasis *n* infection caused by the protozoon *Trichomonas vaginalis*. It is usually, but not exclusively, sexually transmitted. In females it may cause a foul-smelling, frothy green-yellow vaginal discharge with inflammation and intense itching, but may be asymptomatic. It may be asymptomatic in males, but can cause urethritis. ⇒ vaginitis.

trichophytosis *n* infection with a species of the fungus *Trichophyton*, e.g. ringworm of the hair or skin.

trichuriasis *n* infestation with the worm *Trichuris trichiura*, caused by ingesting contaminated soil or food. There are few symptoms but a heavy infestation may cause diarrhoea with bleeding, anaemia and rectal prolapse. Treatment is with an anthelmintic, e.g. mebendazole.

Trichuris *n* a genus of parasitic nematode worms. *Trichuris trichiura* the whipworm. ⇒ trichuriasis.

tricuspid *adj* having three cusps. *tricuspid valve* that between the right atrium and ventricle of the heart. ⇒ atrioventricular.

tricyclic antidepressants (TCAs) *npl* group of widely prescribed antidepressants, e.g. clomipramine, amitriptyline etc. They act by blocking the uptake of the neurotransmitters 5-hydroxytryptamine (serotonin) and noradrenaline (norepinephrine). They take 2–4 weeks to be effective and have unpleasant side-effects that include a dry mouth, constipation and urinary retention.

trigeminal *adj* triple; separating into three sections, e.g. the trigeminal nerves, the fifth and largest cranial nerves, which divide into three divisions: ophthalmic, maxillary and mandibular. They are sensory to the skin of the face, the tongue and teeth, and contain motor fibres that innervate the muscles of chewing. *trigeminal neuralgia* spasms of excruciating pain (of unknown aetiology) in the distribution of the trigeminal nerve. May be precipitated by simple stimuli, such as chewing or cold air on the face. Also known as tic douloureux.

trigger finger a condition in which the finger can be actively bent but cannot be straightened without help; usually due to a thickening on the tendon which prevents free gliding.

triglyceride *n* a lipid comprising a glycerol molecule and three fatty acids. The major source of stored energy in the body as the adipose tissue. Also known as triacylglycerol. ⇒ fat.

trigone *n* a triangular area, especially applied to the bladder base, bounded by the openings of the ureters at the back and the urethral opening at the front — **trigonal** *adj*.

triiodothyronine (T₃) *n* a thyroid hormone required for growth and metabolism. Formed from the conversion of thyroxine, it contains three atoms of iodine.

trimester *n* a period of 3 months. Used particularly to distinguish the three trimesters of pregnancy.

triple duty nurse in the UK, where there are many outlying rural areas, one nurse is employed. Qualified as a community nurse, a midwife and a health visitor.

triple test blood test offered to pregnant women. It measures alpha-fetoprotein, unconjugated oestriol and total hCG in maternal serum and is used early in pregnancy to predict the estimated risk of conditions such as Down's syndrome and neural tube defects. For example, a reduced alpha-fetoprotein and oestriol with an elevated hCG would indicate an increased risk for Down's syndrome. This test is a fairly crude screening of risk which is calculated in conjunction with age, gestation and weight. The test for Down's syndrome does produce false positives and negatives. Where the risk prediction is 1 in 250, the couple are offered more specific tests. ⇒ amniocentesis. ⇒ chorionic villus sampling.

triple vaccine contains diphtheria, tetanus and pertussis (whooping cough) antigens. Given as part of the routine immunization programme for infants. ⇒ DTPer. ⇒ immunization. ⇒ vaccines.

triplet *n* the three sequential bases in the DNA structure that code for an amino acid in a new polypeptide chain during protein synthesis.

triploid *adj* possessing three chromosomal sets (3n). In the case of humans that would be a chromosome number of 69. ⇒ genome. ⇒ haploid. ⇒ polyploidy.

triquetral *n* one of the carpals or wrist bones.

trismus *n* lockjaw. Spasm in the muscles of mastication, such as that seen in tetanus.

trisomy *n* the presence in triplicate of a chromosome that should normally be present only in duplicate. This increases the chromosome number by one (single trisomy), e.g. to 47 in man. *trisomy 18* ⇒ Edward syndrome. *trisomy 21* ⇒ Down's syndrome.

trivalent in chemistry, a substance with a valence of three.

trocar *n* a pointed rod which fits inside a cannula.

trochanters *npl* two processes, the larger one (*trochanters major*) on the outer, the other (*trochanters minor*) on the inner side of the femur between the shaft and neck; they serve for the attachment of muscles. Also known as greater and lesser trochanters respectively — **trochanteric** *adj*.

trochlea *n* any part which is like a pulley in structure or function — **trochlear** *adj* pertaining to a pulley. *trochlear nerves* the fourth pair of cranial nerves. They supply the muscle that moves the eyeball out and downwards.

trophoblastic tissue the cell layer covering the blastocyst stage of the developing ovum. The trophoblast cells secrete the hormone hCG that maintains the corpus luteum, invade the endometrium to allow ovum implantation and are concerned with the nutrition of the embryo. The trophoblastic tissue eventually forms the placenta.

tropomyosin *n* one of the proteins located in the thin filaments of a muscle myofibril.

troponin *n* one of the proteins located in the thin filaments of a muscle myofibril.

Trousseau's sign a sign of latent tetany: forearm muscle spasm is seen, within 3 to 4 minutes, of inflating a cuff on the upper arm to a pressure greater than systolic blood pressure. ⇒ carpopedal spasm. ⇒ hypocalcaemia.

Trypanosoma *n* a genus of protozoa responsible for human disease, e.g. *Trypansoma brucei gambiense.* ⇒ trypanosomiasis.

trypanosomiasis *n* disease produced by infection with *Trypanosoma*. In humans, this may be with *Trypanosoma rhodesiense* in Central and East Africa, or *Trypanosoma brucei gambiense* which is widely distributed in Central and West Africa, both transmitted by the bite of infected tsetse flies. The bite of the fly is painful with immediate signs of inflammation which returns after about 10 days. The disease caused by *T. brucei gambiense* tends to be chronic over months or years with enlarged lymph nodes and bouts of fever. It then affects the central nervous system to cause headache, confusion, insomnia, daytime sleepiness, altered behaviour, and eventual coma and death. ⇒ sleeping sickness. Infection with *T. rhodesiense* is more acute with a petechial rash, hepatitis, myocarditis, pleural effusion and central nervous system involvement, characterized by altered consciousness, tremors and death. In South America, it is also known as Chaga's disease and is caused by *Trypanosoma cruzi*, transmitted via the faeces of bugs.

trypsin *n* active proteolytic enzyme secreted by the pancreas as a precursor.

trypsinogen *n* inactive form of trypsin. Activated by enterokinase.

tryptophan *n* one of the essential (indispensable) amino acids. The B vitamin nicotinamide is synthesized from tryptophan and it is the precursor substance of serotonin. ⇒ pellagra.

tsetse fly a fly of the genus *Glossina*, the vector of *Trypanosoma* in Africa. The *Trypanosoma* live part of their life cycle in the flies and are transferred to new hosts, including humans, in the salivary juices, when the fly bites for a blood meal.

TSS *abbr* toxic shock syndrome.

tsubos ⇒ meridians.

T-suppressor cell *n* a T-cell that stops or slows the activity of B lymphocytes and other T-cells once the immune response has dealt with the antigen. They normally keep the immune response within appropriate limits (also known as T8 or CD8 cells).

T-tube T-shaped tube which is used to drain the common bile duct after surgery. ⇒ wound drains.

tubal *adj* pertaining to a tube. *tubal abortion* ⇒ abortion. *tubal ligation* tying of both uterine tubes as a means of sterilization. *tubal pregnancy* ⇒ ectopic pregnancy.

tubegauz *n* a soft tubular woven bandage available in a variety of sizes – may be used as a protective covering on limbs or digits.

tubercle *n* 1. a small rounded prominence, usually on bone. 2. the specific lesion produced by *Mycobacterium tuberculosis*.

tuberculide, tuberculid *n* a small lump. Metastatic manifestation of tuberculosis, producing a skin lesion, e.g. papulonecrotic tuberculide, rosacea-like tuberculide.

tuberculin *n* a sterile extract of either the crude old tuberculin or refined PPD (purified protein derivative) products prepared from *Mycobacterium tuberculosis*. Used in skin testing for tuberculosis or prior to BCG. ⇒ Heaf test. ⇒ Mantoux reaction.

tuberculoid *adj* resembling tuberculosis. Describes one of the two types of leprosy.

tuberculoma *n* a walled-off region of caseating tuberculosis, usually large, its size suggesting a tumour.

tuberculosis (TB) *n* a chronic granulomatous infection caused by *Mycobacterium tuberculosis* (human type), an acid-fast bacillus (AFB). Other types include: *M. bovis* (cattle) and atypical mycobacteria, e.g. *M. avium intracellulare (MAI)* and *M. kansasii*. Tuberculosis infection is increasing in: (a) travellers to Africa and Asia; (b) the socially disadvantaged, especially the homeless and malnourished; (c) people with AIDS and those who are immunocompromised or debilitated for some other reason. *bovine tuberculosis* endemic in cattle and transmitted to humans via the ingestion of infected milk. Prevented by the pasteurization of milk, and stringent regulations and controls to deal with infection in dairy herds. *miliary tuberculosis* widespread disease which spreads via the blood to all areas of the body. *multidrug resistant tuberculosis (MDR-TB)* a serious event where the *M. tuberculosis* develops resistance to antituberculosis drugs. It is a particular problem in patients with AIDS and in certain countries, e.g. Russia. *primary tuberculosis* occurring in childhood, there is lung involvement, fever and skin rash. *post primary tuberculosis* the most common form which affects the lung but other sites may be affected. Tuberculosis is charaterized by systemic effects such as fever, night sweats and weight loss, plus those dependent upon the site, e.g. cough in pulmonary disease, haematuria in renal TB and infertility if the uterine tubes are affected. Diagnosis is made on: clinical signs, X-rays, skin tests and the presence of acid-fast bacilli in sputum, urine etc. Treatment is based on antituberculosis drugs in combination over a period of months. The first-line drugs include: rifampicin, ethambutol, isoniazid and pyrazinamide. Where these drugs are ineffective or cause side-effects, patients are prescribed the second-line drugs, e.g. capreomycin, cycloserine and streptomycin. Immunization with BCG is used to protect vulnerable individuals, usually detected by skin testing. ⇒ Heaf test — **tubercular, tuberculous** adj.

tuberculostatic adj inhibiting the growth of Mycobacterium tuberculosis.

tuberosity n a bony prominence.

tuberous sclerosis (syn epiloia) an inherited condition (autosomal dominant) characterized by multiple tumours of the brain with progressive deterioration in mental functioning, facial adenomas and tumours of the retina and kidneys. Epilepsy is an early feature of the disease.

tubo-ovarian adj pertaining to or involving both tube and ovary, e.g. tubo-ovarian abscess.

tubular necrosis acute necrosis of the renal tubules. It is caused by ischaemia as in shock, or toxic chemicals and bacterial toxins. The urine flow is greatly reduced (oliguria) and acute renal failure develops with uraemia and hyperkalaemia.

tubule n a small tube. collecting tubule straight tube in the kidney medulla conveying urine to the kidney pelvis. convoluted tubule coiled tube in the kidney cortex. renal tubule the tubular portion of a nephron. seminiferous tubule ⇒ seminiferous.

tularaemia n an infection caused by Francisella tularensis; transmitted by biting insects and acquired by humans either in handling infected animal carcasses, such as rabbits, or by the bite of an infected insect. Skin ulceration at the inoculation site is followed by painful lymphadenopathy and fever with constitutional upset. Rarely it causes septicaemia with high temperature, limb pain, vomiting, diarrhoea, mental changes and complications that include pneumonia. Treatment is with antibiotic drugs, gentamicin or streptomycin — **tularaemic** adj.

tumescence n a state of swelling; turgidity.

tumor n swelling; usually used in the context of being one of the four classical signs of inflammation, the others being calor, dolor, rubor.

tumour n a swelling. A mass of abnormal tissue which resembles the normal tissues in structure, but which fulfils no useful function and which grows at the expense of the body. Benign, simple or innocent tumours are encapsulated, do not infiltrate adjacent tissue or cause metastases and are unlikely to recur if removed. A malignant tumour is not encapsulated and will infiltrate adjacent tissue and cause metastases. ⇒ cancer. ⇒ tumour marker — **tumorous** adj.

tumour lysis syndrome (TLS) may occur after intensive chemotherapy treatment for some haematological cancers. There is rapid release of cellular breakdown products as the cancer cells are destroyed by the drugs. It is characterized by metabolic problems, e.g. hypocalcaemia, hyperuricaemia, hyperphosphataemia, with renal failure and possibly circulatory and respiratory failure.

tumour marker n a substance detected in the serum that may be associated with the presence of a specific cancer or sometimes nonmalignant diseases. They include: alpha-fetoprotein, carcinoembryonic antigen and prostate specific antigen. They are useful for monitoring the progress of disease and efficacy of treatment, but are of limited use for population screening.

tumour necrosis factor (TNF) n a cytokine that is toxic to cancer cells and activates other leucocytes and increases their killing ability. It is responsible for profound metabolic effects that include: inflammatory responses, pyrexia and weight loss.

tumouricidal any agent that is lethal to cancer cells; ionizing radiation, cytotoxic drugs.

tunica n a lining membrane; a coat. tunica adventitia the outer coat of an artery or vein. tunica intima the endothelial lining of an artery or vein. tunica media the middle muscular coat of an artery or vein. tunica vaginalis the outer covering of the testis and epididymis.

tunnel reimplantation operation a surgical procedure used to reimplant the ureter.

turbinate *adj* shaped like a top or inverted cone. *turbinate bones* or nasal conchae. Three on either side forming the lateral nasal walls. They increase mucosal surface area within the nose and cause air turbulence.

turbinectomy *n* removal of turbinate bones.

turgid *adj* swollen; firmly distended, as with blood by congestion — **turgidity** *n*.

Turner's syndrome ovarian dysgenesis. An anomaly of female sex chromosomes; usually there is only one X chromosome (XO with a total number of chromosomes of 45). It is characterized by underdevelopment of the genital tract and secondary sexual characteristics, short stature, webbed neck, aortic coarctation and other abnormalities.

TURP/TUR *abbr* transurethral resection of prostate. ⇒ prostatectomy.

tussis *n* a cough.

tylosis ⇒ keratosis.

tympanic *adj* pertaining to the tympanum or eardrum. *tympanic cavity* middle ear. *tympanic membrane* ⇒ eardrum. *tympanic thermometer* electronic probe introduced into the external auditory canal to record body temperature.

tympanites, tympanism *n* (*syn* meteorism) abdominal distension due to accumulation of gas in the intestine.

tympanitis inflammation of tympanic membrane, otitis media.

tympanoplasty *n* any reconstructive operation on the middle ear (tympanic membrane or ossicles) designed to improve hearing. Normally carried out to correct damage caused by chronic suppurative otitis media with associated conductive deafness — **tympanoplastic** *adj*.

tympanotomy *n* elevation of eardrum to inspect the middle ear.

tympanum describes either the middle ear cavity or the tympanic membrane (eardrum).

type A behaviours behaviours characterized by high competitiveness resulting in compulsive working schedules; believed by some to be associated with an increased risk of coronary heart disease.

type B behaviours behaviours which display minimal aggression and hostility; not highly competitive and believed to have a lower risk of heart disease.

type I and type II errors in research, a type I error (alpha error) is rejecting a null hypothesis that is true, and a type II error (beta error) is not rejecting a null hypothesis that is false. See Box – Type I and Type II errors.

typhoid fever an infectious enteric fever caused by the bacterium *Salmonella typhi*, transmitted by contaminated food, milk or water. Contamination occurs directly by sewage, indirectly by flies or by faulty personal hygiene. It is commonly associated with a lack of clean water and poor sanitation, but outbreaks occur in other areas, usually by food contamination by carriers. Asymptomatic carriers, harbouring the micro-organism in the gallbladder and excreting it in their stools, are the main source of outbreaks of disease in the UK. The average incubation period is 10–14 days. There is bacteraemia and inflammation of small bowel lymphoid tissue (Peyer's patches)

Type I and Type II errors

The possibility of obtaining the results by chance alone is returned by the *P* value. However small it may be, there is always a finite chance that the results were purely due to chance. A *P* value of 0.05 means that one time in twenty you could expect such a result by chance, or that the null hypothesis is rejected when it is true. The occasions where the data did in fact occur due to chance can be considered to be in error if the *P* value is accepted as showing the null hypothesis is false. This is known as a Type I error.

Type II error is the opposite of Type I error, and is seen when you accept that the results were due to chance, when in fact this is not true, i.e. you accept the null hypothesis when it should be rejected.

Clearly the lower we set the α level (threshold at which we reject the null hypothesis) the more likely are Type II errors, and the less likely there are Type I errors, so a compromise is needed, typically α is set to 0.05.

which ulcerates and may perforate or bleed. The onset is characterized by a 'stepladder' rise in temperature, slow pulse, headache, drowsiness and cough. Later there is a 'rose red' spot rash on the abdomen, splenomegaly and typical pea-soup diarrhoea with abdominal tenderness, delerium and bronchitis. Immunization is available for those travelling to areas where typhoid is endemic; however, it is not a substitute for careful hygiene measures. ⇒ paratyphoid.

typhus *n* ⇒ rickettsial fevers.

tyramine *n* an amine present in several foodstuffs, especially mature cheese, yeast extract, broad beans, bananas and some red wines. It has a similar effect in the body to catecholamines, such as adrenaline (epinephrine); consequently people taking drugs in the monoamine oxidase inhibitor (MAOI) group should not eat these foods, otherwise a dangerously high blood pressure may result.

tyrosine *n* an amino acid. Several hormones are synthesized from tyrosine: the catecholamines adrenaline (epinephrine) and noradrenaline (norepinephrine), and it combines with iodine to form triiodothyronine and thyroxine.

tyrosinosis *n* an inborn error of amino acid metabolism inherited as an autosomal recessive condition. There is abnormal metabolism of phenylalanine into tyrosine. Large amounts of toxic intermediates are excreted in the urine. Leads to severe liver disease.

U

UHBI *abbr* upper hemibody irradiation.

UKCC *abbr* United Kingdom Central Council for Nursing, Midwifery and Health Visiting.

UKU side effect rating scale a scale that measures the side effects of neuroleptics. The scale breaks side effects into distinct groupings: psychic; neurological; autonomic; and other. It also assesses global interference of side effects on daily performance, and includes action planning.

ulcer *n* a break in the continuity of either the mucous membrane or skin from whatever cause, producing a crater or indentation. An inflammatory reaction occurs and, if it penetrates a blood vessel, bleeding ensues. There may be infection. If the ulcer is in the lining of a hollow organ it can perforate through the wall. ⇒ arterial ulcer. ⇒ Curling's ulcer. ⇒ peptic ulcer. ⇒ pressure ulcer (decubitus). ⇒ rodent ulcer. ⇒ venous ulcer.

ulcerative *adj* pertaining to or of the nature of an ulcer.

ulcerogenic *adj* capable of producing an ulcer.

ulna *n* the inner long bone of the forearm — **ulnar** *adj* pertaining to the ulna, such as the artery and nerve.

ultrafiltration filtration under pressure. The use of very fine filters to remove minute particles from a solution, such as the technique used in haemofiltration where the blood is filtered under pressure.

ultrasonography *n* production of a visible image from the use of ultrasound. A controlled beam of sound is directed into the body. The reflected ultrasound is used to build up an electronic image of the various structures of the body. Routinely offered during pregnancy to detect fetal and placental abnormalities. ⇒ ultrasound. *diagnostic ultrasonography* information is derived from echoes which occur when a controlled beam of sound energy crosses the boundary between adjacent tissues of differing physical properties. *real-time ultrasonography* an ultrasound imaging technique involving rapid pulsing to enable continuous viewing of movement to be obtained, rather than stationary images — **ultrasonographically** *adv*.

ultrasound *n* sound waves with a frequency of over 20 000 Hz and inaudible to the human ear. *diagnostic ultrasound* ⇒ ultrasonography — **ultrasonic** *adj* pertaining to sound waves of very high frequency.

ultraviolet rays *n* (UV). Electromagnetic rays of short wavelength outside the visible spectrum.

umbilical cord *n* the cord which connects the fetus to the placenta. It contains two arteries and a vein and gelatinous embryonic connective tissue called Wharton's jelly.

umbilical hernia ⇒ hernia.

umbilicated *adj* having a central depression.

umbilicus *n* (*syn* navel) the abdominal scar left by the separation of the umbilical cord after birth — **umbilical** *adj* pertaining to the umbilicus. *umbilical hernia* ⇒ hernia.

unconscious insensible to stimuli. *unconscious mind* that part of the mind which contains feelings, instincts and experiences of which the individual is not normally aware, although they influence behaviour.

unconsciousness *n* state of being unconscious; insensible. Not responding to stimuli, such as after a stroke or during general anaesthesia. ⇒ Glasgow coma scale.

underclass describes a group who are deprived, disenfranchised and marginalized in society, such as the homeless. ⇒ social exclusion.

underwater seal a closed system of drainage used to drain air and fluid from the pleural space following surgery or trauma and to allow lung expansion after a spontaneous pneumothorax. A chest tube is anchored in the pleural cavity and connected to a long tube which, after passing through a cork, has its other end under water in a bottle. Another short tube through the cork introduces air on to the water surface, thus air can escape from the pleural cavity and bubble through the water, but air cannot enter the pleural cavity, as long as the bottle is lower than the cavity and the integrity of the closed system is maintained. (See Figure 64).

undine *n* a small, thin glass flask used for irrigating the eyes.

undulant fever ⇒ brucellosis.

unemployment *n* unable to gain paid employment. There are two groups to be considered – those who have previously been employed, and school-leavers who have been unable to get a job. It has enormous social consequences. More than one member of a family may be unemployed; there may be inadequate income; unstructured daytime living; lack of purpose and self-esteem; and hopelessness may result as succeeding applications are rejected. These factors, together with many others, contribute to an increase in poor general health, parasuicides, premature deaths and suicides. *structural unemployment* longterm unemployment caused by fundamental changes in the economy and the nature of industry, such as the loss of jobs in mining, defence industry and ship building.

unguentum *n* ointment.

unicellular *adj* consisting of only one cell, such as protozoa.

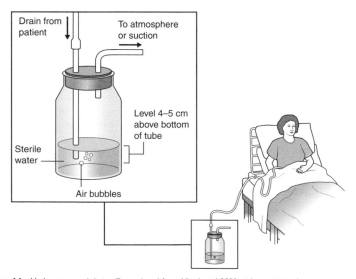

Figure 64 Underwater seal drain. (Reproduced from Nicol et al 2000 with permission.)

unilateral *adj* relating to or on one side only — **unilaterally** *adv*.

uniocular *adj* pertaining to, or affecting, one eye.

uniovular *adj* (*syn* monovular) pertaining to or derived from one ovum, as uniovular twins (identical). ⇒ binovular *ant*.

unipolar depression ⇒ depression.

unit cost an average cost for a specific activity, e.g. a surgical procedure, a diagnostic scan or a home visit. It is calculated by dividing the total cost of the service by the number of outputs.

United Kingdom Central Council (UKCC) for Nursing, Midwifery and Health Visiting the Council was established by an act of Parliament in 1979, and resulted in the formation of the UKCC and the four national boards for England, Northern Ireland, Scotland and Wales. These statutory bodies had certain functions, including the establishment and maintenance of a professional register for all nurses and midwives, the power to remove individuals from the register in cases of misconduct, and the establishment and maintenance of education and training regulations and standards. The UKCC consisted of 60 members from across the relevant professions and with lay membership. Some members being elected to post and others being nominated by the Secretary of State for Health. Following a review of the UKCC in 1999, the UK government recommended that a new and smaller council be established with the end of the four national boards. ⇒ Nursing and Midwifery Council (NMC).

univalent having a valence of one, such as hydrogen.

univariate statistics descriptive statistics that analyse a single variable, such as the mean.

universal precautions *npl* the routine precautions taken during contact, or the possibility of contact, with blood and body fluids, e.g. wearing plastic aprons and gloves. ⇒ infection.

unstable bladder *n* instability of the detrusor muscle leads to powerful contractions of the urinary bladder that cannot be controlled. A common cause of loss of continence with frequency, urgency and urge incontinence.

upper respiratory tract infections (URTI) the upper respiratory tract is the commonest site of infection in all age groups. The infections include the common cold, influenza, rhinitis – usually viral, sinusitis, tonsillitis, laryngitis, pharyngitis, otitis media, croup (acute laryngotracheobronchitis) and acute bronchitis. Care at home is generally symptomatic; rest, analgesia, antipyretics, adequate hydration, steam inhalations (steamy bathroom), humidification and antibiotics only where bacterial infection is present. Complications may include the development of pneumonia, bronchitis, chronic sinusitis, hearing loss, worsening of existing respiratory disease with respiratory failure. URTIs seldom require hospital treatment, with the exception of croup and epiglottitis which can cause asphyxia and death. These patients may require endotracheal intubation or tracheostomy.

urachus *n* the stemlike structure connecting the bladder with the umbilicus in the fetus; in postnatal life it is represented by a fibrous cord situated between the apex of the bladder and the umbilicus, known as the median umbilical ligament. It can persist and give rise to a fistula between the bladder and umbilicus or cyst formation — **urachal** *adj*.

uracil *n* nitrogenous base derived from pyrimidine. A component of ribonucleic acid (RNA).

uraemia *n* azotaemia. A syndrome characterized by high levels of urea and other toxic nitrogenous substances in the blood, with disturbance of electrolytes and acid-base balance. It occurs when renal function is impaired, either from kidney disease or events occurring elsewhere in the body, e.g. hypotension associated with hypovolaemia. Depending on the cause it may or may not be reversible. The fully developed syndrome is characterized by nausea, vomiting, headache, hiccough, pruritus, lethargy, weakness, dimness of vision, arrhythmias, convulsions and altered consciousness. ⇒ renal failure — **uraemic** *adj*.

uraemic snow ⇒ uridrosis.

urate *n* any salt of uric acid; such compounds are present in the blood, urine and tophi; deposits of sodium urate.

urea *n* the chief nitrogenous end-product of protein metabolism; it is produced in the liver and excreted in urine, of which it is the main nitrogenous constituent. May be used as an osmotic diuretic to reduce intracranial and intraocular pressure, but has been largely replaced by other diuretics. Also used topically to moisturize, soften and smooth dry, rough skin. *urea cycle* biochemical cycle in the liver whereby ammonia from amino acid metabolism is combined with carbon dixide to produce urea.

urease *n* bacterial enzyme that breaks down urea.

ureter *n* the tube passing from each kidney to the bladder for the conveyance of urine; its average length is from 25–30 cm — **ureteric, ureteral** *adj* pertaining to the ureter. *ureteric catheter* very fine tube used to introduce contrast medium for a retrograde urogram (pyelogram) or for drainage. ⇒ urography. *ureteric colic* ⇒ renal colic. *ureteric transplantation* ⇒ ileal conduit. ⇒ ileoureterostomy.

ureterectomy *n* excision of a ureter.

ureteritis *n* inflammation of a ureter.

ureterocolic *adj* pertaining to the ureter and colon, usually indicating anastomosis of the two structures.

ureterocolostomy *n* surgical transplantation of the ureters from the bladder to the colon so that urine is passed by the bowel.

ureteroileal *adj* pertaining to the ureters and ileum as the anastomosis necessary in ureteroileostomy (ileal conduit). ⇒ ileoureterostomy.

ureteroileostomy *n* ⇒ ileal conduit. ⇒ ileoureterostomy.

ureterolith *n* a calculus in the ureter.

ureterolithotomy *n* surgical removal of a stone from a ureter.

ureterosigmoidostomy *n* ureterocolostomy.

ureterostomy *n* the formation of a permanent fistula through which the ureter discharges urine. *cutaneous ureterostomy* the ureters are brought out onto the skin surface from where they drain urine. ⇒ ileoureterostomy.

ureterovaginal *adj* pertaining to the ureter and vagina. *ureterovaginal fistula* abnormal communication between the ureters and vagina. May be congenital or secondary to disease, such as advanced cervical cancer.

ureterovesical *adj* pertaining to the ureter and urinary bladder.

urethra *n* the passage from the bladder to the outside through which urine is excreted — **urethral** *adj*.

urethritis *n* inflammation of the urethra. *nonspecific urethritis* ⇒ nongonococcal urethritis.

urethrocele *n* prolapse of the urethra, usually into the anterior vaginal wall.

urethrography *n* radiological examination of the urethra. Can be an inclusion with cystography, either retrograde (ascending) or during micturition — **urethrographically** *adv*.

urethrometry *n* measurement of the urethral lumen using a urethrometer — **urethrometrically** *adv*.

urethroplasty *n* any plastic operation on the urethra — **urethroplastic** *adj*.

urethroscope *n* an instrument designed to allow visualization of the interior of the urethra — **urethroscopically** *adv*.

urethrostenosis *n* urethral stricture.

urethrotomy *n* incision into the urethra; usually part of an operation for stricture.

urgency *n* a strong desire to pass urine, which, if not responded to immediately, may lead to urge incontinence. ⇒ incontinence.

uric acid a derivative of purine metabolism, which is a component of nucleic acids and some foods and beverages. It is excreted in the urine and can form kidney stones. Blood levels may rise when purine intake is high, where there is abnormal breakdown of cells, such as with some leukaemias, and where uric acid excretion is impaired. ⇒ gout.

uricosuric agents *npl* drugs that increase the amount of uric acid excreted in the urine, e.g. probenicid which is used in the management of gout. Probenicid also inhibits the excretion of penicillin and may be used in this way. ⇒ gout.

uridrosis *n* (*syn* uraemic snow) excess of urea in the sweat; it may be deposited on the skin as fine white crystals.

urinalysis *n* analysis of urine. Visual, physical, chemical or microbiological examination of urine. Usually involves commercially prepared test sticks/strips or tablets.

urinary *adj* pertaining to urine. *urinary bladder* a muscular distensible bag situated in the pelvis. It receives urine from the kidneys via two ureters and stores it until the volume causes reflex evacuation through the urethra. Once bladder control has been achieved during childhood the person is able to voluntarily inhibit these nerve impulses to delay bladder emptying. However, once the volume of urine reaches a critical level the bladder will reflexly empty whether it is convenient or not. *urinary catheter* used to drain urine from the bladder. *urinary system* comprises two kidneys, two ureters, one urinary bladder and one urethra. The kidneys produce urine of variable composition to maintain homeostasis; the ureters convey the urine to the bladder, which stores it until there is sufficient volume to elicit the desire to pass urine and it is then conveyed to the exterior by the urethra. *urinary tract infection (UTI)* a very common cause of hospital-acquired infection. It occurs most frequently in the presence of an indwelling catheter. The most common infecting agent is *Escherichia coli*, suggesting that autogenous infection via the periurethral route is the commonest pathway. (See Figure 65).

urination *n* ⇒ micturition.

urine *n* the clear amber-coloured fluid which is excreted from the kidneys at the rate of about 1500 mL every 24 h in the adult, but this depends on fluid intake, activity and age. It normally contains water, nitrogenous waste and electrolytes. The pH is around 6.0 (slightly acid), but

varies between 4.5–8.0. The specific gravity is usually within the range 1005–1030. Both pH and specific gravity vary according to homeostatic need.

urinometer *n* an instrument for estimating the specific gravity of urine.

URL *abbr* uniform resource locator. Used to identify specific web site locations, such as http://www.doh.gov.uk/dhhome. htm

urobilin *n* a brownish pigment formed by the oxidation of urobilinogen and excreted in the faeces. Sometimes found in urine left standing in contact with air.

urobilinogen *n* (*syn* stercobilinogen) pigment formed from bilirubin in the intestine by the action of bacteria. Some is excreted in the faeces. It is reabsorbed into the circulation and converted back to bilirubin in the liver and re-excreted in the bile or urine. Elevated levels in urine may indicate liver abnormalities and haemolysis. Levels are decreased in obstructive jaundice.

urobilinuria *n* the presence of increased amounts of urobilin in the urine. Evidence of increased production of bilirubin in the liver, e.g. after haemolysis.

urochrome *n* the yellow pigment which gives urine its normal colour.

urodynamics *n* the use of sophisticated equipment to measure bladder function. Particularly useful in diagnosing the cause of urinary incontinence.

uroflometry noninvasive technique for assessing urinary flow rates by voiding into a receptacle incorporating a transducer that records rates electronically. ⇒ urodynamics.

urogenital, urinogenital *adj* pertaining to the urinary and the genital organs.

• Being female (short urethra)	• Urinary stasis, e.g. immobility, urinary obstruction, or residual urine left in the bladder after voiding such as with pelvic floor weakness, or neurological conditions
• Poor perineal hygiene (leads to colonization with micro-organisms)	
• Use of some irritant toiletries	• Urinary tract abnormalities, e.g. prostatic enlargement, or ureteric reflux of urine
• Urethral trauma during intercourse and childbirth	• Reduced immune function, e.g. extremes of age, immunodeficient individuals and during immunosuppression
• Pregnancy	
• Catheterization and bladder instrumentation, e.g. cystoscopy	• Diabetes mellitus and any debilitating condition

Figure 65 Risk factors for urinary tract infection.

urogram radiographic image of the urinary tract. ⇒ urography.

urography *n* (*syn* pyelography) radiographic visualization of the renal pelvis and ureter by injection of a contrast medium. The medium may be injected into the bloodstream whence it is excreted by the kidney (intravenous urography) or it may be injected directly into the renal pelvis (anterograde via percutaneous injection) or ureter by way of a fine catheter introduced through a cystoscope (retrograde or ascending urography). *intravenous urography (IVU)* demonstration of the urinary tract following an intravenous injection of a contrast medium — **urographically** *adv.*

urokinase *n* a thrombolytic (fibrinolytic) enzyme. A plasminogen activator produced by the kidney. It is used therapeutically in vitreous haemorrhage (eye), thrombosed arteriovenous shunts and other thromboembolic conditions.

urolithiasis *n* urinary calculi.

urologist *n* a person who specializes in disorders of the female urinary tract and the male genitourinary tract.

urology *n* that branch of science which deals with disorders of the female urinary tract and the male genitourinary tract — **urologically** *adv.*

uropathy *n* disease in any part of the urinary system.

urostomy *n* an opening or stoma that drains urine, such as cutaneous ureterostomy, ileoureterostomy, ureterocolostomy.

URTI *abbr* upper respiratory tract infection.

urticaria *n* (*syn* nettlerash, hives) an allergic skin eruption characterized by multiple, circumscribed, smooth, raised, pinkish, itchy weals, developing very suddenly, usually lasting a few days and leaving no visible trace. Common provocative agents in susceptible subjects are ingested foods, such as shellfish, injected sera and contact with, or injection of, antibiotics such as penicillin and streptomycin. ⇒ angiooedema. ⇒ dermographia.

uterine *adj* pertaining to the uterus. *uterine prolapse* ⇒ prolapse. *uterine supports* the uterus is held in an anteverted and anteflexed position by the muscles of the pelvic floor, the pelvic peritoneum and various ligaments: transverse cervical ligaments (also known as Mackenrodt's or cardinal ligaments), uterosacral ligament, the pubocervical ligament and the round ligaments.

uterine tubes *n* (*syn* fallopian tubes, oviducts) two tubes opening out of the upper part of the uterus. Each measures 10 cm and the distal end is fimbriated and lies near the ovary. They provide the site for fertilization and convey the ovum into the uterus.

uteroplacental *adj* pertaining to the uterus and placenta.

uterorectal *adj* pertaining to the uterus and the rectum.

uterosacral *adj* pertaining to the uterus and sacrum. *uterosacral ligament* extend backwards from the cervix to the sacrum. Part of the supports of the uterus.

uterosalpingography *n* (*syn* hysterosalpingography) radiological examination of the uterus and uterine tubes involving retrograde introduction of a contrast medium during fluoroscopy. Used to investigate patency of uterine tubes.

uterovaginal *adj* pertaining to the uterus and the vagina.

uterovesical *adj* pertaining to the uterus and the urinary bladder.

uterus *n* the womb; a hollow pear-shaped muscular organ in the pelvic cavity (see Figure 54). It has three parts: the top or fundus, the body and the cervix. It connects bilaterally with the uterine tubes and opens inferiorly into the vagina. Its three layers are: (a) an outer serous coat called the perimetrium; (b) the myometrium, a thick layer of interlocking smooth muscle fibres; (c) the endometrium, a mucosal lining of highly vascular glandular epithelium which, during the reproductive years, is influenced by the cyclical secretion of hormones. ⇒ menstrual cycle. ⇒ menstruation. The uterus receives the fertilized ovum and provides the environment for implantation and fetal development, and expels the fetus through the vagina. When the ovum is not fertilized, the endometrial lining of the uterus is shed, resulting in menstrual flow. ⇒ bicornuate.

UTI *abbr* urinary tract infection.

utilitarianism ethical theory that supports the view that an action should always produce more benefits than harm. It aims to provide the greatest good for the majority of people. ⇒ deontological.

utricle *n* a fluid-filled sac in the internal ear. Part of the vestibular apparatus, it contains the hair cells and otoliths: the receptors for static equilibrium that respond to head position relative to gravity and to linear changes in speed and direction. ⇒ saccule.

uvea *n* the pigmented part of the eye, including the iris, ciliary body and choroid. The uveal tract — uveal *adj*.

uveitis *n* inflammation of the uveal tract (uvea).

uvula *n* the central, tag-like structure hanging down from the free edge of the soft palate.

uvulectomy *n* excision of the uvula.

uvulitis *n* inflammation of the uvula.

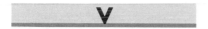

vaccination *n* originally described the process of inoculating persons with discharge from cowpox to protect them from smallpox. Now applied to the inoculation of any antigenic material for the purpose of producing active artificial immunity to specific diseases.

vaccines *npl* suspensions or products of infectious agents, used chiefly for producing active immunity. ⇒ BCG. ⇒ DTPer. → Hib vaccine. → immunization. → MMR vaccine. ⇒ Sabin. → Salk.

vaccinia *n* a pox virus causing disease in cattle. It is used to confer immunity against smallpox in people whose work puts them at risk of contact with pox viruses, such as laboratory staff.

vacuum a space from which the gas or air has been withdrawn. *vacuum aspiration* a method of terminating a pregnancy up to the 14th week of gestation. *vacuum extraction (Ventouse)* an assisted delivery where a vacuum is used to attach a cap to the fetal head and exert gentle traction synchronized with contractions of the uterus.

vacuum drainage system/tube a closed suction drainage system used for the drainage of wounds in the postoperative period. The amount and type of wound drainage or exudate is visible in the drainage container. ⇒ wound drains.

VADAS *abbr* voice activated domestic appliance system.

vagal *adj* pertaining to the vagus nerve.

vagina *n* literally, a sheath; the muscular, membranous passage extending from the cervix uteri to the vulva. The mucosa is arranged in rugae (folds) that allow for distention — vaginal *adj* pertaining to the vagina. *vaginal hysterectomy* ⇒ hysterectomy. *vaginal prolapse* ⇒ cystocele. → prolapse. → rectocele.

vaginismus *n* involuntary spasm of the muscles around the vagina whenever the vulva is touched, during sexual activity or medical examination. It results in dyspareunia and makes sexual intercourse difficult or impossible.

vaginitis *n* inflammation of the vagina. It may be caused by micro-organisms that include: *Trichomonas vaginalis*, *Chlamydia trachomatis*, *Gardenerella vaginalis*, *Neisseria gonorrhoeae* and yeasts, particularly *Candida albicans*. There should be adequate history taking at the initial assessment, followed by physical examination and microbiological tests so that a correct diagnosis of the cause can lead to appropriate treatment. *atrophic vaginitis* thinning of the vaginal mucosa and the reduced acid secretions associated with decreased oestrogen secretion after the menopause make the vagina more prone to infection. Candidiasis is particularly common in older women. The atrophic changes affecting the vaginal mucosa may cause inflammation, dryness, itching and dyspareunia even when infection is not present. Treatment with topical oestrogens may be prescribed, but only after any postmenopausal bleeding has been investigated.

vaginosis bacterial infection of the vagina. ⇒ *Gardnerella vaginalis*.

vagolytic *adj* that which neutralizes the effect of a stimulated vagus nerve.

vagotomy *n* surgical division of the vagus nerves to reduce gastric acid production in peptic ulceration. It may be truncal or selective, both of which are combined with a procedure to improve gastric emptying, such as gastroenterostomy or pyloroplasty, or highly selective, where only the nerve fibres supplying the acid-producing areas of the stomach are divided. Vagotomy generally causes fewer problems associated with eating than gastrectomy, such as dumping syndrome, but diarrhoea can be a problem and the risk of recurrent ulcer is higher.

vagus nerve the parasympathetic pneumo-gastric nerve; the 10th cranial nerve, composed of both motor and sensory fibres, with a wide distribution in the neck, thorax and abdomen, sending important branches to the heart, lungs, oesophagus, stomach, liver, spleen, intestine and kidney. ⇒ vagotomy — **vagal** *adj*.

valence valency. The combining power of an element or radical.

valgus, valga, valgum *adj* exhibiting angulation away from the midline of the body, e.g. hallux valgus.

validity a term in research which indicates the degree to which a method or test measures what it intends to measure. See Box – Validity.

valine *n* one of the essential (indispensable) amino acids.

Valsalva's manoeuvre a forced expiration against a closed glottis. It increases pressure in the thorax and abdomen, and reduces venous return to the heart. Occurs naturally when straining to move/lift heavy objects, changing position or defaecating.

value for money (VFM) see Box – Value for money.

values *npl* the individual and personal view of the worth of an idea or way of behaving. Principles of living which are distilled from life's experience; they guide behaviour and, in a nursing context, are manifested in the integrity of a nurse's work. *value systems* an accepted set of values, conduct and way of behaving in a particular social group. ⇒ beliefs. ⇒ secular beliefs.

valve *n* a fold of membrane in a passage or tube permitting the flow of contents in one direction only, such as those in veins, heart and the ileocaecal valve. *valve replacement* surgical procedure to replace a heart valve — **valvular** *adj*.

valvoplasty *n* a plastic operation on a valve, usually reserved for the heart; to be distinguished from valve replacement or valvotomy — **valvoplastic** *adj*.

Validity

Validity refers to whether you are measuring, recording, observing or assessing the appropriate data. There are several forms of validity:

- Content validity – where each item is examined to see whether it is relevant, often by reference to the literature, or previous studies. One method of achieving content validity is to ask experts in the field to examine the items;
- Construct validity – where the ability to measure some trait is assessed;
- Criterion-related validity – refers to how well a new instrument compares to some well tried older measure;

- Concurrent validity – where the researcher employs a test on groups known to differ and in a way relevant to the concept under study;
- Predictive validity – where a test is applied and the group followed up to determine whether the test can predict those subjects who will develop some condition;
- Convergent validity – this is a more general term that includes the above measures of validity, and refers to the process whereby the measure is tested for harmonization with some pre-existing measure.
- Divergent validity – where measures of different concepts should not correspond with each other, in other words the measures discriminate.

Value for money

Value for money (VFM) is a means of obtaining the best quality of service within resource. The term embraces 'the three Es': economy, efficiency and effectiveness. Economy means that as little resource as possible is spent, whilst still maintaining the appropriate quality of service. Efficiency is the term which describes the relationship between resource input and workload output. Efficiency can be improved by either increasing outputs whilst using the same amount of resource, or by maintaining the output whilst reducing the amount of resources used. Effectiveness describes using the resources to achieve the intended outcome.

valvotomy, valvulotomy *n* incision of a stenotic valve, by custom referring to the heart, to restore normal function.

valvulitis *n* inflammation of a valve, particularly in the heart.

valvulotomy *n* ⇒ valvotomy.

vancomycin-resistant enterococci (VRE) *n* enterococci that have developed resistance to the antibiotic vancomycin, such as *Enterococcus faecium*. ⇒ Enterococcus.

Van den Bergh's test estimation of serum bilirubin. Both the conjugated and unconjugated bilirubin are estimated. Direct positive reaction (conjugated) occurs in obstructive and hepatocellular jaundice. Indirect positive reaction (unconjugated) occurs in haemolytic jaundice and bilirubin transport problems.

vanillylmandelic acid (VMA) *n* a metabolite of adrenaline (epinephrine) which is excreted in the urine. Levels of VMA detected in a 24-hour collection of urine can be used to assess the function of the adrenal medulla.

Vaquez's disease primary proliferative polycythaemia (polycythaemia vera).

variables *npl* in research, any factor or circumstance which is part of the study. *con founding variable* a variable that affects the conditions of the independent variables unequally. *dependent variable* one that depends on the experimental conditions. The factor being studied. *independent variable* the variable conditions of an experimental situation, e.g. experimental or control. *random variable* background factors, e.g. noise, which may affect any conditions of the independent variable conditions equally.

variance a mathematical term used in statistics. The distribution range of a set of results around the mean. Standard deviation is the square root of variance.

varicella *n* ⇒ chickenpox — **varicelliform** *adj*.

varicella/zoster immunoglobulin (VZIG) a blood product which, when injected, produces immunity to varicella and zoster. Used for neonates exposed to infection and immunocompromised individuals.

varicella/zoster virus the herpesvirus that causes chickenpox (varicella) and shingles (herpes zoster).

varices *npl* dilated, tortuous (or varicose) veins. ⇒ oesophageal varices. ⇒ varicose veins — **varix** *sing*.

varicocele *n* varicosity of the veins of the spermatic cord.

varicose dilated or swollen. *varicose veins* tortuous, dilated veins where the valves are incompetent so that blood flow may be reversed. May be caused by a congenital valve defect, obesity, pregnancy and thrombophlebitis. Most commonly found in the superficial veins of lower limbs where they can result in aching and pain, swelling, unacceptable appearance changes, and venous insufficiency (poor venous return) that may lead to the formation of a venous ulcer. Management includes: advice about avoiding standing, resting with legs elevated, exercise and support stockings/tights, injection of sclerosing agent into the veins or surgical stripping or ligation. ⇒ haemorrhoids. ⇒ oesophageal varices.

variola *n* ⇒ smallpox.

varix *n* ⇒ varices.

varus, vara, varum *adj* displaying displacement or angulation towards the midline of the body, e.g. coxa vara. ⇒ talipes.

vas *n* a vessel or duct. *vas deferens* the excretory duct of the testis. It is continuous with the epididymis and conveys spermatozoa to the ejaculatory ducts. *vasa vasorum* the minute nutrient vessels of the artery and vein walls — **vasa** *pl*.

vascular *adj* supplied with vessels, especially referring to blood vessels.

vascularization *n* the acquisition of a blood supply; the process of becoming vascular. Occurs during the healing process.

vasculitis *n* (*syn* angiitis) inflammation of a blood vessel.

vasculotoxic *adj* any substance which brings about harmful changes in blood vessels.

vasectomy *n* surgical excision of part of the vas deferens, usually for sterilization.

vasoactive intestinal peptide (VIP) *n* an intestinal regulatory peptide hormone that inhibits gastric motility. ⇒ enterogastric reflex.

vasoconstriction contraction or narrowing of the lumen of blood vessels.

vasoconstrictor *n* any agent which causes a narrowing of the lumen of blood vessels, e.g. phenylephrine used as a nasal congestant.

vasodilatation, vasodilation dilatation of blood vessels.

vasodilator *n* any agent which causes a widening of the lumen of blood vessels, such as alcohol, the calcium antagonists and nitrates.

vasoepididymostomy *n* anastomosis of the vas deferens to the epididymis.

vasomotor pertaining to the nerves and muscles concerned with vessel lumen size. *vasomotor centre (VMC)* part of the cardiovascular centre, located in the medulla oblongata. It controls the lumen size of peripheral arterioles and operates through sympathetic activity in response to baroreceptors signals. The size of these vessels controls peripheral resistance which is a factor contributing to arterial blood pressure.

vasomotor rhinitis *n* rhinitis resulting from a hypersensitivity of the nasal mucosa that may be triggered by a variety of factors: environmental changes, physical or chemical stimuli and stress. There is excessive sneezing, profuse watery rhinorrhoea and swelling causing nasal obstruction.

vasopressin *n* formed in the hypothalamus. Passes down the nerves in the pituitary stalk to be stored in the posterior lobe of the pituitary gland. It is the antidiuretic hormone (ADH). A synthetic preparation, desmopressin, is available, which can be given intranasally or by injection in diabetes insipidus.

vasopressor *n* a drug which increases blood pressure, usually, but not always, by vasoconstriction of arterioles.

vasospasm *n* constricting spasm of vessel walls — **vasospastic** *adj*.

vasovagal attack syncope due to bradycardia and peripheral vasodilation due to vagal activity. It may be accompanied by pallor, sweating and nausea. It may be caused by fright, pain, unpleasant sights, standing for prolonged periods and fluid loss.

VBI *abbr* vertebrobasilar insufficiency.

VC *abbr* vital capacity.

VDRL test *abbr* Venereal Disease Research Laboratory test.

VDU *abbr* visual display unit. The monitor screen attached to a computer.

vector *n* 1. a carrier of disease. Animal that conveys an organism from one host to another, e.g. mosquito, tick. 2. a quantity that has both direction and magnitude.

vegan *n* a vegetarian, who excludes all animal products from his or her diet. Nutritional deficiencies can occur without careful selection of foods, with particular attention to obtaining the essential amino acids, minerals and vitamins, such as vitamin B_{12}.

vegetations *npl* growths or accretions composed of micro-organisms, fibrin and platelets, occurring on the edge of the cardiac valves in infective endocarditis.

vegetative *adj* 1. pertaining to the nonsporing stage of a bacterium. 2. in psychiatry, describes a state of lethargy and passivity.

vehicle *n* an inert substance in which a drug is administered, e.g. water in mixtures.

vein *n* a vessel conveying blood from the capillaries back to the heart. It has the same three coats as an artery. ⇒ tunica. The lining coat of veins in the limbs is modified to form valves that allow flow in one direction and prevent pooling of blood in the limbs — **venous** *adj* pertaining to veins. *venous pressure* the pressure within the veins. ⇒ central venous pressure. *venous sinuses* channels that convey venous blood, such as in the heart and brain. *venous thrombosis* ⇒ deep vein thrombosis. ⇒ thromboembolism.

vellus hair *n* fine, 'fluffy' soft hair that forms the body hair of women and children. Also appears on the scalp when the hair thins. ⇒ lanugo.

Velpeau's bandage an arm to chest bandage for a fractured clavicle.

vena *n* a vein — **venae** *pl*.

vena cava *n* one of two large veins (inferior and superior) which return venous blood to the right atrium of the heart.

venepuncture (venipuncture) *n* puncture of a vein for introduction of a drug or fluid or withdrawal of blood. When performed on children, a topical anaesthetic cream (EMLA) may be applied in advance. Research has revealed that the traditional method of flexing the arm after venepuncture is more likely to cause bruising than maintaining pressure over a swab with the arm extended. ⇒ intravenous.

venereal *adj* pertaining to or caused by sexual intercourse. *venereal disease* ⇒ sexually transmitted infection. ⇒ contact tracer.

Venereal Disease Research Laboratory (VDRL) test *n* a specific serological test for syphilis.

venereology *n* the study and treatment of sexually transmitted infections.

venesection *n* (*syn* phlebotomy) a clinical procedure, formerly by opening the cubital vein (in the forearm/elbow) with a scalpel, but now usually by venepuncture. Used to collect blood and as a treatment for polycythaemia and haemochromatosis.

venoclysis *n* the introduction of nutrient or medicinal fluids into a vein.

venography *n* (*syn* phlebography) radiological examination of the venous system involving injection of a contrast medium — **venographically** *adv*.

venom *n* a poisonous fluid produced by some scorpions, snakes and spiders.

venotomy *n* incision of a vein. ⇒ venesection.

venous ulcer (*syn* gravitational ulcer) an indolent ulcer with a venous aetiology. They are usually near the ankle or between the ankle or knee. The surrounding skin is often pigmented (brown staining) and there may be varicose (gravitational stasis) eczema and contact dermatitis; ulcers tend to be large and shallow with copious amounts of exudate. Patients often have a history of varicose veins or deep vein thrombosis, and complain of local tenderness and aching legs. ⇒ dermatitis ⇒ eczema.

ventilation the supply of fresh air. Also used to describe the mechanical process of breathing. *ventilation perfusion imaging* used to detect pulmonary emboli. It involves imaging of the lungs following the inhalation of a radioactive gas and an intravenous injection of radioactive albumen. ⇒ alveolar ventilation. ⇒ mechanical ventilation. ⇒ pulmonary ventilation.

ventilation perfusion ratio (V/Q) *n* the ratio between gases in the alveoli (alveolar ventilation) and blood flow in the pulmonary capillaries (pulmonary perfusion). The ratio is subject to homeostatic regulation that ensures that gas exchange proceeds efficiently in the lungs. In healthy individuals there is normally a small mismatch between ventilation and perfusion in different parts of the lungs, but the V/Q is 1.

ventilator *n* device for providing assisted ventilation. Built-in controls can vary the mode of ventilation and monitor some aspects of respiratory function. ⇒ mechanical ventilation.

Ventouse ⇒ vacuum extraction.

ventral *adj* pertaining to the abdomen or the anterior surface of the body — **ventrally** *adv*.

ventricle *n* a small belly-like cavity. *ventricle of the brain* four cavities filled with cerebrospinal fluid within the brain. *ventricle of the heart* the two lower muscular chambers of the heart that pump blood into the circulation (systemic and pulmonary) — **ventricular** *adj* pertaining to the ventricles. *ventricular arrhythmias* abnormal cardiac rhythm arising in the ventricle. ⇒ arrhythmia. ⇒ extrasystole. ⇒ fibrillation. ⇒ supraventricular. *ventricular septal defect (VSD)* ⇒ ventricular septal defect.

ventricular fibrillation a ventricular arrhythmia. The commonest cause of sudden death. There is an uncoordinated rhythm in the ventricles which is ineffective in pumping blood around the circulation. ⇒ cardiac arrest. ⇒ cardiopulmonary resuscitation.

ventricular puncture a highly skilled method of puncturing a cerebral ventricle for a sample of cerebrospinal fluid.

ventricular septal defect (VSD) an abnormal communication between the right and left ventricles of the heart.

ventricular tachycardia a ventricular arrhythmia. There is a rapid ventricular rate of 140–200 per minute, a very serious arrhythmia that may progress to cardiac arrest, ventricular fibrillation or pulseless ventricular tachycardia.

ventriculoatrial shunt *n* a surgical procedure where excess cerebrospinal fluid from a cerebral ventricle is diverted to the right atrium via a plastic shunt. Used in the treatment of hydrocephalus.

ventriculocisternostomy *n* artificial communication between cerebral ventricles and the cisterna magna that normally receives cerebrospinal fluid via the roof of the fourth ventricle. One of the drainage operations for hydrocephalus.

ventriculoperitoneal shunt *n* a surgical procedure where excess cerebrospinal fluid from a cerebral ventricle is diverted to the peritoneal cavity via a plastic shunt. Used in the treatment of hydrocephalus.

ventriculostomy *n* an artificial opening into a ventricle. Usually refers to a drainage operation for hydrocephalus.

ventrosuspension *n* fixation of a displaced uterus to the anterior abdominal wall.

Venturi effect *n* a principle of gas behaviour utilized in certain medical equipment for the mixing and delivery of gases, such as Venturi oxygen masks.

Venturi mask *n* an oxygen therapy mask designed to entrain atmospheric air to mix it with a given flow of prescribed oxygen. Various proprietary masks are available that allow the administration of different oxygen concentrations: 24%, 28% or 35% according to individual needs. (See Figure 66).

venule *n* a small vein.

verbigeration repetition of words or phases which are meaningless.

Veress needle a sharp needle with a blunt-ended trochar which has a lateral hole; it is used for a pneumoperitoneum. When the trochar projects from the needle the gut is pushed safely away from the needle point.

vermicide *n* an agent which kills intestinal worms — **vermicidal** *adj*.

vermiform *adj* wormlike. *vermiform appendix* the vestigial, hollow, wormlike structure attached to the caecum.

vermifuge *n* an agent which expels intestinal worms.

vermis *n* a wormlike structure that joins the two hemispheres of the cerebellum.

vernix caseosa the fatty substance which covers and protects the skin of the fetus in utero. This becomes absorbed in the postmature fetus, leading to drying and cracking of the newborn's skin.

verocytotoxin *n* enterotoxin produced by enterohaemorrhagic *Escherichia coli* (EHEC), e.g *E. coli* 0157. ⇒ Escherichia.

verruca *n* wart. ⇒ condyloma. *verruca necrogenica* (postmortem wart, prosector's wart) develops as result of accidental innoculation with tuberculosis while carrying out a postmortem. *verruca plana* the common multiple, flat, tiny warts often seen on children's hands, knees and face. *verruca plantaris* a flat wart on the sole of the foot. Highly contagious. *verruca seborrhoeica* the brown, greasy wart seen in seborrhoeic subjects, commonly on the chest or back, which increase with ageing. *verruca vulgaris* the common wart of the hands or feet, of brownish colour and rough pitted surface, caused by human papillomavirus type 2 — **verrucous, verrucose** *adj*.

version *n* turning applied to the manoeuvre to alter the presentation of the fetus in utero to facilitate labour. *bipolar version* the version is performed by acting on both fetal poles. *cephalic version* turning the fetus so that the head or vertex presents. *external cephalic version (ECV)* the turning of the fetus with both hands on the abdomen. The technique is safer with the use of ultrasound and tachographic monitoring. *internal version* is turning the fetus by one hand in the vagina, and the other on the woman's abdomen. *podalic version* turning the fetus to a breech presentation. This version may be external or internal. *spontaneous version* one that occurs naturally, such as a breech to vertex presentation or a transverse lie to a cephalic or podalic one.

vertebra *n* one of the 33/34 irregular bones making up the spinal column — **vertebrae** *pl* — **vertebral** *adj* pertaining to the vertebrae. *vertebral arteries* a pair of major arteries which form the basilar artery which contributes to the circular arrangement of arteries at the base of the brain (circle of Willis). *vertebral canal* ⇒ spinal canal. *vertebral column* (*syn* spinal column) made up of 33/34 vertebrae. There are 24 individual bones and 9 or 10 fused bones. The vertebral column articulates with the skull above and the pelvic girdle below. The vertebrae are so shaped that they enclose a cavity (spinal canal, neural canal) which houses the spinal cord.

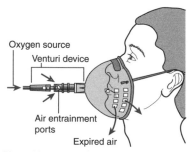

Oxygen source
Venturi device
Air entrainment ports
Expired air

Figure 66 Venturi mask. (Reproduced from Nicol et al 2000 with permission.)

vertebrobasilar insufficiency (VBI) a syndrome caused by lack of blood to the hindbrain. May be progressive, episodic or both. Clinical manifestations include giddiness and vertigo, nausea, ataxia, drop attacks and signs of cerebellar disorder such as nystagmus.

vertex *n* the top of the head. ⇒ presentation.

vertical transmission disease passing from mother to fetus, via the placenta, at delivery or through breast milk, e.g. HIV.

vertigo *n* giddiness, dizziness; a subjective sense of imbalance, often rotary — **vertiginous** *adj*.

very-low-density lipoprotein (VLDL) ⇒ lipoprotein.

vesical *adj* pertaining to the urinary bladder.

vesicant *n* a blistering substance.

vesicle *n* 1. a small bladder, cell or hollow structure. 2. a small skin blister containing serum — **vesiculation** *n*.

vesicoenteric *adj* vesicointestinal. Pertaining to the bladder and intestine, such as a fistula.

vesicostomy *n* ⇒ cystostomy.

vesicoureteric *adj* pertaining to the urinary bladder and ureter *vesicoureteric reflux (VUR)* can cause pyelonephritis.

vesicovaginal *adj* pertaining to the urinary bladder and vagina, such as a fistula.

vesiculitis *n* inflammation of a vesicle, particularly the seminal vesicles.

vesiculopapular *adj* pertaining to vesicles and papules, such as a rash containing both.

vesiculopustular *adj* pertaining to vesicles and pustules, such as a rash containing both.

vessel *n* a tube, duct or canal, holding or conveying fluid, especially blood and lymph.

vestibule *n* 1. part of the bony labyrinth of the inner ear, lying between the semicircular canals and the cochlea. 2. the triangular area between the labia minora. 3. the area of the mouth between the gums/teeth and the lips — **vestibular** *adj* pertaining to the vestibule. *vestibular apparatus* the structures of the inner ear: semicircular canals and the saccule and utricle in the vestibule. They are concerned with balance and position. *vestibular centre* areas in the brain that contain the nuclei that receive impulses from the vestibular apparatus of the ear. *vestibular glands* two pairs of mucus-secreting glands that open into the vestibule of the female external genitalia. ⇒ Bartholin's glands. ⇒ Skene's glands.

vestibulocochlear *adj* pertaining to the vestibule and the cochlea. *vestibulocochlear nerve* the eighth pair of cranial nerves. It has two branches. The vestibular branch carries impulses from the vestibular apparatus to the cerebellum. The cochlear branch coveys impulses from the cochlea to the auditory cortex in the temporal lobe of the cerebrum. Also known as the auditory nerve.

vestigial *adj* rudimentary; indicating a remnant of something formerly present.

VFM *abbr* Value For Money.

VGA *abbr* video graphics array. A screen display supporting high resolution (but less so than SVGA) colour images.

viable *adj* capable of living or surviving independently. Usually applied to a fetus of 24 weeks gestation or more — **viability** *n*.

vibration a massage manipulation; a fine tremor transmitted through the hands and finger tips to body cavities in order to displace gases and fluids.

Vibrio *n* a genus of curved, motile Gram-negative bacteria. *Vibrio cholerae*, or the *comma vibrio*, causes cholera.

vicarious *adj* substituting the function of one organ for another.

vicarious liability the liability of an employer for the wrongful acts of an employee committed whilst in the course of employment.

villus *n* a microscopic fingerlike process projecting from the surface of some cells. *chorionic villus* ⇒ chorionic villi. *intestinal villus* found in the small intestine where they greatly increase the surface area. Concerned with the absorption of nutrients — **villi** *pl*.

vinca alkaloids *npl* cytotoxic drugs extracted from the periwinkle plant, e.g. vincristine, vinblastine. They work by preventing microtubule formation needed for mitosis and cell division. Other drugs derived from plants include: etoposide from mandrake root and paclitaxel from yew bark, which is used in the management of ovarian and some breast cancers.

Vincent's angina (*syn* ulcerative stomatitis) bacterial (spirochaetes and bacilli) infection of the gums with necrosis and ulceration which may spread to other structures, such as the palate and throat. It is treated with penicillin or metronidazole.

viraemia *n* the presence of virus in the blood — **viraemic** *adj.*

viral haemorrhagic fevers *npl* viral fevers which occur mainly in the tropics; they may be transmitted by mosquitoes or ticks. Examples are chikungunya, dengue, Ebola, Lassa fever, Marburg disease and yellow fever.

viral hepatitis ⇒ hepatitis.

virement a financial term meaning to move money from one expenditure category to another.

viricidal *adj* lethal to a virus — **viricide** *n.*

virilism *n* the appearance of secondary male characteristics in the female. ⇒ masculinization.

virology *n* the study of viruses and the diseases caused by them — **virological** *adj.*

virulence *n* infectiousness; the pathogenicity (disease-producing power) of a micro-organism; the power of a micro-organism to overcome host resistance — **virulent** *adj.*

virus *n* any of a diverse group of microorganisms which are only visible using electron microscopy. They contain either DNA or RNA, and can only replicate within the host cell. Viruses infect humans, animals, plants and other microorganisms (bacteriophages). The families of viruses include: adenoviruses, arboviruses, arenaviruses, coronaviruses, filoviruses, hepadnaviruses, herpesviruses, myxoviruses, papovaviruses, picornaviruses, poxviruses, reoviruses, retroviruses, rhabdoviruses and togaviruses. Diseases caused by viruses in humans include: colds, rubella, influenza, measles, rabies, hepatitis, chickenpox, shingles, poliomyelitis, yellow fever, dengue and AIDS. There is increasing evidence to support the view that some viruses are carcinogenic and some are associated with cancer of the cervix, Burkitt's lymphoma and some types of leukaemia. ⇒ Epstein-Barr virus. ⇒ human T-cell lymphotropic virus. ⇒ human papilloma virus.

viscera *npl* the internal organs — **visceral** *adj.*

visceroptosis *n* downward displacement or falling of the abdominal organs.

viscid, viscous *adj* sticky, thick; may be used to describe mucus, sputum etc.

vision the faculty of sight. ⇒ binocular vision. ⇒ diplopia. ⇒ stereoscopic vision.

visiting *v* refers to the time at which visitors can visit patients in hospital. It varies from stipulated periods to a more liberal policy. Visiting can provide psychological support and help to prevent boredom, institutionalization and to encourage rehabilitation. In sick children's units, open visiting is usually allowed and parents enabled to be resident with their child. Visitors of terminally-ill patients, children and people in long-stay wards are encouraged to participate in the nursing of their relatives to relieve their feelings of helplessness.

visual *adj* pertaining to vision. *visual acuity* ⇒ acuity. *visual field* the area within which objects can be seen. *visual impairment* ⇒ blindness. *visual purple* ⇒ rhodopsin.

vital capacity (VC) the maximum amount of air expelled from the lungs after greatest inspiratory effort. ⇒ forced vital capacity. ⇒ respiratory function tests.

vital signs *npl* signs indicating life; pulse, temperature and respiration. Within the context of observations made on patients, it is usual to include blood pressure.

vitallium *n* an alloy which can be left in the tissues in the form of nails, plates, tubes, etc.

vitalograph *n* ⇒ spirometer.

vitamin A (*syn* retinol) a fat-soluble vitamin found in liver, egg yolk and full fat dairy products. In its provitamin form, βcarotene, it is present in carrots, cabbage, lettuce, tomatoes and other fruits and vegetables; in the body it is converted into retinol. It is essential for healthy skin and mucous membranes; it aids night vision. Deficiency can result in stunted growth and night blindness. ⇒ xerophthalmia.

vitamin B refers to any one of a group of water-soluble vitamins of the vitamin B complex. They often occur in the same foods and include: biotin, cobalamins, folates, niacin (nicotinic acid and nicotinamide), pantothenic acid, pyridoxine, riboflavin and thiamine. The B vitamins all act as coenzymes in metabolic processes.

vitamin B₁ thiamine.

vitamin B₆ pyridoxine.

vitamin B₁₂ cobalamins. Sometimes called the extrinsic factor. ⇒ intrinsic factor.

vitamin C ascorbic acid.

vitamin D a fat-soluble vitamin that exists in two forms: ergocalciferol (vitamin D₂) or cholecalciferol (vitamin D₃). The most important source is that produced in the body by the action of ultraviolet on the provitamin 7-dehydrocholesterol. Good dietary sources are oily fish, dairy produce and fortified margarine. Vitamin D is a precursor of active substances, such as 1,25-dihydroxycholecalciferol produced by the kidney, concerned with calcium homeostasis. Deficiency leads to rickets in children and osteomalacia in adults.

vitamin E a group of chemically related compounds known as tocopherols and tocotrienes. A fat-soluble vitamin which functions as an antioxidant, it protects polyunsaturated fatty acids and hence helps maintain cell membranes. Deficiency seen in infants who are premature or small for gestational age may manifest as haemolytic blood disease.

vitamin K essential in the formation of blood clotting factors. Menaquinones are synthesized by bacteria of large intestine and phylloquinones are obtained from plant foods. ⇒ haemorrhagic disease of the newborn.

vitamins *npl* a group of organic compounds required in small amounts by the body. They are vital for many metabolic processes in which they act as coenzymes. Most are obtained from dietary sources, but some can be synthesized in the body, e.g. vitamin D. Vitamins may be: (a) fat-soluble – A, D, E, K, or (b) water-soluble – C and the B complex which includes: thiamine (vitamin B₁), riboflavin (vitamin B₂), niacin (nicotinamide and nicotinic acid), pyridoxine (vitamin B₆), folates, cobalamins (vitamin B₁₂), biotin and pantothenic acid.

vitiligo *n* a skin disease characterized by areas of complete loss of pigmentation. There is an absence of melanocytes in affected areas. The disease is associated with autoimmune conditons that include pernicious anaemia and endocrine disorders and there may be a family history. Exposure to excessive sunlight may be a predisposing factor.

vitrectomy *n* surgical removal of the vitreous humor from the vitreous chamber of the eye.

vitreous *adj* resembling glass. *vitreous chamber* the cavity inside the eyeball and behind the lens. *vitreous humor* the clear jelly-like substance contained in the vitreous chamber where it contributes to intraocular pressure. It is a closed system and is formed during embryonic development.

VLDL *abbr* very-low-density lipoprotein.

VMA *abbr* ⇒ vanillylmandelic acid.

vocal cords the vocal folds. Two membranous folds stretched anteroposteriorly across the larynx. Sound is produced by their vibration as air from the lungs passes between them. Pitch or frequency of the voice changes with the tension (length) of the cords. ⇒ glottis.

vocational assessment *n* appraisal of an individual's ability to perform a particular job (previous or future) It may include the identification of training needs, the need for special equipment or environmental adaptations. Also known as work assessment.

voice activated domestic appliance system computerised system for switching on or off domestic appliances such as lights, kettle, telephone, each 'instruction' to the computer being controlled by the user's voice. Enables severely impaired individuals, e.g. someone with a high spinal fracture, to live as independently as possible, without relying on interventions by helpers.

voiding *n* emptying, usually of the urinary bladder *timed voiding* a fixed voiding schedule, determined by the baseline frequency/volume chart. Often used for older people who may be debilitated or for those with neurogenic bladder.

volatile *adj* evaporating rapidly.

volition *n* the will to act.

Volkmann's ischaemic contracture a flexion deformity of the wrist and fingers from fixed contracture of the flexor muscles in the forearm. The cause is ischaemia of the muscles by injury or obstruction to the brachial artery, near the elbow. ⇒ supracondylar fracture.

volt (v) *n* >the derived SI unit (International System of Units) for electromotive force (also called electrical potential or potential difference).

voluntary *adj* under the control of the will; free and unrestricted; as opposed to reflex or involuntary.

voluntary organizations a group of people who join in an unpaid capacity to serve a particular cause, such as providing a library service to inpatients, running a hospital shop, taking a trolley shop to the wards, organizing a coffee shop in the outpatients' department. Other voluntary organizations are concerned with providing help to patients suffering from a particular condition, and their families.

voluntary sector comprises the groups and organizations run by and controlled by volunteers, e.g. Samaritans, MIND. Many have charitable status, some have grants from local and central government, and some employ professionals and other paid staff to assist in their activities. They provide considerable support to publicly and privately funded health and social care.

volvulus *n* a twisting of a section of bowel (small bowel or sigmoid colon) with its mesentery. Causes gangrene and intestinal obstruction.

vomit *n* ejection of the stomach contents through the mouth; sickness. ⇒ projectile vomiting.

vomiting the disagreeable experience occurring when stomach contents are reflexly expelled through the mouth, it is often accompanied by feelings of nausea. It may be effortless, associated with abdominal pain, or projectile, such as with pyloric stenosis. A person who is vomiting generally needs: privacy and support, a suitable receptacle and a denture container if appropriate, facilities for teeth cleaning, a mouthwash and a wash and bedding/ clothing change as appropriate. Postoperatively, people should be encouraged to support wounds with their hands. The vomit and type of vomiting, e.g. projectile, should be observed and accurate records of fluid balance kept. Apart from these simple measures, nurses should ensure that the most appropriate antiemetic drugs, e.g. metoclopramide, are administered as prescribed. Antiemetics should always be given in anticipation of expected vomiting, such as with cancer chemotherapy with cytotoxic drugs. *vomiting reflex* vomiting is initiated and co-ordinated by two centres in the brain (medulla) – the vomiting (emetic) centre which has overall control, and the chemoreceptor trigger zone (CTZ) which responds to chemical stimuli in the blood and impulses from the cerebral cortex, gastrointestinal tract and the vestibular pathways (vestibular apparatus and centres). (See Figure 67). ⇒ antiemetic. *vomiting of pregnancy* occurs commonly during the first trimester. Excessive or prolonged vomiting is abnormal and may lead to dehydration, electrolyte imbalance and ketosis. ⇒ hyperemesis gravidarum.

vomiting centre *n* a centre in the medulla of the brain that has overall control of vomiting. It responds to stimuli from the chemical trigger zone, higher centres, e.g. emotion, and from visceral afferents in the gastrointestinal tract.

vomiting of pregnancy ⇒ hyperemesis gravidarum. ⇒ vomiting.

vomitus *n* vomited matter.

von Gierke's disease a glycogen storage disease. An inherited condition where the enzyme glucose-6-phosphatase (G6P) is absent.

von Recklinghausen's disease *n* a name given to two conditions: (a) osteitis fibrosa cystica, the result of primary hyperparathyroidism resulting in decalcification of bones and formation of cysts; (b) multiple neurofibromatosis, the tumours can be felt beneath the skin along the course of nerves. There may be pigmented spots (café au lait) on the skin, and neurofibromas may develop in the gastrointestinal tract and endocrine glands. ⇒ neurofibromatosis.

von Willebrand's disease an inherited bleeding disease due to deficiencies relating to the factor VIII proteins in plasma. The inheritance is autosomal dominant, affecting both sexes, and is essentially a disorder of the primary haemostatic mechanism with disordered platelet-endothelial component interaction, such as that involving collagen. In severe cases the clotting defect resembles haemophilia.

voyeurism a psychosexual disorder where individuals derive sexual gratification from watching the sexual behaviour of others.

VRE *abbr* vancomycin-resistant enterococci.

VSD *abbr* ventricular septal defect.

vulva *n* the external genitalia of the female — **vulval** *adj*.

vulvectomy *n* excision of the vulva, usually for cancer.

vulvitis *n* inflammation of the vulva.

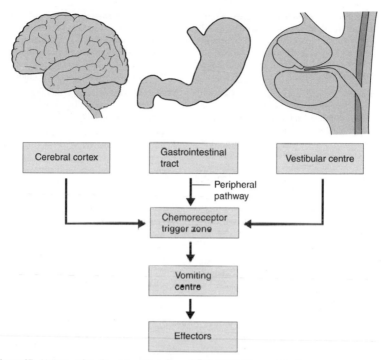

Figure 67 Vomiting reflex. (Reproduced from Bruce & Finlay 1997 with permission.)

vulvovaginal *adj* pertaining to the vulva and the vagina.

vulvovaginitis *n* inflammation of the vulva and vagina.

vulvovaginoplasty *n* operation devised for congenital absence of the vagina, or acquired disabling stenosis — **vulvovaginoplastic** *adj*.

VUR *abbr* vesicoureteric reflux.

VZIG *abbr* varicella/zoster immunoglobulin.

VZV *abbr* varicella/zoster virus.

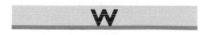

Waldenström's disease *n* ⇒ macroglobulinaemia.

Waldeyer's ring *n* a lymphoid tissue circle surrounding the pharynx. It consists of the palatine, lingual and pharyngeal tonsils.

walking aids *npl* sticks, crutches, tripods and various types of metal frame that allow people to regain or retain independence for walking.

Wallace's rule of nine chart for calculating the percentage of body surface area affected by a burn in adults. ⇒ Lund and Browder's chart.

WAN *acr* for Wide Area Network. A multi-site network where LANs are linked, via modem and the telephone system or high speed data links, to LANs in other locations to enable the sharing of files and resources. ⇒ LAN.

ward rounds traditionally refers to doctors' rounds when e.g. a consultant, registrar and house officer visit each patient to monitor response to treatment. The ward manager (sister or charge nurse) may accompany these rounds. Where primary nursing is being practised, the primary nurse accompanies the round.

wart *n* ⇒ condyloma. ⇒ genital warts. ⇒ verruca.

Wasserman test an obsolete complement fixation test for syphilis.

waterbrash *n* a sudden filling of the mouth with saliva. It is associated with upper gastrointestinal disease, such as peptic ulceration. ⇒ heartburn. ⇒ pyrosis.

Waterhouse-Friderichsen syndrome syndrome resulting from bilateral adrenal haemorrhage accompanying the purpura of septicaemia, usually meningococcal. It is characterized by severe shock and has a high mortality rate.

Waterlow scale *n* a pressure ulcer risk scale developed in the UK by Waterlow in the 1980s. It is more comprehensive than earlier risk scales and includes six main criteria: build/weight for height, continence, skin type/visual risk areas, mobility, sex/age and appetite, and a number of special risks: tissue malnutrition, neurological deficit, major surgery/trauma and medication.

Waterston's operation *n* palliative procedure for Fallot's tetralogy where the right pulmonary artery is anastomosed to the aorta.

watt (W) *n* the derived SI unit (International System of Units) for electrical power.

wavelength *n* the distance between two adjacent wave crests of a wave motion.

WBC *abbr* white blood cell. ⇒ blood. ⇒ leucocyte.

weal *n* a superficial swelling on the skin surface, characteristic of urticaria, nettle-stings, etc.

weaning *v* describes the process that involves the gradual addition of solid food to the milk-only diet of babies. It should not start before the baby is 4 months old, but should start before 6 months, because it is not possible to provide the full nutritional needs after this age, and it becomes more difficult to teach the baby to accept and/or chew lumpy solid foods. The word 'weaning' is also used in the sense of helping to withdraw a person from something on which he is dependent, e.g. assisted ventilation.

web site *n* a collection of one or more pages that can be accessed via the internet or an intranet by using the specific URL. ⇒ home page. ⇒ internet. ⇒ intranet. ⇒ URL.

Weber's test a tuning fork (512 Hz) is used to test hearing by placing the base (after the tuning fork has been struck) on the forehead. When the person hears the sound in the midline, Weber's test is described as being central and normal. ⇒ Rinne's test.

Wegener's granulomatosis a rare chronic inflammatory vasculitis. It causes granulomatous lesions in the respiratory tract, blood vessel necrosis and glomerulonephritis. Treatment is with corticosteroids and the cytotoxic drug cyclophosphamide.

Weil-Felix test a nonspecific agglutination reaction used in the diagnosis of rickettsial disease, such as the typhus group of fevers.

Weil's disease serious disease caused by bacteria (spirochaetes) of the genus leptospira, e.g. *Leptospira icterohaemorrhagiae*, carried by rats who transmit it via infected urine, and other animal hosts. Treatment is with penicillin or a tetracyline. ⇒ leptospirosis.

Welfare of Children in Hospital (Platt Report 1959) a government report that highlighted the detrimental effects caused by the hospitalization of children. It made recommendations about children being cared for by specialist practitioners in suitable environments. A further government report (Welfare of children and young people in hospital 1991) reiterated the principles, and made specific recommendations about involving parents in the care of their children in hospital and the level of staffing in paediatric areas.

welfare state a political system where the state takes responsibility for the provision of various welfare benefits.

well baby clinic mothers are encouraged to bring their new babies during the early years for monitoring by health visitors. General advice and information, and immunization are available.

well man clinic a clinic, usually at the GP's surgery, where men are encouraged to have an annual health check which might include measurement of blood pressure, weight, urinalysis, assessment of diet, smoking, alcohol use and exercise and health promotion. ⇒ risk factor. ⇒ testicular self-examination.

well woman clinic a clinic, usually at the GP's surgery, where women are encouraged to have an annual health check which might include measurement of blood pressure, weight, urinalysis, breast awareness education, cervical smear, assessment of diet, smoking, alcohol use and exercise and health promotion. ⇒ breast awareness. ⇒ Papanicolaou test. ⇒ risk factor.

wen *n* ⇒ sebaceous cyst.

Wernicke's encephalopathy *n* a syndrome occurring in association with the polyneuritis of longterm alcohol misuse. It is characterized by vertigo, nystagmus, ataxia and stupor. A manifestation of thiamine deficiency. ⇒ Korsakoff's psychosis, syndrome.

Wertheim's hysterectomy extended hysterectomy. An extensive operation for removal of carcinoma of the cervix, where the uterus, cervix, upper vagina, tubes, ovaries, peritoneum, fatty tissue and regional lymph nodes are removed.

West nomogram used to calculate body surface area in children.

Western blot a method of testing for HIV infection. The test is usually not carried out until two positive results have been gained from the less specific ELISA test.

Wharton's jelly a jelly-like embryonic connective tissue contained in the umbilical cord.

wheezing *n* a type of dyspnoea audible as a whistling sound, often only detectable by stethoscope, and usually present on inspiration and expiration. Associated with the bronchospasm of asthma and other conditions.

Whipple's operation *n* radical surgery for carcinoma of the head of pancreas. It involves: partial pancreatectomy, excision of the bile duct, duodenum and pylorus, a gastrojejunostomy with the pancreas and gallbladder joined to the jejunum.

whipworm *n* *Trichuris trichiura*. ⇒ trichuriasis.

white asphyxia → asphyxia.

white leg (*syn* phlegmasia alba dolens) thrombophlebitis occurring in women after childbirth.

white matter white nerve tissue of the central nervous system, the myelinated nerve fibres. ⇒ grey matter.

white papers government report/plans that result from a consultation exercise, e.g. Department of Health (1999) *Saving Lives: our healthier nation*. London: The Stationery Office. ⇒ green papers.

whitlow *n* ⇒ paronychia.

whole body vibration an occupational disease which affects drivers of certain vehicles, e.g. tractors, helicopters and some ships. There is discomfort from interference with the natural resonance of organs and may lead to osteoarthritis of the spine.

whooping cough ⇒ pertussis.

Widal test an agglutination reaction for typhoid fever that detects antibodies in the blood.

Wilcoxon test *n* a nonparametric alternative to Student's paired t test.

Wilms' tumour ⇒ nephroblastoma.

Wilson's disease hepaticolenticular degeneration. A rare inherited autosomal recessive condition where copper metabolism and excretion is abnormal. Copper is deposited in the liver, basal nuclei, kidneys, bone and the eye. It is characterized by tremor, choreic movements, dementia, hepatitis, cirrhosis, hepatic portal hypertension and liver failure. It is treated with penicillamine, a copper-binding drug. The bound copper is then excreted in the urine. Family members should be investigated and treated if they have the condition, even if they are asymptomatic. ⇒ Kayser-Fleischer ring.

windpipe *n* ⇒ trachea.

withdrawal *n* 1. a particular group of signs and symptoms experienced by people when giving up a substance such as alcohol, prescribed tranquillizers and antidepressants, illegal drugs, tobacco or solvents to which they have been addicted. 2. a negative coping behaviour when a person becomes increasingly socially isolated. 3. an unreliable method of contraception. ⇒ coitus interruptus.

Wolff-Parkinson-White (WPW) syndrome *n* a supraventricular ectopic rhythm caused by the presence of an abnormal portion of atrioventricular conducting fibres (bypass tract). It is characterized by a shortening of the PR interval, a change in the QRS complex, tachycardia and the risk of life-threatening ventricular arrhythmias. The treatment of choice is destruction of the bypass tract with laser or radiofrequency techniques, but drugs, such as disopyramide, can be used to slow conduction. ⇒ ablation.

wolffian ducts *npl* primitive embryonic ducts which give rise to the male genitourinary structures in the genetically male embryo, under the influence of testosterone from the gonads. ⇒ mullerian ducts.

womb *n* the uterus.

Wood's light special ultraviolet light used for the detection of fungal infections, e.g. ringworm.

woolsorters' disease ⇒ anthrax.

word processor a program which provides for text to be entered, edited, corrected and printed prior to storage. The majority of word processing packages contain features such as spell checking, cut and paste blocks of text and the production of contents and index pages. Advanced programs support printers that produce different fonts, graphics and even full 'desk top publishing' facilities. ⇒ font. ⇒ graphics.

word salad describes the jumble of disconnected words characteristic of the speech of psychotic patients, such as those with schizophrenia.

work physical or mental activities performed for a specific social or productive purpose that has a desired outcome.

work related upper limb disorder ⇒ repetitive strain injury.

working memory ⇒ short term memory.

World Health Organization (WHO) an agency of the United Nations affiliated with other organizations concerned with health promotion, epidemiology, environmental conditions and access to health facilities on a regional and global scale. For administrative purposes, the world is divided into 6 regions, each having a regional office. The headquarters is in Geneva, Switzerland.

worms *npl* invertebrate animals, many of which are parasitic in humans. ⇒ cestode. ⇒ nematodes. ⇒ trematodes.

wound *n* most commonly used when referring to injury to the skin or underlying tissues or organs by a blow, cut, missile or stab. It also includes injury to the skin caused by chemicals, cold, friction, heat, pressure and radiation. Wounds may be acute or chronic. ⇒ abrasion. ⇒ contusion. ⇒ fungating wound. ⇒ incision. ⇒ infection. ⇒ lacerated wound. ⇒ penetrating wound (puncture). Wounds may be classified as: *clean* certain surgical procedures, e.g. hysterectomy, where aseptic technique is maintained; *clean contaminated* surgical operations involving the respiratory or gastrointestinal tract; *contaminated* acutely inflamed without pus, or where leakage from a hollow organ has occurred, or clean procedures where aseptic techniques were breached and recent traumatic wound; *dirty* presence of pus, perforated internal organs and non-recent traumatic wounds. *wound measurement* a vital part of initial and ongoing assessment of healing progress and the efficacy of management. Methods include: simple contact such as use of tracing paper, gauges to measure depth, measuring wound volume using fluids or moulding material, surface contour tracing, and more complex (three dimensional) noncontact methods, such as structured light or laser triangulation, that are accurate but not generally available.

wound closure strips sterile skin closure strips that can be used in place of sutures; wound edges are brought within 3 mm (to allow for drainage); the strips are placed across the wound with space between. Lastly, a strip is placed on either side, parallel to the wound.

wound drains most commonly used in surgical wounds. They may be inserted as a therapeutic measure, e.g. to drain an abscess, or prophylactically, e.g. to prevent blood clotting and forming a haematoma, or in case of the escape of bile. Drainage may be active where the drain is attached to a vacuum system or suction apparatus producing a 'closed wound suction'. ⇒ T-tube. ⇒ underwater seal.

wound dressings proprietary materials of different substances applied to surgical or medical wounds. Modern dressings aim to be permeable to water vapour and gases but not to bacteria or liquids; this retains serous exudate which is actively bactericidal. They do not adhere to the wound surface and, on removal, do not damage new tissue. (See Figure 68). ⇒ alginates. ⇒ deodorants. ⇒ foam dressings. ⇒ hydrocolloid dressings. ⇒ hydrogel dressings. ⇒ iodine. ⇒ paraffin gauze dressing. ⇒ semipermeable films. ⇒ silicone.

wound healing normal wound healing has four overlapping phases: haemostasis, inflammation, proliferative and maturation, which may take many months. The healing process may be prolonged by local factors, e.g. poor blood supply, drying of wound bed, mechanical stress, necrotic tissue/foreign body etc, or general factors that include: ageing, nutritional state, dehydration, stress, drugs such as corticosteroids and cytotoxic drugs etc. ⇒ angiogenesis. ⇒ epithelialization. ⇒ granulation. Wound healing may take place by: *first/primary intention* when the edges of a clean wound are accurately held together, healing occurs with the minimum of scarring and deformity; *second* *intention* when the edges of a wound are not held together, the gap is filled by granulation tissue before epithelium can grow over the wound; or by *third intention* when a wound is left open until infection has been treated or a foreign body removed, and then the wound edges are brought together. ⇒ moist wound healing.

WPW *abbr* Wolff-Parkinson-White syndrome.

wrist *n* the joint between the hand and forearm; the carpus.

wrist drop paralysis of the muscles which raise the wrist, because of damage to the radial nerve.

writ *n* ⇒ claim form.

wryneck *n* → torticollis

WTEs *abbr* Whole Time Equivalents. ⇒ establishment.

www *abbr* worldwide web. A term for the information stored on computer web sites and accessed via the internet. ⇒ internet. ⇒ web site.

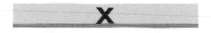

xanthelasma *n* a variety of xanthoma *xanthelasma palpebrarum* small yellowish plaques appear on the eyelids.

xanthine *n* dioxypurine found in liver, muscle, pancreas and urine. An intermediate metabolite formed from the degradation of nucleic acids to uric acid, excreted in the urine.

xanthochromia *n* yellow discoloration of the CSF. It may be caused by degraded haemoglobin following a subarachnoid haemorrhage.

xanthoderma yellow discoloration of the skin.

xanthoma *n* a collection of fatty substances, such as cholesterol under the skin producing a plaque and yellow discoloration — **xanthomata** *pl.*

xanthopsia visual disorder where all objects appear to be yellow.

xanthosis *n* yellow discoloration of the skin caused by ingesting high levels of certain foods, such as carrots.

X chromosome *n* sex chromosome that is paired in the homogametic sex (genetic female). It is present in every female gamete and in half of the male gametes. Carries many major genes. ⇒ sex-linked. ⇒ Y chromosome.

xenograft *n* heterograft. A graft with material obtained from a donor of different species.

xenon (Xe) *n* a rare gas that is chemically inert.

Xenopsylla *n* a genus of fleas. *Xenopsylla cheopis* is the rat flea that transmits typhus and bubonic plague.

xeroderma *n* (xerodermia) dryness of the skin. → ichthyoses. *xeroderma pigmentosum* (Kaposi's disease) a familial dermatosis characterized by extreme photosensitivity. There are freckles and telangiectases. Pathological changes give rise to keratosis and potentially fatal neoplastic growth.

xerophthalmia *n* dryness and ulceration of the cornea which may lead to blindness. Associated with lack of vitamin A

xerosis *n* dryness. *xerosis conjunctivae* excessively dry conjunctiva with thickening. An early sign of vitamin A deficiency, especially in children → Bitôt's spots.

xerostomia *n* dry mouth.

- Maintains high humidity at the wound
- Removes excess exudate and toxic substances from the wound
- Permits the exchange of gases
- Insulates the wound
- Impermeable to bacteria
- Free of any particles, fibres or toxic wound components
- Nonadherent–allows removal without wound trauma

- Nonallergenic and nontoxic
- Comfortable and conformable
- Protects the wound from further damage
- Needs only infrequent dressing changes
- Long shelf-life
- Cost-effective
- Easily available

Figure 68 Characteristics of an ideal wound dressing. (Adapted from Bale and Jones 1997 with permission.)

xiphoid sword-shaped cartilage attached to the sternum. Also known as ensiform cartilage.

X-rays short rays of electromagnetic spectrum. The word is popularly used for radiographs.

XXY syndrome ⇒ Klinefelter syndrome.

xylose absorption test an investigation for malabsorption. Xylose 5 g (a pentose sugar) is given orally and its urinary excretion is measured. Excretion of at least 2 g is considered normal, and reduced amounts indicate malabsorption syndrome. Xylose labelled with radioactive carbon (^{14}C-xylose) can be given orally and the amount of exhaled carbon dioxide ($^{14}CO_2$) can also be used.

XYY syndrome genetic anomaly in males where the cells have an extra Y chromosome, bringing the total to 47, or occasionally two extra XYYY. Affected individuals tend to be tall, may have mild learning disability and behavioural problems such as aggressive tendencies.

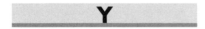

Y

yaws *n* a tropical granulomatous disease caused by *Treponema pertenue*. It resembles syphilis, but is not sexually transmitted and is modified by differences of climate, social habit and hygiene. Lesions affect the skin and bones. ⇒ bejel. ⇒ pinta.

Y chromosome *n* sex chromosome found only in the heterogametic sex (genetic male). It carries fewer major genes and is shorter than the X chromosome.

yeast *n* a unicellular fungus. Some are pathogenic in humans, e.g. *Candida albicans*, *Cryptococcus neoformans*. Other yeasts are used to make bread and in the brewing industry.

yellow card reporting in the UK, a system by which prescribers report suspected adverse drug reactions to the Committee on Safety of Medicines (CSM), the body responsible for monitoring drug safety and advising on the licensing of new drugs.

yellow fever an acute febrile illness of tropical areas, caused by a virus of the togavirus family. It is spread by mosquitoes. Characteristic features are fever,

headache, backache, nausea and vomiting, jaundice, petechial haemorrhages, gastrointestinal bleeding and anuria. Treatment is supportive, such as, fluid replacement and dialysis. The nonpathogenic strain of the virus, known as 17D, is prepared as vaccine for immunization.

Yersinia *n* a genus of Gram-negative bacilli. *Yersinia pestis* is the causative organism of plague.

yin and yang *n* the philosophical concepts underlying complementary therapies, such as acupuncture and shiatsu. Yin and yang describes a dynamic, symbiotic relationship between active and passive energy forces said to be present in the universe and the human body. In order for health to be maintained, equilibrium between these two aspects should be maintained. Universal energy is referred to as true Qi and in the body termed Qi.

yoga a discipline that uses breathing techniques, exercises and postures to relax, reduce stress and generally enhance physical, psychological and spiritual well-being.

yolk *n* the stored nutrient of the ovum. *yolk sac* early embryonic structure formed from endodermal cells. A site for early blood cell production.

Young's syndrome *n* a ciliary dysfunction syndrome with abnormal movement of the respiratory cilia. It causes repeated infection leading to bronchiectasis.

yttrium-90 (^{90}Y) a radioactive isotope of yttrium. Used in the treatment of malignant effusions.

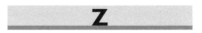

Z

Ziehl-Neelsen stain *n* a staining technique used in the microscopic identification of acid-fast bacilli, such as *Mycobacterium tuberculosis*.

ZIFT *abbr* zygote intrafallopian transfer.

zinc (Zn) *n* a metallic element required in small amounts (trace element) by the body. It is required as a cofactor for certain enzyme reactions and is essential for cell multiplication and successful wound healing. Zinc is involved with insulin storage. Its absorption from the diet is reduced by phytates in wholemeal cereals.

zinc oxide a widely used mild astringent, present in many dermatological applications.

Zollinger-Ellison syndrome *n* the presence of ectopic gastrin producing tissue, usually a pancreatic tumour. Gastric acid secretion increases in response to the hormone release, resulting in peptic ulceration and the inactivation of intestinal enzymes with diarrhoea.

zona *n* a zone or a girdle. *zona facialis* applied to herpes zoster (shingles) affecting the face. *zona fasiculata, glomerulosa and reticularis* the three zones of the adrenal cortex. *zona pellucida* the membrane surrounding the oocyte.

zonula ciliaris suspensory ligament attaching the periphery of the lens of the eye to ciliary body.

zonule *n* small zone, belt or girdle. Also called a zonula.

zonulolysis *n* breaking down the zonula ciliaris – sometimes necessary before intracapsular extraction of the lens — **zonulolytic** *adj.*

zoonosis *n* a disease transmitted from animals to humans, e.g. rabies, anthrax, psittacosis — **zoonoses** *pl.*

zoophilia abnormal liking for animals. The term includes a psychosexual disorder in which the individual derives sexual gratification from fantasy involving animals, sexual or other close contact with animals.

zoster ⇒ herpes zoster. ⇒ shingles.

Z-track an intramuscular injection technique used to prevent leakage and staining such as with iron preparations. (See Figure 69).

zwitterion *n* a molecule that has both positively and negatively charged regions, such as an amino acid in a neutral solution.

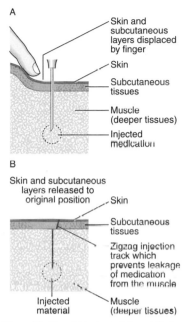

Figure 69 Z track injection technique. A During injection. B After injection. (Reproduced from Brooker 1996 with permission.)

zygoma *n* the cheekbone — **zygomatic** *adj.*

zygote *n* the fertilized ovum. The diploid cell produced by the fusion of the male and female nuclei. *zygote intra-fallopian transfer* process used in assisted conception. Mature ova are retrieved. After mixing with sperm, fertilization is awaited and the resultant zygote placed within the uterine tube.

zymogen *n* a proenzyme. An inactive precursor of a proteolytic enzyme, such as digestive enzymes and clotting factors. *zymogen cells* ⇒ chief cells.

APPENDICES

Contents

APPENDIX 1

Anatomical illustrations

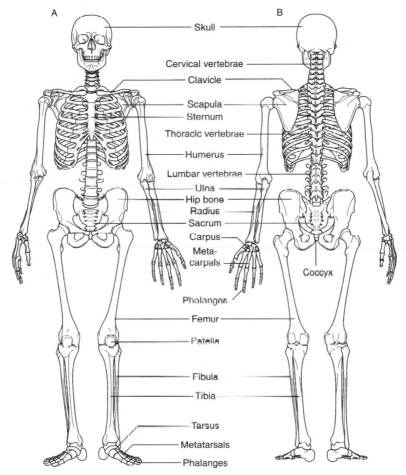

A

B

Skull

Cervical vertebrae

Clavicle

Scapula
Sternum

Thoracic vertebrae

Humerus

Lumbar vertebrae

Ulna

Hip bone

Radius

Sacrum

Carpus

Meta-
carpals

Coccyx

Phalanges

Femur

Patella

Fibula

Tibia

Tarsus

Metatarsals

Phalanges

Figure 70 Skeleton. A Front view. B Back view.

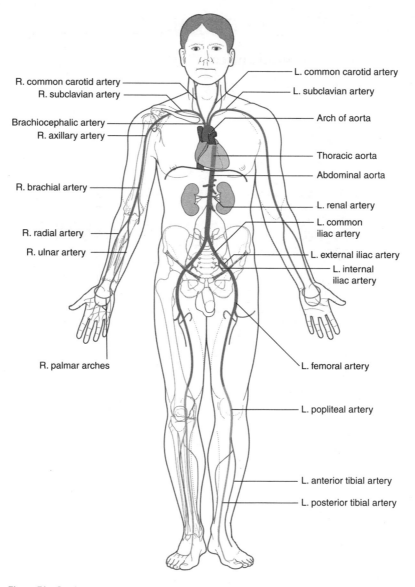

R. common carotid artery
R. subclavian artery
Brachiocephalic artery
R. axillary artery
R. brachial artery
R. radial artery
R. ulnar artery
R. palmar arches

L. common carotid artery
L. subclavian artery
Arch of aorta
Thoracic aorta
Abdominal aorta
L. renal artery
L. common iliac artery
L. external iliac artery
L. internal iliac artery
L. femoral artery
L. popliteal artery
L. anterior tibial artery
L. posterior tibial artery

Figure 71 Circulatory system – arteries.

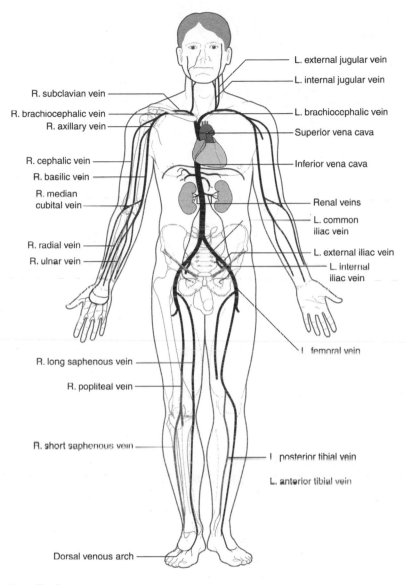

R. subclavian vein

R. brachiocephalic vein
R. axillary vein

R. cephalic vein
R. basilic vein

R. median
cubital vein

R. radial vein
R. ulnar vein

L. external jugular vein
L. internal jugular vein

L. brachiocephalic vein
Superior vena cava

Inferior vena cava

Renal veins
L. common
iliac vein

L. external iliac vein
L. internal
iliac vein

L. femoral vein

R. long saphenous vein
R. popliteal vein

R. short saphenous vein

L. posterior tibial vein

L. anterior tibial vein

Dorsal venous arch

Figure 72 Circulatory system – veins.

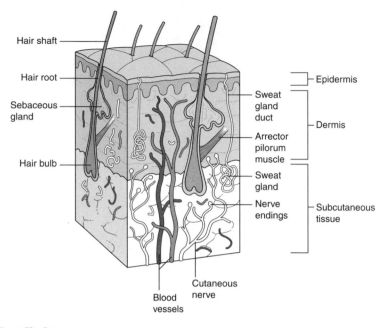

Figure 73 Skin.

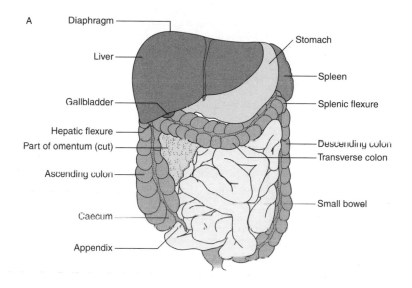

A

Diaphragm

Stomach

Liver

Spleen

Gallbladder

Splenic flexure

Hepatic flexure

Descending colon

Part of omentum (cut)

Transverse colon

Ascending colon

Small bowel

Caecum

Appendix

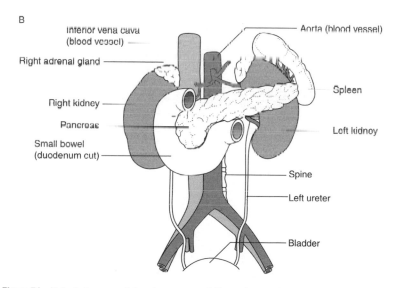

B

Inferior vena cava (blood vessel)

Aorta (blood vessel)

Right adrenal gland

Right kidney

Spleen

Pancreas

Left kidney

Small bowel (duodenum cut)

Spine

Left ureter

Bladder

Figure 74 Abdominal contents. A Anterior structures. B View with most of the organs of digestion removed.

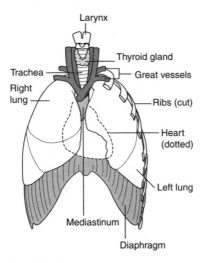

Figure 75 Thoracic contents.

APPENDIX 2

Units of measurement

Units of measurement — International System of Units (SI), the metric system, and conversions

The International System of Units (SI) or Système International d'Unités is the measurement system used for scientific, medical and technical purposes in most countries. In the United Kingdom SI units have replaced those of the Imperial System, e.g. the kilogram is used for mass instead of the pound (in everyday situations, both mass and weight are measured in kilograms although weight, which varies with gravity, is really a measure of force).

The SI comprises seven base units with several derived units. Each unit has its own symbol and is expressed as a decimal multiple or submultiple of the base unit by using the appropriate prefix, e.g. millimetre is one thousandth of a metre.

Base units

Quantity	Base unit and symbol
length	metre (m)
mass	kilogram (kg)
time	second (s)
amount of substance	mole (mol)
electric current	ampere (A)
thermodynamic temperature	kelvin ($^\circ$K)
luminous intensity	candela (cd)

Derived units

Derived units for measuring different quantities are reached by multiplying or dividing two or more base units.

Quantity	Derived unit and symbol
work, energy, quantity of heat	joule (J)
pressure	pascal (Pa)
force	newton (N)
frequency	hertz (Hz)
power	watt (W)
electrical potential, electromotive force, potential difference	volt (v)
absorbed dose of radiation	gray (Gy)
radioactivity	becquerel (Bq)
dose equivalent	sievert (Sv)

Factor, decimal multiples and submultiples of SI units

Multiplication factor	Prefix	Symbol
10^{12}	tera	T
10^9	giga	G
10^6	mega	M
10^3	kilo	k
10^2	hecto	h
10^1	deca	da
10^{-1}	deci	d
10^{-2}	centi	c
10^{-3}	milli	m
10^{-6}	micro	μ
10^{-9}	nano	n
10^{-12}	pico	p
10^{-15}	femto	f
10^{-18}	atto	a

Rules for using units and writing large numbers and decimals

- The symbol for a unit is unaltered in the plural and should not be followed by a full stop except at the end of a sentence:
  5 cm not 5 cm. or 5 cms.
- Large numbers are written in three-digit groups (working from right to left) with spaces not commas (in some countries the comma is used to indicate a decimal point):
  fifty thousand is written as 50 000
  five hundred thousand is written as 500 000
- Numbers with four digits are written without the space, e.g. four thousand is written as 4000.
- The decimal sign between digits is indicated by a full stop positioned near the line, e.g. 50.25. If the numerical value of the decimal is less than 1, a zero should appear before the decimal sign:
  0.125 not .125
  Decimals with more than four digits are also written in three-digit groups, but this time working from left to right, e.g. 0.000 25.
- 'Squared' and 'cubed' are expressed as numerical powers and not by abbreviation:
  square centimetre is cm^2 not sq. cm.

Commonly used measurements requiring further explanation

- Temperature — although the SI base unit for temperature is the kelvin, by international convention temperature is measured in degrees Celsius (°C).
- Energy — the energy of food or individual requirements for energy are measured in kilojoules (kJ); the SI unit is the joule (J). In practice many people still use the kilocalorie (kcal), a non-SI unit, for these purposes.

  1 calorie = 4.2 J.
  1 kilocalorie (large calorie) = 4.2 kJ.

- Volume — volume is calculated by multiplying length, width and depth. Using the SI unit for length, the metre (m), means ending up with a cubic metre (m³), which is a huge volume and is certainly not appropriate for most purposes. In clinical practice the litre (L or l) is used. A litre is based on the volume of a cube measuring 10 cm × 10 cm × 10 cm. Smaller units still, e.g. millilitre (mL) or one thousandth of a litre, are commonly used in clinical practice.
- Time — the SI base unit for time is the second (s), but it is acceptable to use minute (min), hour (h) or day (d). In clinical practice it is preferable to use 'per 24 hours' for the excretion of substances in urine and faeces: g/24 h
- Amount of substance — the SI base unit for amount of substance is the mole (mol). The concentration of many substances is expressed in moles per litre (mol/L) or millimoles per litre (mmol/L) which replaces milliequivalents per litre (mEq/L). Some exceptions exist and include haemoglobin and plasma proteins in grams per litre (g/L); and enzyme activity in International Units (IU, U or iu).
- Pressure — the SI unit of pressure is the pascal (Pa), and the kilopascal (kPa) replaces the old non-SI unit of millimetres of mercury pressure (mmHg) for blood pressure and blood gases. However, mmHg is still widely used for measuring blood pressure. Other anomalies include cerebrospinal fluid, which is measured in millimetres of water (mmH$_2$O); and central venous pressure, which is measured in centimetres of water (cmH$_2$O).

Measurements, equivalents and conversions (SI or metric and imperial)

Length

1 kilometre (km)	= 1000 metres (m)
1 metre (m)	= 100 centimetres (cm) or 1000 millimetres (mm)
1 centimetre (cm)	= 10 millimetres (mm)
1 millimetre (mm)	= 1000 micrometres (μm)
1 micrometre (μm)	= 1000 nanometres (nm)

Conversions

1 metre (m)	= 39.370 inches (in)
1 centimetre (cm)	= 0.3937 inches (in)
30.48 centimetres (cm)	= 1 foot (ft)
2.54 centimetres (cm)	= 1 inch (in)

Volume

1 litre (L)	= 1000 millilitres (mL)
1 millilitre (mL)	= 1000 microlitres (μL)

NB The millilitre (mL) and the cubic centimetre (cm³) are usually treated as being the same.

Conversions

1 litre (L)	= 1.76 pints (pt)
568.25 millilitres (mL)	= 1 pint (pt)
28.4 millilitres (mL)	= 1 fluid ounce (fl oz)

Weight or mass

I kilogram (kg)	= 1000 grams (g)
I gram (g)	= 1000 milligrams (mg)
I milligram (mg)	= 1000 micrograms (µg)
I microgram (µg)	= 1000 nanograms (ng)

NB To avoid any confusion with milligram (mg) the word microgram (µg) should be written in full on prescriptions.

Conversions

I kilogram (kg)	= 2.204 pounds (lb)
I gram (g)	= 0.0353 ounce (oz)
453.59 grams (g)	= I pound (lb)
28.34 grams (g)	= I ounce (oz)

Temperature conversions

To convert Celsius to Fahrenheit:
multiply by 9, divide by 5, and add 32 to the result,
e.g. 36°C to Fahrenheit:
$36 \times 9 = 324 \div 5 = 64.8 + 32 = 96.8°F$
therefore 36°C = 96.8°F

To convert Fahrenheit to Celsius:
subtract 32, multiply by 5, and divide by 9,
e.g. 104°F to Celsius:
$104 - 32 = 72 \times 5 = 360 \div 9 = 40°C$
therefore 104°F = 40°C

Temperature comparison

°Celsius	°Fahrenheit
100	212
95	203
90	194
85	185
80	176
75	167
70	158
65	149
60	140
55	131
50	122
45	113
44	112.2
43	109.4
42	107.6
41	105.8
40	104
39.5	103.1
39	102.2
38.5	101.3
38	100.4

°Celsius	°Fahrenheit
37.5	99.5
37	98.6
36.5	97.7
36	96.8
35.5	95.9
35	95
34	93.2
33	91.4
32	89.6
31	87.8
30	86
25	77
20	68
15	59
10	50
5	41
0	32
-5	23
-10	14

NB Boiling point = 100°C = 212°F
Freezing point = 0°C = 32°F

APPENDIX 3

Normal values

The values below represent an 'average' reference range, in adults, for blood, cerebrospinal fluid, urine and faeces. These ranges should be used as a guide only. Reference ranges vary between individual laboratories and readers should consult their own laboratory for those used locally. This is especially important where reference values depend upon the analytical equipment and temperatures used.

Blood (haematology)

Test	Reference range
Activated partial thromboplastin time (APTT)	30–40s
Bleeding time (Ivy)	2–8 min
Erythrocyte sedimentation rate (ESR)	
Adult women	3–15 mm/h
Adult men	1–10 mm/h
Fibrinogen	1.5–4.0 g/l
Folate (serum)	4–18 µg/L
Haemoglobin	
Women	115–165 g/L (11.5–16.5 g/dL)
Men	130–180 g/L (13–18 g/dL)
Haptoglobins	0.3–2.0 g/L
Mean cell haemoglobin (MCH)	27–32 pg
Mean cell haemoglobin concentration (MCHC)	30–35 g/dL
Mean cell volume (MCV)	78–95 fl
Packed cell volume (PCV or haematocrit)	
Women	0.35–0.47 (35–47%)
Men	0.4–0.54 (40–54%)
Platelets (thrombocytes)	150–400×10^9/L
Prothrombin time	12–16 s
Red cells (erythrocytes)	
Women	3.8–5.3×10^{12}/L
Men	4.5–6.5×10^{12}/L
Reticulocytes (newly formed red cells in adults)	25–85×10^9/L
White cells total (leucocytes)	4.0–11.0×10^9/L

Blood-venous plasma (biochemistry)

Test	Reference range
Alanine aminotransferase (ALT)	10–40 U/L
Albumin	36–47 g/L
Alkaline phosphatase	40–125 U/L
Amylase	90–300 U/L
Aspartate aminotransferase (AST)	10–35 U/L
Bicarbonate (arterial)	22–28 mmol/L
Bilirubin (total)	2–17 µmol/L
Caeruloplasmin	150–600 mg/L
Calcium	2.1–2.6 mmol/L
Chloride	95–105 mmol/L
Cholesterol (total)	ideally below 5.2 mmol/L
HDL–Cholesterol	
Women	0.6–1.9 mmol/L
Men	0.5–1.6 mmol/L
$PaCO_2$ (arterial)	4.4–6.1 kPa
Copper	13–24 µmol/L
Cortisol (at 08.00 h)	160–565 nmol/L
Creatine kinase (total)	
Women	30–150 U/L
Men	30–200 U/L
Creatinine	55–150 µmol/L
Gamma-glutamyl-transferase (γGT)	
Women	5–35 U/L
Men	10–55 U/L
Globulins	24–37 g/L
Glucose (venous blood, fasting)	3.6–5.8 mmol/L
Glycosylated haemoglobin (HbA_1)	4–6%
Hydrogen ion concentration (arterial)	35–44 nmol/L
Iron	
Women	10–28 µmol/L
Men	14–32 µmol/L
Iron-binding capacity total (TIBC)	45–70 µmol/L
Lactate (arterial)	0.3–1.4 mmol/L
Lactate dehydrogenase (total)	230–460 U/L
Lead (adults, whole blood)	<1.7 µmol/L
Magnesium	0.7–1.0 mmol/L
Osmolality	275–290 mmol/kg
PaO_2 (arterial)	12–15 kPa
Oxygen saturation (arterial)	>97%
pH	7.36–7.42
Phosphate (fasting)	0.8–1.4 mmol/L
Potassium (serum)	3.6–5.0 mmol/L
Protein (total)	60–80 g/L
Sodium	136–145 mmol/L
Transferrin	2–4 g/L
Triglycerides (fasting)	0.6–1.8 mmol/L
Urate	
Women	0.12–0.36 mmol/L
Men	0.12–0.42 mmol/L

Test	Reference range
Urea	2.5–6.5 mmol/L
Uric acid	
Women	0.09–0.36 mmol/L
Men	0.1–0.45 mmol/L
Vitamin A	0.7–3.5 µmol/L
Vitamin C	23–57 µmol/L
Zinc	11–22 µmol/L

Cerebrospinal fluid

Test	Reference range
Cells	0–5 mm³
Chloride	120–170 mmol/L
Glucose	2.5–4.0 mmol/L
Pressure (adult)	50–180 mm/l H_2O
Protein	100–400 mg/L

Urine

Test	Reference range
Albumin/creatinine ratio	<3.5 mg albumin/mmol creatinine
Calcium (diet dependent)	<12 mmol/24 h (normal diet)
Copper	0.2–0.6 µmol/24 h
Cortisol	9–50 µmol/24 h
Creatinine	9–17 mmol/24 h
5-Hydroxyindole-3-acetic acid (5HIAA)	10–45 µmol/24 h
Magnesium	3.3–5.0 mmol/24 h
Oxalate	
Women	40–320 mmol/24 h
Men	80–490 mmol/24 h
pH	4–8
Phosphate	15–50 mmol/24 h
Porphyrins (total)	90–370 nmol/24 h
Potassium (depends on intake)	25–100 mmol/24 h
Protein (total)	no more than 0.3 g/L
Sodium (depends on intake)	100–200 mmol/24 h
Urea	170–500 mmol/24 h

Faeces

Test	Reference range
Fat content (daily output on normal diet)	<7 g/24 h
Fat (as stearic acid)	11–18 mmol/24 h

APPENDIX 4

Nutrients

Helen Barker

The nutrients necessary for supplying energy and the production of the molecules needed for cell growth and repair are divided into two groups: (a) the energy-yielding macronutrients — protein, fat and carbohydrate (including nonstarch polysaccharide); and (b) the micronutrients — vitamins and minerals (including trace elements).

Macronutrients

Protein

- RNI: 55.5 g/d male; 45 g/d female (DoH 1991).
- Sources: Meat, fish, nuts, pulses, dairy products, tofu, quorn and eggs.
- Functions: Essential component of all body tissues; source of energy (in some circumstances).
- Deficiency: Retarded growth; poor wound healing; impaired immune system; weight loss and muscle wasting; fatty deposits in liver.
- Excess: Has been linked to bone demineralization and age-related decline in renal function.
- Additional information: Western diets usually have a protein content that is higher than the RNI.

Fat

- RNI: Should not exceed 33% of total daily energy intake and of this no more than 10% should be saturated fatty acids (DoH 1991).
- Sources: Cooking oils, fried foods, full-fat dairy products, ghee, margarine, meat, oily fish, seeds, nuts, pastry, chocolate, cakes, biscuits and crisps.
- Functions: Energy source, energy storage, insulation, synthesis of steroid hormones, nerve and cell membrane structure; absorption of fat-soluble vitamins.
- Deficiency: Weight loss; deficiency of essential fatty acids can cause neurological damage.
- Excess: Obesity; increased risk of many conditions including cardiovascular disease and some cancers.
- Additional information: There are two essential fatty acids — linoleic acid and alpha linolenic acid — which are necessary for the normal development of the nervous system.

Carbohydrate

- RNI: A minimum of 47% of total daily energy intake should be provided by carbohydrate. This should include no more than 10% as nonmilk extrinsic sugars (DoH 1991).

- Sources: Rice, pasta, noodles, chapatti, bread, breakfast cereals, yam, plantain and potato.
- Functions: Source of energy for metabolic processes.
- Deficiency: Weight loss; ketosis.
- Excess: Obesity; hypertriglyceridaemia (high level of triglycerides in the blood).
- Additional information: Diets that are high in carbohydrate are usually low in fat.
- RNI: Nonstarch polysaccharide 18 g/d (DoH 1991).

Micronutrients
Vitamins
Vitamins are divided into two groups — fat-soluble and water-soluble.

Fat-soluble vitamins
Vitamin A (retinol)
- RNI: 700 µg/d male; 600 µg/d female (DoH 1991).
- Sources: As retinol in liver, kidney, oily fish, egg yolk, full-fat dairy produce. As the provitamin carotenes in green, yellow, orange and red fruit and vegetables, for example broccoli, carrots, apricots, mangoes, sweet potatoes and tomatoes.
- Functions: Normal growth and development of tissues; essential for healthy skin and mucous membranes; aids night vision; acts as an antioxidant.
- Deficiency: Poor growth; rough, dry skin and mucous membranes, encouraging infection; xerophthalmia and eventual blindness; increased susceptibility to infection; poor night vision.
- Excess: High doses are teratogenic.
- Additional information: Synthesized in the body from carotenes present in the diet.

Vitamin D (cholecalciferol and ergosterol)
- RNI: 10 µg/d for the housebound (DoH 1991).
- Sources: Oily fish, egg yolk, butter, fortified margarine; action of ultraviolet rays of sunlight (see below).
- Functions: Assists absorption and metabolism of calcium and phosphorus.
- Deficiency: Rickets in children; osteomalacia in adults.
- Excess: Rare; weight loss and diarrhoea.
- Additional information: Produced in the body by action of sunlight on a provitamin in the skin, deficiency develops in those who are not exposed to sun, for example the housebound.

Vitamin E (tocopherols and tocotrienes)
- RNI: Not set.
- Sources: Wheatgerm, egg yolk, milk, cereals, liver, green vegetables.

- Functions: An antioxidant which may protect against cancer and heart disease.
- Deficiency: Haemolytic anaemia can develop in premature infants; malabsorption syndrome.
- Excess: breast pain; muscle weakness; gastrointestinal disorders.
- Additional information: Requirement is increased with increased intake of polyunsaturated fatty acids.

Vitamin K (phylloquinones and menaquinones)
- RNI: Not set.
- Sources: Green leafy vegetables, fruit and dairy products.
- Functions: Essential for the production of prothrombin and other coagulation factors.
- Deficiency: Delayed clotting time; liver damage.
- Excess: Not yet observed from naturally occurring vitamin.
- Additional information: Synthesized by intestinal bacteria so deficiency unusual; can occur in newborns (haemorrhagic disease of the newborn) and those on anticoagulant therapy.

Water-soluble vitamins

Vitamin B group
(i) Thiamin(e) (B_1)
- RNI: 0.4 mg/1000kcal (DoH 1991).
- Sources: Milk, liver, eggs, pork, fortified breakfast cereals, vegetables, fruit, wholegrain cereals.
- Functions: Important for metabolism of carbohydrate, fat and alcohol.
- Deficiency: Beri-beri; neuritis; mental confusion; fatigue; poor growth in children; Wernicke's encephalopathy and Korsakoff's syndrome when deficiency occurs with alcohol misuse.
- Excess: Headache; insomnia; irritability; contact dermatitis.
- Additional information: Requirement increases with increase in carbohydrate intake.

(ii) Riboflavin (B_2)
- RNI: 1.3 mg/d male; 1.1 mg/d female (DoH 1991).
- Sources: Milk, milk products, offal, fortified breakfast cereals.
- Functions: Metabolism of carbohydrate, fat and protein.
- Deficiency: Fissures at corner of mouth; tongue inflammation; vascularization of cornea.
- Excess: Large quantities are not absorbed, thus preventing toxicity.
- Additional information: Destroyed by sunlight.

(iii) Niacin (nicotinic acid and nicotinamide) (B_3)
- RNI: 6.6 mg/1000kcal, as nicotinic acid equivalents (DoH 1991).
- Sources: Meat, fish, pulses, wholegrains, fortified breakfast cereals.

- Functions: Energy metabolism, as part of coenzymes NAD and NADP which are involved in oxidation and reduction reactions.
- Deficiency: Pellagra — dermatitis, diarrhoea and dementia.
- Excess: skin irritation; liver damage.
- Additional information: Can be synthesized from the amino acid tryptophan.

(iv) Pantothenic acid (B_5)
- RNI: Not set.
- Sources: Liver, eggs, yeast, vegetables.
- Functions: Protein, fat, carbohydrate and alcohol metabolism.
- Deficiency: vomiting; insomnia.
- Excess: Not reported.

(v) Pyridoxine (B_6)
- RNI: 1.4 mg/d male; 1.2 mg/d female (DoH 1991).
- Sources: Meat, fish, wholegrains, eggs.
- Functions: Protein metabolism.
- Deficiency: Rare; metabolic abnormalities and convulsions.
- Excess: Peripheral nerve damage.
- Additional information: Used therapeutically for a range of conditions; requirement is related to protein intake.

(vi) Biotin
- RNI: Not set.
- Sources: Widely distributed in many foods, for example egg yolk, legumes; can be synthesized by intestinal bacteria.
- Functions: Protein, fat and carbohydrate metabolism.
- Deficiency: Rare; dermatitis, hair loss, nausea, fatigue and anorexia. May be seen in patients having longterm total parenteral nutrition and where large quantities of raw egg are eaten.
- Excess: None known.

(vii) Cobalamins (B_{12})
- RNI: 1.5 µg/d (DoH 1991).
- Sources: Animal products, meat, eggs, fish, dairy products.
- Functions: Essential for red blood cell formation and nerve myelination.
- Deficiency: Megaloblastic anaemia; irreversible neurological damage.
- Excess: Not reported.
- Additional information: Requires intrinsic factor secreted by gastric cells for absorption; only found in foods of animal origin, therefore strict vegetarians and vegans require a dietary supplement.

(viii) Folates (folic acid)
- RNI: 200 µg/d (DoH 1991).
- Sources: Green vegetables, fortified breakfast cereals, yeast extract, liver, oranges.

- Functions: Assists production of red blood cells and protein synthesis.
- Deficiency: Megaloblastic anaemia; growth retardation.
- Excess: Can mask the megaloblastic anaemia of B_{12} deficiency.
- Additional information: Supplement recommended prior to conception and during first 3 months of pregnancy to reduce the incidence of neural tube defects.

Vitamin C (ascorbic acid)

- RNI: 40 mg/d (DoH 1991).
- Sources: Citrus fruits, kiwi fruit, blackcurrants, green leafy vegetables, potato, strawberries, tomatoes. Content decreases with storage.
- Functions: Formation of bones, connective tissue, teeth and red blood cells; acts as an antioxidant.
- Deficiency: Sore mouth and gums; capillary bleeding; scurvy; delayed wound healing; breaking down of scars.
- Excess: Diarrhoea, oxalate stones in kidneys.
- Additional information: Destroyed by cooking in the presence of air and by plant enzymes released when cutting and grating raw food.

Minerals

Details are given below of some of the minerals required by the body. In addition to these there is a requirement for other minerals and trace elements (needed in minute quantities) that include chloride, copper, chromium, fluoride, phosphorus as phosphates, manganese, molybdenum and selenium.

Calcium

- RNI: 700 mg/d (DoH 1991).
- Sources: Milk, dairy products, green leafy vegetables, white bread and hard water.
- Functions: Formation of bones and teeth; blood coagulation; normal muscle and nerve function.
- Deficiency: Osteomalacia; rickets; tetany.
- Excess: Calcium deposits in soft tissue; hypercalcaemia.
- Additional information: Absorption helped by vitamin D and parathyroid hormone.

Iodine

- RNI: 140 µg/d (DoH 1991).
- Sources: Sea food; iodized salt; milk.
- Functions: Synthesis of the thyroid hormones; thyroxine and triiodothyronine.
- Deficiency: Goitre; retarded growth; impaired brain development; congenital abnormalities.
- Excess: Goitre and hyperthyroidism.

- Additional information: Radioisotope used in scanning; some vegetables contain goitrogens which inhibit iodine absorption.

Iron

- RNI: 8.7 mg/d male; 14.8 mg/d female (DoH 1991).
- Sources: Liver, kidney, red meat, egg yolk, wholegrains, dark green vegetables, raisins, treacle, cocoa, molasses.
- Functions: Component of haemoglobin, myoglobin and many enzymes.
- Deficiency: Anaemia; fatigue; lethargy; poor growth; impaired intellectual development.
- Excess: Liver damage.
- Additional information: Absorption is aided by vitamin C and inhibited by phytates and tanins.

Magnesium

- RNI: 300 mg/d male; 270 mg/d female (DoH 1991).
- Sources: Cereals and green vegetables.
- Functions: Influences many enzymes; essential for carbohydrate and protein metabolism; important role in calcium homeostasis.
- Deficiency: Unlikely, mainly in cases of chronic malabsorption and chronic renal failure when it will accompany hypocalcaemia.
- Excess: Unlikely from dietary sources.
- Additional information: Absorption inhibited by phytate.

Potassium

- RNI: 3500 mg/d (DoH 1991).
- Sources: Fruit, vegetables, meat, wholegrains.
- Functions: Principal intracellular electrolyte; influences muscle contraction and nerve excitability
- Deficiency: Muscular weakness; depression; confusion; arrhythmias; cardiac arrest.
- Excess: Hyperkalaemia, cardiac arrest.
- Additional information: Kidney controls secretion and absorption, deficiency is rare due to poor dietary intake but can occur following prolonged use of diuretics and purgatives.

Sodium

- RNI: 1600 mg/d (DoH 1991).
- Sources: Table salt, milk, meat, vegetables, pre-prepared foods, cheese.
- Functions: Principal extracellular electrolyte; important for regulating water balance.
- Deficiency: Weakness; abdominal cramps; faintness.
- Excess: Oedema, hypertension.
- Additional information: Lost through fever, sweat and diarrhoea.

Zinc

- RNI: 9.5 mg/d male; 7.0 mg/d female (DoH 1991).
- Sources: Red meats, eggs, wholegrains.
- Functions: Structural role in some proteins; wound healing; functioning of immune system; sexual and physical development.
- Deficiency: Fatigue; retarded growth and sexual maturity.
- Excess: Nausea, vomiting, fever, or anaemia with chronic excess.
- Additional information: Present in all tissues.

Reference

Department of Health (DoH). 1991 Report on Health and Social Subjects 41. Dietary Reference values for Food energy and Nutrients for the United Kingdom. London: HMSO.

APPENDIX 5

Drugs — the law, measurement and calculations
Jennifer Kelly

Drugs and the law
The main acts governing the use of medicines are the Medicines Act 1968, the Misuse of Drugs Act 1971 and the Medicinal Products: Prescription by Nurses Act 1992.

The Misuse of Drugs Act 1971
This act imposes controls on those drugs liable to produce dependence or cause harm if misused. It prohibits the possession, supply and manufacture of medicinal and other products, except where this has been made legal by the Misuse of Drugs Regulations 1985. The Misuse of Drugs Act categorizes drugs into five separate schedules according to different levels of control. Nurses, midwives and health visitors should be familiar with regulations governing Schedule 2 and 3 medicines. The substance cited in Schedule 2 of the act are known as 'Controlled Drugs' (CDs) and include:

- amfetamine (amphetamine)
- cocaine
- codeine injection
- dexamfetamine (dexamphetamine)
- dextromoramide
- diamorphine
- dihydrocodeine injection
- dipipanone
- fentanyl
- methadone
- methylphenidate
- morphine
- pethidine
- phenazocine.

Schedule 3 includes medicines such as barbiturates, buprenorphine and temazepam, which are also controlled drugs.

Registered medical practitioners and registered dentists may prescribe preparations containing controlled drugs. However, the Misuse of Drugs (Notification of and Supply to Addicts) Regulations 1973 state that medical practitioners may not prescribe, administer or supply controlled drugs to addicted persons as a means of treating their addiction, unless specifically licensed to do so. This is to ensure that addicts will be referred for treatment to a hospital or clinic.

A prescription involving controlled drugs must fulfil the following conditions:

- Patient's name and address specified in ink.
- Signed and dated by prescriber.
- Dose and dosage form, e.g. tablets, capsules, to be specified.
- Total quantity to be supplied written in words and figures.

N.B. All above in the doctor's handwriting (computer-generated prescriptions are not permitted).

Accurate records must be kept by general practitioners, dentists and hospital staff of all purchases, amounts of drugs issued and dosages given. In hospital the following controls are imposed:

- Special double-locked cupboard for controlled drugs alone.
- Key kept and carried by Nurse-in-Charge.
- Supplies can be obtained by prescription signed by a medical officer, and the drugs can only be given under such written instructions. Ward stocks of controlled drugs in frequent use can also be ordered in special Controlled Drugs Order Books. Each order must be signed by the Nurse-in-Charge.
- Written record of each dose is made stating date, patient's name, time administered and dosage. This record is signed by the nurse giving the drug and another nurse who has checked the source of the drug as well as the dosage against the prescription.

All containers used for controlled drugs must bear special labels to distinguish them clearly. The hospital pharmacist checks the contents of the CD cupboard at regular intervals against the record books. Any discrepancies require full investigation.

The Medicines Act 1968

Under this act, medicines are divided into three groups:

- Prescription Only Medicines (POM) (apart from Controlled Drugs) — includes most of the potent drugs in common use, from antibiotics to hypnotics. These are drugs that may only be supplied or administered to a patient on the instructions of the appropriate practitioner (a doctor or dentist) and from an approved list for a nurse prescriber.
- Pharmacy Only Medicines (P) — drugs supplied under the control and supervision of a registered pharmacist. Representative drugs include ibuprofen and antihistamines.
- General Sales List Medicines (GSL) — include commonly used drugs such as aspirin and paracetamol, available through any retail outlet.

These distinctions of POM, P and GSL medicines do not apply to hospitals where it is accepted practice that medicines are supplied only on prescription.

Medicinal Products: Prescription by Nurse Act 1992

This act together with subsequent amendments to the Pharmaceutical Services regulations allows registered health visitors and district nurses, who have their qualification recorded on the UKCC register, to become nurse prescribers after completing appropriate educational programmes. Practitioners whose prescribing status is denoted on the register, and who are approved within their employment setting, may prescribe from the Nurse Prescribers' Formulary (NPF), which can be found in the British National Formulary. Nurse prescribers must comply with the current legislation and be accountable for their practice.

Further reading and information sources

British Medical Association and the Royal Pharmaceutical Society of Great Britain *British National Formulary*. London (revised twice yearly)

Department of Health 1999 *Review of Prescribing, Supply and Administration of Medicines. Final Report*. Department of Health, London

United Kingdom Central Council for Nursing, Midwifery and Health Visiting (UKCC) 2000 *Guidelines for the Administration of Medicines*. UKCC, London

www.bnf.org.uk

Drug and measurement calculations

The International System of Units (SI) is used for drug doses and concentrations and patient data (including weight and body surface area), drug levels in the body and other measurements (see Appendix 2 for more information).

Weight

Grams (g) and milligrams (mg) are the units most often encountered in drug dosages. Doses of less than 1 g should be expressed in milligrams, e.g. 250 mg rather than 0.25 g. Similarly, doses less than 1 mg should be expressed in micrograms, e.g. 200 micrograms rather than 0.2 mg. Whenever drugs are prescribed in microgram dosages, the units should be written in full, e.g. digoxin 250 micrograms, as the use of the contracted terms μg or mcg may in practice be mistaken for mg and, as this dose is one thousand times greater, disastrous consequences may follow.

Drug dosages are often described in terms of unit dose per kg of body weight, i.e. mg/kg, μg/kg, etc. This method of dosage is frequently used for children and allows dosages to be tailored to the individual patient's size.

Volume

Litres (L or l) and millilitres (mL or ml) account for almost all measurements expressed in unit volume for the prescription and administration of drugs.

Concentration

When expressing concentration of dosages of a medicine in liquid form, several methods are available:

- Unit weight per unit volume — describes the unit of weight of a drug contained in unit volume, e.g. 1 mg in 1 mL, 40 mg in 2 mL. Examples of drugs in common use expressed in these terms: pethidine injection 100 mg in 2 mL; chloral hydrate mixture 1 g in 10 mL; phenoxymethylpenicillin oral solution 250 mg in 5 mL.
- Percentage (weight in volume) — describes the weight of a drug expressed in grams (g) which is contained in 100 mL of solution, e.g. calcium gluconate injection 10% which contains 10 g in each 100 mL of solution, or 1 g in each 10 mL or 100 mg (0.1 g) in each 1 mL.
- Percentage (weight in weight) — describes the weight of a drug expressed in grams (g) which is contained in 100 g of a solid or semi-solid medicament, such as ointments and creams, e.g. fusidic acid ointment 2% which contains 2 g of fusidic acid in each 100 g of ointment.
- Volume containing '1 part' — a few liquids and to a lesser extent gases, particularly those containing drugs in very low concentrations, are often described as containing 1 part per 'x' units of volume. For liquids, 'parts' are equivalent to grams and volume to millimetres, e.g. adrenaline injection 1 in 1000 which contains 1 g in 1000 mL or expressed as a percentage (w/v) — 0.1%.
- Molar concentration — only very occasionally are drugs in liquid form expressed in molar concentration. The mole is the molecular weight of a drug expressed in grams and a one molar (1 M) solution contains this weight dissolved in each litre. More often the millimole (mmol) is used to describe a medicinal product, e.g. potassium chloride solution 15 mmol in 10 mL indicates a solution containing the molecular weight of potassium chloride in milligrams × 15 dissolved in 10 mL of solution.

Body height and surface area

Drug doses may be expressed in terms of microgram, milligram or gram per unit of body surface area. This is frequently the case where precise dosages tailored to individual patients' needs are required. Typical examples may be seen in cytotoxic chemotherapy or in drugs given to children. Body surface area is expressed as square metres or m^2 and drug dosages as units per square metre or units/m^2, e.g. cytarabine injection 100 mg/m^2.

Formulae for calculation of drug doses and drip rates

Oral drugs (solids, liquids)

$$\text{Amount required} = \frac{\text{Strength required} \times \text{Volume of stock strength}}{\text{Stock strength}}$$

Parenteral drugs

(a) Solutions (IM, IV injections)

$$\text{Volume required} = \frac{\text{Strength required} \times \text{Volume of stock strength}}{\text{Stock strength}}$$

(b) Powders

It is essential to follow the manufacturer's directions for dilution, then use the appropriate formula.

(c) IV infusions

$$\text{Rate (drops/min)} = \frac{\text{Volume of solution (mL)} \times \text{Number of drops/mL}}{\text{Time (min)}}$$

Macrodrip (20 drops/mL) — clear fluids

1. $$\text{Rate (drops/min)} = \frac{\text{Volume of solution (mL)} \times 20}{\text{Time (min)}}$$

2. Macrodrip (15 drops/mL) — blood

$$\text{Rate (drops/min)} = \frac{\text{Volume of solution (mL)} \times 15}{\text{Time (min)}}$$

(d) Infusion pumps

$$\text{Rate (mL/h)} = \text{Volume (mL)} \div \text{Time (h)}$$

(e) IV infusions with drugs

$$\text{Rate (mL/h)} = \frac{\text{Amount of drug required (mg/h)} \times \text{Volume of solution (mL)}}{\text{Total amount of drug (mg)}}$$

NB After selecting the appropriate formula, ensure that all strengths are in the same units, otherwise convert.

1% solution contains 1 g of solute dissolved in 100 mL of solution.

1:1000 means 1 g in 1000 mL of solution, therefore 1 g in 1000 mL is equivalent to 1 mg in 1 mL.

Other useful formulae

Children's dose (Clarke's Body Weight Rule)

$$\text{Child's dose} = \frac{\text{Adult dose} \times \text{Weight of child (kg)}}{\text{Average adult weight (70 kg)}}$$

Children's dose (Clarke's Body Surface Area Rule)

$$\text{Child's dose} = \frac{\text{Adult dose} \times \text{Surface area of child (m}^2)}{\text{Surface area of adult (1.7 m}^2)}$$

Acknowledgements

The measurement section was adapted from Henney C R et al 1995 Drugs in Nursing Practice, 5th edn. Churchill Livingstone, Edinburgh, with permission; and the formulae from Havard M 1994 A Nursing Guide to Drugs, 4th edn. Churchill Livingstone, Edinburgh, with permission.

APPENDIX 6

Useful addresses

Action for Sick Children
300 Kingston Road
London SW20 8LX
www.actionforsickchildren.org

Age Concern (England)
1268 London Road
London SW16 4ER
www.ace.org.uk

Alcoholics Anonymous
PO Box 1
Stonebow House
Stonebow
York YO1 2NJ
www.alcoholics-anonymous.org.uk

Alzheimer's Society
Gordon House, 10 Greencoat Place
London SW1P 1PH
www.alzheimers.org.uk

Arthritis Care
18 Stephenson Way
London NW1 2HD
www.arthritiscare.org.uk

Association of British Paediatric Nurses (ABPN)
PO Box 14
Ashton-Under-Lyne
Lancashire OL5 9WW

Association of Carers
20–25 Glasshouse Yard
London EC1A 4JS

Breast Cancer Care
Kiln House
210 New King's Road
London SW6 4NZ
www.breastcancercare.org.uk

British Association for Cancer United Patients BACUP
3 Bath Place
Rivington Street
London EC2 3JR
www.cancerbacup.org.uk

British Colostomy Association
15 Station Road
Reading RG1 1LG
www.bcass.org.uk

British Deaf Association
1–3 Worship Street
London EC2A 2AB
www.bda.org.uk

British Epilepsy Association
New Anstey House
Gate Way Drive
Leeds LS3 1BE
www.epilepsy.org.uk

British Heart Foundation
14 Fitzharding Street
London W1H 4DH
www.bhf.org.uk

British Pregnancy Advisory Service
Austy Manor
Wootton Wawen
Solihull
West Midlands B95 6BX
www.bpas.org

British Red Cross
9 Grosvenor Crescent
London SW1X 7EJ
www.redcross.org.uk

Capability (formerly Spastics Society)
12 Park Crescent
London W1N 4EQ

Chartered Society of Physiotherapy
14 Bedford Row
London WC1R 4ED
www.csphysio.org.uk

Coeliac Society
PO Box 220
High Wycombe
Buckinghamshire HP11 2HY
www.coeliac.co.uk

College of Occupational Therapists
106–114 Borough High Street
Southwark
London SE1 1LB
www.cot.co.uk

Commission for Racial Equality
Elliot House
10–12 Allington Street
London SW1E 5EH
www.cre.gov.uk

Commonwealth Nurses Federation
c/o International Department
Royal College of Nursing
20 Cavendish Square
London W1M 0AB

Cruse
Cruse House
126 Sheen Road
Richmond, Surrey TW9 1UR
www.crusebereavementcare.org.uk

Department of Health
(Northern Ireland)
Dundonald House
Upper Newtownards Road
Belfast BT4 3SB

Department of Health
Richmond House
79 Whitehall
London SW1A 2NS
www.doh.gov.uk

Diabetes UK (formerly British Diabetic Association)
10 Queen Anne Street
London W1M 0DD
www.diabetes.org.uk

Disabled Living Foundation
380–384 Harrow Road
London W9 2HU
www.dlf.org.uk

Equal Opportunities Commission
Arndale House
Arndale Centre
Manchester M4 5EQ
www.eoc.org.uk

Haemophilia Society
Chesterfield House
385 Euston Road
London NW1 3AU
www. haemophilia.org.uk

Health & Safety Executive
Rose Court
2 Southwark Bridge
London SE1 9HS
www.hse.gov.uk

Health Development Agency
Trevelyan House
30 Great Peter Street
London SW1P 2HW
www. hea.org.uk

Health Service Commissioner
13th Floor Millbank
Millbank Tower
London SW1P 4QP
www.health.ombudsman.org.uk

Health Visitors' Association
50 Southwark Street
London SE1 1UN

Ileostomy & Internal Pouch Support Group
Amblehurst House
PO Box 23
Mansfield NG18 4TT

Institute of Complementary Medicine
PO Box 194
London SE15 1QZ

International Confederation of Midwives
10 Barley Mow Passage
London W4 4PH

International Council of Nurses (ICN)
3 Place Jean Marteau
1201 Geneva
Switzerland
www.icn.ch

King's Fund
11–13 Cavendish Square
London W1M 0AN

Leukaemia Society
14 Kingfisher Court
Venny Bridge
Pinhoe
Exeter EX4 8JN

Macmillan Cancer Relief
89 Albert Embankment
London SE1 7UQ
www.macmillan.org.uk

Malcolm Sargent Cancer Fund for Children
14 Abingdon Road
London W8 6AF

MIND — National Association for Mental Health
Granta House
15–19 Broadway
London E15 4BQ
www.mind.org.uk

Multiple Sclerosis Society
National Centre
372 Edgware Road
London NW2 6ND
www.mssociety.org.uk

National Aids Trust
New City Cloisters
188/196 Old Street
London EC1V 9FR
www.nat.org.uk

National Association of Theatre Nurses
Daisy Ayris House
6 Grove Park Court
Harrogate
North Yorkshire HG1 5DP

National Asthma Campaign
Providence House
Providence Place
London N1 0NT
www.asthma.org.uk

National Childbirth Trust (NCT)
Alexandra House
Oldham Terrace
London W3 6NH

National Society for the Prevention of Cruelty to Children (NSPCC)
42 Curtain Road
London EC2A 3NH
www.nspcc.org.uk

Nurses Welfare Service
Victoria Chambers
16/18 Strutton Ground
London SW1P 2HP

Nursing and Midwifery Council (replacing the UK Central Council for Nursing, Midwifery & Health Visiting)
23 Portland Place
London W1N 3AF
www.ukcc.org.uk

Royal College of Midwives
15 Mansfield Street
London W1M 0BE

Royal College of Nursing
(Northern Ireland)
28 Howard Street
Belfast BT1 6PH

Royal College of Nursing
(Scottish Board)
37 Frederick Street
Edinburgh EH2 1EP

Royal College of Nursing
(Welsh Board)
4 Cathedral Road
Cardiff CF1 9LJ

Royal College of Nursing of the United Kingdom
20 Cavendish Square
London W1M 0AB
www.rcn.org.uk

Royal Commonwealth Society
18 Northumberland Avenue
London WC2N 5BJ

Royal National Institute for the Blind (RNIB)
224 Great Portland Place
London W1N 6AA
www.rnib.org.uk

Royal National Institute for the Deaf (RNID)
19–23 Featherstone Street
London EC1Y 8SL
www.rnid.org.uk

Royal Society of Health
38a St Georges Drive
London SW1Y 4BH

St John Ambulance Association & Brigade
1 Grosvenor Crescent
London SW1X 7EF
www.sja.org.uk

Scottish Health Department
St Andrew's House
Regent Road
Edinburgh EH1 3DE
www.scotland.gov.uk

Sickle Cell Society
54 Station Road
Harlesden
London NW10 4UA
www.sicklecellsociety.org

Society of Chiropodists & Podiatrists
53 Welbeck Street
London W1M 7HE

Society & College of Radiographers
2 Carriage Row
183 Eversholt Street
London NW1 1BU

Stillbirth & Neonatal Death Society (SANDS)
28 Portland Place
London W1N 4DE

Stroke Association
123–127 Whitecross Street
London EC1Y 8JJ
www.stroke.org.uk

Terrence Higgins Trust
52–54 Grays Inn Road
London WC1X 8JU
www.tht.org.uk

UNISON (Head Office)
1 Mabledon Place
London WC1H 9HA

VSO
317 Putney Bridge Road
London SW15 2PN

World Health Organization
Avenue Appia
1211 Geneva 27
Switzerland
www.who.org

APPENDIX 7

Abbreviations in Nursing

Nursing/Medical Abbreviations, Degrees, Diplomas and Organizations

AA	Alcoholics Anonymous
AAA	abdominal aortic aneurysm
ABGs	arterial blood gases
ac	ante cibum (Latin abbreviation previously used in prescriptions), before food
ACE	angiotensin-converting enzyme
ACTH	adrenocorticotrophic hormone
ADH	antidiuretic hormone
ADHD	attention deficit hyperactivity disorder
ad lib	ad libitum (Latin abbreviation previously used in prescriptions), to the desired amount
ADLs	Activities of Daily Living
ADP	adenosine diphosphate
ADRs	adverse drug reactions
AF	atrial fibrillation
AFB	acid-fast bacilli
AFP	alpha-fetoprotein
AGA	appropriate for gestational age
AHF	antihaemophilic factor
AID	artificial insemination using donor semen
AIDS	acquired immune deficiency syndrome
AIH	artificial insemination using husband's (partner's) semen
AIMSW	Associate of the Institute of Medical Social Workers
ALD	adrenoleucodystrophy
ALL	acute lymphoblastic leukaemia
ALs	Activities of Living
ALS	advanced life support
ALT	alanine aminotransferase
AMI	acute myocardial infarction
AML	acute myeloid leukaemia
AMP	adenosine monophosphate
ANOVA	analysis of variance
anti-HBc	antibody against hepatitis B core antigen
anti-HBe	antibody against hepatitis B e antigen
anti-HBs	antibody against hepatitis B surface antigen
ANP	atrial natriuretic peptide

APEL	Accreditation (Assessment) of Prior Experiential Learning
APL	Accreditation (Assessment) of Prior Learning
APKD	adult polycystic kidney disease
arboviruses	arthropod-borne viruses
ARC	AIDS-related complex
ARDS	acute respiratory distress syndrome
ARF	(1) acute renal failure (2) acute respiratory failure
ASCII	American standard code for information interchange
ASD	atrial septal defect
ASO	antistreptolysin O
ASOM	acute suppurative otitis media
AST	aspartate aminotransferase
ATD	Alzheimer's type dementia
ATN	acute tubular necrosis
ATP	adenosine triphosphate
ATS	anti-tetanus serum
ATT	anti-tetanus toxoid
A-V	atrioventricular (1) node (2) bundle
AVP	vasopressin
BA	Bachelor of Arts
BACUP	British Association of Cancer United Patients
BAI	Beck Anxiety Inventory
BASIC	Beginner's All-purpose Symbolic Instruction Code
BBA	born before arrival
BBB	(1) blood-brain barrier (2) bundle branch block
BBVs	blood-borne viruses
BCC	basal cell carcinoma
BCG	Bacille-Calmette-Guérin
bd	bis die (Latin abbreviation previously used in prescriptions), twice daily
BDI	Beck Depression Inventory
BEd	Bachelor of Education
BHS	Beck Hopelessness Scale
BID	(1) brought in dead (2) twice daily (see bd)
BIOS	Basic Input/Output System
BIT	binary digit
BLS	basic life support

BMA	British Medical Association	**CF**	cystic fibrosis
BMI	body mass index	**CFT**	complement fixation test
BMR	basal metabolic rate	**CFTR gene**	cystic fibrosis transmembrane
BMT	bone marrow transplant		regulator gene
BN	Bachelor of Nursing	**CGLI**	City and Guilds of London
BNF	British National Formulary		Institute
BP	(1) blood pressure (2) British	**CHC**	Community Health Council
	Pharmacopoeia	**CHD**	coronary heart disease
BPD	bronchopulmonary dysplasia	**CHF**	congestive heart failure
BPH	benign prostatic hyperplasia	**CHI**	(1) Commission for Health
BPRS	Brief Psychiatric Rating Scale		Improvement (2) creatinine
Bq	becquerel		height index
BRCS	British Red Cross Society	**CIN**	cervical intraepithelial
BRM	biological response modifier		neoplasia
BSA	body surface area	**CINAHL**	Cumulative Index to Nursing
BSc	Bachelor of Science		and Allied Health Literature
BSc (Soc Sc-Nurs)	Bachelor of Science	**CJD**	Creutzfeldt-Jakob disease
	(Nursing)	**CLL**	chronic lymphatic leukaemia
BSE	(1) bovine spongiform	**CML**	chronic myeloid leukaemia
	encephalopathy (2) breast self-	**CMRS**	Case Managers Rating Scale
	examination	**CMV**	(1)Cytomegalovirus (2)
BSS	Beck Scale for Suicide Ideation		controlled mandatory ventilation
		CNS	(1) central nervous system (2)
CABG	coronary artery bypass graft		clinical nurse specialist
CAD	coronary artery disease	**COAD**	chronic obstructive airways
CAH	(1) congenital adrenal		disease
	hyperplasia (2) chronic active	**COMA**	The Committee on Medical
	hepatitis		Aspects of Food Policy
CAL	computer assisted learning	**COPD**	chronic obstructive pulmonary
CAN	Camberwell Assessment of		disease
	Need	**COSHH**	control of substances
CAPD	continuous ambulatory		hazardous to health
	peritoneal dialysis	**CPA**	care programme approach
CAPE	Clifton Assessment Procedures	**CPAP**	continuous positive airways
	for the Elderly		pressure
CAT	(1) computed axial	**CPD**	Continuing Professional
	tomography (2) computer		Development
	assisted tomography	**CPH**	Certificate of Public Health
CATS	Credit Accumulation Transfer	**CPK**	creatine phosphokinase
	Scheme	**CPN**	Community Psychiatric Nurse
CBF	cerebral blood flow	**CPR**	cardiopulmonary resuscitation
CCETSW	Central Council for the	**CPU**	central processing unit
	Education and Training in	**CRC**	Cancer Research Campaign
	Social Work	**CRF**	(1) chronic renal failure (2)
CCF	congestive cardiac failure		corticotrophin releasing factor
CCU	coronary care unit	**CSF**	(1) cerebrospinal fluid (2)
CD	(1) controlled drug (2)		colony stimulating factor
	curriculum development	**CSI**	Caregiver Strain Index
CDC	Centres (centers) for Disease	**CSM**	Committee on Safety of
	Control and Prevention		Medicines
CDH	congenital dislocation of the	**CSOM**	chronic suppurative otitis
	hip		media
CD-ROM	Compact Disk Read-Only	**CSSD**	central sterile supplies
	Memory		Department
CDS	Calgary Depression Scale	**CSSU**	central sterile supply unit
CDSC	Communicable Disease	**CT**	(1) cerebral tumour (2)
	Surveillance Centre		computed tomography (3)
CEA	carcinoembryonic antigen		coronary thrombosis

CTG	cardiotocograph	DSH	deliberate self-harm
CTZ	chemoreceptor trigger zone	DTPer	diphtheria, tetanus and
CUSA	Cavitron ultrasonic surgical		pertussis vaccine
	aspirator	DU	duodenal ulcer
CV	curriculum vitae	DVT	deep vein thrombosis
CVA	cerebrovascular accident		
CVP	central venous pressure	EAB	extra-anatomic bypass
CVS	(1) cardiovascular system (2)	EAR	estimated average
	chorionic villus sampling		requirement
CVVH	continuous venous-venous	EB	epidermolysis bullosa
	haemofiltration	EBM	(1) evidence-based medicine
CVVHD	continuous venous-venous		(2) expressed breast milk
	haemodiafiltration	EBP	Evidence-based Practice
CXR	chest X-ray	EBV	Epstein-Barr Virus
		ECF	extracellular fluid
DADL	Domestic Activities of Daily	ECG	electrocardiogram
	Living	ECI	Experience of Caregiving
DC	direct current		Inventory
D and C	dilatation and curettage	ECMO	extracorporeal membrane
DCD	Diploma of Child		oxygenator
	Development	ECT	electroconvulsive therapy
DCH	Diploma in Child Health	ECV	external cephalic version
DDH	developmental dysplasia of	EDD	expected date of delivery
	the hip	EDV	end-diastolic volume
DEO	disability employment officer	EEG	electroencephalography
DI	donor insemination	EFAs	essential fatty acids
DIC	disseminated intravascular	EHEC	enterohaemorrhagic
	coagulation		*Escherichia coli*
DIDMOAD	diabetes insipidus, diabetes	EIA	exercise induced asthma
	mellitus, optic atrophy, and	EIEC	enterovasive *Escherichia coli*
	deafness	ELISA	enzyme-linked immunosorbent
DipHE	Diploma in Higher Education		assay
DipEd	Diploma in Education	E-mail	electronic mail
DipN	Diploma in Nursing	EMD	electromechanical
DipNEd	Diploma in Nursing Education		dissociation
DIMS	disorders of initiating and	EMG	electromyography
	maintaining sleep	EMLA	eutetic mixture of local
DKA	diabetics ketoacidosis		anaesthetics
DM	diabetes mellitus	EMS	Emergency Medical Service
dmft	decayed missing and filled	ENT	ear, nose and throat
	teeth (deciduous)	EOG	electro-oculogram
DMFT	decayed missing and filled	EPEC	enteropathic *Escherichia coli*
	teeth (permanent)	ERASMUS	European Community Action
DN	(1) Diploma in Nursing (2)		Scheme for the Mobility of
	district nurse		University Students
DNA	deoxyribonucleic acid	ERCP	endoscopic retrograde
DNE	Diploma in Nursing Education		cholangiopancreatography
DNT	district nurse teacher	ERG	electroretinogram
DOA	dead on arrival	ERPC	evacuation retained products
DOES	disorders of excessive		of conception
	somnolence	ERV	expiratory reserve volume
DoH	Department of Health	ESP	extrasensory perception
DPH	Diploma in Public Health	ESPs	extended scope physiotherapy
DPhil	Doctor of Philosophy		practitioners
DRS	Delusions Rating Scale	ESR	erythrocyte sedimentation rate
DRV	dietary reference values	ESRD	end stage renal disease
DSA	digital subtraction	ESS	early signs scale
	angiography	ESV	end-systolic volume

ESWL	extracorporeal shock wave lithotripsy
ET	(1) embryo transfer (2) endotracheal
ETEC	enterotoxigenic *Escherichia coli*
EUA	examination under anaesthetic
FAS	fetal alcohol syndrome
FBC	full blood count
FBS	fasting blood sugar
FET	forced expiratory technique
FETC	Further Education Teaching Certificate
FEV	forced expiratory volume
FFA	free fatty acids
FFP	fresh frozen plasma
FHS	Family Health Service
FPA	Family Planning Association
FPCert	Family Planning Certificate
FQ	Fear Questionnaire
FRC	functional residual capacity
FRcn	Fellow of the Royal College of Nursing
FSF	fibrin stabilizing factor
FSH	follicle stimulating hormone
FSHRH	follicle stimulating hormone releasing hormone
FTA-abs test	fluorescent treponemal antibody absorbed test
FVC	forced vital capacity
GABA	gamma aminobutyric acid
GAS	general adaptation syndrome
GCS	Glasgow coma scale
GCSF	granulocyte colony stimulating factor
GFR	glomerular filtration rate
GGT	gamma-glutamyl-transferase
GH	growth hormone
GHIH	growth hormone inhibiting hormone
GHQ	General Health Questionnaire
GHRH	growth hormone releasing hormone
GI	gastrointestinal
GIFT	Gamete Intrafallopian Transfer
GM	genetically modified
GMC	General Medical Council
GMS	General Medical Services
GN	glomerulonephritis
GnRH	gonadotrophin releasing hormone
GOR	gastro-oesophageal reflux
GP	general practitioner
GPI	general paralysis of the insane
GSL	general sales list
GTN	glyceryl trinitrate

GUM	genitourinary medicine
GUS	genitourinary system
GVHD	graft versus host disease
HAI	hospital acquired infection
HAV	hepatitis A virus
HAVS	hand-arm vibration syndrome
HAZ	Health Action Zone
Hb	haemoglobin
HBcAg	hepatitis B core antigen
HBeAg	Hepatitis B e Antigen
HBIG	hepatitis B immunoglobulin
HBsAg	hepatitis B surface antigen
HBV	hepatitis B virus
HC	head circumference
HCA	healthcare assistant
HCG(hCG)	human chorionic gonadotrophin
HCV	hepatitis C virus
HD	Huntington's disease
HDL	high density lipoprotein
HDSU	Hospital Sterilization and Disinfection Unit
HDU	high dependency unit
HDV	hepatitis delta virus
HEV	hepatitis E virus
HFEA	Human Fertilization and Embryology Authority
HGP	Human Genome Project
HHNK	hyperglycaemic hyperosmolar nonketotic
Hib vaccine	*Haemophilus influenzae* type B vaccine
HImP	Health Improvement Programme
HIV	human immunodeficiency virus
HLA	human leucocyte antigens
HMG(hMG)	human menopausal gonadotrophin
HOCM	hypertrophic obstructive cardiomyopathy
HoNOS	Health of the Nation Outcome Scale
HPV	human papilloma virus
HR	heart rate
HRS	Hallucinations Rating Scale
HRT	hormone replacement therapy
HSA	human serum albumin
HSDU	Hospital Sterilization and Disinfection Unit
HSV	herpes simplex virus
HTLV	human T-cell lymphotrophic viruses
HTML	hyper text markup language
HUS	haemolytic uraemic syndrome

HV	health visitor	IVP	intravenous pyelogram
HVCert	Health Visitor's Certificate	IVT	intravenous therapy
HVT	health visitor teacher	IVU	intravenous urogram
IAA	indispensable amino acid	JCA	juvenile chronic arthritis
IABP	intra-aortic balloon pump	JVP	jugular venous pressure
IADL	Instrumental Activities of Daily		
	Living	KASI	Knowledge About
IBD	inflammatory bowel disease		Schizophrenia Interview
IBS	irritable bowel syndrome	KP	keratitic precipitates
IC	inspiratory capacity	KS	Kaposi's sarcoma
ICD	International Classification of	KUB	kidneys ureters and bladder
	Disease		
ICE	ice, compress and elevate	LAD	left axis deviation
ICF	intracellular fluid	LAN	Local Area Network
ICN	(1) Infection Control Nurse (2)	LASER	Light Amplification by
	International Council of		Stimulated Emission of
	Nurses		Radiation
ICP	intracranial pressure	LDH	lactic dehydrogenase
ICSH	interstitial cell stimulating	LDL	low-density lipoprotein
	hormone	LDQ	Leeds Dependence
ICSI	intracytoplasmic sperm injection		Questionnaire
ICU	Intensive Care Unit	LEA	Local Education Authority
ID	(1) identity (2) intradermal	LFT	liver function test
IDDM	insulin dependent diabetes	LGA	large for gestational age
	mellitus	LGLs	large granular lymphocytes
IGT	impaired glucose tolerance	LGVCFT	lymphogranuloma venereum
IHD	ischaemic heart disease		complement fixation test
IM	(1) infectious mononucleosis	LH	luteinizing hormone
	(2) intramuscular	LHBI	lower hemibody irradiation
IM&T	information management and	LHG	Local Health Group
	technology	LHRH	luteinizing hormone releasing
IMV	intermittent mandatory		hormone
	ventilation	LMP	last menstrual period
INR	Index of Nursing Research	LOA	left occipitoanterior
IOL	intraocular lens	LOC	level of consciousness
IOP	intraocular pressure	LOP	left occipitoposterior
IPD	intermittent peritoneal dialysis	LP	lumbar puncture
IPP	intermittent positive pressure	LRNI	lower reference nutrient
IPPV	intermittent positive pressure		intake
	ventilation	LRTI	lower respiratory tract
IQ	intelligence quotient		infection
IRV	inspiratory reserve volume	LSD	lysergic acid diethylamide
IS	insight scale	LTM	long term memory
ISO 9000/BS 5750	International and	LUNSERS	Liverpool University
	British Standards in Quality		Neuroleptic Side-Effect Rating
	Systems		Scale
IT	information technology	LVAD	left ventricular assist device
ITU	intensive therapy unit	LVEDP	left ventricular end-diastolic
IUCD	intrauterine contraceptive		pressure
	device	LVF	left ventricular failure
IUD	intrauterine device		
IUGR	intrauterine growth retardation	MA	Master of Arts
IUI	intrauterine insemination	MAC	mid-arm circumference
IV	intravenous	MADEL	Medical and Dental Education
IVC	inferior vena cava		Levy
IVF	in vitro fertilization	MAI	*Mycobacterium avium*
IVI	intravenous infusion		*intracellulare*

MAMC	mid-arm muscle circumference	**MT**	midwifery teacher
MAOI	monoamine oxidase inhibitor	**MTD**	Midwife Teachers Diploma
MAST	(1) Michigan Alcoholism Screening Test (2) military antishock trousers	**NACNE**	National Advisory Committee on Nutrition Education
		NAD	nicotinamide adenine dinucleotide
MBA	Master of Business Administration	**NADP**	nicotinamide adenine dinucleotide phosphate
MBC	maximal breathing capacity	**NAI**	nonaccidental injury
MBIM	Member of the British Institute of Management	**NAMCW**	National Association for Maternal and Child Welfare
MCA	Medicine Control Agency	**NAS**	no added salt
MCH	mean cell haemoglobin	**NAWCH**	National Association for the Welfare of Children in Hospital
MCHC	mean cell haemoglobin concentration		
MCV	mean cell volume	**NBM**	nil (nothing) by mouth
MDA	Medical Devices Agency	**NCVs**	nerve conduction velocities
MDM	mental defence mechanism	**NCVQ**	National Council for Vocational Qualifications
MDMA	methylenedioxymethamphet amine		
		NDN	National District Nurse Certificate
MDR-TB	multidrug resistant tuberculosis		
ME	myalgic encephalopathy	**NEC**	necrotizing enterocolitis
MEd	Master of Education	**NG**	nasogastric
MEN	multiple endocrine neoplasia	**NGU**	nongonococcal urethritis
MHC	major histocompatability complex	**NHL**	nonHodgkin's lymphoma
		NHS	National Health Service
MI	myocardial infarction	**NICE**	National Institute for Clinical Excellence
MIND	National Association for Mental Health		
		NICU	neonatal intensive care unit
MLNS	mucocutaneous lymph node syndrome	**NIDDM**	noninsulin dependent diabetes mellitus
mmHg	millimetres of mercury	**NIPPV**	noninvasive positive pressure ventilation
mmol	millimole		
MMR	measles, mumps and rubella vaccine	**NK**	natural killer (cells)
		NMC	Nursing and Midwifery Council
MMV	mandatory minute volume		
modem	modulator/demodulator	**NMET**	Nonmedical Education and Training
MODS	multiple organ dysfunction syndrome		
		NMR	nuclear magnetic resonance
MODY	maturity onset diabetes of the young	**NPF**	nurse prescribers' formulary
		NRDS	neonatal respiratory distress syndrome
MPhil	Master of Philosophy		
MPQ	McGill pain questionnaire	**NREM**	nonrapid eye movement (sleep)
MRC	Medical Research Council	**NSAIDs**	nonsteroidal anti-inflammatory drugs
MRI	magnetic resonance imaging		
mRNA	messenger ribonucleic acid	**NSFs**	National Service Frameworks
MRSA	multiple resistant *Staphylococcus aureus*	**NSP**	nonstarch polysaccharides
		NST	nonshivering thermogenesis
MS	(1) multiple sclerosis (2) musculoskeletal system	**NSU**	nonspecific urethritis
		NT	nurse teacher
MSAFP	maternal serum alpha-fetoprotein	**NVQ**	National Vocational Qualification
MSc	Master of Science		
MSH	melanocyte stimulating hormone	**OAE**	otoacoustic emission
		OBS	organic brain syndrome
MSP	Munchausen syndrome by proxy	**OCD**	obsessive compulsive disorder
		od	omni die (Latin abbreviation previously used in prescriptions), daily
MSU	midstream specimen of urine		
MSW	medical social worker		

ODA	operating department assistant	**PCT**	Primary Care Trust
OECD	Organization for Economic Co-operation and Development	**PCV**	packed cell volume
		PCWP	pulmonary capillary wedge pressure
OGD	oesophagogastroduodenoscopy	**PDA**	patent ductus arteriosus
OHE	Office of Health Economics	**PDP**	Personal Development Plan
OHNC	Occupational Health Nursing Certificate	**PE**	pulmonary embolus
		PEEP	positive end expiratory pressure
om	omni mane (Latin abbreviation previously used in prescriptions), in the morning	**PEFR**	peak expiratory flow rate
		PEG	percutaneous endoscopic gastrostomy
on	omni nocte (Latin abbreviation previously used in prescriptions), at night	**PEM**	protein-energy malnutrition
		PET	positron emission tomography
		PFI	Private Finance Initiative
ONC	Orthopaedic Nurses' Certificate	**PGL**	persistent generalized lymphadenopathy
OND	Ophthalmic Nursing Diploma	**pH**	hydrogen ion concentration
OPCS	Office of Population Censuses and Surveys	**PHC**	primary health care
		PhD	Doctor of Philosophy
ORS	oral rehydration solution	**PHLS**	Public Health Laboratory Services
ORT	oral rehydration therapy		
OT	(1) occupational therapy (2) operating theatre	**PICC**	peripherally inserted central catheter
OTC	over-the-counter (remedies)	**PICU**	paediatric intensive care unit
OU	Open University	**PID**	(1) pelvic inflammatory disease (2) prolapsed intervertebral disc
PABA	para-aminobenzoic acid	**PIs**	performance indicators
PAC	premature atrial contraction	**PKU**	phenylketonuria
PACT	Prescribing Analysis And Costs	**PMB**	postmenopausal bleeding
PADL	Personal Activities of Daily Living	**PMRAFNS**	Princess Mary's Royal Air Force Nursing Service
PAFC	pulmonary artery flotation catheter	**PMS**	premenstrual syndrome
		PMT	premenstrual tension
PAL	physical activity level	**PNI**	psychoneuroimmunology
PALS	paediatric advanced life support	**POAG**	primary open angle glaucoma
PANSS	Positive and Negative Syndrome Scale	**POM**	prescription only medicine
		POP	(1) plaster of Paris (2) progestogen only pill
Pap	Papanicolaou smear test		
PAP	primary atypical pneumonia	**POSSUM**	Patient-Operated Selector Mechanism
PAR	physical activity ratio		
PAT	paroxysmal atrial tachycardia	**PPD**	purified protein derivative
PAWP	pulmonary artery wedge pressure	**PPLO**	pleuropneumonia-like organism
PBC	primary biliary cirrhosis	**PPS**	plasma protein solution
PBM	peak bone mass	**PPV**	positive pressure ventilation
PC	personal computer	**PR**	per rectum
pc	post cibum (Latin abbreviation previously used in prescriptions), after food	**PREP**	Postregistration Education and Practice
		PRH	prolactin-releasing hormone
PCA(S)	patient controlled analgesia (system)	**PRL**	prolactin
		prn	pro re nata (Latin abbreviation previously used in prescriptions), when required
PCEA	patient controlled epidural analgesia		
PCG	Primary Care Group	**PSA**	prostate specific antigen
PCM	protein-calorie malnutrition	**PSCT**	pain and symptom control team
PCNL	percutaneous nephrolithotomy	**PSD**	personal and social development
PCP	*Pneumocystis carinii* pneumonia	**PSV**	pressure support ventilation

PT	(1) physiotherapist	REM	rapid eye movement (sleep)
	(2) prothrombin	RES	reticuloendothelial system
PTA	plasma thromboplastin	RF	rheumatic fever
	antecedent	RG	remedial gymnast
PTC	percutaneous transhepatic	RGN	Registered General Nurse
	cholangiography	Rh	rhesus
PTCA	percutaneous transluminal	RHA	Regional Health Authority
	coronary angioplasty	RHD	rheumatic heart disease
PTH	parathyroid hormone	RHV	Registered Health Visitor
PTSD	post traumatic stress disorder	RICE	rest, ice, compress, elevate
PTT	partial thromboplastin time	RIF	right iliac fossa
PUFA	polyunsaturated fatty acid	rINN	Recommended International
PUO	pyrexia of unknown origin		Nonproprietary Name
PUVA	psoralen + ultraviolet light	RIP	raised intracranial pressure
	A (long wavelength)	RIST	radioimmunosorbent test
PV	per vagina	RM	Registered Midwife
PVD	peripheral vascular disease	RMN	Registered Mental Nurse
PVR	pulmonary vascular resistance	RN	Registered Nurse
PVS	persistent vegetative state	RNA	ribonucleic acid
		RNI	reference nutrient intake
QALYs	quality-adjusted life years	RNIB	Royal National Institute for
QARANC	Queen Alexandra's Royal		the Blind
	Army Nursing Corps	RNMH	Registered Nurse for the
QARNNS	Queen Alexandra's Royal		Mentally Handicapped
	Naval Nursing Service	RNT	Registered Nurse Tutor
qds	quater die sumendus (Latin	RO	reality orientation
	abbreviation previously used in	ROA	right occipitoanterior
	prescriptions), four times daily	ROM	(1) range of movement
QIDN	Queen's Institute of District		(exercises) (2) Read-only
	Nursing		Memory
qqh	quarta quaque hora (Latin	ROP	right occipitoposterior
	abbreviation previously used in	RPCF	Reiter protein complement
	prescriptions), every four hours		fixation
		RPE	retinal pigment epithelial (cells,
RAD	right axis deviation		layer)
RADAR	Royal Association for	RPR	rapid plasma reagin
	Disability and Rehabilitation	rRNA	ribosomal ribonucleic acid
RAI	Relatives Assessment Interview	RS	respiratory system
RAISSE	Relatives Assessment Interview	RSCN	Registered Sick Children's
	for Schizophrenia in a secure		Nurse
	environment	RSI	repetitive strain injury
RAM	Random Access Memory	RSV	respiratory syncytial virus
RAS	reticular activating system	RTA	(1) renal tubular acidosis (2)
RAST	radioallergosorbent test		road traffic accident
RBC	red blood cell	RV	(1) residual volume (2) right
RCC	red cell concentrate		ventricle
RCM	Royal College of Midwives	RVF	right ventricular failure
RCN	Royal College of Nursing and		
	National Council of Nurses of	SA	(1) sinus arrhythmia (2)
	the United Kingdom		sinoatrial (node)
RCNT	Registered Clinical Nurse	SACD	subacute combined
	Teacher		degeneration
RCT	randomized controlled trial	SAD	seasonal affective disorder
RDA	recommended daily allowance	SaFFs	Service and Financial
REHAB	Rehabilitation Evaluation of		Frameworks
	Hall and Baker	SAH	subarachnoid haemorrhage
RELATE	National Marriage Guidance	SANS	Schedule for Assessment of
	Council		Negative Symptoms

SBE	subacute bacterial endocarditis	STD	sexually transmitted disease
SBS	short bowel syndrome	STI	sexually transmitted infection
SCAT	sheep cell agglutination test	STM	short term memory
SCBU	special care baby unit	SVGA	super video graphics array
SCC	(1) spinal cord compression (2) squamous cell carcinoma	SVQs	Scottish Vocational Qualifications
SCD	sequential pneumatic compression device	SVR	systemic vascular resistance
		SVT	supraventricular tachycardia
SCM	State Certified Midwife	SWS	slow wave sleep
SCOTEC	Scottish Technical Education Council	T_3	triiodothyronine
SD	standard deviation	T_4	thyroxine
SDAT	senile dementia Alzheimer's type	TB	tuberculosis (tubercle bacillus)
		TBI	total body irradiation
SDH	subdural haematoma	TBW	total body water
SE	standard error	TCA	tricyclic antidepressant
SERMs	selective (o)estrogen receptor modulators	TCP	thrombocytopenia
		tds	ter die sumendus (Latin abbreviation previously used in prescriptions), three times daily
SFS	Social Functioning Scale		
SGA	small for gestational age		
SGOT	serum glutamic oxaloacetic transaminase, now aspartate aminotransferase		
		TEDs	ThromboEmbolic Deterrent (stockings)
SHHD	Scottish Home and Health Department	TEN	toxic epidermal necrolysis
		TENS	transcutaneous electrical nerve stimulation
SHO	senior house officer		
SI Units	Système International d'Unités	TIA	transient ischaemic attack
SIADH	syndrome of inappropriate antidiuretic hormone	TIBC	total iron binding capacity
		TIPSS	transjugular intrahepatic portasystemic stent shunting
SIB	self-injurious behaviour		
SIDS	sudden infant death syndrome	TLC	total lung capacity
SIMV	synchronized intermittent mandatory ventilation	TLS	tumour lysis syndrome
		TMJ	temporomandibular joint syndrome
SLA	Service Level Agreement		
SLE	systemic lupus erythematosis	TNF	tumour necrosis factor
SLT	speech and language therapist	TNM	tumour, node, metastasis
SLS	social and life skills	TOP	termination of pregnancy
SMO	senior medical officer	tPA	recombinant tissue-type plasminogen activator
SNAP	Schizophrenia Nursing Assessment Protocol		
		TPHA	Treponema pallidum haemagglutination assay
SPECT	single photon emission computed tomography		
		TPN	total parenteral nutrition
SPF	sun protection factor	TPR	temperature, pulse, respiration
SPOD	The Association to Aid the Sexual and Personal Relationships of People with a Disability	TQM	Total Quality Management
		TRH	thyrotropin-releasing hormone
		TRIC	trachoma inclusion conjunctivitis
SPSS	Statistical Package for Social Sciences	tRNA	transfer ribonucleic acid
		TSF	triceps skinfold thickness
SRN	State Registered Nurse	TSH	thyroid-stimulating hormone
SSPE	subacute sclerosing panencephalitis	TSS	toxic shock syndrome
		TT	(1) tetanus toxoid (2) thrombin clotting time
SSRC	Social Science Research Council		
SSRI	selective serotonin re-uptake inhibitors	TURP	transurethral resection of the prostate gland
stat	statim (Latin abbreviation previously used in prescriptions), at once	TURT	transurethral resection of tumour
		TV	tidal volume

UC	ulcerative colitis	VGA	video graphic array
UGH	uveitis + glaucoma + hyphaema syndrome	VLDL	very-low-density lipoprotein
		VMA	vanillylmandelic acid
UHBI	upper hemibody irradiation	VRE	vancomycin-resistant enterococci
UKCC	United Kingdom Central Council for Nursing, Midwifery and Health Visiting	VRS	verbal rating scale
		VSD	ventricular septal defect
URL	uniform resource locator	VSO	Voluntary Service Overseas
URT	upper respiratory tract	VT	ventricular tachycardia
URTI	upper respiratory tract infection	VUR	vesicoureteric reflux
		VZIG	varicella/zoster immunoglobulin
USS	ultrasound scan		
UTI	urinary tract infection	VZV	varicella/zoster virus
UVA	ultraviolet light A		
UVB	ultraviolet light B	WAN	Wide Area Network
		WBC	white blood cells/count
VADAS	voice activated domestic appliance system	WHO	World Health Organization
		WPW	Wolff-Parkinson-White syndrome
VAS	visual analogue scale		
VBI	vertebrobasilar insufficiency	WRVS	Women's Royal Voluntary Service
VC	vital capacity		
VDRL	Venereal Disease Research Laboratory	WTE	Whole Time Equivalent
		www	worldwide web
VDU	visual display unit		
VF	ventricular fibrillation	ZIFT	zygote intrafallopian transfer
VFM	value for money	ZN	Ziehl-Neelsen stain

APPENDIX 8

Enhancing and developing your career via your curriculum vitae (CV), personal development planning and networking
Julie Hyde

Over the past decade, the pattern of work for everyone within and outside the healthcare sector has changed. Structures have been flattened and management responsibility pushed further down the hierarchy, and there are fewer posts which give an opportunity to 'try out' the job. Many 'support posts' and middle management posts have disappeared, with the end result that the more senior you become, the fewer posts there are. Writers have described 'a career climbing frame' rather than 'a career ladder'. This implies that individuals may make lateral career moves, as well as career steps 'up the ladder'. Whilst this has been happening in nonclinical posts in the NHS (as well as outside the healthcare industry), paradoxically the introduction of the nurse grading system, along with the move towards specialism as opposed to generalism (as in the medical career model), tended to confound this pattern. Nurses were discouraged from taking sideways moves into another specialty once they were beyond a D grade, as this would 'dilute' their specialty expertise, and the grade promotion system depended upon this expertise. Whilst for the organization this is a legitimate way of managing scarce resources, for many individual nurses who wished to stay in clinical posts it felt like a barrier to progression. The recent introduction of nurse consultant posts aims to address this concern.

The introduction of formalized human resource practices into the NHS does mean that formal job application processes are now well established. Gone are the days (for nurses) when a little chat with matron would suffice. Thus, from day one, we need to be developing the skills and tools to 'sell' ourselves in the marketplace, as the exciting concept of portfolio careers gains ground.

Apart from the obvious things, like being able to do the job, and holding the relevant licence to practise, there are a number of 'career skills' to collect in your personal development toolbox. Three of the key skills are the ability to produce a focused and 'living' curriculum vitae (CV); the ability to carry out proactive personal development planning via your Personal Development Plan (PDP); and the ability to undertake structured networking.

Preparing your curriculum vitae

An up-to-date CV is an important tool for us all. It serves three purposes:

- it acts as a focal point to assist you to capture your skills, knowledge and achievements
- it serves as a basis for your PDP and thus is likely to inform your appraisal process at work
- it acts as a marketing tool to 'sell' you when you are seeking new opportunities, whether that be a particular new job, or just testing the market.

The preparation of this important document follows a number of stages. Most people, however, find that one CV is not enough. That is not to say that your CV represents someone other than yourself — quite the reverse. Your CV gives you the opportunity to add emphasis to your experience and to show transferability of your knowledge and skills. Clearly, a number of circumstances unique to you will inform your CV and CV preparation. If you qualified last week and entered nursing straight from school, you will have less material to include in your CV than someone who has been in the profession for many years. The important fact to remember is that the principles and processes involved in crafting a CV are the same. Your CV is not a fixed document; it grows and develops and evolves with your growth, development and evolution.

An effective CV puts the right emphasis upon your experience, and clearly, that emphasis is informed and shaped by the purpose for which the CV is prepared. As a means of illustrating this, we will assume that individuals might want to have three current CVs. CV1 will be a baseline, a collection of information capturing their uniqueness as a professional and as a person.

Subsequent CVs will take the same material as in CV1 and address the emphasis to match the purpose. If an individual were applying for a clinical post, then the emphasis in CV2 would be his or her clinical experience. Even then there could be two ways of dealing with this clinical experience. If he or she were applying for a job requiring very specialized clinical expertise in, for example, clinical nurse specialist in renal nursing, he or she would need to highlight in CV2 a detailed clinical focus. If, however, the role/job required a more general focus, then the way the skills would be packaged would be different. There would be less emphasis on the clinical expertise in renal nursing, rather the individual would generalize the clinical experience to a broader perspective, for example to enable him or her to manage a medical unit. The nurse would not be expected to be expert in all specialities represented in the medical unit, but would draw on his or her overall experience to manage the unit as a whole.

In preparing the CV it would be necessary to make a judgement about the culture and values of the organization. An aggressively business oriented organization may want to see a different emphasis in a CV than a charitable organization. All CVs will include the individual's professional and educational qualifications, as well as professional and personal experiences. In the two hypothetical scenarios above (i.e. renal nursing and medical unit), it is more likely that clinical/management experience will be the crucial focus.

However, if the individual was applying for an academic post, in preparing CV3 he or she will need to include more detail about the types and levels of academic courses, and include details of publications, conference papers, etc. This is not to say that these are not of interest in CV1 and CV2, but it is a matter of emphasis. An emphasis on the number and range of academic courses when applying for a job in a business culture might cause the manager looking at the CV to worry that the individual is more interested in courses than doing the job. It is all a matter of organizational culture and core values.

Conversely, the organizational culture of an academic establishment values as currency the academic processes and achievement the applicant can offer, and thus these must be given in detail. A word of warning here though: the level of detail must be appropriate — from present times, backwards. A two-hour inhouse course completed twenty years ago is unlikely to have currency value today.

The one thing that all versions of the CV can have in common is the structure. One structure is offered here, but this is not the only one. Some readers may be surprised that it appears, at first glance, the wrong way round. Most people, on the front page of the CV, include all personal details, name, address, etc. Pause for a moment to think about this. In a job application, the purpose of the CV is to get you an interview (the interview then gets you the job!). When the person shortlisting for the post is reading the CV, they are looking for a vignette of the person and his/her ability, not their address etc. Capitalize on this; use the first page for impact and include:

On page 1
- Name, qualifications, and current post.
- Any roles/experiences that are unique to you outside your post, for example adviser to another organization, chair of a professional group.
- Key personal skills, strengths and attributes which describe you. Word these to match the organizational culture in which the job is based, for example effective communicator; understands the importance of working within resource; effective change agent; can work within a team, etc. Present these in a bullet-pointed list to give impact and to catch the eye of the reader.
- Two or three sentences that capture what you have to offer to the profession/organization. For example, 'I can bring to the organization in-depth knowledge of 'x', enthusiasm and ability to get the job done through motivating my staff.'

On page 2

- Current post .... (wef 1st June 1997)

Responsibilities and achievements include:

Try to write these as outcome statements, rather than just describing a part of your role. For example: (a) initiated and co-ordinate a journal club within the Unit. As a result the unit has a collection of review notes on relevant topics which act as a resource; or (b) led an outreach service to support renal patients in the community. As a result, the number of readmissions to the unit has decreased by 20% over a period of 6 months.

Finish with ....

My current post gives me .... one or two sentences

- Previous post .... 1st July 1995 – 31st May 1997

Responsibilities and achievements

You can include a little less detail here. The detail will get less as you move backwards in time.

Finish with ....

The focus of this post was ....

- Previous post .... 1st August 1991 – 30th June 1995

Responsibilities and achievements

Finish with a sentence highlighting the key issue of this experience.

If your career spans more than 10–15 years, it is usually only necessary to refer to the earliest experience in brief terms, for example January 1970 – – March 1976 — various posts at staff nurse grade.

- Career breaks

A great deal of debate has been generated about whether career breaks (usually in relation to women) should be recorded in CVs. The feminist view may believe that there is no need to explain or apologize for a break. A more pragmatic view is to include a statement something like: 'during the period January 1980 to May 1985 I took a career break.' This allows the potential employer to track your experience and this is important in ensuring safety for patients and clients. Many organizations positively welcome those people with life experience, as this brings an added dimension and balance to the workplace.

On the final page

This should include the 'nut and bolts' about you. A layout is suggested below:

- Personal details

Name	Date of birth
Address (home)	Tel/fax, e-mail
Business address (optional)	Tel/fax, e-mail

- Educational and professional qualifications (in reverse order)
- Professional body membership
  e.g. Member — Royal College of Nursing
- Publications
- Current studies
- Personal interests and activities include .... Two or three sentences usually suffice.
- You may also like to include your referees here, with their contact details, having first alerted them to your intentions.

The first rule of CV writing is to have 'one you prepared earlier'. Often, when you decide to apply for a job, the turnaround date for applications is quite tight. You need that time to gather information about the particular organization, so having a CV ready to adjust, rather than having to start from scratch, is a real bonus.

Prepare your CV on good-quality white or cream paper and use a basic, plain typeface and black ink. Resist the temptation to use graphics and colour. Unless you are in the world of the arts and media, this is considered inappropriate and it can cause problems in reproducing your CV. Many organizations now scan CVs to copy them and colours and graphics do not survive this process well.

Proactive personal development planning

The value of preparing and maintaining a PDP has never been more apparent than today. In the healthcare industry, as in others, the picture of career profile, career portfolio and career development has changed dramatically. It is a more complex process than many believe.

Every bit of your work and life experience can contribute to your future career. Activities undertaken during career breaks, or when working abroad or outside health care can offer something of value to your future. The structure of the 'portfolio' career has been formalized and is now valued for its eclecticism, rather than being labelled fragmented and piecemeal.

However, the important thing is for you to take charge of your career — don't assume someone else will do it for you. For example, if you see an opportunity at work, once you have done your homework about what it entails and how it might fit into the 'big picture', put yourself forward and suggest how you might tackle it. In this way, your own personal development is contributing to the well-being of the organization and vice versa. Development is about doing things 'on the job', as well as formal study.

PDPs should be congruent with the organizational development plan — in that way, the optimum outcome results from the effort everyone puts in to a project.

The timeframe for your PDP is important. Five years is now considered long term, normally three years is considered to be medium term and one year is a short-term view. This has arisen because of the rapid and continuous pace of change in the world of work. It is too easy to be shell-shocked by this and think that planning is futile because by the time you have developed a plan, it is irrelevant because the world has changed. This gives the clue to how to prepare your PDP. Keep it flexible and responsive. The portfolio of experience you, as a nurse, are required to produce in order to remain on the live register is an excellent basis for your PDP. Preparing this gives you the opportunity to reflect on what you have done, what you enjoyed and what you think you do well. Remember to capture your experience as well as courses.

When looking ahead, try not to think in defined roles. For example, it is not helpful to think that in three to five years time 'I want to be a xx'. The way things are changing, it is unlikely that there will be a post called xx, and in any case, different organizations call the same post different things. Be open to opportunities that present themselves. One danger of planning too far ahead is that you overlook exciting things available now. The thing to do is to record the sort of things you would like to be doing in your role in one, three and five years time. For example, you may say you want to work in a team, or in an autonomous post. You may prefer a big hospital or a remote community. When you have collected this information, you may find it helpful to skim the job advertisements in a number of professional journals. Look at the description of the job rather than the title and match it to your 'wish list'. You may be surprised and begin to look at different roles in different contexts.

Another important activity when working on your PDP is to consider, objectively, your strengths and development needs. Brainstorming these on paper allows you to consider ways to capitalize on strengths and develop those skills and knowledge areas you have identified as priority. Be careful not to fall into the trap of thinking that you must do a course for everything. Some areas of development are best achieved by shadowing a colleague. For example, if you think you are weak on chairing meetings, ask a colleague whom you feel is good at chairing if you can sit in. Then watch the process of meeting management. Normally we concentrate on the content of the meeting. Make notes on what you felt worked well and why, and try it out for yourself.

A mentor can be a good resource to help you to consider different career opportunities. This is not the same sort of relationship you may have had with your allotted mentor or preceptor on the ward. Clearly it is important that you feel comfortable with your mentor, so take time choosing the right person. They do not have to be from the same professional background as yourself — in fact, sometimes someone outwith your professional group can provide a fresh perspective. You may only need to visit this person two or three times a year, so you may choose someone from another area of the country. You may meet your mentor as a result of networking.

Structured networking

Structured networking is an excellent and cost-effective way of developing your career and tapping into a plethora of resources relevant to your area of practice. Most people find that they are networking automatically but you may find it helpful to consider one or two basic activities as a way to develop your networking skills further. Always keep a note of telephone numbers, and e-mail and postal addresses of people you meet. This may be from conferences, visitors to your place of work, or people with a high professional profile you feel could contribute to your development. Providing you have a focused objective, you will find that the majority of professionals are happy to give time to others and many more senior or experienced people see this as an overt responsibility. Should you wish to contact someone whom you do not know personally, either write to him or her or telephone the personal assistant, explaining who you are and how you feel the person can help you. You must be very focused and succinct. Ask for a 30-minute appointment. Be on time, have your questions ready and conclude the interview within the · allotted time. Be sure to follow up the meeting with a thank you letter.

Keep contact details of those who have published an interesting journal article. If you feel you would like to ask a question, write to them. Professional groups, such as the RCN specialist fora, offer a good way of networking with people who have similar professional interests.

The key points to remember are: be proactive, be focused, be reliable and be prepared to give your time to others when approached.

APPENDIX 9

Research, evidence-based practice, libraries, literature searching, reference and citation systems and referencing and web sources
Denis Anthony

This appendix discusses (briefly) how research is undertaken. However, dissemination is vital if research is not to simply gather dust in libraries. A short discussion follows of the barriers and bridges to implementing research.

The use of libraries to obtain research-based information is discussed. The need for clinical practice to use research as its base, with reference to literature reviews is outlined. The main referencing systems, Harvard and Vancouver, are covered.

Finally a list of Web resources is offered that cover the areas in greater detail.

Research
Research has many definitions, for example it is 'any systematic activity designed to develop or contribute to generalizable knowledge' (http://home.mwo.edu/research/query7.html) and it is 'an organized and systematic way of finding answers to questions' (http://humanities.byu.edu/ Linguistics/ Henrichsen/ResearchMethods/RM_1_01.html). According to Dempsey and Dempsey (1996) it is 'a scientific process of inquiry and/or experimentation that involves purposeful, systematic, and rigorous collection of data'.

There are several research paradigms, and the methodology employed will depend on the nature of the enquiry. Broadly there are two types of research, qualitative and quantitative. For a discussion of the various strengths of the two broad types of methods see 'Quantitative vs. qualitative research' on http://www.windsor.igs.net/~nhodgins/quant_qual.html.

Implementation of research
There is an acknowledged theory–practice gap in nursing (and other disciplines). Key aspects are (Tierney 1997):

- research education
- research activity
- dissemination
- national nursing organizations' support
- funding.

These are inter-related. For if nurses are to value research, they need to understand the process through education. A knowledge of research methods allows the nurse to understand papers and thus dissemination will be more effective. Some nurses will undertake research, requiring institutional support and funding. National nursing organizations can take a lead in providing support for research.

Barriers to research implementation are the perception of research as remote, and absence of supporting infrastructure (Wuest 1995). Highest rated barriers in a further study have been understanding of research and acquisition of research skills; lowest rated were a need for research as basis for nursing practice (Lynn & Moore 1997). In nurse education, with a history of teaching rather than research, teachers worry about neglect of teaching excellence (Lorentzon et al 1998).

Funding is an issue, and nurses have not been as successful in gaining research funds as other professional groups, in particular medical staff. In one study regional R&D applications showed limited applications from nurses, and proposals were withdrawn voluntarily, typically after insensitively worded referees' comments, but vigorously pursued nursing proposals rated higher than medical-led proposals (Mead et al 1997). It may be thought that nurses should adopt the strategies employed by doctors, performing quantitative studies (typically RCTs), working in partnership with doctors, and working with other organizations. All these may be useful but none should be adopted without good reason.

Projects in one study were more likely to succeed if the method was qualitative and the lead researcher was a nurse (Brooker et al 1997), and no more likely to succeed if a medical collaborator, a statistician or a health economist was involved, or if there were more than three collaborators, or if they came from more than one university (Brooker et al 1997).

Bridges from the literature have included:

- Staff recruitment and retention, funding, contracts, support and publication (Cleverly 1998).
- Funding councils, the NHS (e.g. DoH, Region, Training Consortia), professional bodies, medical charities (e.g. Help the Aged), industry (e.g. Smith & Nephew) and nursing charities (e.g. Foundation of Nursing Studies).
- Nonfunding bridges have included creating agenda of agreed problems (e.g. interprofessionalism, community health), issues of communication and dissemination and methodological mix (Watson 1998).
- Dissemination/communication bridges include practice development nurses, clinical nurse specialists, link nurses, tutorial series, study days, nursing journals, clinical guidelines, research networks (e.g. RCN), clinical networks (e.g. Tissue viability society) and local groups (Brooks & Anthony 2000).

Local initiatives have been shown to be effective. Bridges implemented in one trust include a research development facilitator, a centre for nursing research and partnership between trust and university (Martin et al 1998). An example from Australia is Sydney, where a reward system for research productivity (funding-designated research groups/faculty support units), the creation of a nursing clinical development unit, and a leadership programme (new clinical chairs) and nursing research seminars were considered success-ful initiatives in research implementation (Greenwood & Gray 1998).

Research can be effective in stimulating clinical staff, for example research is greater in nursing development units than comparators, and networking higher, though the number of audits was the same (Redfern & Murrells 1998). Networking facilitates research, promotes quality, quantity and usefulness of research, and places research into patient care (Leighton-Beck 1997).

Strategies to implement and encourage research include communication with top management, provision of development opportunities, technical research support, building on completed research and use of multidisciplin-ary teams (Gaynor & Verdin 1973).

Thus nurses can do quality research, and this research does not have to be quantitative. For research to be successful support, education and profes-sional development are needed. Clinical nurse specialists have a special role to play as they are opinion leaders, and nurse consultants are likely to have a similar or stronger role. Dissemination and networking is helpful, and both traditional and electronic modes should be considered, for example email lists, newsgroups as well as newsletters and conferences.

Thus, having shown that research is needed and nurses are capable of con-ducting or using research, we shall discuss some types of research.

Quantitative research methods
Quantitative research deals with data that may be counted or measured in numerical format. This may be further split into:

- Descriptive studies — where the data are recorded in tables, graphs or measures of central tendency (mean, mode, median) and spread of data (e.g. variance, range).
- Inferential studies — where hypotheses are proposed and these are tested with statistical tests. An example would be: there is no significant differ-ence in serum albumin between two groups, those with a pressure ulcer and those with none.
  Typical quantitative research designs include:
- Surveys using either interviews or questionnaires to obtain data that can be expressed in numerical terms, for example number of nurses with a degree, age of student nurses in training.
- Quasi-experimental studies, for example comparing the pressure sore incidence in two hospitals with different treatment regimens.

- Parallel double-blind randomized studies, for example comparing two barrier creams randomly allocated to patients, where neither researcher nor patient knows which cream is allocated to each patient.
- Double-blind randomized controlled trials (RCTs), the 'gold standard', where a placebo is compared with an active treatment, where neither researcher nor patient knows whether the patient has received a treatment or placebo (control).

Qualitative research methods
In qualitative studies, the data are richer, often not capable of being expressed in numerical form, and typically using small numbers of subjects, from whom large quantities of data are obtained. Typical qualitative studies might include:

- Historical studies, where primary and secondary sources are examined and analysed to uncover patterns, trends, political and economic outcomes, etc., 'Studying the past facilitates understanding of the present and future.' (Hewitt 1997)
- Focus groups, where a group of subjects are interviewed together.
- Phenomenological studies, where it is attempted to capture the lived experience of the subjects.
- Interviews and surveys using open-ended questions that do not lend themselves to numerical coding.

Evidence-based practice
Research should be the basis behind clinical practice: this is evidence-based practice. As far as is possible, practice should be evidence-based. Increasingly clinical guidelines are employed that have a specific defined research base. The Scottish Intercollegiate Guidelines Network (SIGN), Cochrane and NHS Centre for Reviews and Dissemination (York) all use some variant of a numerical classification system that gives most weight to studies with strong evidence. In this scheme a meta-analysis of many RCTs is the best form of evidence, and expert opinion at the other extreme.

Libraries
Where do you find the research articles on which to base your practice? Typically libraries are the best source, but these may not be local and thus can be difficult to access.

Libraries can be accessed via universities, schools of nursing and hospitals. However, increasingly these are accessed via the Internet. In the university sector many universities use the OPAC system, making titles and booking available on the Internet. COPAC (www.copac.ac.uk) is a system where several university libraries are combined, so you may identify for example the nearest library that has a book you need.

Bibliographic databases are available at libraries, typically on CD-ROM. However, many of these are available on the Internet, some for free. For example, Medline is available via the National Library of Medicine (among others) for no charge.

Literature search

Research is cumulative, and any study is likely to be a step in a series of work and itself to add to that body of knowledge. Thus any research report will probably need to refer to earlier work using a review of relevant literature. Ideally a review should be systematic, that is, performed according to a specific set of criteria. These include a search strategy, inclusion and exclusion criteria for studies, and methods of evaluation of studies. A systematic review can form the basis for a clinical guideline.

In practice, owing to resource constraints, reviews are often narrative rather than systematic. However, some components of a systematic method increase rigour at low cost, for example specification of the search strategy employed.

The use of a systematic approach aids in maintaining validity by ensuring as far as possible that relevant articles are located, and the use of assessment criteria further help by ranking the quality of material.

Referencing and citation systems

The previous work, upon which any study is built (or sometimes which it is attempting to replace) needs to be referenced, so the reader may know from where the evidence derives and locate the original if required.

There are several forms of referencing, but most are based on two types, Harvard and Vancouver. Each academic journal or textbook is likely to have a house style, and these are usually at most minor variants of either of these two systems. Increasingly material is referenced from the Internet, especially the Web.

The order of items will depend on the reference style used, for example Harvard will have the date immediately after the author. In Harvard material is cited in the text using the author and date, and the reference list is in ascending order alphabetically. In Vancouver a number is used to cite material, and the reference list is in order of appearance. Thus a sentence in Harvard might be:

The UK Department of Health (DoH) has issued several documents which support clinical governance and clinical guidelines (Mann 1996, Department of Health 1999)

Department of Health (1999) *Steps towards clinical governance.* Department of Health, London.

Mann, T (1996) *Clinical guidelines: Using clinical guidelines to improve patient care within the NHS.* NHS Executive, Leeds.

And in Vancouver:

The UK Department of Health (DoH) has issued several documents which support clinical governance and clinical guidelines[1,2].

1. Mann T. Clinical guidelines: Using clinical guidelines to improve patient care within the NHS. 1996. Leeds, NHS Executive.
2. Department of Health. Steps towards clinical governance. 1999. London, Department of Health.

There are many places with information on how to reference articles from the Web, either articles placed on the Web but available on paper, and those available only on the Web. The important points are that the type of medium could be the Web, not simply paper publications, and that the date you access such a Web-based article should be given on the grounds that Web-based material can evolve over time and the accession date is thus the equivalent of the edition in a book.

Summary

We have seen that research is needed but that there is a gap between theory and practice. To ensure practice is research based (evidence based), appropriate access to library material, often via the Internet, is vital. Dissemination of research does not occur simply by publication, and strategies should be employed by clinical leaders, such as education, use of link nurses, etc.

There is a huge variety of research methods but these fall mainly into two groups, qualitative and quantitative. The best research is valid research, and the most valid approach (qualitative or quantitative) will depend on the context of the study. All research should build on prior work and this needs to be referenced in a clear and consistent fashion. Web resources are an excellent way of accessing all sorts of research, bibliographic databases and centres with advice on carrying out research, though they should be quality assessed in a similar way as any printed material.

Web resources

Clinical guidelines, dissemination centres and other clinical resources

Resource	URL
Agency for Health Care Policy and Research (USA)	http://www.ahcpr.gov
Canadian Medical Association	http://www.cma.ca/cpgs/index.htm
Center for Disease and Control (CDC) Prevention Guidelines (USA)	http://aepo-xdv-www.epo.cdc.gov/wonder/prevguid/prevguid.htm
Clinical Practice Guidelines (USA)	http://www.dfwhc.org/clinical.htm
Cliniweb (USA)	http://www.ohsu.edu/cliniweb/
Guidelines Project (IHS)	http://www.ihs.ox.ac.uk/guidelines/
National Electronic Library for Health (UK)	http://www.nelh.nhs.uk

table continues

Resource	URL
National Guideline Clearing House (USA)	http://www.guideline.gov
National Guideline ClearinghouseTM (USA)	http://www.guideline.gov
National Institute of Clinical Excellence (UK)	http://www.nice.org.uk/clin_guide/clingud_ind.htm
New Zealand Guidelines Group	http://www.nzgg.org.nz/index.htm
Royal College of Nursing Clinical Guidelines (UK)	http://www.rcn.org.uk/services/promote/clinical/clinical guidelines.htm
Scottish Intercollegiate Guidelines Network	http://www.sign.ac.uk
US National Library of Medicine	http://text.nlm.nih.gov
Virtual Hospital: Clinical Guidelines (USA)	http://www.vh.org/Providers/ClinGuide/CGType.html

Evidence-based health

Resource	URL
Centre for evidence based medicine	http://cebm.jr2.ox.ac.uk
NHS Centre for Reviews and Dissemination	http://agatha.york.ac.uk/welcome.htm
NHS Executive Trent Research & Development Group	http://nhstrent.users.netlink.co.uk/trentrd/role.htm and http://www.nhsetrent.gov.uk/trentrd/rd.html
The National Research Register	http://www.doh.gov.uk/nrr.htm
Trent Institute for Health Services Research	http://www.trentinstitute.org.uk
UK Department of Health Research and Development	http://www.doh.gov.uk/research/index.htm

Referencing

Resource	URL
'How do you cite URLs in a bibliography?'	http://www.nrlssc.navy.mil/meta/bibliography.html
Harvard referencing guide	http://www.shef.ac.uk/~lib/libdocs/hsl-dvc1.html
Harvard system	http://www.lmu.ac.uk/lss/ls/docs/harv.htm
Harvard system	http://www.lmu.ac.uk/lss/ls/docs/harvfron.htm
Reference styles: Harvard and Vancouver systems	http://www.library.bma.org.uk/html/refsystem.html
Vancouver system	http://www.le.ac.uk/library/teach/irsm/irsm71.html
Vancouver system style tutorial	http://www.lib.monash.edu.au/vl/cite/citeprvr.htm

Qualitative research

Resource	URL
Qualitative Nursing Research Methodology	http://www.arkanar.minsk.by/medicine/91/Nursing_Research_Qualitative_Perspective.htm
Qualitative Research Methods Bibliography	http://www.unm.edu/~gamradt/courses/qualbib.htm and http://www.art.ttu.edu/arted/syllabi/res%20biblio/qual.html
Qualitative Research Resources on the Internet	http://www.nova.edu/ssss/QR/qualres.html
Qualitative Research Web Ring Home Page	http://www.irn.pdx.edu/~kerlinb/qr/
Qualitative Research Web Sites	http://www.nova.edu/ssss/QR/web.html
Qualitative Research: an Overview	http://www.thatnursingsite.com/research/content/tns-r0002f.asp
QualPage: Resources for qualitative research for nurses (papers, conferences, links to other sites, electronic journals etc.)	http://www.ualberta.ca/~jrnorris/qual.html

Quantitative research

Resource	URL
'Quantitative Research Proposal Guidelines' from Western Kentucky University, Department of Nursing offers a structure for a proposal, and includes sample size as determined by power analysis	http://www.wku.edu/Nursing/n510quant.htm
The Royal Windsor Society for Nursing Research has links to many research centres and documents and web resources dealing with referencing, data analysis and ethics	http://royalwindsor.homepage.com

References

Brooker C, Read S, Morrell C J, Repper J, Jones R, Akehurst R 1997 Coming in from the cold? An analysis of research proposals submitted by the Nursing Section at ScHARR, 1994–1997. NT Research 423; 2(6):405–413

Brooks N, Anthony D 2000 Clinical guidelines in community hospitals. Nursing Standard 15(1):35–39

Cleverly D 1998 Nursing research — taking an active interest. Nurse Education Today 18(4):267–272

Dempsey P, Dempsey D 1996 Nursing Research: Text and workbook, 4th edn. Little, Brown and Company, Boston

Gaynor S, Verdin J A 1973 Conducting unit-based research to improve quality of care. Journal of Nursing Care Quality 12(2):63–71

Greenwood J, Gray G 1998 Developing a nursing research culture in the university and health sectors in Western Sydney, Australia. Nurse Education Today 18(8):642–648

Hewitt L C 1997 Historical research in nursing: standards for research and evaluation. Journal of the New York State Nurses Association 28(3):16–19

Leighton-Beck L 1997 Research networking. Networking: putting research at the heart of professional practice. British Journal of Nursing 6(2):120–122

Lorentzon M, Gass L, Wimpenny P, Gibb S 1998 Protectionism or competition in managing British nursing research? Current debate among nurse and midwifery teachers. Journal of Nursing Management 6(1):29–35

Lynn M R, Moore K 1997 Research utilization by nurse managers: current practices and future directions. Seminars for Nurse Managers 5(4):217–223

Martin C R, Bowman G S, Knight S, Thompson D R 1998 Progress with a strategy for developing research in practice. Including commentary by Bartlett H. NT Research 3(1):28–35

Mead D, Moseley L, Cook R 1997 The performance of nursing in the research stakes: lessons from the field. NT Research 2(5):335–344

Redfern S, Murrells T 1998 Occasional paper. Research, audit and networking: who's in the lead? Nursing Times 94(28):57–60

Tierney A J 1997 Organization report. The development of nursing research in Europe. European Nurse 2(2):73–84

Watson D 1998 Developing the capacity of nursing and midwifery research: the view from higher education. NT Research 3(2):93–99

Wuest J 1995 Breaking the barriers to nursing research. Canadian Nurse 91(4):29–33